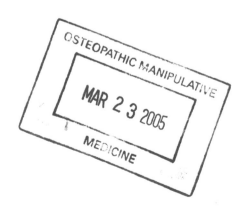

Clinical Pain Management
Chronic Pain

Series editors

Andrew S C Rice MB BS MD FRCA
Senior Lecturer in Pain Research, Department of
Anaesthetics, Faculty of Medicine, Imperial College,
Chelsea & Westminster Hospital Campus, London,
UK

Carol A Warfield MD
Edward Lowenstein Professor of Anesthesia,
Harvard Medical School; Chairman, Department of
Anesthesia and Critical Care, Beth Israel Deaconess
Medical Center, Boston, Massachusetts, USA

Douglas Justins MB BS FRCA
Pain Management Centre, St Thomas' Hospital,
London, UK

Christopher Eccleston PhD
Director, Pain Management Unit, University of Bath
and The Royal National Hospital for Rheumatic
Diseases, Bath, UK

Acute Pain
Edited by David J Rowbotham and
Pamela E Macintyre

Chronic Pain
Edited by Troels S Jensen, Peter R Wilson, and
Andrew S C Rice

Cancer Pain
Edited by Nigel Sykes, Marie T Fallon, and
Richard B Patt

Practical Applications and Procedures
Edited by Harald Breivik, William Campbell, and
Christopher Eccleston

Clinical Pain Management
Chronic Pain

Edited by

Troels S Jensen MD DMSci
Professor, Experimental and Clinical Pain Research,
Department of Neurology and Danish Pain Research
Center, Faculty of Health Sciences, Aarhus University,
Aarhus, Denmark

Peter R Wilson MB BS PhD FFPMANZCA
Professor of Anesthesiology and Pain Medicine, Mayo
Graduate School of Medicine, Rochester, USA

and

Andrew S C Rice MB BS MD FRCA
Senior Lecturer in Pain Research, Department of
Anaesthetics, Faculty of Medicine, Imperial College,
Chelsea & Westminster Hospital Campus, London, UK

A member of the Hodder Headline Group
LONDON

First published in Great Britain in 2003 by
Arnold, a member of the Hodder Headline Group,
338 Euston Road, London NW1 3BH

http://www.arnoldpublishers.com

Distributed in the United States of America by
Oxford University Press Inc.,
198 Madison Avenue, New York, NY10016
Oxford is a registered trademark of Oxford University Press

Whilst the advice and information in this book are believed to
be true and accurate at the date of going to press, neither the
authors nor the publisher can accept any legal responsibility
or liability for any errors or omissions that may be made. In
particular (but without limiting the generality of the preceding
disclaimer) every effort has been made to check drug dosages;
however it is still possible that errors have been missed.
Furthermore, dosage schedules are constantly being revised
and new side-effects recognized. For these reasons the reader
is strongly urged to consult the drug companies' printed
instructions before administering any of the drugs recommended
in this book.

British Library Cataloguing in Publication Data
A catalogue record for this book is available from the British
Library

Library of Congress Cataloging-in-Publication Data
A catalog record for this book is available from the Library of
Congress

ISBN 0 340 80993 0 (Chronic Pain)

ISBN 0 340 73154 0 (2-vol set: Chronic Pain/Practical
Applications and Procedures)

ISBN 0 340 70635 X (4-vol set: Acute Pain/Chronic Pain/Cancer
Pain/Practical Applications and Procedures)

1 2 3 4 5 6 7 8 9 10

Commissioning Editor: Joanna Koster
Development Editor: Sarah Burrows
Production Editor: James Rabson
Production Controller: Martin Kerans
Project Manager: Lindsey Williams
Cover Designer: Terry Griffiths

Typeset in 10 on 12 pt Minion by Prepress Projects Ltd, Perth

Printed and bound in Italy by Giunti Industrie Grafiche

Contents

Contributors

Praveen Anand MA MD FRCP
Professor of Clinical Neurology, Head, Peripheral
Neuropathy Unit, Division of Neuroscience and
Psychological Medicine, Imperial College School of
Medicine, London, UK

Rob Atcheson MD FRCA
Consultant in Anaesthesia and Pain Management,
Department of Anaesthesia and Pain Management, Royal
Hallamshire Hospital, Sheffield, UK

Carol Banks RN MSC
Nurse Specialist in Pain Management, Orsett Hospital,
Grays, Essex, UK

Antonio Barbieri MD
Resident in Neurosurgery, Modena State University, and
Fellow in Clinical Pain Research, Pain Medicine Center,
Scientific Institute and Hospital San Raffaele, Milan, Italy

Miles Belgrade MD
Medical Director, Fairview Pain Management Center,
Fairview University Medical Center, Minneapolis, MN, USA

Nikolai Bogduk MD PhD DSc Dip Pain Med FFPM (ANZCA)
Professor of Pain Medicine, University of Newcastle,
Department of Clinical Research, Newcastle Hospital,
Newcastle, New South Wales, Australia

Fiona Campbell BSc MD FRCA
Consultant in Anaesthesia and Pain Management, Pain
Management Centre, University Hospital Trust, Queen's
Medical Centre, Nottingham, UK

Kenneth L Casey MD
Professor of Neurology and Professor of Physiology,
University of Michigan, and Chief, Neurology Service,
Veteran's Affairs Medical Center, Ann Arbor, MI, USA

Edmond Charlton MB BS FRCA DobstRCOG
Consultant in Pain Management and Anaesthesia, Royal
Victoria Infirmary, Newcastle upon Tyne, UK

Emma Chojnowska MB BChir MA FRCA
Consultant in Pain Management and Anaesthesia,
Worthing Hospital, Worthing, UK

Alf Collins FRCA
Consultant Anaesthestist, Department of Anaesthetics,
Musgrove Park Hospital, Taunton, UK

Daniel M Doleys PhD
Director, Pain and Rehabilitation Institute, Birmingham,
AL, USA

Rose Dotson
Department of Neurophysiology, Mayo Clinic, Rochester,
MN, USA

Christopher Eccleston PhD
Pain Management Unit, University of Bath, Bath, UK

Ayman Eissa MBBCh FRCA MD
Special Registrar in Anaesthetics, Northern Schools of
Anaesthesia, Pain Management Unit, The James Cook
University Hospital, Middlesborough, UK

G Allen Finley MD FRCPC
Professor of Anesthesia and Psychology, Dalhousie
University, IWK Health Centre, Halifax, Nova Scotia,
Canada

David Fishbain MD
Professor of Psychiatry, Neurological Surgery, and
Anesthesiology, Comprehensive Pain and Rehabilitation
Center, University of Miami School of Medicine, South
Shore Hospital, Miami Beach, FL, USA

Fabio Formaglio MD
Neurologist and Anaesthesiologist, Director, Cancer
Pain Unit, Pain Medicine Center, Scientific Institute and
Hospital San Raffaele, Milan, Italy

James Fricton DDS MS
Professor, University of Minnesota, School of Dentistry,
Minneapolis, MN, USA

Gilbert R Gonzales MD
Pain and Palliative Care Service, Department of
Neurology, Memorial Sloan-Kettering Cancer Center, New
York, NY, USA

Hanne Gottrup
Department of Neurology and Danish Pain Research
Centre, Aarhus Kommunehospital, Aarhus C, Denmark

C Roger Goucke MB ChB FANZCA FFPMANZCA
Consultant in Pain Medicine, Department of Pain
Management, Sir Charles Gairdner Hospital, Perth,
Western Australia, Australia

Paul J Graziotti MBBS FFARACS FFARCS FFPMANZCA
Consultant in Pain Medicine, West Australian Pain
Management Centre, Nedlands, Western Australia,
Australia

Nortin M Hadler MD FACP FACR FACOEM
Professor of Medicine and Microbiology/Immunology,
University of North Carolina at Chapel Hill, and Attending
Rheumatologist, University of North Carolina Hospitals,
Department of Medicine, University of North Carolina at
Chapel Hill, Chapel Hill, NC, USA

Sheelah D Harrison BSc (Hons) BDS PhD FDSRCS
Specialist Registrar Oral Maxillofacial Surgery, The
Eastman Dental Hospital, London, UK

Samuel J Hassenbusch MD PhD
Professor, Department of Neurosurgery, University of
Texas M.D. Anderson Cancer Center, Houston, TX, USA

Hamid Hekmat PhD
Psychology Department, University of Wisconsin, WI, USA

Robert D Helme MBBS PhD FRACP FFPMANZCA
Consultant Neurologist, Barbara Walker Centre for Pain
Management, St Vincent's Hospital, Fitzroy, Victoria,
Australia

Ross Hetherington PhD CPsych
Assistant Professor of Psychology, University of Toronto,
and Psychologist, Hospital for Sick Children, Toronto,
Ontario, Canada

John Hughes MB BS FRCA
Consultant in Anaesthetics and Pain Management, The
James Cook University Hospital, Middlesborough, UK

Ali Jawad FRCP
Honorary Senior Lecturer and Consultant, The Royal
London Hospital, London, UK

Troels S Jensen MD PhD
Professor, Department of Neurology and Danish Pain
Research Centre, Aarhus Kommunehospital, Aarhus C,
Denmark

Rigmor Jensen MD
Assistant Professor, Department of Neurology, University
of Copenhagen, Glostrup Hospital, Glostrup, Denmark

Benny Katz MB BS FRACP FFPMANZCA
Director, Pain Management Clinic, Melbourne Extended
Care and Rehabilitation Service, Parkville, Victoria,
Australia

Bruce L Kidd DM FRCP FRACP
Professor of Clinical Rheumatology, Bone and Joint
Research Unit, Barts and The London School of Medicine
and Dentistry, London, UK

Steven A King MD
Professor of Psychiatry, Department of Psychiatry, Temple
University School of Medicine, Philadelphia, PA, USA

Erik Kinnman MD PhD
Department of Anaesthesiology, Pain Section, Karolinska
Institute, Stockholm, Sweden

Jens D Kristensen MD PhD
Vice President Clinical Development, Melacure
Therapeutics, Uppsala, Sweden

Marco Lacerenza MD
Neurologist and Anaesthesiologist and Director,
Neuropathic Pain Unit, Pain Medicine Center, Scientific
Institute and Hospital San Raffaele, Milan, Italy

Philip A Low MD
Department of Neurophysiology, Mayo Clinic, Rochester,
MN, USA

Patrick J McGrath PhD FRCS
Professor of Psychology, Pediatrics and Psychiatry,
Department of Psychology, Dalhousie University, Halifax,
Novia Scotia, Canada

Paolo Marchettini MD
Neurologist and Orthopaedic Surgeon and Chairman,
Pain Medicine Center, Scientific Institute and Hospital San
Raffaele, Milan, Italy

Tricia E Markusen MD
Department of Obstetrics and Gynecology, UCLA School of
Medicine, Los Angeles, CA, USA

Malvern May MRCP FRCA
Consultant in Pain Management, Basildon Hospital,
Basildon, UK

George Mendelson MB BS MD FRANZCP FFPMANZCA
Honorary Clinical Associate Professor, Department of
Psychological Medicine, Monash University, and Clinical
Director and Consultant Psychiatrist, Caulfield Pain
Management and Research Centre, Caulfield General
Medical Centre, Melbourne, Victoria, Australia

Danuta Mendelson MA PhD LLM
Senior Lecturer, School of Law, Deakin University,
Burwood, Victoria, Australia

Stephen Morley PhD
Professor of Clinical Psychology, Academic Unit of
Psychiatry and Behavioural Sciences, School of Medicine,
University of Leeds, Leeds, UK

David B Morris PhD
Writer/Adjunct Professor of Medicine, University of New
Mexico, Albuquerque, NM, USA

Paul R Nandi MRCP FRCA
Consultant Anaesthetist, University College London
Hospitals Pain Management Centre, The National Hospital
for Neurology and Neurosurgery, London, UK

Timothy J Ness MD PhD
Associate Professor of Anesthesiology, Research Division,
Department of Anesthesiology, University of Alabama at
Birmingham, Birmingham, AL, USA

Toby R O Newton-John BA (Hons) MPsychol PhD
Consultant Clinical Psychologist, Department of Pain
Management, National Hospital for Neurology and
Neurosurgery, London, UK

Turo J Nurmikko MD
Pain Relief Foundation Professor of Pain Science, Pain
Research Institute, Department of Neurological Science,
Clinical Science Centre, University of Liverpool, Liverpool,
UK

Christopher O'Brien MD
Vice President Medical Affairs, Elan Biopharmaceuticals,
San Diego, CA, USA

Akiko Okifuji PhD
Associate Professor, Department of Anesthesiology, Pain
Research and Management Center, University of Utah,
Salt Lake City, UT, USA

Janine Pernak de Gast MD PhD
Director, Center of Pain Medicine, Institute of Mother and
Child, Warsaw, Poland

Andrea Rapkin MD
Professor of Obstetrics and Gynecology, Department of
Obstetrics and Gynecology, UCLA School of Medicine, Los
Angeles, CA, USA

Andrew S C Rice MB BS MD FRCA
Senior Lecturer in Pain Research, Department of
Anaesthetics, Faculty of Medicine, Imperial College,
Chelsea & Westminster Hospital Campus, London, UK

Ben A Rich JD PhD
Associate Professor, Bioethics Program, Department of
Internal Medicine, University of California-Davis Medical
Center, Sacramento, CA, USA

James P Robinson MD PhD
Multidisciplinary Pain Center, University of Washington,
Seattle, WA, USA

Steven R Sabers MD
Institute for Low Back and Neck Care, Minneapolis, MN,
USA

Paola Sandroni MD PhD
Neurology and Autonomic Disorders Center, Mayo Clinic,
Rochester, MN, USA

Lauren C Seeberger MD
CNI Movement Disorder Center, Colorado Neurological
Institute, Englewood, CO, USA

Prafulla Shembalkar MD DM
Clinical Research Fellow, Division of Neurosciences and
Psychological Medicine, Peripheral Neuropathies Unit,
Imperial College School of Medicine, Hammersmith
Hospital, London, UK

Richard A Sherman PhD
Chief Research Consultant, Orthopedic Surgery, Madigan
Army Medical Center, Tacoma, WA, USA

Søren H Sindrup MD
Consultant Neurologist, Department of Neurology, Odense
University Hospital, Odense C, Denmark

Christopher D Sletten PhD
Comprehensive Pain Rehabilitation Unit, Mayo Clinic,
Rochester MN, USA

Alf Sollevi MD PhD
Professor at Karolinska Institute, Head of the Department
of Anaesthesia and Intensive Care, Huddinge University
Hospital, Stockholm, Sweden

Anna Spacek MD
Associate Professor of Anaesthesiology, Department of
Anaesthesiology and General Intensive Care, University of
Vienna, Vienna General Hospital, Vienna, Austria

Peter S Staats MD
Division of Pain Medicine, Johns Hopkins Medical Center,
Baltimore MD, USA

Arthur W Staats PhD
Professor (Emeritus) of Psychology, Department of
Psychology, University of Hawaii, Honolulu, HI, USA

Catherine Stannard MB ChB FRCA
Consultant in Pain Medicine, Pain Clinic, Macmillan
Centre, Frenchay Hospital, Bristol, UK

Peer Tfelt-Hansen PhD
Consultant, Department of Neurology, University of
Copenhagen, Glostrup Hospital, Glostrup, Denmark

Simon Thomson MB BS FRCA
Director of Pain Management Services, Basildon and
Thurrock NHS Trust, Nethermayne, Basildon, UK

Glyn R Towlerton BSc MRCP FRCA
Consultant Anaesthetist and Honorary Senior
Lecturer, Magill Department of Anaesthetics and Pain
Management, Chelsea & Westminster Hospital, London,
UK

Dennis C Turk PhD
John and Emma Bonica Professor of Anesthesiology and
Pain Research, Department of Anaesthesiology, University
of Washington, Seattle, WA, USA

C Peter N Watson MD FRCP
1 Sir William's Lane, Toronto, Ontario, Canada

Zsuzsanna Wiesenfeld-Hallin PhD
Professor, Karolinska Institute, Department of Medical
Laboratory Sciences and Technology, Division of
Clinical Neurophysiology, Huddinge University Hospital,
Stockholm, Sweden

Amanda C de C Williams MSc PhD CPsychol
Senior Lecturer in Clinical Health Psychology, GKT School
of Medicine and Dentistry, University of London, and
Consultant Clinical Psychologist, INPUT Pain Management
Unit, Guy's and St Thomas' Hospital NHS Trust, London,
UK

Peter R Wilson MB BS PhD FFPMANZCA
Professor of Anesthesiology and Pain Medicine, Mayo
Graduate School of Medicine, Rochester, MN, USA

Xiao-Jun Xu MD PhD
Associate Professor, Department of Medical Laboratory
Science and Technology, Division of Clinical
Neurophysiology, Karolinska Institute, Huddinge
University Hospital, Huddinge, Sweden

Joanna M Zakrzewska MB BChir BDS MD FDSRCS FFDRCSI
Department of Oral Medicine, Barts and the London,
Queen Mary's School of Medicine and Dentistry, London,
UK

Series preface

Clinical Pain Management is a brand new reference text, providing comprehensive coverage of this broad discipline for those training and practicing in pain management and related specialties. The work comprises four volumes, three covering the three major clinical disciplines of pain relief (acute, chronic, and cancer pain) accompanied by a fourth complementary volume discussing practical aspects of clinical management and clinical research that share a greater or lesser degree of communality with all three disciplines.

We believe that practice should be firmly based on the best available evidence. However, as things currently stand, a truly evidence-based textbook of pain management would be a relatively scant affair. We were anxious not to exclude discussion of clinical management strategies that are thought to represent reasonable practice by an appreciable body of clinicians, but for which there is currently a lack of evidence to either support or refute such a practice. Nevertheless, we were also concerned that the reader should be instantly aware of the quality of evidence that supports any recommendation for a clinical intervention. Therefore, we have encouraged authors to use a universal system for scoring quality of evidence. If no score is included in the text then the implication is that the supporting evidence is of very low quality.

As befits the multidisciplinary nature of modern pain management, both the authorship and editorship of *Clinical Pain Management* is drawn from a wide range of medical and paramedical clinical specialties. The team of contributors is truly international in nature, with a total of over 200 authors and editors practicing in approximately 16 different countries. While we have attempted to ensure that each author has contributed a balanced discussion that crosses national boundaries, inevitably in a few chapters the authors' views will predominantly reflect the viewpoint as seen from a particular country or system of health care delivery.

Although the textbook of *Clinical Pain Management* is extensively referenced, we are also keen that the reader can easily identify key references. Accordingly, in the reference list at the end of each chapter important and seminal papers and key reviews are highlighted with special symbols.

Clinical Pain Management is not intended to replace the most prestigious and well-known textbook edited by Ronald Melzack and the late Patrick Wall. Instead it represents a complementary work, addressing the practical clinical aspects immediately relevant to those working on the 'factory floor' of clinical pain management rather than the equally important cutting edge of laboratory research into pain. We believe that there is a proper place for both titles on the bookshelves of pain management clinicians.

Finally, we are greatly indebted to the volume editors and chapter authors, without the considerable efforts of whom publication would not have been possible. We are also most grateful to the publishing team at Arnold, particularly the publisher, Joanna Koster, without whose Herculean efforts in holding together a team of editors and authors spanning the globe none of this would have seen the light of day. Thanks are also due to her predecessor, Annalisa Page, who was instrumental in conceiving and administering the early stages of the project, and to the production and project management teams.

Andrew S C Rice
Carol Warfield
Douglas Justins
Christopher Eccleston
London, Boston, and Bath
August 2002

Introduction to Clinical Pain Management: Chronic Pain

Until recently, the term "chronic pain" has often had the negative connotation of psychogenic etiology and an arbitrary time domain. It has also been a pejorative term to the extent that Chronic Pain Syndrome was omitted from the IASP Taxonomy of Chronic Pain Syndromes. This new volume begins to gather together the scientific and clinical evidence that confirms chronic pain as the final common path of many etiologies, and shows that it does indeed have the characteristics of an identifiable syndrome.

As is consistent with a syndrome, there are common neurophysiological, neuroanatomical, and functional changes regardless of the precipitating factors. These changes are addressed in the early chapters of this volume. In addition, there is physical, psychological, and psychiatric deconditioning that may be attributed to this central and peripheral nervous system dysfunction. Socioeconomic impairment and reduction in quality of life almost invariably accompany these changes.

There has also been a recent paradigm shift from the curative medical model of pain in which symptoms are expected to resolve once the underlying pathologic process is treated medically or surgically. This volume addresses this aspect of chronic pain in those specific conditions where applicable. It also explores the conceptually distinct rehabilitation model in which it is recognized that the underlying pathology may be incurable or untreatable. The goals of this latter model involve minimizing the adverse effects of the pain and maximizing function and quality of life.

Fundamental changes in practitioners' responsibilities to patients and society are occurring as a result of philosophical and legal advances related to chronic pain. Previously implied rights of patients now have been formalized in various intractable pain acts of several jurisdictions. The classical doctrine of *primum non nocere* (first do no harm) is being challenged ethically and legally under these circumstances. Experts in these fields explore these changing ethical and legal climates in early chapters.

This volume contains 47 chapters in three parts. The first part, *Basic Considerations,* comprises 14 chapters that cover subjects ranging from basic neurophysiology through clinical evaluation to the ethical, legal, and societal aspects of this disease as described above. Part 2, entitled *Management – therapies,* contains 12 chapters that address pharmacological, psychological, behavioral, interventional (invasive) and alternative/complementary/placebo issues. Part 3 has 21 chapters that describe both specific and nonspecific pain syndromes and their management. The subjects discussed include general neuropathic pain syndromes, specific pain syndromes and regional pain (neck, back, joints, chest, abdomen, and pelvis), and issues related to pain at the extremes of age.

Chronic pain now covers a vast scientific and clinical arena, and the scientific background and therapeutic options are much better described now than at any time in the past. This volume gathers the available evidence-based information in a useful format without overwhelming detail. Where such data are not available, the authors provide thoughtful advice based on scientific experience and clinical wisdom. It is inevitable in a volume such as this that there will be omissions, for which we must accept responsibility. Nevertheless, we believe that this volume will become essential for chronic pain clinicians and scientists.

Troels S Jensen, Peter R Wilson,
and Andrew S C Rice

Cross-references, evidence scoring, and reference annotation

The four volumes of *Clinical Pain Management* incorporate the following special features to aid the readers' understanding and navigation of the text.

Cross-references

Cross-references to other chapters within *Clinical Pain Management* are prefixed by a code indicating the volume in which the chapter referred to is to be found. The codes are as follows:

A   Acute Pain
Ch   Chronic Pain
Ca   Cancer Pain
P   Practical Applications and Procedures

Evidence scoring

In chapters in which recommendations for surgical, medical, psychological and complementary treatment, and diagnostic tests are presented, the quality of evidence supporting authors' statements relating to clinical interventions is graded by insertion of the following symbols into the text:

***   systematic review or meta-analysis
**   one or more well designed randomized controlled trials
*   nonrandomized controlled trials, cohort study etc.

Where no * is inserted, the quality of supporting evidence, if any exists, is of low grade only (e.g. case reports, clinical experience).

Other textbooks devoted to the subject of pain include a tremendous amount of anecdotal and personal recommendations, and it is often difficult to distinguish these from those with an established evidence base. This text is thus unique in allowing the reader the opportunity to do this with confidence.

Reference annotation

The reference lists are annotated, where appropriate, to guide readers to key primary papers and major review articles as follows:

Key primary papers are indicated by a ◆
Major review articles are indicated by a ●

We hope that this feature will render extensive lists of references more useful to the reader and will help to encourage self-directed learning among both trainees and practicing physicians.

PART I

Basic considerations

The challenges of pain and suffering

DAVID B MORRIS

> The work which you are accomplishing is immensely important for the good of humanity, as you seek the ever more effective control of physical pain and of the oppression of mind and spirit that physical pain so often brings with it.
>
> Pope John Paul II (26 July 1987)[1]

Pain medicine arose during the last half of the twentieth century and accompanied the rise of new clinics and treatment centers devoted specifically to pain. Change accelerated after Ronald Melzack and Patrick Wall published their landmark gate-control theory of pain in 1965,[2] which was rapidly absorbed into mainstream biomedical thinking despite unresolved questions that eventually led Melzack to look beyond spinal gates.[3] Organizational developments kept pace. In 1973, John Bonica invited some 300 participants to a conference outside Seattle, where they discussed founding a worldwide medical–scientific association focused on pain.[4] Soon, several agencies within the US National Institutes of Health assigned priority to pain research and control, creating incentives and guidelines for progress, and many academic medical centers responded by setting up pain teams. Public health systems and private insurers debated who would pay, how much, and for what. Multinational corporations invested huge sums to market powerful over-the-counter and prescription analgesics. Pain was big business. As the century ended, the organization that emerged from the now famous Seattle–Issaquah Conference – the International Association for the Study of Pain (IASP) – had an impressive 6,675 individual members in 93 countries.[5]

The proliferation of specialized journals and annual meetings on pain, together with new technologies for research and communication, maintains a fast pace of change. In 1991, for example, Melzack criticized the lack of serious interest in cortical dimensions of pain.

"What happens in the brain after cortical activation," he observed, "is a question most people want to avoid."[6] The same year saw publication of the first studies that use positron emission tomography (PET) to examine the human brain, showing activation in the anterior cingulate cortex of subjects exposed to acutely painful heat.[7,8] Almost instantly, brain imaging contributed remarkable new insights to pain research.[9] The mere expectation of pain, as magnetic resonance images (MRIs) show, corresponds to activation of a specific area within the human brain.[10] A 1999 topical review declared that "the cortical representation of pain has become one of the most active areas in pain research."[11] As in other fields of science and medicine, one formidable challenge is simply to keep up with the speed and trajectory of change.

The challenges extend in many directions, especially as researchers examine pain processes at the cellular level. In tissue cultures from newborn rats, for example, specific neurons from the sympathetic nervous system grow axons that make contact with sensory neurons, which suggests possibilities of interaction between the two separate pain systems.[12] Advances in genetics have opened up fruitful areas of pain research that were unknown 50 years ago. We recently learned that certain strains of mice possess genetic variance in nociception and in morphine-induced analgesia.[13] Strains of rats possess a congenital hypersensitivity that makes them, in effect, prone to pain.[14] Despite the disclaimers about animal models, we will soon see huge advances in understanding genetic components of the human pain process, even as advances in pharmacology reveal how pain-killers ranging from nonsteroidal anti-inflammatory drugs (NSAIDs) to opioids operate with different effects on multiple sites within the nervous system, permitting better use of drugs in combination.[15,16] Optimists believe that this accumulating knowledge will ultimately lead to the full-scale control or eradication of pain. Perhaps governments will lock away a few last pains for research purposes in case of national emergencies.

Unfortunately, pain is not likely to surrender its power during our lifetimes, and suffering is an ineradicable part of the human condition. Indeed, as social services and medical systems focus on pain, they find more pain that needs relief. Among adults, the prevalence of chronic benign pain – in which a nociceptive substrate is difficult to find – ranges between 2% and 40% of the population, depending on the study.[17] In the Netherlands, the cost of back pain alone equals 1.7% of the gross national product, and lost work as a result of back pain costs the Netherlands on average $1.5 million per hour.[18,19] In the USA, the rate of disability claims associated with low back pain has increased over the rate of population growth by 1,400%.[20] Such massive costs and complex clinical dilemmas help to explain why an IASP Task Force in 1995 recommended that nonspecific low back pain be reconceived not as a medical condition but as "activity intolerance."[21] The controversial recommendation – linking low back pain, jobs, and disability insurance – stands as a reminder that neither pain nor suffering can be wholly reduced to a universal biology of nerves, neurotransmitters, and brain states. In what follows, pain and suffering in their implicit complications pose four specific challenges that are indirectly but firmly related to treatment: how to define them, how to classify them, how to understand them, and how to confront the implicit ethical dilemmas they encompass.

PAIN AND SUFFERING: WHAT ARE THEY?

Scientific and medical definitions are tools. Even when we recognize them as imperfect or provisional, awaiting replacement by an improved version, they perform work that cannot be accomplished by less precise instruments. It was thus a serious matter when in 1979 the subcommittee on taxonomy appointed by the newly formed IASP published its now familiar definition of pain as "an unpleasant sensory and emotional experience associated with actual or potential tissue damage, or described in terms of such damage."[22] This brief definition – reaffirmed in a 1994 second edition[23] – has made it possible for researchers and clinicians working in many different countries, in various languages, and in far-flung disciplines to possess at least a basic mutual understanding of what they mean (and, equally important, do *not* mean) by the all-purpose, ragtag, everyday English word *pain*.

The IASP definition recognizes that tissue damage remains for most people – patients especially – the gold standard for pain. It also recognizes, however, that pain may occur when tissue damage is not present. The IASP definition even allows that tissue damage sometimes simply generates the language we apply to various unpleas-

ant or traumatic sensory and emotional experiences. The extended "note" accompanying the IASP definition states clearly that pain is *not* equivalent to nociception, the process by which a signal of tissue injury is transmitted through the nervous system: "Activity induced in the nociceptor and nociceptive pathways by a noxious stimulus," the IASP authors insist, "is not pain, which is always a psychological state …." As a psychological state, pain is irreducible to objective signs. The extended annotation begins with the blunt and unequivocal statement that "Pain is always subjective."

It is fascinating how much matter for controversy has been packed into the brief IASP definition of pain. The definition and its supporting annotations gently but surely dissolve any necessary connection between pain and tissue damage. Extensive tissue damage may occur without pain, as Henry K. Beecher showed in his classic study of soldiers wounded in World War II.[24,25] Pain may also occur in the total absence of tissue damage, as researchers recently confirmed.[26] Most important, with a daring that merits repetition, the IASP definition recognizes that pain is always a subjective, psychological state. No purely pathophysiological model of pain can encompass such recognitions. At the same time, the task force authors also state in the annotation what is surely true: that pain, despite its psychological and subjective nature, "most often has a proximate physical cause." In short, the IASP definition proves to be concise, flexible, and accurate. It has served the community of pain medicine very well. Naturally, there are voices today arguing that we should get rid of it.

Recent objections to the IASP definition emphasize two claims: it is Cartesian, and it neglects the ethical dimensions of pain. Cartesian today is often a synonym for wrong. As the best-known proponent of mind/body dualism, Descartes has erroneously been identified as the precursor or progenitor of any theory that separates body from mind. Complaints that the IASP definition of pain is Cartesian, however, ignore several facts. The definition implies no such thing. It implies, on the contrary, that minds as well as bodies are necessarily involved in the experience of pain, an experience that is multidimensional, not the straight-forward projection of sensory impulses that Descartes had described. Moreover, Descartes did not separate body from mind as neatly as his modern critics assume.[27] The bodily mechanism responsible for pain in humans was ineffectual when disengaged from the mind or soul, which is why Descartes could argue that animals (soulless, by definition) do not feel pain. We should stop referring to all medical mind/body dualisms as Cartesian: most are not the direct legacy of Descartes but flow from nineteenth century positivist science.[28] True, Descartes sees the mind as a passive receiver of sensory impulses, not as an active participant in the pain process. This justifiable criticism of Descartes, however, does not underwrite unjustified criticism of the IASP definition. Mind–body interrelations are indispensable in any definition that views pain as "always psychological," since even painful psychological states distinct from nociception require our personal and cultural histories of tissue damage in order to generate the language in which such psychological states are described and perceived.

A second criticism of the IASP definition is that it ignores ethical concerns implicit in pain and thus indirectly sustains or promotes unethical practices. One critic observes that the definition fails to highlight pain among disempowered and neglected minorities such as women, blacks, children, and the elderly.[29] Certainly, we need to pay increased attention to pain in minority or marginalized groups, and a vigorous biomedical literature is beginning to address this lapse. The IASP definition, however, neither supports nor promotes social injustice: reform must find more effective and appropriate expressions. It is equally short-sighted to claim, as another critic observes, that the IASP definition makes pain dependent upon "full linguistic competence," ignoring pain in neonates, for example, and in animals.[30] Animal pain is not identical to human pain, and the IASP definition deals with pain in humans. More important, the IASP account treats linguistic competence not as a philosophical prerequisite for pain but as a clinical resource. Its most radical implication lies in valuing the patient's subjective self-report – still too often devalued or dismissed by doctors unable to find an objectively verifiable lesion. We know that self-reports are imperfect, influenced by variables such as memory, mood, and the questions posed to patients or research subjects.[31] Like objective data, they must be evaluated within the context of a full medical record. The IASP definition, however, makes it clinically irresponsible to dismiss the patient's subjective account of pain, accounts that today go beyond verbal reports to include visual analog scales, drawings, and even electronic diaries that record numerical estimates of pain intensity.

One can criticize the IASP definition on various grounds – such as a circularity in defining pain as "unpleasant" – but pain is a complex state, resistant to language, and the IASP definition provides a solid, workable, valuable tool. It was created specifically, as subcommittee chair Harold Merskey writes, "for use in clinical practice."[23] Nobody ever claimed it was perfect or eternal. Moreover, a definition is exactly the wrong place to address serious ethical issues (some of which will be addressed later in this chapter). The burden lies on critics to provide a better tool capable of achieving widespread use. They should also come clean about what submerged medical, social, or philosophical agendas their own new definitions advance. A workable definition of pain need not be – and should not be – a theory of pain. We still lack a fully agreed-upon theory of pain that accounts for all the multiple combinations of causes and effects in numerous different diseases, syndromes, and cries for help. Thanks to the IASP definition, researchers and clinicians, even if they cannot always explain or treat it, mostly agree on what they do and do not mean by pain. General agreement disappears when we turn from pain to suffering.

There is no consensus about whether suffering falls within the boundaries of pain medicine – or even within medicine – but the medical neglect of suffering is palpable. Suffering rarely gets an entry in medical textbooks, and only a few authors with medical training discuss it directly.[32,33] In a practical sense, health professionals confront every day the problems of suffering – as suffering emerges during the course of illnesses that range from cancer and depression to Alzheimer's disease. This practical, everyday approach, however, fails to tell us what suffering is – and suffering as a distinctive state (a state that transcends specific illnesses) tends to be ignored. Paradoxically, the demands of everyday patient care often manage to insulate biomedicine from any real contact with suffering, which may be regarded as a nonmedical consequence of illness and thus reassigned to pastoral care, a discipline where suffering is taken seriously.[34] The standard institutional separation between theologians and physicians only deepens medical unawareness of suffering. Despite some welcome signs of change, the stark question remains as to whether pain medicine will come to view suffering – at least suffering directly related to pain – as a condition that demands serious thought and effective responses. If so, we must begin (as the IASP did with pain) to define what we mean by suffering.

Suffering is sometimes employed as a synonym for pain – as if pain were the cause, suffering the effect, and their linguistic relation interchangeable[35] – but they are theoretically distinct. A broken bone may bring pain without suffering; a broken heart may bring suffering without pain. Suffering and pain thus cannot be exactly identical or synonymous. This theoretical difference, however, often collapses in practice, where suffering and pain may occur together in ways that not only undermine hypothetical distinctness but also alter their relationship. The special complications that mark the unstable relations between pain and suffering have received attention from psychologist C. Richard Chapman and pain specialist Jonathan Gavrin.[36] They define suffering as "threat or damage to the integrity of the self" – following physician and bioethicist Eric J. Cassell[32] – and they specify that the threat or damage entails "a disparity between what one expects of one's self and what one does or is." Persistent pain, they observe, often causes "serious disruption" of a human life, and such disruption may constitute a crisis of identity that is experienced as suffering and perpetuated by physiological processes similar to the maladaptive stress response. Chapman and Gavrin do not set out to propose a solution to the problem of suffering, but they assert that physicians who understand suffering can learn how to prevent the predictable damage to the self that often accompanies persistent pain.

The medical discussion of suffering is at such an early stage that any account must remain incomplete, valuable especially for the questions it raises. Chapman and Gavrin offer an appropriately complex account of human selfhood in its neurological, behavioral, cognitive, and developmental aspects. Such complexity, however, also raises questions about whether most selves ever manage to possess a wholeness or harmony that would constitute the "integrity" presumed lost in suffering. Sociologists write about normative human identity today as characterized by a "destabilization" in which selves are not understandable as private inner cores but rather as a fluid *mélange* of public roles, performances, and appearances.[37,38] In private communication, Chapman emphasizes his view that the self is "not so much an entity as a process of constant redefinition in reaction to a changing world." He describes the loss of integrity as a failure of "coherence," noting that "awareness of incoherence within one's self is a powerful negative experience." He observes that there is perhaps no more powerful source of human incoherence than the failure or loss of the relationships that bind us to others, including not only family and loved ones but also peoples, nations, deities, or even cherished abstract versions of otherness such as justice and freedom. Suffering understood as an experience of radical incoherence may prove ultimately to be a more useful concept than selfhood regarded as the possession of integrity, wholeness, or harmony.

The work of Chapman and Gavrin invites us to ask why some pain patients suffer when others who face serious disruption of their lives seem to prosper under adversity? Suffering, in the view of some social scientists, is not only an individual experience but also a cultural practice that certain societies or subcultures or ethnic groups code quite differently.[39] The differences in individual responses to disruption may reflect different ways of "coding" adversity that are learned from families or cultures. We might also understand more about suffering from studies in "learned helplessness."[40] Suffering is by definition a state of helplessness, as few people would choose to suffer if they could avoid it. The helplessness typical of suffering, however, is also learned and reinforced by repeated failures to find aid. The repeated failure of efforts to find assistance is not the same as suffering conceived as a state of helpless passivity. In an analysis of how suffering is learned, the therapeutic value lies in active interventions designed to break the self-reinforcing cycle of helplessness – as demonstrated in feminist responses to battered women, for example – through specific techniques designed to empower the disempowered. Responses to the helplessness intrinsic to suffering allow sufferers to recognize the (limited) power they do not know they possess, which creates a basis for small steps forward.[41] From this perspective, suicide is less a product of suffering than suffering transformed to a state in which helplessness is absolute, immutable, and toxic.

A clinical definition of suffering, in addition to acknowledging threats to the self from incoherence and helplessness, will need to account for an elusive quality within suffering that resists any probe that seeks to lay it bare to objective analysis. Pope John Paul II acknowledged this elusiveness when he wrote about the "oppression of mind and spirit" that often accompanies pain. Suffering encompasses, like pain, an irreducible subjective dimension, but it is distinctive in shattering the norms of life in which even pain can be understandable and thus bearable. For contemporary philosopher Emanuel Levinas, suffering is "the *impasse* of life and being"; what he calls "the explosion and most profound articulation of absurdity."[42] We must not expect a crystal clear account of suffering when it constitutes an experience that plunges our most basic assumptions about life into utter chaos and absurdity. Suffering is like a text that suddenly plunges into an unknown language – or outside language. We do not so much know suffering (in ourselves or in others) as much as suffer or witness it. Yet, granted this resistance to understanding, a new challenge is emerging in connections between pain medicine and palliative care.[43] When cure is impossible, palliative care focuses on the alleviation of symptoms and on the relief of suffering.[44] Fear of pain is a regular source of suffering, especially among patients who fear dying in pain, and pain medicine is thus an indispensable resource for assisting hospices in the effort to relieve suffering at the end of life.

CLASSIFICATION EXCESS: THE MULTIPLICITY OF PAIN AND SUFFERING

Pain and suffering are especially resistant to definition because they are plural concepts. The history of pain is a record of pain's multiple *re*-inventions.[45] The English word *pain* refers to innumerable different experiences linked together not by a common essence (or by an immutable shared core) but by what philosopher Ludwig Wittgenstein calls "family resemblances."[46] Pain (an abstract concept) exists only through concrete, multiple, and very distinctive pains. Even if we exclude metaphorical applications of pain to unhappiness and disappointment, as when coaches talk about the "agony" of defeat, it is now clear that the pain of migraine differs from cancer pain, that cancer pain differs from the pain of arthritis, that arthritis pain differs from the pain of fibromyalgia. Such differences go beyond variations in the quality, length, and intensity of sensation. They may correspond to distinctive biological processes and to particular experiences. As neuroscientist Tony Yaksh said in 1992: "At this moment, we're becoming just barely sufficiently sophisticated to say that all pain is not the same, and therefore to know why some analgesics may be very effective in some pain states and less effective in others. We need to learn the precise nature and mechanism of all the pain producers."[47]

The invention of pain medicine rests upon an awareness that pain is never a simple unity. The centers and clinics emerging in the late 1960s and the 1970s were mostly committed to a bedrock distinction between acute and chronic pain. The distinction is not trouble free, but the basic principle won rapid acceptance. Chronic pain differs in kind – not in degree – from acute pain, and neither holds its traditional status as a symptom. Ronald Dubner, another neuroscientist who focused on pain, summed up changes that constitute a thorough challenge to traditional biomedical thinking. "We know now that pain is not merely a passive symptom of disease," he stated in 1992, "but an aggressive disease in itself, producing changes in the brain that underlie the pathology of persistent or chronic pain."[48] Soon it became necessary to abandon even the ancient medical truism that nobody ever died from pain. Psychologist John Liebeskind showed in laboratory animals that pain depresses the immune system and destroys cancer-fighting cells. As the title of his seminal essay puts it bluntly, pain *can* kill.[49]

The specific syndromes discussed in the IASP *Classification of Chronic Pain* tabulate almost as many kinds of pain as there are strains of roses, from the steady sharp or throbbing ache of gout to the sudden severe stab of trigeminal neuralgia.[23] There is visceral pain in the neck, chest pain, vascular disease of the limbs, abdominal pain of neurological origin, pain in the bladder and rectum, lumbar spine syndromes, pain syndromes of the hip and thigh, musculoskeletal syndromes of the leg, and multiple pains of the foot, as well as burns to the skin, arthritis in the joints, nerve damage, and lesions to the central nervous system (called central pain). There is stiff man syndrome, sickle cell arthropathy, and the pain of acquired immunodeficiency syndrome (AIDS). No single sensory process underlies all these diverse forms of affliction, but the last place where most patients would expect to find a common source for their pains is in a region devoid of sensory neurons. This, however, is exactly the paradox that neurosurgeon John Loeser confronts us with. "The brain," he writes, "is the organ responsible for all pain. All sensory input, including nociception, can be altered by conscious or unconscious mental activity."[50]

The brain, as the organ responsible for all pain, holds a dual function. One function is biological and internal. The brain is crucial not only to the cortical activities that process nociceptive impulses from the periphery but also to painful experiences generated in the absence of nociceptive input. You do not need a leg to feel pain in your leg – as patients with phantom limbs know, all you need is a working brain. The other function of the brain connects us with the external, interpersonal world of human culture. In effect, the brain is a natural interface between culture and biology. Your pain and my pain (even when evoked by nearly identical tissue damage) may differ significantly owing to variations in our social backgrounds and personal histories, including differences in our individual memories, beliefs, and emotional states.

The multiplicity of pain and suffering has no clear limit because our brains situate us within an open-ended matrix of biology and culture. Gender, for example, plays a significant role in pain. The relationship between gender and pain is complex, since identifiable patterns change with different medical conditions and across the life cycle.[51] Men and women, however, show quantitative differences in sensitivity to pain and to analgesia that suggest differences in neural processing. Women also compose the majority of chronic pain patients, although it is unclear whether women face greater risk of pain or merely use health care services more often.[52] Women are certainly more likely to experience a variety of recurrent pains, to report more severe levels of pain, more frequent pain, and pain of longer duration.[53] While good evidence suggests that females exhibit greater sensitivity to noxious stimuli than do males, other studies suggest that women are better at coping with discomfort and that they complain less over time.[54] Biological differences are important in this gender-influenced pain. Kappa opioids work twice as well for women as for men.[55] Migraine affects about 6% of men and 15–18% of women.[56] (The diminished frequency of migraines during pregnancy suggests a link with estrogen.) A significant implication of this research on gender differences in pain is that we should also expect gender differences in suffering. Women are overrepresented among battered spouses, whose suffering often combines physical injury with emotional trauma. A woman's position as caregiver in dysfunctional or chaotic families also suggests that suffering may be inflected by the social distribution of gender roles. Social beliefs about gender certainly affect clinical decisions regarding pain treatment.[57] We should expect that suffering too, both inside and outside medical contexts, will reveal significant biocultural differences associated with gender.

The multidimensional quality of pain and suffering – situated within cultures as well as within nervous systems – implies a need to resist the temptation to eliminate from research and from treatment all the messy local variations that come with living in societies. Low back pain is simply not the same experience in the USA as it is in Japan. In one study, Japanese patients proved significantly less impaired in psychological, social, vocational, and avocational function.[58] Research comparing 10 American cancer patients with 10 cancer patients from India found significant differences in quality of life and in the meaning of the pain experience.[59] Indian patients, who sought medical assistance only after their pain became intolerable, saw their suffering as the fulfillment of a "higher good," whereas American patients interpreted their own suffering as a form of "punishment." The authors of a review article focusing on numerous cross-cultural investigations conclude that more such studies are needed to explore the diverse "social and psychological variables that govern pain perceptions, beliefs, and reactions."[60] The culture-inflected character of pain is well illustrated in the reflections, commentaries, and essays collected in the Canadian–American anthology *When Pain Strikes*, with its self-conscious resolve to speak from and to the condition known as postmodernity.[61] Suffering and pain are persistent features of human life, but not timeless states. We cannot fully understand them apart from an awareness of how the human brain situates us inescapably within the modifying environment of a particular time and place and culture.

UNDERSTANDING: THE MATRIX OF BIOLOGY AND CULTURE

Human pain is always a biocultural condition – a composite experience requiring a biology of brain states and of neural processes negotiated within a social space where individuals interact with the surrounding culture, including the culture of medicine. One major challenge is to understand how the biological processes associated with pain are influenced directly and indirectly by individual beliefs, social institutions, and cultural forces. We continue to learn about the neuroanatomy of the human pain system and its modulating pathways.[62] It remains unclear, however, how this complex neuroanatomy is set in motion or modified by thoughts and emotions, which are influenced in turn by external and interpersonal forces such as medical systems, disability insurance, religious beliefs, and cultural attitudes. There is also a crucial role in human pain played by human consciousness. We know more about what disability insurance and religious beliefs contribute to pain than about the slippery contributions of human consciousness.

The importance of psychosocial factors in pain has been demonstrated recently in numerous articles and books. Psychologists Dennis Turk and Robert Gatchell contend that post-1960 attention to the cognitive and behavioral psychology of pain constitutes nothing less than a "revolution," and they argue for the continuing relevance of a clinical model that recognizes the mutual interdependence of biological and psychosocial processes.[63] One fascinating illustration of this mutual interdependence concerns the role of memory in pain. A patient's recollection of pain is most closely related to the intensity of pain during the inciting episode, and severe pain that persists for more than a day creates changes in the structure and function of sensory neurons.[64] The memory of severe pain thus differs from other, more casual memories, both at the cortical level and at the level of altered sensory neurons. Preemptive analgesia now commonly prescribed for postoperative patients not only prevents short-term discomfort but also avoids long-term complications that can accompany the memory of pain.

Beliefs about pain illustrate a broader interdependence between biology and culture, i.e. human pain implies continuous processes of conscious and nonconscious interpretation.[65,66] (Nonconscious interpretation occurs for example when we process traffic signals without awareness.) Meaning helps to constitute pain, even if only in the nonconscious acknowledgment that a scratch is usually meaningless. We cannot name or discuss pain except by employing a language that exists only at a specific moment in its historical development and inevitably colors our understanding.[67] Pain thus always comes already interpreted by the social world we inhabit. Meanings not only encompass articulate beliefs, such as the conviction that pain is a punishment, but they also interpenetrate in less obvious ways our inarticulate attitudes, unexpressed emotions, habitual behavior, and even nonconscious knowledge. Pain-killing drugs may temporarily circumvent conscious meaning-making processes, but meaning does not therefore go away. A patient's knowledge of drugs – like the equally widespread fear of opioids – is not innate but requires extensive, if largely nonconscious, cultural learning. In difficult cases of chronic pain, patients' beliefs and attitudes may impede, complicate, or entirely undermine treatment.

Recent research into pain beliefs challenges the entrenched opinion (still popular among patients) that pain is an electrochemical impulse triggered by tissue damage. Nociception is neither a necessary nor a sufficient condition for pain. Beliefs that help to shape the experience of pain include our convictions about cause, control, duration, outcome, and blame.[68,69] Such beliefs affect not only chronic pain but also acute and postoperative pain.[61] Further, emotion is an intrinsic part of the pain experience – saturated with and shaped by cognitive processes – rather than a mere reaction to pain.[70,71] Many beliefs about pain are directly linked to strong emotions: anger toward a negligent employer, fear of catastrophe, hope for financial gain, love for a spouse. Specific pain beliefs can predict pain intensity.[72] Beliefs also influence the ability to cope with pain. Researchers have found that patients function better when they believe they have some control over their pain, when they believe in the value of medical services, when they believe that family members care for them, and when they believe that they are not severely disabled.[73] A study of 100 patients showed that specific pain beliefs correlate directly with treatment outcomes.[74] Such research has clear implications for clinical practice, where the interdependence between culture and biology challenges us to consider new approaches to the ethics of pain and suffering.

THE ETHICS OF PAIN AND SUFFERING: NARRATIVE ANALYSIS

"Man by his very nature," wrote Cicely Saunders in 1962, "finds that he has to question the pain he endures and seek meaning in it."[75] For patients, the drive to find meaning in pain often takes the form of narrative – from extended personal stories to compressed beliefs. The belief that all pain and suffering are sent or sanctioned by God, for example, constitutes a compressed mini-narrative that regularly occurs within larger accounts of divine providence throughout world religions. Although medicine officially distrusts narrative as mere anecdotal evidence far inferior to science or fact, medical education and practice are bursting with narrative, whether in formal case studies and patient histories or in casual tales swapped around the water cooler.[76] In 1999, the *British Medical Journal*, defying the culturally coded devaluation of narrative as no more than entertainment, ran a five-part series entitled "narrative-based medicine." The title, evoking a deliberate contrast with "evidence-based medicine," expresses a conviction that narrative in medical contexts constitutes useful (if limited) evidence and a valuable (if selective) tool that might complement traditional biomedical practices. The British Medical Journal Press republished the articles along with additional contributions in a book-length study (*Narrative Based Medicine: Dialogue and Discourse in Clinical Practice*) that includes an essay by Sir Richard Bayliss entitled "Pain narratives."[77]

What are pain narratives and how might they help clinicians address urgent issues of bioethics? Pain, we might say, is the ancient antagonist of which the brain must perpetually make sense, and one way we make sense of pain is through narrative. Moreover, individual narratives are never wholly unique but share basic features with other stories circulating inside a culture. We understand any text ultimately because we have learned the narrative conventions that govern it, from case studies to *Star Wars*. Further, we inhabit cultures that surround us with prepackaged narratives. "Country" music specializes in miniature erotic narratives of pain and suffering, as do standard rock anthems such as John Mellancamp's *Hurts So Good*. (In edgier performance narratives, the American rock band Genitorturers draws spectators on stage at live concerts to have needles jammed into their groins.) Popular culture is awash with pain narratives. Televised talk-shows have added the newest variant with their tales of nonstop victimization. We all live out our lives, as philosopher Alasdair MacIntyre tells us, in terms of narrative.[78] It is rash to believe that the pain narratives circulating within popular culture have no impact on how people live. The study of pain beliefs shows the damage that ensues when patients anxiously imagine catastrophic outcomes. The challenge is to study the harmful or helpful consequences of pain beliefs that are enfolded within more fully developed social and personal narratives. Such research holds implications not only for medical treatment but also for medical ethics.

One helpful approach to narratives of pain and suffering comes from sociologist Arthur W. Frank in *The Wounded Storyteller: Body, Illness, and Ethics*.[79] Frank offers a typology of four narrative structures that reappear when contemporary patients write about their illnesses. It would be useful for pain specialists to recognize instantly, almost as a diagnostic category, what Frank identifies as the recurrent type of "chaos" narrative. It would also be useful to develop an extended typology of the narratives that patients bring to a pain center. We know that chronic pain often constitutes a threat to individual identity.[80] If

individual identity is inseparable from the tacit narratives of self-hood that we construct or accept, then the dilemmas of chronic pain and suffering include an inescapable narrative dimension. Frank argues that the self cannot be reconstructed in healing without the reconstruction of a new personal narrative. The Greek term *ethos* originally referred to a person's settled disposition or character, and the narrative reconstruction of a human life, in healing, is a profoundly ethical matter.

The skills developed through narrative are relevant enough to medical education to fit comfortably within the prevailing language of competencies.[81] Some narrative competencies are especially relevant to pain, including the basic clinical act of listening. As a low-technology virtue that everyone praises but few take seriously, listening is a skill that needs to be relearned inside medical contexts for professional purposes, much as a competitive swimmer must relearn how to breathe. One famous study showed that doctors listened on average for just 18 s before interrupting patients in order to take control.[82] Later studies indicate that the situation is not quite so one-sided, but listening is a skill that, for various reasons, comes hard in medical settings.[83] If a health maintenance organization (HMO) requires physicians to spend on average no more than 7 min per patient, listening to pain narratives may seem an unaffordable luxury. A sounder approach, however, might regard skilled listening to patients as necessary for accurate medical understanding. Accurate medical understanding thus would require skills in listening. Failure to obtain skills necessary for medical practice is not merely unprofessional but unethical.

Skills in listening to patient narratives are sometimes crucial to pain medicine. For example, pain entails special problems for the elderly, who may suffer serious side-effects from medications or hold erroneous pain beliefs that make any treatment less effective. The IASP study *Pain in the Elderly* recommends exploring nondrug therapies.[84] The practice of skilled listening to patient narratives, like the practice of writing in narrative form for patients, can have therapeutic value. Narrative can help pain specialists learn how to listen and what to listen for. Speech and story are never wholly transparent. As bioethicist Tod Chambers writes: "Every telling of a story – real or imagined – encompasses a series of choices about what will be revealed, what will be privileged, and what will be concealed: there are no artless narrations."[85] There is no need to pump up claims for skilled listening or for the uses of narrative. They are not the answer to pain. But nothing *else* is either, including morphine. Skilled listening is one more useful tool in a multidisciplinary approach to the multiple dimensions of pain, and research with hospice patients has shown, at least in selected circumstances, the value of narrative-based therapies such as structured life review.[86]

Narrative helps to illuminate the ethical issues always implicit in pain. The mere act of paying attention, so basic to the reception of narrative, is a moral as well as cognitive state: in turning a deaf ear, we demonstrate how little we value the speaker. Narrative also helps us to recognize and respond to the ethical significance of unnoticed, everyday acts, such as the pain treatment accorded to ethnic minorities. Moreover, because narrative is among the ancient and enduring forms of moral knowledge, from *Aesop's Fables* to *Schindler's List*, it provides a resource for exploring the ways in which pain and suffering make a claim on us as moral beings. A cry of pain places us always, implicitly, under an ethical obligation. Its inevitable subjectivity is not impenetrable but belongs to social, interpersonal codes as instantly comprehensible as SOS. We may not be able personally to answer every SOS, but it is self-deception to pretend that we do not know what it means or what response it asks from us. Narrative is a resource for developing skills in the recognition and interpretation of ethical dilemmas intrinsic to pain. Even an unresolved dilemma, if we recognize it for what it is, at least invites future resolution. An unrecognized ethical dilemma in medical settings, especially a dilemma that centers on pain and suffering, is a potentially harmful form of ignorance.

The medical undertreatment of pain has been well documented for over 20 years.[87] Its ethical implications, however, are not often recognized or addressed.[88] One prominent study, for example, shows that 50% of hospitalized dying patients in the USA spent at least half their time (according to family members) in moderate to severe pain.[89] The method that researchers employed to redress this undertreatment of pain in dying patients centered on staff education, not on ethics and certainly not on narrative, and it yielded no improvement. As an alternative method for recognizing and addressing the ethical implications of undertreatment for pain, narrative can hardly do worse. Consider the 1999 *New York Times* story about Mrs Ozzie Chavez.[90] Mrs Chavez, a California Medicaid patient, was refused proper anesthesia in childbirth because she had not paid an additional (illegal) fee required by the anesthesiologist. "The anesthesiologist wouldn't even come into the room until she got her money," Mrs Chavez was reported saying. "I was lying there having contractions, and they wouldn't give me an epidural. I felt like an animal."

Narrative will not get us to the bottom of the story – to expose the truth about what really happened in Mrs Chavez's room – but it helps us to unfold the ethical implications of the patient's experience. It illustrates too how the ethical implications of everyday acts often go unnoticed in our emphasis on megawatt, headline-grabbing, life-and-death bioethical issues.[91] When this story ran in the newsletter of the American Society of Anesthesiologists, it evoked the following commentary from one doctor: "Poor people can't expect to drive a Rolls Royce, so why should they expect to receive the Cadillac of analgesics for free." As if to head off a looming public relations disaster, the president of the American Society of Anes-

thesiologists, John B. Neeld Jr, vaulted directly to first principles. "It is unethical," he said, "to withhold services because of reimbursement." End of story?

A narrative on bioethics would not consider the story to have finished when one character, no matter how eminent, denounces the behavior of another character as unethical. Just as there are no artless narrations, narrative theory reminds us to consider what is unsaid or even unsayable. Neeld, for example, does not mention (is it unsayable?) that medical services are withheld every day in America because of inability to pay. Nor is the USA alone in withholding services. Further, as in the dilemma of hospitalized dying patients, medical services for pain are routinely withheld for causes apparently *unconnected* with cost.[28] These causes – reflected in what William Breitbart has called the "dramatically undertreated" pain of AIDS patients[67] – express bias as well as economics. Sex and race, as one (disputed) study shows, affect a medical decision as seemingly neutral as recommendations for cardiac catheterization.[92] Sickle cell pain, with its predominant impact on people of African heritage, is not untroubled by issues of race. Within this cultural mix, as it applies to Mrs Chavez, we must consider the substandard payment policies of certain government agencies. Finally, in a narrative analysis which assumes that language matters, we should note that Mrs Chavez did not say she felt pain. She said she felt like an animal. Pain for Mrs Chavez evokes a down-to-earth ethics of respect and degradation. Narrative analysis does not say who is right or wrong, but it helps us to understand and to unfold the ethical implications of neglected everyday acts.

One benefit of a renewed attention to narrative would be an emphasis on the ethical – rather than on the strictly regulatory – aspects of undertreatment. Of course, we need effective institutional guidelines and review processes in place to combat the long-standing neglect and medical myths that prevent patients from receiving adequate pain medication.[93] We need political action to combat the negative influence that licensing boards, disciplinary groups, and drug enforcement agencies exert on the medical use of opioid analgesics.[94] Such pragmatic changes, however, are not enough. The distinguished philosopher of medicine Edmund D. Pellegrino has recently insisted in a discussion of emerging ethical issues in palliative care that – given the availability of effective medications – not to relieve pain optimally is "tantamount to ethical and legal malpractice."[95] Serious inquiry into the ethics of undertreatment may avoid a deluge of legal challenges.

We lack medications to relieve suffering that are as effective as opioids in relieving pain. There is, however, an equally serious issue to face. The best medical approach to suffering is not always aggressive action. Although medicine prefers action and thrives on problem-solving, sometimes little or nothing can be done. Surgeon Sherwin B. Nuland writes: "The diagnosis of disease and the quest for overcoming it with his intellect are the challenges that motivate every specialist who is any good at what he does. He is fascinated with pathology. When faced by the certainty of his own impotence to treat it, the would-be healer too often turns away."[96] This is unfortunate, but not surprising. When medical practice becomes preeminently an arena of action, inaction is usually misinterpreted as failure. Yet sometimes suffering will run its terrible course regardless of any intervention. In such cases, there is great value in openly discussing the role of witness.

An almost inescapable logic drives professional disciplines to remove human experience from its flow in everyday local worlds and to reshape it in accordance with the needs of the profession that addresses it.[97] This logic proves dangerous when it comes to the experience of suffering. Therefore, as a complement to the preferred medical stance of active, even heroic, practice, it is important to consider the role of witness. *Witness* comes from an Old English verb meaning "to know." The witness is someone who knows firsthand, and such knowing is not a passive possession, mere looking or seeing, opposed to practice. Witnessing is an action. The witness is one who – in the medical term derived from a Latin root that means "to bend to, to notice" – "attends," and such vigilant "attending" requires far more than physical presence. The witness cannot erase suffering, prevent tragedy, or defeat death. When suffering is inescapable, however, the active role of witnessing opens up possibilities that can in part offset or redeem sheer loss. The decision to be present, as witness, is an ethical choice. Moreover, the presence of the witness can comfort the person who suffers, and there is no higher act, inside or outside medicine, that we are called upon to perform.

REFERENCES

1. Pope John Paul II. Letter handed to John Bonica on the occasion of the Fifth World Congress on Pain. In: Benedetti C, Chapman CR, Giron G eds. *Opioid Analgesia: Recent Advances in Systemic Administration* (*Advances in Pain Research and Therapy*, vol. 14). New York, NY: Raven Press, 1990.
2. Melzack R, Wall PD. Pain mechanisms: a new theory. *Science* 1965; **150:** 971–9.
3. Melzack R. Gate control theory: on the evolution of pain concepts. *Pain Forum* 1996; **5:** 128–38.
4. Baszanger I. *Inventing Pain Medicine: from the Laboratory to the Clinic*. New Brunswick, NJ: Rutgers University Press, 1998; first published in French in 1995.
5. IASP, 27 June 1999: http://www.halcyon.com/iasp.
6. Melzack R. Central pain syndromes and theories of pain. In: Casey KL ed. *Pain and Central Nervous System Disease: the Central Pain Syndromes*. New York, NY: Raven Press, 1991: 59–64.
7. Jones AKP, Brown WD, Friston KJ, *et al*. Cortical and sub-cortical localization of response to pain in man using positron emission tomography. *Proc R Soc Lond B* 1991; **244:** 39–44.
8. Talbot JD, Marrett S, Evans AC, *et al*. Multiple representations of pain in human cerebral cortex. *Science* 1991; **251:** 1355–8.
9. Derbyshire SWG. Imaging the brain in pain. *Am Pain Soc Bull* 1999; **9** (3): 7–9.
10. Ploghaus A, Tracey I, Gati JS, *et al*. Dissociating pain from its anticipation in the human brain. *Science* 1999; **284:** 1979–81.
11. Treede R-D, Kenshalo DR, Gracely RH, Jones AKP. The cortical representation of pain. *Pain* 1999; **79:** 105–11.
12. Belenky M, Devor M. Association of postganglionic sympathetic neurons with primary afferents in sympathetic-sensory co-cultures. *J Neurocytol* 1997; **26:** 715–31.
13. Elmer GI, Pieper JO, Negus SS, Woods JH. Genetic variance in nociception and its relationship to the potency of morphine-induced analgesia in thermal and chemical tests. *Pain* 1998; **75:** 129–40.
14. Devor M, Raber P. Heritability of symptoms in an experimental model of neuropathic pain. *Pain* 1990; **42:** 51–67.
15. Yaksh TL. Pharmacology and mechanisms of opioid analgesic activity. *Acta Anaesthesiol Scand* 1997; **41:** 94–111.
16. Yaksh TL, Dirig DM, Malmberg AB. Mechanism of action of nonsteroidal anti-inflammatory drugs. *Cancer Invest* 1998; **16:** 509–27.
17. Verhaak PFM, Kerssens JJ, Dekker J, *et al*. Prevalence of chronic benign pain disorder among adults: a review of the literature. *Pain* 1998; **77:** 231–9.
18. van Tulder MW, Koes BW, Bouter LM. A cost-of-illness study of back pain in The Netherlands. *Pain* 1995; **62:** 233–40.
19. Linton SJ. The socioeconomic impact of chronic back pain: is anyone benefiting? *Pain* 1998; **75:** 163–8.
20. Robertson JT. The rape of the spine. *Surg Neurol* 1993; **39:** 5–12.
21. Fordyce WE ed. *Back Pain in the Workplace: Management of Disability in Nonspecific Conditions*. Seattle, WA: IASP Press, 1995.
22. Pain terms: a list with definitions and notes on usage. *Pain* 1979; **6:** 249–52.
23. Merskey H, Bogduk N eds. *Classification of Chronic Pain: Descriptions of Chronic Pain Syndromes and Definitions of Pain Terms*, 2nd edn. Seattle, WA: IASP Press, 1994.
24. Beecher HK. Pain in men wounded in battle. *Bull US Army Med Dept* 1946; **5:** 445–54.
25. Blank JW. Pain in men wounded in battle: Beecher revisited. *IASP Newsletter* 1994; **Jan/Feb:** 2–4.
26. Bayer TL, Baer PE, Early C. Situational and psychophysiological factors in psychologically induced pain. *Pain* 1991; **44:** 45–50.

27. Duncan G. Mind–body dualism and the biopsychosocial model of pain: what did Descartes really say? *J Med Philos* 2000; **25:** 485–513.

28. Sullivan M. In what sense is contemporary medicine dualistic? *Cult Med Psychiatry* 1986; **10:** 331–50.

29. Cunningham N. Primary requirements for an ethical definition of pain. *Pain Forum* 1999; **8:** 93–9.

30. Rollin BE. Some conceptual and ethical concerns about current views of pain. *Pain Forum* 1999; **8:** 78–83.

31. Jensen MP. Validity of self-report and observation measures. In: Jensen TS, Turner JA, Wiesenfeld-Hallin Z eds. *Proceedings of the 8th World Congress on Pain. Progress in Pain Research and Management*, vol. 8. Seattle, WA: IASP Press, 1997: 637–61.

32. Cassell EJ. *The Nature of Suffering and the Goals of Medicine*. New York, NY: Oxford University Press, 1991.

33. Kleinman A. *The Illness Narratives: Suffering, Healing, and the Human Condition*. New York, NY: Basic Books, 1988.

34. Bowker J. *Problems of Suffering in Religions of the World*. Cambridge: Cambridge University Press, 1970.

35. Wall PA. *Pain: the Science of Suffering*. London: Weidenfeld, 1999.

◆ 36. Chapman CR, Gavrin J. Suffering: the contributions of persistent pain. *Lancet* 1999; **353:** 2233–7.

37. *The Hedgehog Review: Critical Reflections on Contemporary Culture* 1999; **1:** 5–102; the entire issue is devoted to sociological reflections on "identity."

38. Turkle S. *Life on the Screen: Identity in the Age of the Internet*. New York, NY: Simon and Schuster, 1995.

39. Kleinman A, Das V, Lock M eds. *Social Suffering*. Berkeley, CA: University of California Press, 1997.

40. Peterson C, Maier SF, Seligman MEP. *Learned Helplessness: a Theory for the Age of Personal Control*. New York, NY: Oxford University Press, 1993.

41. Candib LM. Power-in-relation. In: *Medicine and the Family: a Feminist Perspective*. New York, NY: Basic Books, 1995: 240–53.

42. Levinas E. Useless suffering. In: Bernasconi R, Wood D eds. *The Provocation of Levinas: Rethinking the Other*. London: Routledge, 1988: 156–67; first published in French in 1982 and translated by R. Cohen.

43. Portenoy RK. Palliative care: an opportunity for pain specialists. *Am Pain Soc Bull* 1999; **9** (3): 2–5.

44. Gawande A. A queasy feeling: why can't we cure nausea? *The New Yorker* 1999; **5 July:** 34–41.

45. Rey R. *The History of Pain*. Wallace LE, Cadden JA, Cadden SW trans. Cambridge, MA: Harvard University Press, 1993; first published in French in 1993.

46. Sullivan MD. Pain in language: from sentience to sapience. *Pain Forum* 1995; **4:** 3–14.

47. Yaksh TL. Pain speaking – and anesthesiologists answer. *JAMA* 1992; **267:** 1578–9.

48. Dubner R. Pain speaking – and anesthesiologists answer. *JAMA* 1992; **267:** 1578–9.

49. Liebeskind JC. Pain *can* kill. *Pain* 1991; **44:** 3–4.

50. Loeser JD. What is chronic pain? *Theor Med* 1991; **12:** 213–25.

51. LeResche L. Gender considerations in the epidemiology of chronic pain. In: Crombie IK, Croft PR, Linton SJ, *et al*. eds. *Epidemiology of Pain*. Seattle, WA: IASP Press, 1999: 43–52.

52. Weir R, Browne G, Tunks E, *et al*. Gender differences in psychosocial adjustment to chronic pain and expenditures for health care services used. *Clin J Pain* 1996; **12:** 277–90.

● 53. Unruh AM. Gender variations in clinical pain experience. *Pain* 1996; **65:** 123–67.

54. Fillingim RB, Maixner W. Gender differences in the responses to noxious stimuli. *Pain Forum* 1995; **4:** 209–21.

55. Gear RW, Miaskowski C, Gordon NC, *et al*. Kappa-opioids produce significantly greater analgesia in women than in men. *Nature Med* 1996; **2:** 1248–50.

56. Lipton RB, Stewart WF. Prevalence and impact of migraine. *Neurol Clin* 1997; **15:** 1–13.

57. Vallerand AH. Gender differences in pain. *Image J Nurs Scholarship* 1995; **27:** 235–7.

58. Brena SF, Sanders SH, Motoyama H. American and Japanese low back pain patients: cross-cultural similarities and differences. *Clin J Pain* 1990; **6:** 113–24.

59. Kodiath MF, Kodiath A. A comparative study of patients who experience chronic malignant pain in India and the United States. *Cancer Nurs* 1995; **18:** 189–96.

60. Cross-cultural investigations of pain. In: Crombie IK, Croft PR, Linton SJ, *et al*. eds. *Epidemiology of Pain*. Seattle, WA: IASP Press, 1999: 53–80.

61. Burns B, Busby C, Sawchuk K eds. *When Pain Strikes*. Minneapolis, MN: University of Minnesota Press, 1999.

62. Willis WD, Westkund KN. Neuroanatomy of the pain system and of the pathways that modulate pain. *J Clin Neurophysiol* 1997; **14:** 2–31.

63. Gatchell RJ, Turk DC eds. *Psychosocial Factors in Pain: Critical Perspectives*. New York, NY: Guilford Press, 1999.

64. Song S-O, Carr DB. Pain and memory. *Pain Clin Updates* 1999; **7:** 1–4.

65. Morris DB. *The Culture of Pain*. Berkeley, CA: University of California Press, 1991.

66. Morris DB. *Illness and Culture in the Postmodern Age*. Berkeley, CA: University of California Press, 1998.

67. Stephenson J. Experts say AIDS pain "dramatically undertreated." *JAMA* 1996; **276:** 1369–70.

68. Williams DA, Thorn BE. An empirical assessment of pain beliefs. *Pain* 1989: **36:** 351–8.

● 69. Jensen MP, Turner JA, Romano JM, Karoly P. Coping with chronic pain: a critical review of the literature. *Pain* 1991; **47:** 249–83.

70. Bromm B. Consciousness, pain, and cortical activity. In: Bromm B, Desmedt JD eds. *Pain and the Brain: from*

Nociception to Cognition. Advances in Pain Research and Therapy, vol. 22. New York, NY: Raven Press, 1995: 35–59.

71. Chapman CR. The affective dimension of pain: a model. In: Bromm B, Desmedt JD eds. *Pain and the Brain: from Nociception to Cognition. Advances in Pain Research and Therapy*, vol. 22. New York, NY: Raven Press, 1995: 283–301.

72. Williams DA, Keefe FJ. Pain beliefs and the use of cognitive–behavioral coping strategies. *Pain* 1991; **46:** 185–90.

73. Jensen MP, Karoly P. Pain-specific beliefs, perceived symptom severity, and adjustment to chronic pain. *Clin J Pain* 1992; **8:** 123–30.

74. Shutty MS Jr, DeGood DE, Tuttle DH. Chronic pain patients' beliefs about their pain and treatment outcomes. *Arch Phys Med Rehabil* 1990; **71:** 128–32.

75. Saunders C. And from sudden death …. *Nursing Times* 1962; **17 August:** 1045–6.

76. Hunter KM. *Doctors' Stories: the Narrative Structure of Medical Knowledge*. Princeton, NJ: Princeton University Press, 1991.

77. Bayliss R. Pain narratives. In: Greenhalgh T, Hurwitz B eds. *Narrative Based Medicine: Dialogue and Discourse in Clinical Practice*. London: British Medical Journal Press, 1998: 75–82.

78. MacIntyre A. *After Virtue: a Study in Moral Theory*. Notre Dame, IN: University of Notre Dame Press, 1981.

79. Frank AW. *The Wounded Storyteller: Body, Illness, and Ethics*. Chicago, IL: University of Chicago Press, 1995.

80. Eccleston C, Williams ACdeC, Rogers WS. Patients' and professionals' understandings of the causes of chronic pain: blame, responsibility and identity protection. *Soc Sci Med* 1997; **45:** 699–709.

81. Hunter KM, Charon R, Coulehan JL. The study of literature in medical education. *Acad Med* 1995; **70:** 787–94.

82. Beckman HB, Frankel RM. The effect of physician behavior on the collection of data. *Ann Intern Med* 1984; **101:** 692–6.

83. Lown B. *The Lost Art of Healing*. Boston, MA: Houghton-Mifflin, 1996.

84. Ferrell BR, Ferrell BA eds. *Pain in the Elderly*. Seattle, WA: IASP Press, 1996.

85. Chambers T. From the ethicist's point of view: the liter-ary nature of ethical inquiry. *Hastings Cent Rep* 1996; **26:** 25–33.

86. Haight BK. The therapeutic role of a structured life review process in homebound elderly subjects. *J Gerontol* 1988; **43:** 40–4.

87. American Pain Society Quality of Care Committee. Quality improvement guidelines for the treatment of acute pain and cancer pain. *JAMA* 1995; **274:** 1874–80.

88. Rich BA. A legacy of silence: bioethics and the culture of pain. *J Med Humanities* 1997; **18:** 233–59.

89. SUPPORT Principal Investigators. A controlled trial to improve care for seriously ill hospitalized patients. *JAMA* 1995; **274:** 1591–8.

90. Pear R. Mothers on Medicaid overcharged for pain relief. *New York Times* 8 March 1999; http://archives/nytimes.com/archives.

91. Komasaroff PA. From bioethics to microethics: ethical debate and clinical medicine. In: Komasaroff PA ed. *Troubled Bodies: Critical Perspectives on Postmodernism, Medical Ethics, and the Body*. Durham, NC: Duke University Press, 1995: 62–86.

92. Schulman KA, Berlin JA, Harless W, *et al*. The effect of race and sex on physicians' recommendations for cardiac catheterization. *N Engl J Med* 1999; **340:** 618–26; see also erratum (*N Engl Med J* 1999; **340:** 1130) and critical responses (*N Engl J Med* 1999; **341:** 285–7).

93. Hill Jr CS. When will adequate pain treatment be the norm? *JAMA* 1995; **274:** 1881–2.

94. Hill CS Jr. The negative influence of licensing and disciplinary boards and drug enforcement agencies on pain treatment with opioid analgesics. *J Pharm Care Pain Sympt Control* 1993; **1:** 43–62.

95. Pellegrino ED. Emerging ethical issues in palliative care. *JAMA* 1998; **279:** 1521–2.

96. Nuland SB. *How We Die: Reflections on Life's Final Chapter*. New York, NY: Alfred A. Knopf, 1994.

97. Kleinman A, Kleinman J. Suffering and its professional transformation: toward an ethnography of interpersonal experience. *Cult Med Psychiatry* 1991; **15:** 275–301.

98. Williams, DA. Acute pain management. In: Gatchel RJ, Turk DC eds. *Psychological Approaches to Pain Management: a Practitioner's Handbook*. New York, NY: Guilford Press, 1996: 55–77.

Epidemiology of chronic pain

EMMA CHOJNOWSKA AND CATHERINE STANNARD

Chronic pain is a multidimensional experience produced by a combination of host, causative agent, and environmental factors undergoing temporal variation. By studying pain within the general population, epidemiology can not only provide quantitative information but can *also* serve as a powerful analytical tool to unravel the complex nature of pain and act as a guide to management. Despite this great potential, only since the 1990s have large numbers of papers been published on the epidemiology of pain.[1] The increasing costs of pain within affluent industrialized nations, particularly within the workforce, have led to increasing interest in the management and prevention of persistent or chronic pain.

The International Association for the Study of Pain (IASP) Task Force on Epidemiology was established in 1994 to improve the quality of epidemiological studies relevant to pain and to provide a definitive review.[2]

Owing to the huge diversity and, often, poor quality of reported studies, aggregation of data for specific chronic pain conditions was found to be generally unreliable and unhelpful. Much work is required on primary research. Therefore, this chapter provides an overview of epidemiology methodology and a consideration of important population factors (gender, age, and culture), and highlights what epidemiology can tell us about some common pain problems (e.g. chronic postsurgical pain and low back pain).

THE ROLE OF EPIDEMIOLOGY

- Frequency of disease.
- Natural history of disease.
- Understanding disease etiology.
- Disease prevention: primary, secondary, and tertiary.
- Planning health care services.

Epidemiology studies the frequency of disease and its natural history in the general population, exploring how disease frequency varies by age, gender, race, and location and how frequency changes with time. Direct comparative studies between various subgroups within society contribute to the understanding of disease etiology and identification of risk factors. Determining the extent and distribution of medical problems can be used for planning health care services. Prevention of disease by removing or reducing exposure to these risk factors is the ultimate aim of epidemiological study. The final step is investigation of the effectiveness of health care service and success of preventative measures. Hence, Last[3] defined epidemiology as the study of the distribution and determinants of disease in the population and the application of this study to the control of health problems.

Three types of prevention may be considered. *Primary prevention* aims to stop the occurrence of pain. History has demonstrated that the precise pathology of disease is not necessary to discover preventative measures that control disease. The pioneering physician John Snow ended a local outbreak during the 1854 cholera epidemic in London by dismantling a pump in Broad Street, Soho. Further studies confirmed that water contaminated with sewage was the source of the disease and led to laws governing the safe disposal of sewage and supply of clean drinking water. Joseph Goldberger, an American epidemiologist working in the early part of this century, demonstrated that pellagra was caused by dietary deficiency (niacin) and not infection in poor communities reliant on maize. Whole-population prevention of vitamin deficiency is now achieved by fortifying basic foods, for example cornflakes, with vitamins.

Secondary prevention aims to prevent continuing illness by early intervention. An example is acute back pain, in which prompt treatment aims to prevent the development of chronic pain.[4] *Tertiary prevention* tries to minimize the effects of chronic pain on physical and psychological well-being, and on employment.[1]

EPIDEMIOLOGICAL ENQUIRY

Disease definition

A requirement of any epidemiological investigation is to define pain. Infectious disease and trauma present the researcher with clear diagnostic tests. Pain presents special problems. The subjective definition of pain as "an unpleasant sensory and emotional experience associated with actual or potential tissue damage or described in terms of such damage"[5] makes measurement problematic. It is essential that some consensual validated criteria are used to describe groups of individuals with similar chronic pain syndromes to enable the reproducibility and comparability of epidemiological studies. An extensive classification of pain was produced by the International Association for the Study of Pain (IASP) Subcommittee on Taxonomy in 1986,[5] and later revised by Merskey and Bogduk.[6] The IASP taxonomy is based largely on clinical grounds, rather than causal criteria assigning patients to specific diagnostic categories based on combinations of characteristics, including body site, system involved, symptoms, signs, and test results. Such classification systems may be difficult to use, e.g. Bruehl *et al.*[7] have raised concerns regarding current IASP criteria for complex regional pain syndrome (CRPS). Although sensitivity was high, poor specificity led to overdiagnosis. Increasing the number of signs and symptoms required to make a diagnosis of CRPS optimized diagnostic efficiency. The absence of objective findings in almost all cases of low back pain has forced investigators to rely on a diverse range of symptoms. Numerous definitions and diagnostic classifications of low back pain render comparison of studies difficult. The IASP classification has considerable potential, but further research is needed to improve diagnostic efficiency.

A further consideration is the multidimensionality of pain and the importance of functional, psychosocial, and behavioral characteristics (in addition to symptoms and signs) in classification. Turk and Rudy's empirical approach uses psychosocial and behavioral data to distinguish three profiles (dysfunctional, interpersonally distressed, and adaptive coper) as a complementary taxonomy to IASP classification.[8] The usefulness of combining different taxonomies for epidemiological study has not been fully assessed.

Identifying the onset of chronicity also requires consensus. Without a suitable time period for each pain condition, findings from different studies cannot be compared. The episodic nature of pain makes determination of onset of chronicity difficult.

Disease occurrence

Having defined the pain condition, epidemiological investigation can measure occurrence. Detailed study uncovers differences in occurrence between sexes and across age groups, over time, and between different geographical populations. Age and sex effects on pain, as with other diseases, may be so strong that, without such data, the occurrence of pain cannot be compared between populations and within the same population over time.

Incidence or prevalence

Incidence records disease onset. *First-ever incidence* may include only those subjects who present with the first pain episode during a particular time period. Alternatively, *episode incidence* records onset of all episodes regardless of whether the episode is the first or a recurrence. Measures of incidence can quantify the probability of occurrence of a pain state, i.e. onset of a pain condition or of disability related to a pain condition. The episode incidence can also provide useful information on the probability of recurrence of pain, e.g. migraine, which can be clearly defined with periods of disease absence.

Prevalence records disease states and quantifies the proportion of the population in a specified pain state, e.g. chronic pain or pain-related disability. *Point prevalence* describes occurrence of a particular condition at any given moment. However, chronic pain is often characterized by insidious onset, episodic course, and a broad spectrum of severity. Prevalence takes this variability into account. For episodic conditions, prevalence is a function of incidence, episode duration, and probability of recurrence.[9] *Period prevalence* describes the occurrence at any time within a defined period, usually a year, but *cumulative prevalence* extends the time period to include all those who have been in a disease state during their lives between two specific points in time, e.g. between the ages of 30 and 60. The extended time period will include people with a single resolved episode some years previously as well as those with continuing disease.

The consequences of using different definitions of pain when estimating prevalence has been demonstrated by Von Korff *et al.*[10] In response to a postal questionnaire, 37% of health maintenance organization enrollees reported recurrent or persistent pain, but only 5.4% had severe and persistent pain and 2.7% severe and persistent pain with 7 or more days of limited activity in the preceding 6 months. Similarly, prevalence surveys of back pain, counting as cases all individuals who have experienced any back pain at all during the reporting period, will produce markedly different prevalence rates than surveys defining a case as individuals with severe back pain or activity limitation.

Standardized definitions need to focus on disabling conditions rather than including the whole spectrum of pain severity in order to identify the relevant risk factors.

Disease causation and outcome

By quantifying the strength of association between various etiological factors and pain conditions, causation of pain and outcome may be determined. Identification of cause or risk factors permits the development of preventative strategies. Prevention is particularly important in chronic pain because for many patients treatment is not always effective.

For most chronic pain conditions, etiology is complex and may be considered under three headings: agent, host, and environment.[11] The interaction between these factors is often represented as a triangle of the web of causation (Fig. 2.1)

An example of these factors interacting in low back pain have identified sociodemographic (age, gender, education), clinical (obesity, height, comorbidity), occupational (physical workload, bending and lifting, vibrating equipment, mental stress, psychosocial, job satisfaction), and psychological (depression, self-confidence, somatization) factors.

The multifactorial nature of pain means that most risk factors investigated are neither sufficient, i.e. they will not cause pain on their own, nor necessary, i.e. the condition can occur in the absence of that exposure. For example, not all patients with lung cancer have smoked, and not all smokers develop lung cancer.

Etiological factors may also show multiplicity of effect – producing different pain states – and equifinality of effect, with different etiological factors producing the same outcome. If pain behavior alters environmental factors, for example unemployment and/or divorce, there may be further alterations in the person's pain perception and behavior. The variability in the effects of etiological factors between individuals may cause difficulties in epi-

demiological study, particularly in determining outcome. Because most reports are from cross-sectional studies, it is unclear whether psychological association precedes or follows the onset of back problems.[12] Compensation has a negative influence on the length of disability.

Disease management and disease prevention

The intervention trial aims to prove causative links between suspected exposure factors and disease. The intervention trial can be applied to a comparison of health service policies and can be used to assess the effectiveness of a population-wide preventative strategy. Questions such as these require the same rigorous epidemiological approach as those investigating disease occurrence and natural history.

EPIDEMIOLOGICAL METHODOLOGY

Study design determines analytical power. Problems in population selection are one of the major reasons for a study's conclusion being invalid. Further problems may arise from information gathering, analysis, interpretation of results (can the results be explained by bias or associations explained by confounding factors and are they applicable to the whole population), and logistics (ethics and cost). These problems are outside the scope of this chapter. An introduction to epidemiological methodology may be found in practical guides by Silman[13] and Barker and Rose.[14]

Study design

- Descriptive.
- Analytical.

In *descriptive* studies, the frequency of occurrence of disease in different communities or subgroups within a community is described. *Analytical* studies test hypotheses about the influence of risk factors on the development of disease in a population or in individuals within a population and, unlike descriptive studies, usually demand

Figure 2.1 *The pain triangle.*

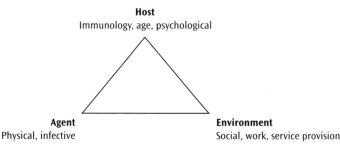

Host
Immunology, age, psychological

Agent
Physical, infective

Environment
Social, work, service provision

the use of controls. The same study design may then be used to test hypotheses by showing whether or not the frequency of a disease may be changed by altering exposure to a suspected risk factor.

Descriptive studies

Descriptive studies include the simple descriptive survey, cross-sectional population study, and longitudinal population study.

Simple descriptive survey

Unlike clinical surveys, which describe patients, epidemiological surveys describe patients in relation to a population. Simple descriptive surveys describe a disease by relating the characteristics, such as age, sex, and occupation of a group of cases, to those of the population.

Cross-sectional population study

These studies or surveys measure disease and exposure to determinants of disease states at a point in time or over a short period of time. A cross-sectional population study is a single examination of a cross-section of population, whereas longitudinal studies trace changes in a population over a period of time. The study group is a sample of a complete population: people with and without pain are caught in the survey net and are not distinguished until results are examined, hence the cases represent the disease in the whole community and there is no selection or assessment bias as with a case series assembled from hospital records.

The measure of disease frequency that cross-sectional studies yield is prevalence (the terms cross-sectional study or survey and *prevalence survey* are sometimes used interchangeably).

The measurement of risk factor status usually relies on self-reported information or on simple objective measurements. Association between risk factor and disease must be interpreted with caution. Bias may arise from questionnaires. For example, in a survey of back pain in nursing staff, if nurses with back pain sought alternative employment they would be excluded from a cross-sectional study, thus lowering the observed prevalence rate.

A cross-sectional study may also make it difficult to establish what is cause and what is effect, e.g. if a pain condition results in unemployment this may affect the person's subjective experience of pain. Because of these difficulties, cross-sectional surveys of etiology are best suited to diseases that produce little disability and the presymptomatic phases of more serious disorders. It should be noted that only exceptionally does association reveal etiology, e.g. association of childhood lymphoma and malaria. More often, information from the study can test etiological hypotheses by comparing characteristics of the sick and healthy.

Longitudinal population studies

Descriptive studies in which subjects are followed over prolonged periods with continuous or repeated monitoring of risk factors, health outcome, or both are termed longitudinal studies. These studies can specifically measure incidence, follow natural history, and examine the association between initial characteristics and risk of future disease. The fluctuating course of pain may be followed, i.e. remission, recurrence, and progression.

Observation over a period of time can explain associations found in cross-sectional studies. Von Korff and Simon[15] used longitudinal data to examine the relationship between pain and depression. Among primary care pain patients, depressive symptoms were elevated. Subsequent improvement in pain was associated with depressive symptoms returning to normal levels. No improvement in pain and significant activity limitation was associated with continuing depressive symptoms at 1 year but depressive symptoms did not increase with time, suggesting continuing pain does not necessarily worsen depression.

Analytical studies

The purpose of analytical study is to study the association of a putative risk factor with disease onset to test hypotheses about the causes of a disease. These studies usually demand the use of a control. Case–control studies compare people with a disease and those without it. Cohort studies compare people exposed to the suspected cause and those not exposed. Some writers use the terms retrospective and prospective instead of case–control and cohort study respectively. The underlying concept is that case–control studies look backward from people with the disease to suspected causes that have already acted. Cohort studies are forward looking in that they start with people exposed to the suspected cause. The terms retrospective and prospective may also apply to the method of recording observations, i.e. before or after the occurrence of disease, for either analytical study. A further source of confusion is that the terms longitudinal study and cohort study are sometimes used interchangeably. In this text, longitudinal study observes a population over a prolonged period and cohort study tests a specific etiological hypothesis.

Case–control studies

Generally, case–control studies are used for exploratory investigation, and a particular strength is the ability of a single study to simultaneously explore several possible risk factors measuring strength of association with disease. In the choice between case–control or cohort methods, their relative feasibility and cost-efficiency is often the dominant consideration. Case–control studies may be carried out quickly and cheaply since clinics offer a ready source of cases.

Case–control studies compare a sample of people with recent onset of the condition under study and a sample of controls selected to avoid sampling bias with respect to risk factors. The strength of association is quantified by the *odds ratio*, which is derived from the ratio of the odds of being exposed to a risk factor if the disease is present compared with those of being exposed if the disease is absent. The odds ratio is a good estimate of relative risk,[8] and can be calculated when data on incidence are not available (most typically in the case–control study). If the odds ratio is greater than unity (>1), the exposure is associated with the disease, and if <1 the exposure is protective.

To calculate odds ratios and relative risks:[16]

If the proportions of subjects experiencing an event in two groups are P^1 (not exposed to risk factor) and P^2 (exposed to risk factor) then the relative risk is P^1/P^2 and the odds ratio is $(1-P^1)/(1-P^2) \times$ relative risk.

For example, LeResche *et al.*[17] found exposure to exogenous hormones in the form of oral contraceptives and hormone replacement therapy was associated with an increased risk of seeking treatment for temperomandibular pain.

Major difficulties lie in selecting a suitable control group.[18] Limitations of case–control studies also derive from potential sources of bias.[19] In the case of chronic pain, by studying prevalence rather than incidence, factors affecting duration may be confused with those influencing risk. The highly selected nature of patients using a pain clinic may result in selection bias. Patients with chronic pain are more likely to recall previous injuries and possible risk factors that a person without pain would have forgotten.

Cohort studies

Cohort studies, usually of prospective longitudinal design (sometimes referred to as *prospective studies*), test precisely formulated hypotheses, with the suspected cause forming the basis for cohort selection. These cohorts are followed over time to detect and date the occurrence of endpoints, for example recurrence of condition, chronicity, and disability, that are compared with a control group not exposed to the risk factors under investigation. These studies tend to be time consuming and costly: low incidence rates require large cohorts and years of follow-up to yield statistically significant findings. If routinely collected data are available, for example hospital records, large cohorts may be studied retrospectively without prohibitive expense.

The strength of a suspected cause can be expressed by its relative risk or incidence ratio (see above):

Incidence in exposed/Incidence in nonexposed

Useful information may be determined relative to time. When Crook *et al.*[20] followed up chronic pain patients for 2 years, they found 13% of patients no longer reported pain as a problem. Magni *et al.*[21] found 32.5% of chronic pain sufferers had become pain free over an 8-year follow-up.

GENDER-RELATED FACTORS IN THE EPIDEMIOLOGY OF PAIN

Epidemiological research into the prevalence of pain complaints in a general population shows that, in general, women are more likely than men to report a variety of temporary and persistent pains.[22] Women also report pain of greater severity, frequency, and duration than do men.[23] The epidemiological review by LeResche[24] observed definite gender differences in the prevalence of many chronic pain conditions as well as differences between age groups, these conditions occurring more frequently in women.

Disease definition may affect the outcome of studies. As an example, headache occurs at a higher rate in women. Scher *et al.*[25] demonstrated in a meta-analysis of studies on headache an almost constant prevalence rate with age in adult men (at about 60% of the population) and a prevalence of 75–80% up to age 45 years in women. The prevalence in women then declines until at age 60 years it is similar to men. However, when specific conditions are considered, the results may be quite different. Cluster headaches predominantly affect males, usually in their fourth decade. The prevalence of migraine in women is up to twice as high as for men at all ages, rising over reproductive years and declining after age 40 years.[26]

Studies of *occurrence* generally find a higher prevalence of pain conditions in women, e.g. temperomandibular disorders (TMD), fibromyalgia, abdominal pain, and, after 50 years old, joint pain. Interestingly, data on back pain present no consistent pattern across the studies, interpreted by Scher *et al.*[25] as geographical, socioeconomic, occupational, and cohort differences (e.g. case definition) being greater than the influence of gender.

An important aspect of study design is the *population selection*. As an example, in patients attending health clinics, chronic orofacial pain related to TMD occurred more frequently (range 2:1 to 9:1) in women than men.[27] In the community, the ratio of prevalence in women versus men is about 2:1.[17] Thus, data drawn from only a clinic population might present a biased picture of gender factors related to pain. Population selection must also consider age groups under investigation as gender-specific factors may vary significantly with age. Pain associated with TMD occurs in approximately 10% of the population over age 18 years, but primarily affects young middle-aged adults rather than children or the elderly.

The gender of the experimenter may create a potential source of error in epidemiological study. Levine *et al.*[28] found that, when the experimenter was female rather than male, men reported less pain.

There has been very little research examining *biological differences* between sexes in the pain pathways. However, gender differences in the action of sex hormones may influence the peripheral and central mechanisms of nociceptive pain transmission, pain sensitivity, and pain perception. Experimental pain response for women varies across the menstrual cycle, with Giamberardino *et al.*[29] concluding that menstrual phases, dysmenorrhea status, segmental site (abdomen more sensitive than limb), and tissue depth all affected pain thresholds to electrical stimulation. A meta-analysis[30] of the perception of experimentally induced pain across the menstrual cycle in healthy females suggests that the menstrual cycle effect is too large to ignore. In clinical studies, the pattern of prevalence for migraine and TMD is consistent with hormonal factors playing an important causative role.[17,26,31] Both conditions are uncommon in children, and incidence rates rise sharply at onset of puberty. The prevalence of migraine is similar for girls and boys before puberty, but increases with puberty for girls. Migraine in adult women may be affected not only by menstruation, pregnancy, and the menopause but also by the oral contraceptive pill.

Pain experiences differ between the sexes.[23] Women are more likely than men to have persistent and recurrent pain due to chronic but not life-threatening conditions. These conditions include normal biological events related to reproductive cycles (i.e. menstruation, menopause) and pathology associated with normal female physiology, e.g. endometriosis, ectopic pregnancy. Hence, women must make distinctions between manageable and excessive physiological pain and separate such pains from potentially pathological sources. In contrast, men are more likely to experience pain from injury and acute and chronic life-threatening diseases. Therefore, men may be more likely to regard pain as insignificant until it becomes severe, unless it is associated with other factors that heighten anxiety, e.g. chest pain.

Psychological and sociological factors may influence pain perception and pain behavior to increase the occurrence of pain presentation but not necessarily as the result of increased pain sensitivity. These factors may combine to further increase the ratio of women–men attending health clinics. Bush *et al.*[27] examined temperomandibular disorder in a clinical population and found no significant difference in pain-related sensitivity, meanings of pain, and pain-related illness behavior. The study concluded that the higher ratio of women seeking treatment was consistent with women's greater health awareness or interest in symptoms. Linton *et al.*[32] in a postal survey of spinal pain in the 35- to 45-year age group found that, although men and women had a similar prevalence of spinal pain, when the pain was at its worst men took sick leave whereas women sought health care. In the review by Unruh examining gender differences,[23] women reported more health care utilization and more short-term disability when they experienced pain, but they also used more coping strategies and sought more social support. Gender differences affect the presentation of pain in a health care setting. Women's greater expression of pain might be perceived by health care providers as exaggeration or dramatization, resulting in pain undermedication.

CROSS-CULTURAL FACTORS

Most of the studies examining cross-cultural factors do not meet the criteria for major high-quality epidemiological study.[33] Poorly defined diagnostic criteria and convenience rather than random sampling make it difficult for prevalence studies to be representative and comparable.

Volinn[34] reported that Western societies have two to four times higher prevalence rates of low back pain than low- and middle-income countries. Within a low-income population, low back pain was not associated with hard physical labor in a rural population, but the association increased in the urban population working in enclosed workshops. A rising incidence of low back pain among workers was associated with urbanization and rapid industrialization, although the disparity in rates indicated a weakness in epidemiological method for a large number of studies.

When comparing patients with low back pain in the USA and New Zealand, Carron *et al.*[35] found that Americans reported greater emotional and behavioral disruption, and a far higher incidence of financial compensation (49% USA versus 17% New Zealand) was associated with a reduction in the likelihood of return to full activity. Although this study had only a 55% follow-up rate, Moore and Brødsgaard[33] reported other prospective studies that support these conclusions.

PEDIATRIC PAIN

Research, particularly in the last decade, has led to a better assessment of pain in children and during therapeutic intervention. Although biological, psychological, social, and environmental aspects of pain clearly interact in pediatric pain, the importance of age-related developmental changes in childhood and gender-related differences are poorly understood. Most studies survey prevalence of pain in children. There has been much less investigation of the natural history of pediatric pain; hence, the influence of childhood factors on pain in adult life has yet to be determined. Discussion of gender- and age-related factors in pediatric pain is influenced by the publication bias to report differences rather than similarities and by the lack of gender-related data analysis.[23]

Gender-specific pain and response to pain may be dramatically affected by the onset of puberty. Eminson[36] reported a significant increase in lifetime prevalence of physical symptoms in girls following menarche. In addition to cramping pain, girls may experience other pains such as headache and backache. Menstrual pain is fairly common among adolescents, ranging from 36% to 93% depending on the age of sample and diagnostic criteria used.[37] Studies examining psychopathology in children and adolescents typically do not inquire about menstrual pain. Gender may affect the type of psychopathology associated with somatic complaints. Egger et al.[38] found in 9- to 16-year-old schoolchildren somatic complaints were strongly associated with emotional disorders in girls and with disruptive behavior disorders in boys. For girls, stomachaches and headaches together and musculoskeletal pains alone were associated with anxiety disorders. For boys, stomach aches were associated with oppositional defiant disorders and attention-deficit hyperactivity disorder. Musculoskeletal pains were associated with depression in both girls and boys.

Gender-related biological differences do not appear to have a substantial influence on the pain experience of infants or young children, but this may reflect strong overriding influences that encourage girls but discourage boys from emotional expression of pain.[37]

Biological effects of sex hormones are subtle until the onset of puberty, which is associated with increasing risk of pain in girls for certain conditions such as migraine and pathological pain conditions including juvenile rheumatoid chronic arthritis. However, more research is needed to delineate the impact of sex hormones on physiological pain mechanisms and the effects of rapid growth changes, particularly during the growth spurt at puberty.

Low back pain is producing an epidemic of chronic disability in industrialized nations,[39] hence the importance of identifying factors in childhood that may influence pain in adult life. McGrath's review of the epidemiology of chronic pain in children observes the lack of diagnostic criteria for nonspecific back pain in children and that most studies are cross-sectional surveys of prevalence based on child or parent self-report.[40] Comparisons between studies are made more difficult by a frequent lack of specification of a minimum duration in the disease definition. The incidence of at least one episode of back pain in adolescents ranges from 25% to 35%,[37] with some studies reporting a significantly higher rate for girls[41,42] and others reporting more back pain for boys.[43] Several studies have identified an increased prevalence of back pain with age. Taimela et al.[44] found the lowest prevalence around 7-year-old (1%) and 10-year-old (6%) schoolchildren in Finland. The prevalence increased to 18% for 14- and 16-year-old adolescents and no gender difference was found. However, although the proportion of reported recurrent and chronic low back pain similarly increased with age, it was significantly higher in girls. Mikkelsson et al.[45] reported no gender difference for low back pain but a significantly higher rate of upper back pain for girls. Investigation of gender-related factors also needs to consider that some backache is associated with menstrual pain for some girls.

Many factors related to the etiology of low back pain have been evaluated in children,[40] of which physical activities (particularly those associated with musculotendinous or ligamentous strains caused by excessive loading), positive family history of pain, and gender are positively correlated with lifetime or period prevalence. Posture and radiographic changes are not correlated with back pain.

Evidence of causative factors is often equivocal, and the predictive value for adult low back pain is not known. Strong predictors of adult back pain may consist of a combination of causative factors. A 25-year prospective cohort study by Harreby et al.[46] interviewed schoolchildren aged 14–16 years and followed up 90% of the initial cohort at age 38 years. Although radiological changes in the spine showed no correlation to pain, the presence of low back pain in adolescence, particularly when combined with familial occurrence of back problems, had predictive value for adult low back pain.

In one of the few studies to examine the health conditions of child workers, Mitra[47] compared boys aged between 7 and 14 years who were working in small-scale leather workshops in the slums of Calcutta with a control group from the same locality and in the same socioeconomic class. Of the children who worked, 30% reported back and ankle pain, but of those not working none reported pain. The particular sitting posture of the child workers for long working hours was a possible cause of pain. The high prevalence of back pain in both children and adults in enclosed workshops suggests that environmental changes associated with industrialization may be more significant than age-related factors and back strength in childhood. Waddell[39] suggests that additional environmental factors, namely modern medicine and social security, are reinforcing and exacerbating chronic low back disability in adults.

PAIN IN THE ELDERLY

The *prevalence* of overall chronic pain increases with age, but this increase does not extend beyond the seventh decade. Brattberg et al.[48] examined the "oldest old" in Sweden and found an overall prevalence of pain of 73% (77+ years) and 68% (> 85 years). This plateau in prevalence may reflect a balance between age-related impairment of the pain pathways and increased pathology of old age.[49] More importantly, the impact of pain has not been systematically evaluated even though it is likely to be a major cause of depression and suffering in the elderly. The low incidence of conditions such as postherpetic neuralgia, although well known to increase with age,[50] has meant that studies have focused primarily on ubiquitous conditions associated with significant morbidity such as joint disease. Sternbach[51] reported 71% prevalence for joint pain during the preceding 12 months in a sample of people over the age of 65 years in the USA.

Reviewing epidemiology of pain in older people, Helme and Gibson[49] found that the frequencies of headache, muscle pains, stomach pain, and dental pain are lower in older (> 65 years) than in younger individuals (18–24 years). The frequency of joint pains are more than double in the older age group (> 65 years). However, there is a wide variation in prevalence figures for chronic pain, and in the case of age-related back pain no definite conclusion can be drawn.[49]

Helme and Gibson[51] have identified many *sources of error in epidemiological study*. Selection of the study population from the general population or institutions, etc., and age distribution of the sample are important factors. Collection of data, whether by personal or telephone interview or by postal survey, may influence results. Postal surveys have a selection bias toward healthier, older people,[10] i.e. if individuals are too frail to complete forms or post letters they are less likely to return a form. The Health Status of Older People project[52] reported a slight increase in pain with age of 4.6% per decade in females if pain occurred daily, but a decrease if the pain occurred one or two times per month to a few times per year. Hence, the same data can be seen to produce both an age-related increase or decrease in pain prevalence depending on the definition of pain used in the study.

Biological factors may be less important in postmenopausal women.[49] Pain conditions occurring more frequently in women after puberty, for example migraine, lose the gender difference after the female menopause, as does headache in general. Abdominal and visceral pain complaints are more common in women aged 18–40 years than men, but are reported equally in older individuals.

CHRONIC POSTSURGICAL PAIN

A wide variety of surgical procedures can produce a diverse range of pain syndromes. Macrae and Davies[53] have suggested a working definition for chronic postsurgical pain (CPSP) using the following criteria:

1 The pain developed after a surgical procedure.
2 The pain is of at least 2 months' duration.
3 Other causes for pain have been excluded (including the preexisting problem).

Examination of CPSP epidemiological studies indicates that patients are frequently dissatisfied with the results of their surgery, and up to 20% of patients in chronic pain clinics have surgery as the main or a contributory cause of their pain.[54,55]

Breast surgery

Macrae and Davies's review[53] reveals that one-quarter or more of women continue to report pain over a 1-year period after surgery. The pain may be phantom breast pain or pain around the operative site. Additional pain symptoms may arise years later, in the arm, from infiltration by cancer or from radiotherapy to the brachial plexus. In a prospective cohort study, Kroner et al.[56] reported at 1 year after mastectomy 13% phantom pain and 23% scar pain. The highest reported rates relate to more invasive surgery. Wallace et al.[57] have shown 49% of those having mastectomy with reconstruction had pain at 1 year compared to 31% of those having mastectomy alone. A common finding was underrecognition of the problem, attributing the pain to psychological factors (although there is no evidence to justify this view).

Hernia repair

A randomized prospective clinical trial, the Cooperative Hernia Study,[58] identified three types of pain:

* somatic – localized to the common ligamentous insertion to the pubic tubercle;
* neuropathic – referable to the ilioinguinal or genitofemoral nerve distribution;
* visceral – ejaculating pain.

The incidence of persistent moderate to severe pain was 12% at 1 year and 11% at 2 years. Callesen et al.[59] recorded an incidence of 6% after open groin hernia repair, with an increased risk in patients who had a high postoperative pain score 1 week after operation and after surgery for a recurrent hernia.

Vasectomy

Despite vasectomy being the second most common operation performed in men (after circumcision), the epidemiology of pain is not clear. Macrae and Davies's review[53] found an incidence of pain or discomfort varying between 5%[60] and 33%[61] occurring spontaneously or at the time of intercourse. Injection of local anesthetic into the vas deferens at the time of surgery may reduce the risk of developing chronic pain.[62]

Thoracotomy

Studies have revealed that chronic post-thoracotomy pain is serious and widespread. Importantly, chronic post-thoracotomy pain is usually continuous from the postoperative period. In a retrospective review, Keller et al.[63] found that patients reporting worsening pain after a period of adequate pain control were found to have recurrence of tumor.

There is some evidence to suggest that postoperative pain relief may influence development of post-thoracotomy pain. In a small but prospective study, Katz et al.[64] have found that early postoperative pain was the only factor that significantly predicted long-term pain, supporting earlier retrospective studies by Matsunaga et al.[65] and Kalso et al.[66] Interestingly, Roxburgh et al.[67] found that cryotherapy to the intercostal nerves did not improve postoperative pain control and possibly increased the risk of long-term pain.

Summary

The lack of well-conducted studies is reflected by the extent to which CPSP is neglected in surgical textbooks. Increased awareness and well-designed studies are required to unravel the importance of such factors as acute postoperative analgesia and type of surgery. Recognition of CPSP will also help to avoid repeat surgery for a surgery-induced problem and recommend modern pain management approaches.

CHRONIC LOW BACK PAIN

Problems with epidemiological study begin with a lack of agreement about definition. Chronic low back pain is sometimes defined as back pain lasting for longer than 3 months, that may not have a well-defined underlying pathological cause, and that may be intermittent over a long period. Many national insurance and industrial sources of data only include individuals associated with work disability, compensation, or time off work. Chronic low back pain may be a convenient diagnostic label for problems related to psychosocial dysfunction as it is a socially more acceptable label. Andersson[68] adds that these problems indicate that caution is needed when examining epidemiological studies.

Occurrence

Dionne's review[12] observed that low back pain affects 58–84% of all adults at some point in their life (lifetime prevalence). A more stringent definition of low back pain used by the US Second National Health and Nutrition Examination Survey reported a lifetime prevalence of 13.8% for "pain in the lower back on most days for at least 2 weeks."[70] Hence, although low back pain is common, it has severe consequences in only a small proportion of those affected. Defining back pain related to work absenteeism, statistics are even more conservative. The 1-year cumulative incidence of compensation claims for back pain (70% in the low back) with a minimum of 1 day work absence has been estimated at 1.4% in Canada.[71]

However, the actual number of people affected by severe low back pain remains large. In the USA, back pain is ranked among the five leading reasons for medical consultation.[71,72]

Interestingly, epidemiological evidence does not support an epidemic of back pain but rather a dramatic increase in reporting low back pain-related disability.[39,74] An estimate of the annual cost of low back pain in society by Waddell[39] was put at US$100 × 10^9 in the USA and at US$9 × 10^9 in the UK. While it is doubtful that any of the cost estimates currently available are entirely accurate, they all emphasize that direct and indirect costs of this disabling complaint are huge.

Etiology

The multifactorial etiology of low back pain raises difficulties in studying individual risk factors. Risk factors include:

- Specific etiological diagnosis.
- Older age.
- Previous back pain.
- Psychiatric problems – anxiety disorder, substance abuse.
- Occupation – involving bending, lifting, and twisting with heavy loads.
- Litigation.

Other factors such as low educational status may be markers for occupational, physical, environmental, and behavioral risk factors. Pure psychological factors have not been found to have predictive value in recovery.

Recovery

Most patients with back pain make a full recovery. Andersson's review[68] found that 60–70% recover by 6 weeks and 89–90% by 12 weeks. Thereafter, return to work rate is only 50% after 6 months and almost 0 at 2 years.[74] Compensation has a negative influence on the length of disability. Sander and Meyers[75] found that the average time off work for an on-duty strain injury was 14.9 months compared with 3.6 months for off-duty injuries.

Rate of surgery

There is substantial variation between countries in rates of back surgery. Cherkin *et al.*[76] looked at 13 countries and found that in the USA the rate is 40% higher than in any other country, and five times higher than in the UK. Andersson[68] considered differences in practice patterns and availability of health care provision the most likely explanation rather than differences in the underlying prevalence.

With increasing rates of disability in developed countries, despite no increase in underlying prevalence rates, preventative measures need to be explored. To date, attempts at primary prevention have been unsuccessful. Secondary prevention may provide a better course of action.

CONCLUSION

Epidemiology is the study of the distribution and determinants of disease. By documenting the nature of medical problems, studies can be used to plan health care services. However, estimates of the prevalence of pain in the community vary widely. This variation results from differences in the period studied and in definition of pain severity and duration. Hence, although surveys demonstrate that pain is a major public health problem, they provide little of the information that is needed to prevent pain problems. Studies are needed which focus on specific pain conditions and assess pain management in order to clearly identify the extent of the unmet needs of people with pain in the community.

Determination of prevalence is further advanced than research into causes of pain and identification of strategies for the prevention of pain. Prevention is conventionally divided into three types: primary prevention aims to stop the occurrence of pain; secondary prevention aims to prevent continuing illness by early intervention; and tertiary prevention aims to minimize long-term disability.

Research into causes is made difficult by the many factors that contribute to the subjective experience of pain. Pain may arise from physical damage, but is also modulated by many psychosocial factors. Understanding this web of causation requires carefully designed studies that focus on groups of pain patients with similar etiological factors. Study design must use methods more powerful than surveys. Case–control and cohort studies of specific patient groups must be the goal of future epidemiological research, together with consistency of definition and method to produce consistency of results and permit useful comparison of studies.

REFERENCES

● 1. Crombie IK. The potential of epidemiology. In: Crombie IK, Croft PR, Linton SJ, *et al.* eds. *Epidemiology of Pain*. Seattle, WA: IASP Press, 1999: 1–5.

● 2. Crombie IK, Croft PR, Linton SJ, *et al.* eds. *Epidemiology of Pain*. Seattle, WA: IASP Press, 1999.

3. Last JM. *A Dictionary of Epidemiology*. Oxford: Oxford University Press, 1988.

4. Jayson MIV. Why does acute back pain become chronic? *Br Med J* 1997; **314**:1639–40.

5. Merskey H, Bogduk N eds. *Classification of Chronic Pain. Descriptions of Chronic Pain Syndromes and Definitions of Pain Terms*. New York, NY: Elsevier, 1994.

6. Merskey H, Bogduk N. *Classification of Chronic Pain: Description of Chronic Pain Syndromes and Definitions of Pain Terms*. Seattle, WA: IASP Press, 1994.

7. Bruehl S, Harden RN, Galer BS, *et al.* External validation of IASP diagnostic criteria for Complex Regional Pain Syndrome and proposed research diagnostic criteria. *Pain* 1999; **81**:147–54.

8. Turk DC, Rudy TE. The robustness of an empirically derived taxonomy of chronic pain patients. *Pain* 1990; **43**: 27–35.

9. Von Korff M, Parker RD. The dynamics of the prevalence of chronic episodic disease. *J Chron Dis* 1980; **33**: 79–85.

10. Von Korff M, Dworkin SF, LeResche L. Graded chronic pain status: an epidemiologic evaluation. *Pain* 1990; **40**: 279–91.

11. Lilienfeld AM, Lilienfeld DE. *Foundations of Epidemiology*. New York, NY: Oxford University Press, 1980.

● 12. Dionne C. Low back pain. In: Crombie IK, Croft PR, Linton SJ, *et al.* eds. *Epidemiology of Pain*. Seattle, WA: IASP Press, 1999: 283–97.

13. Silman AJ. *Epidemiological Studies: a Practical Guide*. Cambridge: Cambridge University Press, 1995.

14. Barker DJP, Rose G. *Epidemiology in Medical Practise*, 4th edn. Edinburgh: Churchill Livingstone, 1992.

15. Von Korff M, Simon G. The relationship of pain and depression. *Br J Psychiatry* 1996; **168** (Suppl. 30): 101–8.

16. Davies HTO, Crombie IK, Tavaakoli M. When can odds ratios mislead? *Br Med J* 1998; **316**: 989–91.

17. LeResche L, Saunders K, Von Korff M, *et al.* Use of exogenous hormones and risk of temperomandibular disorder pain. *Pain* 1997; **69**: 153–60.

18. Marbach JJ, Schwartz S, Link BG. The control group conundrum in chronic pain case/control studies. *Clin J Pain* 1992; **8**: 39–43.

19. Sackett DL. Bias in analytic research. *J Chron Dis* 1979; **32**: 51–63.

20. Crook J, Weir R, Tunks E. An epidemiological follow-up survey of persistent pain sufferers in a group family practise and specialty pain clinic. *Pain* 1989; **36**: 49–61.

21. Magni G, Marchetti M, Moreschi C, *et al.* Chronic musculoskeletal pain and depressive symptoms in the National Health and Nutrition Examination. I. Epidemiological follow-up study. *Pain* 1993; **53**: 163–8.

22. Crook J, Rideout E, Browne G. The prevalence of pain complaints in a general population. *Pain* 1984; **18**: 299–314.

23. Unruh AM. Gender variation in clinical pain experience. *Pain* 1996; **65**: 123–67.

● 24. LeResche L. Gender consideration in the epidemiology of chronic pain. In: Crombie IK, Croft PR, Linton SJ, *et al.* eds. *Epidemiology of Pain*. Seattle, WA: IASP Press, 1999: 43–52.

● 25. Scher AI, Stewart WF, Lipton RB. Migraine and headache: a meta-analytic approach. In: Crombie IK, Croft PR, Linton SJ, *et al.* eds. *Epidemiology of Pain*. Seattle, WA: IASP Press, 1999: 159–70.

26. Stewart WF, Linet MS, Celentino DD, *et al.* Age- and sex-specific incidence rates of migraine with and without visual aura. *Am J Epidemiol* 1991; **134**: 1111–20.

27. Bush FM, Harkins SW, Harington WG, Price DD. Analysis of gender effects on pain perception and symptom presentation in temperomandibular pain. *Pain* 1993; **53**: 73–80.

28. Levine FM, De Simone LL. The effects of experimenter gender on pain report in male and female subjects. *Pain* 1991; **44**: 69–72.

29. Giamberardino MA, Berkley KJ, Iezzi S, *et al.* Pain

Table 3.1 *Characteristics of the curative and palliative models of medicine*

Curative model	Palliative model
Objective	Subjective
Scientific	Humanistic
Rational	Empathic
Impersonal	Personal
Reductionist	Holistic

last 3 days of their lives.[12] SUPPORT simply reconfirmed the persistence of one aspect of a general phenomenon of undertreated pain of all types that has pervaded the medical literature for over 20 years.[13] The primary locus of curative medicine is the tertiary care hospital; the primary locus of palliative medicine is the hospice. When one abandons the hope of a cure, one accepts the tender mercies of hospice. While one continues to strive for a cure or remediation of a disease, which is presumably why one becomes a patient in academic medical centers such as those participating in SUPPORT, one accepts the pain and suffering that attend many of modern medicine's interventions. The hegemony of the curative model in modern medical education and medical practice has, it can be argued, displaced the relief of pain and suffering from its traditional status as a fundamental goal and core value of medicine. If that is not the case, then the pervasive phenomenon of undertreated pain suggests a remarkable and disturbing disconnection between the custom and practice among physicians and the ancient goals and core values of the medical profession.

In 1996, an International Project of the Hastings Center entitled The Goals of Medicine – Setting New Priorities issued its report. The goals of medicine identified by this distinguished panel of physicians are the following:[14]

- The prevention of disease and injury and promotion and maintenance of health.
- The relief of pain and suffering caused by maladies.
- The care and cure of those with a malady, and the care of those who cannot be cured.
- The avoidance of premature death and the pursuit of a peaceful death.

Perhaps the most striking aspect of these goals, in contrast to the hegemony of the curative model, is the remarkable balance between the curative and palliative aspects of medicine. With regard to the relief of pain and suffering in particular, the special report emphasizes that this is by no means a new goal, but rather one of "the most ancient duties of the physician and a traditional goal of medicine." Nevertheless, the report goes on to say that, for a host of reasons, the goal remains largely unfulfilled. While in many underdeveloped countries access to state-of-the-art medications and advanced nonpharmacologic treatment modalities is an important part of the problem, in developed countries even affluent patients encounter formidable barriers to pain relief, barriers which are sociopolitical rather than economic or technological. Moreover, if there is one type of pain that is more frequently or consistently unrelieved than others, it is chronic nonmalignant pain.[15] A rigorous ethical analysis of the phenomenon of undertreated pain requires a detailed examination of these barriers, particularly if they are offered, as they often are, not merely as reasons why physicians undertreat pain but as excuses for such practice. First, however, we should briefly note the pervasiveness of the problem of undertreated pain.

THE INTERNATIONAL SCOPE OF UNDERTREATED PAIN

The international literature examining the phenomenon of undertreated pain is dominated by studies that focus on cancer pain. There is, nonetheless, reason to believe that such findings may indicate the magnitude of the problem of undertreated chronic nonmalignant pain as well. An aggressive approach to pain management, including the use of large, sustained doses of the strongest opioid analgesics, has been advocated by pain management experts when necessary to achieve optimal pain relief for patients with cancer or other conditions in their terminal phase.[16] Quite to the contrary, with regard to the treatment of patients with chronic nonmalignant pain, it has been axiomatic that the long-term use of opioids is inappropriate.[17] Thus, many patients who fail to achieve adequate relief from nonopioid therapies are admonished to live with their pain.

Recent studies indicate that opiophobia among health care professionals is not strictly an American phenomenon, but is widespread in European countries as well.[18] In Germany, for example, it was noted that 98% of cancer patients never received a strong opioid for pain.[19] In France, 51% of cancer patients received inadequate pain relief, and 30% of the patients who reported pain were not receiving any drugs for pain relief.[20] While there are differences among nations in the regulation of physician prescribing practices, drug availability, and educational requirements for professionals with prescribing authority, studies of physicians' attitudes about pain management in a wide variety of countries reveal common barriers to adequate pain control.[21] While any particular barrier may be more of a factor in the undertreatment of pain in one country than another, the frequency with which physicians identify these barriers in each country surveyed strongly suggests that they have achieved a status and exert an influence that transcends political and cultural boundaries.

Although a disproportionate amount of the available data, both regarding the situation in the USA and elsewhere in the world, pertains to opioid availability and use in the care of patients with cancer, the implications of such data for the treatment of chronic nonmalignant pain is inescapable. The 1961 Single Convention on Narcotic

Drugs, as amended by the 1972 Protocol, is the international treaty regulating the availability of opioids. The preamble of this treaty recognizes that "the medical use of narcotic drugs continues to be indispensable for the relief of pain." Of course, the treaty also states that "addiction to narcotic drugs constitutes a serious evil." Thus, the treaty, just as with national drug regulation laws, purports to at one and the same time prevent the abuse of opioids while assuring that they will be available for legitimate medical use.[22] The World Health Organization has urged, with varying degrees of success, that individual countries fashion their regulatory requirements for physicians, nurses, and pharmacists to dispense opioids to patients so as to recognize that "decisions concerning the type of drug to be used, the amount of the prescription and the duration of therapy are best made by medical professionals on the basis of the individual needs of each patient, and not by regulation."[23]

The International Narcotics Control Board (INCB), created by the 1961 Single Convention, compiles statistical data supplied by national governments and publishes an annual report that provides a comprehensive survey of the world drug situation. A 1995 study by the INCB on the availability of opioids for pain management worldwide noted that in many countries opioids are unavailable for medical needs.[24] Remarkably, the study revealed that only 48% of the governments reported that morphine in any form was available in all cancer treatment facilities. In addition to periodic shortages in the availability of opioids that were attributed to insufficient importation, distribution delays, and health system administrative problems, the perennial obstacles of physician concerns about addiction and fears of legal sanctions for prescribing opioids were also offered as partial explanations.[25]

THE BARRIERS TO EFFECTIVE PAIN RELIEF

Certain "barriers" to effective pain relief are so consistently cited in the literature that there would appear to be no genuine dispute about either their existence or their nature. Here are the usual suspects that are rounded up by the advocates of improved pain management practices:

- The failure of clinicians (primarily physicians and nurses) to identify pain relief as a priority in patient care.
- Insufficient knowledge among clinicians about the assessment and management of pain.
- Clinicians' fear of regulatory scrutiny of the prescribing and administering of opioid analgesics.
- The failure of health care institutions and organizations to hold clinicians accountable for effective pain relief.

Other barriers are mentioned with varying degrees of frequency that do not implicate physicians quite so directly, e.g. patient and family concerns about addiction, tolerance, and side-effects, absence of certain narcotics from formularies, and reimbursement problems with pain therapies. However, patients and families must look to physicians for accurate information about opioid analgesics, and formulary and reimbursement issues came about long after the other barriers had been recognized and copiously documented.

There is important information in the use of the term "barrier" to explain the phenomenon of undertreated pain. It suggests that, but for the existence of these barriers, physicians would consistently provide optimal pain relief to their patients. Indeed, these barriers are sometimes described as though they were artifacts of nature, as formidable and immutable as a mountain range. The fact of the matter is, of course, that these barriers are the product of cultural beliefs, attitudes, and prejudices. We have created them, and, if necessary or appropriate, we can remove them. The fact that they have been with us for at least the last 50 years suggests that there is something less than a strong consensus and a concerted effort to bring them down. Perhaps, in scrutinizing each more carefully, we can gain some understanding as to why that might be so.[26]

The failure of clinicians to identify pain relief as a priority in patient care

Accepting as we (at least tacitly) do, the professional obligation of physicians to relieve human suffering, including that which is engendered by severe, persistent pain, this well-recognized failure of health care professionals to make it a priority in their care of patients verges on the inexplicable. There is a "chicken and egg" conundrum about the first two barriers to effective pain management. Do clinicians fail to identify pain relief as a priority because they have not been taught how to provide it? Or is it rather the case that medical schools and residency training programs do not emphasize training in pain management because clinicians, including medical educators, do not consider pain relief to be a priority in patient care? There may be a synergy between the forces that have erected these two barriers that confounds the search for a satisfactory answer to these questions.

Some insight into the problem can be gained by noting that it appears to have been exacerbated by the advent of modern, scientifically based, high-technology medicine that has shaped what we have previously noted to be the curative model of medical practice. As the term suggests, the curative model focuses primarily, if not exclusively, upon the goal of cure, i.e. the eradication or radical reversal of a disease process. Particularly to the extent that curative interventions themselves cause pain, discomfort, temporary dysfunction, or risk of death, the relief of pain and suffering can be interpreted as a conflicting goal, and hence one that must be abandoned during the pursuit of a cure. One commentator suggests that the pain experienced by the patient is subjected to two kinds of forgetting: one psychologic and the other conceptual.[27] The psychologic component arises from a need of the clinician to distance him or herself from the patient's pain as well as to convince the patient that the pain is not really as bad as it seems, or that it is a regrettable byproduct of the necessary means to a desirable clinical outcome. The conceptual component treats pain as a symptom of the underlying disease process, something to be observed but not managed or eliminated. This is particularly the case given the widely held (mis)perception that relieving pain impedes the process of cure. The patient's reports of pain are noted, if at all, as information about the progression of the disease, not as cries of distress giving rise to a duty to provide relief. To the extent that this perspective is accurate, it may call into question the ultimate effectiveness of one proposal by pain specialists to improve pain management in the inpatient setting – charting pain as the "fifth vital sign."[28] The implicit assumption is that pain is more likely to be treated if it is measured and recorded. However, if pain continues to be conceptualized as nothing more than an indicator of the progression of disease, noting its presence and severity in the chart will not necessarily result in interventions to relieve it. For insight into why that might be the case, we need to explore further the nature of the prevailing model of medical practice.

It has been persuasively argued that the pervasiveness and the overemphasis of the curative model in medical education not only results in a particular style of medical practice but also engenders a set of assumptions, attitudes, and values which are inherent in the model.[11] Among these are the focus on the disease process rather than the patient's experience of illness. Such a focus privileges the objective and scientifically verifiable, and discounts the subjective and unverifiable. This focus, of course, has significant implications for the care of patients with chronic, nonmalignant pain. The implicit message of the curative model is that there is no compelling need to know the patient as a person so long as the professional has a firm grasp upon the pathophysiology of their disease and an interventional strategy for reversing it. While the curative model may not pose any significant problems for patients whose pain is of the acute variety and limited in its severity and duration, it has itself been the cause of considerable unnecessary suffering for patients with chronic malignant or nonmalignant pain. The predominance of the curative model of medical education and its obsession with the pathophysiology of disease rather than the patient's subjective experience of illness is "disastrous," according to Arthur Kleinman, to the care of the chronically ill.[29] Indeed, the curative model, in conjunction with rampant opiophobia and an ethic of undertreatment of pain, has resulted in numerous instances of pseudoaddiction among chronic pain patients. Pseudoaddiction is an iatrogenic condition caused by the failure of physicians to provide adequate pain relief that forces the patient to employ (legitimate) drug-seeking behaviors to obtain analgesics they are entitled to.

Kleinman's work with chronic pain patients, as physician, psychiatrist, and medical anthropologist, provides a number of important maxims for those who seek to provide compassionate care to such individuals:

- One of the core tasks in the effective clinical care of the chronically ill is to affirm the patient's experience of illness as constituted by their explanatory models and to use those models in the development of an acceptable therapeutic approach.
- Chronic illness is as distinctive as the lived experience of different individuals because in the end it *is* the lived experience of different individuals.
- One half of all patients with chronic pain syndrome, like many others afflicted with chronic illness, meet the official criteria for major depressive disorder. More than anything else, the depressive mood represents demoralization from the life of pain and the persistent questioning by others, including health care professionals, of the authenticity of the patient's experience of pain.
- The science of pain medicine must include social science interpretations together with biomedical explanations. It must bring to bear knowledge of the economic, political, and social psychologic sides of pain.

The maxims I have gleaned from Kleinman's work describe what he characterizes as a "meaning-centered" model of chronic illness that he deems essential to the compassionate and effective care of such patients. It is a biocultural model that places the emphasis upon the patient's illness experience, as does the palliative model, and in doing so stands in stark contrast to the biomedical model whose exclusive focus is the disease process – its diagnosis and its cure or remediation.[30] While it may be much too simplistic to suggest that restoring some proportionality between the curative and palliative (or biomedical and biocultural) models of medicine in the education and training of physicians would eliminate this and related barriers to effective pain relief, it is also the case that it is naive and unrealistic to suggest that continuing professional education programs on pain management alone can overcome the assumptions, attitudes, and values that have been instilled in physicians by the curative model of medical education. Physician practice styles and patterns are acquired early and thereafter are highly resistant to change. Part of the solution goes not only to the substantive content of medical education but also to the venue. While most physicians practice in settings that would be hospitable to a balance between the curative and palliative approach to patient care, by far most medical education and residency training takes place in the acute, tertiary care setting where the hegemony of the curative model is most complete.[31]

Insufficient knowledge among physicians about pain assessment and management

Critics of medical education in the area of pain – its causes, assessment, and treatment – suggest that the typical medical school curriculum seems almost purposely designed to keep physicians in the dark about pain. In a 1989 interview, John J. Bonica, generally regarded as the founder of the movement toward specialized pain clinics, observed: "No medical school has a pain curriculum."[32] Over 15 years earlier, a study of hospital inpatients revealed significant undertreatment of pain based in part on marked knowledge deficits on the part of physicians with regard to effective does range, duration of action, and risks of addiction for narcotic analgesics.[13] At the conclusion of the study, the authors called for a major educational initiative, beginning in medical school, to improve the knowledge and skills of physicians in the use of narcotic analgesics for the management of pain. Interestingly, in addition to basic medical information, the authors suggested that any program of instruction must take into account the fact that for many physicians these drugs "have a special emotional significance that interferes with their rational use." The term which has been coined to describe this phenomenon is "opiophobia."[33] Like other, more generally recognized phobias, opiophobia cannot be cured or even effectively controlled by classroom education about the groundless nature of the fears. It is a behavior that is modeled and reinforced throughout all levels of medical education, from student clerkships to internship and residency.

The pharmacologist who coined the term "opiophobia" indicates that, after closely observing the opioid analgesic prescribing patterns of physicians in the USA, it would be tempting, but technically incorrect, to declare that "American physicians know nothing of the treatment of severe pain with narcotic opioids." They have learned well, as they progressed through their medical education, the prescribing patterns that are customary. Those patterns, however, are inconsistent with the best current medical knowledge. Indeed, they suggest that the patterns and practices that are at the root of undertreated pain have nothing to do with medical science whatsoever. For example, the belief that chronic pain patients managed with opioids are likely to become addicted (as opposed to physiologically dependent) runs directly counter to the best clinical data, which indicate that the risk of iatrogenic addiction for pain patients is less than 0.01%.[34] Similarly, the widespread fear of severe, perhaps even fatal, episodes of respiratory depression runs directly counter to numerous reports in the medical literature. Although many of these reports pertain to cancer patients, the salient point made therein is that it is only the opioid-naive patient who is at serious risk of respiratory depression.[35] A patient with moderate to severe chronic pain, regardless of whether it is caused by malignancy, whose analgesic level has been titrated upward appropriately, is not at serious risk.

It would be a mistake, however, to assume that opiophobia is entirely an American phenomenon, one secondary to such unique aspects of American culture and social history as the puritan heritage, the "noble" experiment of prohibition, or the contemporary "War on Drugs." Restrictive prescribing laws are common in many European countries, both reflecting and sustaining an international opiophobia among health care professionals as well as patients.[19] It is extremely difficult to measure the extent to which opiophobia is a product of overzealous measures (such as a declared or undeclared "War on Drugs") to deter and detect drug diversion rather than the persistence of myths and misinformation about the risks and benefits of opioid analgesics. Nevertheless, it is a lamentable fact that the rhetoric and *modus operandi* of the regulators in waging the War on Drugs has made physicians conscripts and pain patients noncombatant casualties, and has inflicted grave collateral damage on one of medicine's core values – the duty to relieve suffering. Recently published follow-up studies strongly suggest that state medical licensing board members, who play a pivotal role in the regulation of physician prescribing of opioid analgesics, have been particularly resistant to reeducation on such issues as the nature of addiction and the appropriateness of opioids in the management of some patients with chronic nonmalignant pain.[36] We will consider this issue further in the next section.

In concluding our analysis of this particular barrier to effective pain management, I wish to introduce a concept which I characterize as "the culpability of cultivated ignorance." As we have seen in this brief survey, it has been known and identified as a problem for decades that medical school and residency training program curricula are woefully inadequate with regard to the assessment and management of all types of pain. Yet these institutions have failed or refused to reform themselves. It surely cannot be because pain has not been shown to be a pervasive problem frequently encountered by most physicians in their practice. The continuing absence of a significant pain component in medical education and training is indefensible, and the calling to account of these institutions by society for the persistence of such curricular deficits and their negative impact on patient care is long overdue.

A pain curriculum in medical school that is worth the effort it would take to implement would need to be comprehensive. It must begin in the lecture hall and continue through the role modeling and mentoring by a faculty of senior medical students, interns, and residents. The custom and practice in the institutions where young physicians are enculturated must be consistently based on the latest scientific knowledge and outcome studies of pain treatment modalities, something that the prevailing practice of physicians in most countries presently does not provide.

What is equally troublesome, however, from an ethical

standpoint, is the continuing reliance by practicing physicians upon these curricular deficits as an excuse for why they fail to possess state-of-the-art knowledge and skill in pain assessment and management. While deficiencies in their professional education and training may provide an explanation for substandard care of patients with pain, they do not constitute an excuse. Entering a profession entails the acceptance of a responsibility to engage in life-long learning and the continuing development and refinement of the knowledge and skills essential to the competent practice of that profession. The law can and will hold persons responsible not only for applying their knowledge and skills in a prudent manner but also for a failure to possess the knowledge and skills necessary to adequately engage in their profession or calling.

Fear of regulatory scrutiny of opioid prescribing practices

There is an ongoing debate between the regulators and the regulated about the extent to which the regulations, and/or the manner of their enforcement, do or should have a chilling effect upon the quality of pain relief provided by health care professionals. Physicians in the USA recount horrific tales of armed Drug Enforcement Administration (DEA) agents descending upon physicians' offices in response to a report, often by a local pharmacist, of excessive prescribing practices.[37] Similarly, state medical licensing boards have been known to harshly discipline physicians for deviating from the customary practice of underprescribing opioid analgesics, or for prescribing them at all in the care of patients with chronic, nonmalignant pain. Later in this section, we will consider one such case in detail because it illustrates both the attitudes of many licensing board members and the reason why physician fears of regulatory scrutiny and disciplinary action have some foundation in fact.

The DEA responds to these charges by noting that its *Physicians' Manual* explicitly acknowledges that opioid analgesics can and should be considered one of the primary means of controlling many types of moderate to severe pain, and that such an official pronouncement should provide physicians with all of the reassurance they can legitimately demand that the DEA does not stand between them and proper treatment of their patients' pain problems. Moreover, the mission of the DEA is declared to be the prevention of, or prosecution for, drug diversion. When cases raising issues concerning the appropriate prescribing of controlled substances – and hence physician judgment – arise, the stated policy of the DEA is to refer them to the appropriate state medical board for review. A number of state medical licensing boards, sometimes but not always through the prodding of state legislative initiatives, have begun to issue guidelines or policies with regard to the use of opioid analgesics for the management of chronic pain, especially chronic non-

malignant pain. Rarely do such boards acknowledge that their prior practices in any way justified the undertreatment of pain. Nevertheless, they offer these guidelines as further assurances to physicians that they certainly can no longer point to medical board policies and practices as justification for undertreating pain.

In the USA, the Federation of State Medical Licensing Boards has now adopted "Model Guidelines for the Use of Controlled Substances for the Treatment of Pain," and strongly encourages each state medical licensing board to adopt similar guidelines. Such guidelines accomplish several important goals. First, they make an important public policy statement that licensing boards expect physicians to provide effective pain relief to their patients. Second, they provide general guidelines for the physician to follow in order to document, among other things, that the opioid analgesics prescribed for a particular patient are medically indicated, properly monitored, and demonstrably improve the patient's level of function and/or quality of life. Third, they often incorporate by specific reference the significantly more comprehensive clinical practice guidelines for acute and cancer pain management of the Agency for Health Care Policy and Research. While the precise legal status of such guidelines remains uncertain, and can be expected to vary from one jurisdiction to another, it will become increasingly difficult for physicians who depart frequently and materially from the "best practices" delineated by such guidelines to justify their approach, especially when the outcome is the unnecessary pain and suffering of their patients. Later in this chapter, we will consider two legal cases that may shed further light on the legal implications of substandard pain management practice.

Another question that at this time has not been definitively answered is whether such guidelines will be utilized by state medical licensing boards to discipline physicians who deviate from such statements of accepted practice by underprescribing opioid analgesics for their patients with pain. In 1998, the California medical board declined to take any disciplinary action against a physician whom it found to have provided inadequate pain management to a patient dying of cancer. In 2001, a jury awarded a sizeable judgment to the family of that patient in a lawsuit charging the attending physician with elder abuse. This is one of two cases we will consider in a subsequent section. In 1999, the Oregon Board of Medical Examiners became the first to actually take disciplinary action against a physician for undertreating the pain of his patients.[38] Those who support the Oregon Board do so, at least in part, on the grounds that such actions are the only way to send a clear message to practicing physicians, and indirectly to their patients, that both overprescribing and underprescribing of opioid analgesics constitute unprofessional practice for which there will be genuine accountability. In all other jurisdictions at the present time, the message implicit in licensing board conduct is that, while providing appropriate pain relief is commendable, drug diversion and "overprescribing" will actually place the physician at risk of disciplinary action.

Recent studies reveal that many members of state licensing boards in the USA are ill-equipped by training or experience to evaluate the quality of pain management provided by their licensees.[36] Furthermore, some recent disciplinary actions against physicians who used opioid analgesics for patients with severe, chronic nonmalignant pain suggest that medical boards do not even recognize a need to compensate for their lack of expertise by relying on specialists in the field. A case in point is a disciplinary action by the Florida Medical Licensing Board that was reversed by an appellate court.[39] Katherine Hoover, a board-certified internal medicine physician, was charged with "inappropriately and excessively" prescribing Schedule II narcotics to seven chronic pain patients. The agency's case against Dr Hoover consisted of the testimony of two physicians whom it recognized as experts. Neither of the agency's witnesses had examined any portion of the medical records of any of the seven patients in question. Furthermore, neither of the agency's witnesses specialized in the care of patients with chronic pain. In fact, both testified that they referred all such patients to pain management clinics. The sole basis for the opinions which they offered with regard to the appropriateness of Dr Hoover's care of the seven patients was a review of the computer printouts from the pharmacies which had filled the prescriptions written by Dr Hoover. On that basis alone, they opined, and the agency ultimately determined, that Dr Hoover had prescribed amounts of opioid analgesics that were "excessive, perhaps lethal." It did not seem to influence the agency's assessment of this testimony that none of these seven patients had suffered any adverse effects from these so-called "lethal doses" prescribed by Dr Hoover. In deciding to discipline Dr Hoover for her prescribing practices, the Board disregarded the findings and conclusions of the hearing officer, who had determined that the evidence submitted by Dr Hoover's experts persuasively demonstrated that her care of the patients under consideration was appropriate.

Dr Hoover appealed the adverse ruling by the Board of Medicine to an appellate court, which held that the Board's actions in disregarding the recommendations of the hearing officer were not supported by clear and convincing evidence. Still more disconcerting, however, was the appellate court's references in its written opinion to previous cases in which the Board had disregarded the findings and conclusions of hearing officers as to the weight of the evidence, and forged ahead with disciplinary action against the physician for "overprescribing" Schedule II narcotics. In each of those cases, an appellate court of the State of Florida had chastised the Board for taking disciplinary action against a physician on the basis of sparse and inadequate evidence.

What is particularly revealing about the Board's missionary zeal in policing the prescribing practices of physicians who treat patients with chronic pain, which the court in *Hoover* described as "draconian," is that they continued unabated despite the fact that the Florida legislature had recently enacted an intractable pain statute specifically intended to encourage physicians to provide state-of-the-art care for such patients. Because the statute was not technically applicable to the *Hoover* case owing to the chronology of events, the Board completely disregarded its policy implications. Such intransigence in the face of a clear public policy mandate does not serve to reassure clinicians that state medical licensing boards have embarked upon a new and more enlightened view of the role of opioid analgesics in the care of patients with chronic pain.

One might be tempted to conclude that the philosophy underlying the regulatory strategies of medical licensing boards appears to be that patients who require large, sustained doses of Schedule II narcotics to manage their pain are better off enduring the pain than relying on opioid analgesics for relief. However, as the approach of the board in the *Hoover* case demonstrates, the welfare of the patients was not really a genuine concern of the board. If it had been, some attention might have been paid to the patient records, and to patient testimony about the actual outcomes of Dr Hoover's treatment of their chronic pain, rather than exclusively focusing on pharmacy computer printouts. What we find, instead, is an unreflective, essentially reactionary approach to prescribing practices that are tailored to the needs of the patient rather than to some antiquated and scientifically unsubstantiated set of algorithms that has heretofore defined "good medical practice" with regard to the prescribing of opioid analgesics. Consequently, from an ethical perspective, licensing boards cannot justify their policies by reference to the ancient medical aphorism *primum non nocere*.

There are additional ethical considerations related to this particular barrier to effective pain management. The typical medical board, after all, is not composed of government bureaucrats or the lay public, but rather of practicing physicians. Presumably, they reflect the knowledge, attitudes, and beliefs of their profession. Indeed, one of the perennial concerns about and critiques of such boards is that they are simply a means by which the profession looks out for itself and perpetuates its own values and agenda. Regardless of whether and to what extent that may be true, it is nonetheless the case that organized medicine has yet to initiate any concerted effort to persuade all professional licensing boards to embrace a more scientifically based and patient-friendly approach to their oversight of physician prescribing practices. Instead, the typical physician has allowed opiophobic attitudes of medical licensing boards to establish and maintain a standard, and indeed an ethic of underprescribing. So long as such a standard and ethic prevail, exceptional physicians like Katherine Hoover, who have the moral courage to take on their board when necessary to the welfare of their patients, must become martyrs to the cause of pain relief for their patients.

The failure of health care institutions to hold clinicians accountable for pain relief

Traditionally, health care institutions have been dominated by their organized medical staff, at least with regard to determinations of what constitutes appropriate patient care. It logically follows that if effective pain management is not a priority of the medical staff, neither will it be an institutional priority of the hospital, long-term care facility, or clinic. The notable exception that proves the general rule is hospice. Since the defining role and mission of hospice is to provide palliative care to dying patients, only physicians who share that priority tend to associate themselves with it. However, even hospices and their physicians sometimes fail to make the relief of a patient's pain the cardinal principle of care.[40]

Decades ago, a seminal study of the institutional response (or lack thereof) of hospitals and their medical and nursing staffs framed the issue as the "politics of pain management."[41] The modern hospital is preeminently an acute care facility, typically consisting of an emergency room, diagnostic facilities, surgical suites, one or more intensive care units, and other units where generally short-term therapeutic measures are undertaken. Pain in such settings, as previously noted, is viewed as an important diagnostic tool, a symptom of some more serious underlying condition that must be diagnosed and hopefully cured. Eliminating or significantly mitigating the pain would be (or so it has been assumed) counterproductive to the diagnostic and therapeutic agenda. Similarly, patients who have recently undergone a procedure are monitored closely for complications, one indication of which is pain. Patients who are receiving optimal pain control will be at risk of unnoticed problems. Finally, many of the interventions that are indicated in the pursuit of diagnosis or cure themselves cause pain, only some of which may be alleviated without in some manner compromising its ultimate success.

Anecdotal evidence abounds, and has found its way into plays, motion pictures, and television, of patients and families who are subjected to considerable distress (physical and emotional) by health care professionals who scrupulously titrate pain medications and rigidly adhere to dosages and administration schedules. Complaints of severe pain are met with the staff response that another administration of the prescribed form of pain relief is not due yet, and the patient is then admonished not to complain because everything that can be done has been done. Particularly influential in the care of hospitalized patients are anticipated pain trajectories. When a patient demonstrates an unexpected pain trajectory, particularly one where the pain persists beyond the paradigm or is reported to be more severe than that which is usually reported, the staff may not be organizationally or emotionally equipped to respond appropriately.[41] A not uncommon response of the staff in such situations is to question the accuracy of the patient's complaints of pain, or to dismiss the patient as histrionic or attention-seeking. If the complaints persist, and focus on the need for more pain medication, the patient is at risk for being labeled a drug-seeker or even an addict. Such labeling constitutes the ultimate means of discrediting the patient's complaints, which at bottom constitute a charge that the staff has failed in one of its fundamental responsibilities – to relieve patient suffering.

The study to which we have been referring concludes that "staff is not really accountable … for the actions it takes in regard to the patient in pain." Furthermore, the prognosis for any demonstrable improvement was grim:[41]

> Genuine accountability concerning pain work could only be instituted if the major authorities on given wards or clinics understood the importance of that accountability and its implications for patient care. They would then need to convert that understanding into a commitment that would bring about necessary changes in written and verbal communication systems. This kind of understanding and commitment can probably come about only after considerable nationwide discussion, such as now is taking place about terminal care, but that kind of discussion seems to lie far in the future.

Ironically, phase II of the SUPPORT study undertook precisely such an intervention designed to improve written and verbal communication on wards or clinics with the aim of improving the care of seriously ill patients. The intervention was a notorious failure, and the failure was attributed in significant part to the prevailing culture of medicine, which is driven by the therapeutic rather than the palliative model of care.

Realistically, boards that regulate health care professionals cannot be a patient's first line of defense against substandard medical care. Neither can medical malpractice litigation serve this function. That role and responsibility falls upon the institutions and organizations in which patient care is most commonly provided: the hospital and its clinics, ambulatory care centers, and long-term care facilities. Their tolerance of health care professionals who are unable or unwilling to provide appropriate pain relief to patients is an abrogation of their social and moral responsibility. For example, several of the patients whose inappropriate pain management served as the basis of the Oregon Board of Medical Examiner's ground-breaking disciplinary action against Dr Paul Bilder were receiving their treatment at the same institution. Yet there is no indication that any of the standing committees of the hospital responsible for the monitoring of the quality of patient care, e.g. quality assurance or medical staff credentials, had undertaken any measures to protect future patients from similar instances of unnecessary suffering. Hence, a period of 5 years and a total of six patients had to accrue before the medical board was in a position to initiate corrective action.

Within the last few years, a more concerted effort has been initiated by some leaders in the field, particularly nurses, to institutionalize good pain management and to institute mechanisms for holding the staff accountable for providing it.[42] However, what holds the greatest promise for actually bringing about systematic changes in the way in which pain is managed in most health care institutions are the new standards that have been promulgated and implemented by the Joint Commission for the Accreditation of Health Care Organizations (JCAHO).[43] In order to comply with these standards, institutions must do the following:[44]

- Recognize the right of patients to appropriate assessment and management of their pain.
- Identify patients with pain in an initial screening assessment.
- When pain is identified, perform a more comprehensive pain assessment.
- Record the results of the assessment in a way that facilitates regular reassessment and follow-up.
- Educate relevant providers in pain assessment and management.
- Determine and assure staff competency in pain assessment and management.
- Address pain assessment and management in the orientation of all new staff.
- Establish policies and procedures that support appropriate prescription or ordering of effective pain medications.
- Ensure that pain does not interfere with participation in rehabilitation.
- Educate patients and their families about the importance of effective pain management.
- Address patient needs for symptom management in the discharge planning process.
- Collect data to monitor the appropriateness and effectiveness of pain management.

The expedited introduction of these standards into the JCAHO institutional survey process is a strong indication of the perceived need to bring health care organizations promptly into compliance. Because of the importance that is attached to the JCAHO survey process, these standards create a realistic expectation that we may be in the process of moving from mere rhetoric to genuine reform of pain management practices in the USA.

PAIN AND THE COURTS

In the 10 years from 1991 to 2001, two trial courts and the Supreme Court of the USA addressed the issue of pain management in the care of dying patients. Although one can argue that the ethical, legal, and social issues in the management of chronic nonmalignant pain differ from those in the care of dying patients, there are still important insights to be gained from the disposition of these cases. We will begin with the 1997 Supreme Court decisions in *Washington vs. Glucksberg*[45] and *Vacco vs. Quill.*[46]

These two cases challenged the constitutionality of statutes prohibiting physician-assisted suicide in Washington and New York respectively. The justices ruled 9–0 that there is no constitutional right to physician-assisted suicide, even when such a right is narrowly circumscribed to include only competent patients with a terminal condition who are in great pain and repeatedly request such assistance. However, five of the nine justices wrote or joined in concurring opinions that have been interpreted as recognizing that such patients may well have a constitutional right to effective pain relief, such that any law creating an undue burden on access to such care would be unconstitutional.[47] Because the issue of pain management for such patients was arguably tangential to the issue before the Court for decision, the fact that these justices were moved to write these opinions is a strong indication of the seriousness they attach to the provision of appropriate relief to patients with severe, persistent pain.

In 1991 and again in 2001, juries rendered large damage awards to the families of elderly patient's whose pain associated with a terminal illness was undertreated. What distinguishes these cases – the first was in rural, northeastern North Carolina and was brought against a nurse and the nursing home that employed her; the second was in the Bay Area of northern California and was brought against a physician and an acute care hospital – is less significant than what they have in common. Both cases involved the failure or refusal to provide appropriate doses of opioid analgesics such as morphine to control the pain associated with terminal cancer. The defendants in both cases denied that the care provided was below that which is usually or customarily provided to such patients, and both challenged the plaintiffs' contention that the patient suffered severely and unnecessarily. At both trials, expert witnesses for the plaintiffs testified that the patient's suffering was unnecessary and was proximately caused by the defendant's failure to meet a recognized standard of care for the management of pain for patients in the terminal phase of an illness in which significant pain should be anticipated and promptly and effectively addressed.

In the first case, *Estate of Henry James vs. Hillhaven Corp.,*[48] the jury awarded the plaintiff $7.5 million in compensatory damages and $7.5 million in punitive damages. The case was never reviewed by an appellate court because the parties settled for an undisclosed amount following the trial. In the second case, *Bergman vs. Wing Chin, MD, and Eden Medical Center,*[49] the jury found that the defendant Chin's care constituted elder abuse and awarded $1.5 million in compensatory damages to the patient's family. Eden Medical Center settled with the patient's family prior to trial. In neither case had state authorities taken any disciplinary action against the institutions or individuals involved.

These jury verdicts provide compelling evidence of an observation by Eric Cassell many years ago: "The relief of suffering, it would appear, is considered one of the primary ends of medicine by patients and lay persons, but not by the medical profession."[50] As we reflect upon pain and society, and particularly its ethical and legal dimensions, we must be concerned about this continuing and significant disparity between lay and profession opinion about the duty of health care professionals to relieve suffering and the seriousness that should be attached to a failure to fulfill that duty. Juries are, in a sense, the conscience of the community, and when they award millions of dollars in damages for the failure to properly manage pain, they are sending a clear message to the health professions that a custom and practice of undertreating pain is unacceptable and will not be tolerated.

CONCLUSION

Opiophobia and an ethic of undertreating pain are aspects of clinical practice that are international in scope and negatively impact all patients with pain. While physicians who regularly care for such patients continue to be at risk of close, even chilling regulatory scrutiny, they now have available an unprecedented number of nationally and internationally recognized policy statements, guidelines, texts, and scientific journal articles supporting in the strongest of terms the prompt, effective, and diligent approach to pain management, with opioid analgesics as the often indispensable weapon against severe chronic pain. Clinically appropriate utilization of state-of-the-art pain management techniques, careful monitoring of patients, and scrupulous and thorough documentation should in most instances insure that health care professionals will not be at an unreasonable risk of adverse action when they provide their patients with the kind of sensitive, skillful, and compassionate care that they have a right to expect and that is consistent with the most ancient goal and core values of medicine – the relief of suffering.

REFERENCES

1. Zborowski M. *People In Pain*. San Francisco, CA: Jossey-Bass, 1969.
2. Lipton JA, Marbach JJ. Ethnicity and the pain experience. *Soc Sci Med* 1984; **19:** 1279–98.
3. Bates MS, Edwards W, Anderson K. Ethno-cultural influences on chronic pain perception. *Pain* 1993; **52:** 101–12.
4. Caton D. The secularization of pain. *Anesthesiology* 1985; **62:** 493–501.
5. Morris DB. What we make of pain. *Wilson Q* 1994; **18:** 8–26.
6. Morris DB. *The Culture of Pain*. Berkeley, CA: University of California Press, 1991.
7. Kleinman A. *The Illness Narratives: Suffering, Healing and the Human Condition*. New York, NY: Basic Books, 1988.
8. Cassel EJ. *The Nature of Suffering and the Goals of Medicine*. New York, NY: Oxford University Press, 1991: 32.
9. California Business and Professions Code 2241.5; Florida Statutes 458.326; Missouri Statutes 334.105 *et seq.*; Nevada Revised Statutes 630.3066; North Dakota Century Code 19-03.3-02 *et seq.*; Oregon Revised Statutes 677.470 *et seq.*; Texas Civil Statutes Article 4495c; Virginia Statutes 54.1-3408.1.
10. Cassel EJ. *The Nature of Suffering and the Goals of Medicine*. New York, NY: Oxford University Press, 1991.
11. Fox E. Predominance of the curative model of medical care – a residual problem. *JAMA* 1997; **278:** 761–3.
12. The SUPPORT Principal Investigators. A controlled trial to improve care for seriously ill hospitalized patients. *JAMA* 1995; **274:** 1591–8.
13. Marks RM, Sachar EJ. Undertreatment of medical inpatients with narcotic analgesics. *Ann Intern Med* 1973; **78:** 173–81.
14. The International Project Special Report. The goals of medicine: setting new priorities. *Hastings Center Rep* 1996; special supplement: 1–27.
15. Brena S. *Chronic Pain: America's Hidden Epidemic*. New York, NY: Atheneum/SMI, 1978.
16. World Health Organization. *Cancer Pain Relief and Palliative Care*. Geneva: World Health Organization, 1990.
17. Turk DC, Brody MC, Okifuji EA. Physicians' attitudes and practices regarding the long-term prescribing of opioids for non-cancer pain. *Pain* 1994; **59:** 201–8.
18. Zenz M, Willweber-Strumpf A. Opiophobia and cancer pain in Europe. *Lancet* 1993; **341:** 1075–6.
19. Zenz M, Zenz T, Tryba M, Strumpf M. Severe undertreatment of cancer pain. *J Pain Symptom Manage* 1995; **10:** 187–91.
20. Larue F, Colleau SM, Brasseur L, Cleeland CS. Multicentre study of cancer pain and its treatment in France. *Br Med J* 1995; **310:** 1034–7.
21. Larue F, Colleau SM, Fontaine A, Brasseur L. Oncologists and primary care physicians' attitudes toward pain control and morphine prescribing in France. *Cancer* 1995; **76:** 2375–82.
22. United Nations. *Single Convention on Narcotic Drugs*, 1961 (as amended by the 1972 Protocol). New York, NY: United Nations, 1977.
23. World Health Organization. *Cancer Pain Relief*, 2nd edn. Geneva: World Health Organization, 1996.
24. International Narcotics Control Board. *Availability of Opiates for Medical Needs*. New York, NY: United Nations, 1996.
25. Selva C. International control of opioids for medical use. *Eur J Palliative Care* 1997; **4:** 194–8.
26. Joranson DE, Cleeland CS, Weissman DH. Opioids for chronic cancer and non-cancer pain: a survey of state medical board members. *Fed Bull* 1992; **79:** 15–49.
27. Ruddick W. Do doctors undertreat pain? *Bioethics* 1997; **11:** 244–6.

28. Foley K. Pain relief into practice: rhetoric without reform. *J Clin Oncol* 1995; **13**: 2149–51.

29. Kleinman A. *The Illness Narratives: Suffering, Healing and the Human Condition*. New York, NY: Basic Books, 1988: 254.

30. Morris DB. *Illness and Culture in the Postmodern Age*. Berkeley, CA: University of California Press, 1998: Chapter 4.

31. Billings JA, Block S. Palliative care in undergraduate medical education: status report of future directions. *JAMA* 1997; **278**: 733–8.

32. Weiner RS. An interview with John J. Bonica, MD. *Pain Pract* 1989; **1**: 2.

33. Morgan JP. American opiophobia: customary underutilization of opioid analgesics. *Adv Alcohol Subst Abuse* 1985; **5**: 163–73.

34. Porter J, Jick H. Addiction rare in patients treated with narcotics. *N Engl J Med* 1980; **302**: 123.

35. Walsh TD. Opiates and respiratory function in advanced cancer. *Recent Results Cancer Res* 1984; **89**: 115–17.

36. Gilson AM, Joranson DE. Controlled substances and pain management: changes in knowledge and attitudes of state medical regulators. *J Pain Symptom Manage* 2001; **21**: 227–37.

37. McKinney M, Fintor L. News: how physicians handle drug investigations. *J Natl Cancer Inst* 1991; **83**: 1282–4.

38. Barnett EH. Case marks big shift in pain policy. *The Oregonian* September 2, 1999. Available at http://www.oregonlive.com:80/news/99/09/st090201.-html.

39. Hoover vs. Agency for Health Care Administration, 676 So. 2d 1380 (Fla. Dist. Ct. App. 1996).

40. Webb M. *The Good Death*. New York, NY: Bantam Books, 1997: 63–71.

41. Fagerhaugh S, Strauss A. *Politics of Pain Management: Staff–Patient Interaction*. Menlo Park, CA: Addison-Wesley, 1977: 22–27.

42. Ferrell BR, Dean GE, Grant M. An institutional commitment to pain management. *Am Pain Soc Bull* 1994; **April–May:** 16.

43. Joint Commission for the Accreditation of Health Care Organizations. *Accreditation Manual*. Chicago, IL: JCAHO, 2000.

44. Berry PH, Dahl JL. Making pain assessment and management a healthcare system priority through the new JCAHO pain standards. *J Pharm Care Pain Symptom Control* 2000; **8**: 5–20.

45. 521 US 702 (1997).

46. 521 US 793 (1997).

47. Burt R. The supreme court speaks: not assisted suicide but a constitutional right to palliative care. *N Engl J Med* 1997; **337**: 1234–6.

48. 89 CVS 64 (N.C. Super. Ct. Jan 15, 1991).

49. H205732-1 (Cal. App. Dep't. Super. Ct. Feb. 16, 1999).

50. Cassell EJ. The nature of suffering and the goals of medicine. *N Engl J Med* 1982; **306**: 639–45.

4

Chronic pain, impairment, and disability

JAMES P ROBINSON

Physicians are often called upon to make judgments about the disability status of patients whom they are treating for chronic pain. These judgments are difficult and routinely evoke discomfort on the part of the treating physician. This chapter deals with issues that physicians frequently encounter when they make disability judgments about patients whom they are treating. It is divided into four sections:

1 Problems of disability evaluation.
2 Disability agencies and conceptual models of disability.
3 Strategies for carrying out disability evaluations.
4 Case histories.

A caveat is needed at the outset. This chapter will focus only on disability evaluation as it is carried out in the USA. In particular, the focus will be on the evaluation of patients who are seeking benefits through the Social Security Administration (SSA), or the Washington State Department of Labor and Industries. The Social Security Administration is a federal agency that administers two large disability programs – Social Security Disability Income (SSDI) and Supplemental Security Income (SSI). The Washington State Department of Labor and Industries (DLI) is an agency in Washington that provides workers' compensation benefits for most workers in the state, and regulates workers' compensation programs for all workers in the state. Any statement made in this chapter about workers' compensation is based on the DLI system. This chapter focuses on the SSA programs for two reasons: (1) they are the largest disability systems in the USA and (2) they are the only ones for which extensive public documentation is available. This chapter focuses on the DLI system because the author has worked with it extensively for the past 13 years.

This limitation reflects a basic assumption of the chapter – that disability evaluation can be discussed or understood only in relation to the disability agencies that commission the evaluations. Thus, one can speak of disability evaluation of a candidate for Social Security Disability Income (SSDI), or disability evaluation of an injured worker receiving workers' compensation from the Department of Labor and Industries in Washington State, but it is usually meaningless to talk about disability evaluation in the abstract.

PROBLEMS OF DISABILITY EVALUATION

Physicians play a crucial role in the roughly seven million disability evaluations that are carried out annually in the USA. Sometimes, physicians are hired by insurance companies or disability agencies to perform independent medical examinations on patients whom they are not treating. In other instances, physicians are asked (or required) to make disability judgments about patients whom they are treating. This chapter focuses on the latter setting for disability evaluation.

Physicians have good reason to feel discomfort when they make disability judgments about their patients. In a general way, the process of disability evaluation places a physician in the middle between his/her patient and a variety of insurance companies or disability agencies. In the best of circumstances, this often has the feel of fitting a round peg into a square hole, since the administrative categories established by disability agencies often do not match the clinical realities of patients. In the worst case, clinicians end up feeling caught in the crossfire between warring adversaries. They *may* perceive employees of disability agencies as unenlightened bureaucrats who make excessive demands for documentation and seem to lose the forest for the trees. At the same time, they *may* perceive their patients as reporting extraordinary amounts of incapacitation and as trying to enlist physicians as allies in their battles with disability agencies.

The concerns that treating physicians have about performing disability evaluations fall into two categories – knowledge deficits and ethical concerns.

Knowledge deficits

Many physicians who do not carry out forensic work or independent medical examinations on a regular basis feel uncomfortable because they perceive that they lack skills and knowledge that are crucial to disability determination. For example, they typically lack familiarity with:

- The disability laws that are relevant to their patients, and the disability agencies with which their patients interact. Thus, physicians are uncertain about how the opinions they render will be used.
- Methods for assessing causation in the sense of legal responsibility.
- The mechanics of performing impairment ratings, e.g. following the procedures described in the American Medical Association's *Guides to the Evaluation of Permanent Impairment*.
- Methods for determining whether patients are capable of various kinds of work. For example, they may not be familiar with physical capacities examinations, or categories of work as defined by the *Dictionary of Occupational Titles*.[1]

Ethical concerns

Regardless of their knowledge, treating physicians are often troubled by ethical issues that arise during disability evaluations. These include the following:

- Some physicians are concerned about broad issues related to disability in the aggregate. For example, Nachemson[2] has raised the specter that spiraling disability rates threaten to undermine the ability of western societies to maintain a social support network. Physicians with this perspective may well feel uncomfortable that their decisions about individual patients are aggravating an important social problem.
- Other physicians take the position that their role is to do everything possible to help the individual patients they are treating. Thus, they are able to function as patient advocates without angst about the significance of disability at a societal level. Even within this narrow focus, however, the ethical landscape is rugged and uncertain. Typically, patients applying for disability emphasize their incapacitation and the hardships they face when they work. One option for physicians is to assume the responsibility of communicating this suffering to disability adjudi-

cators, even when the medical pathology underlying patients' complaints is unclear, i.e. physicians might accept the assessments that patients make about their work capacities at face value. Another option is to confront patients' self-assessments. Physicians often do this because they believe that their patients will function better and experience more satisfaction in the long run if they are reintegrated into the work force. In many instances, though, physicians are conflicted about the appropriate stance to take.

- Regardless of whether or not they support their patients' requests regarding disability, many physicians are appropriately concerned that the process of disability evaluation might compromise their relationships with patients, i.e. they are concerned about conflicts between the *clinical* role they normally play when they treat patients, and the *adjudicative* role that is required during a disability evaluation. Informal observation as well as examination of the limited literature on these roles[3–6] suggest the differences shown in Table 4.1. As Sullivan and Loeser[5] have noted, significant ethical issues arise when physicians switch back and forth between these two roles.

As the above points indicate, the intellectual and ethical challenges raised by disability evaluations are multiple and complex. Only some of them can be addressed in this chapter. For example, the mechanics of impairment ratings are discussed in publications such as the American Medical Association's *Guides to the Evaluation of Permanent Impairment*,[7] and will not be reviewed here.

The discussion below focuses on basic concepts in disability evaluation and on the administrative agencies that manage disability programs. Unfortunately, ambiguity abounds in these areas for several reasons:

1 In the USA, there are 50 state workers' compensation systems, three federal workers' compensation systems, two disability programs run by the Social Security Administration (SSA), a Veterans' Administration disability program, and several disability programs offered by private insurance companies. Also, many public assistance (welfare) programs provide benefits for disabled people, and miscellaneous other programs (such as Medicare and Medicaid) deal to some extent with disability.[8–11] Because of the multitude of disability programs, virtually any statement about disability is likely to have exceptions, and it is difficult even to define concepts unambiguously.

2 The conceptual ambiguities surrounding disability are aggravated greatly by the fact that disability agencies create what might be called an "administrative model" of disability. They implicitly communicate the sense that clinicians should understand this model, and should be able to apply it to their patients. As will be discussed below, this "administrative model" is actually quite shaky.

3 The administrative model of disability is particu-

Table 4.1 *Role expectations for physicians: clinical vs. adjudicative*

Clinical role	Adjudicative role
The physician's primary obligation is to their patient. It is appropriate for the physician to be a patient advocate, and to do everything possible to help their patient return to health	The examiner is not a patient advocate, and is not obliged to meet the needs of the patient being evaluated (some critics would assert that independent medical examiners often function as advocates for insurance companies)
A patient's history provides 90% of the clinical information that a physician needs. The physical examination and laboratory tests are important but secondary sources of information	The emphasis in an evaluation should be on objective findings (e.g. on physical examination or imaging findings) rather than on the patient's complaints
Where there is doubt about the accuracy of a patient's statements, the patient is given the benefit of the doubt	Be skeptical of patients' reports
A major task of a physician is to diagnose a patient's problems, i.e. to identify the pathophysiology underlying the patient's symptoms	The focus should be on legal causation of a patient's symptoms
A physician's job is to provide medical or surgical assistance – not to get embroiled in a patient's legal problems	The major job of the independent medical examiner is to relate a patient's clinical condition to applicable laws or administrative regulations that define responsibilities of third-party payors

larly problematic when it is applied to patients who are disabled primarily because of pain. Patients with chronic pain challenge the fundamental premise of the administrative model of disability – that impairments should be objectively observable.

In essence, you should expect to find ambiguity (or outright incoherence) when you attempt to understand concepts related to disability evaluation, and to apply them to your patients. Some of the ambiguity is inevitable, but you can mitigate it by learning as much as you can about the specific disability agencies with which you interact.

DISABILITY AGENCIES AND CONCEPTUAL MODELS OF DISABILITY

Disability as a social status

Disability can be loosely defined as the inability to carry out certain activities because of a medical problem. Disability exists among people throughout the world, but societies differ greatly in how they respond to people with disabilities. In many societies, disability is managed informally within the family of the disabled person. In contrast, the USA and many other industrialized societies have large, formal programs to provide support for disabled people.

The presence of large, formal disability programs – such as the Social Security Disability Income (SSDI) program run by the SSA – changes the dynamics of disability. An individual with activity limitations because of a medical problem must submit an application to an agency that administers a disability program. Adjudicators from the

agency must determine whether the applicant meets eligibility criteria for benefits. In order to make this determination, the adjudicators typically request medical information from the applicant's treating physician. Thus, physicians are routinely drawn into the disability determination process for patients whom they are treating.

Disability agencies have a profound impact on the entire dialog about disability. The reason is simple: to a large extent, disability agencies establish the criteria that individuals must meet in order to get benefits and the procedures that are followed when they apply for benefits. This is fairly obvious when the "disability agency" is a private insurance company. An insurance company has wide latitude regarding the insurance policies it creates and the procedures it uses to determine whether a policy-holder has a legitimate claim to benefits. Governmental agencies such as the SSA are more constrained – by the enabling legislation that permits them to function, by judicial decisions, and by input from the executive branch of the federal government.[12] But these inputs provide only general guidelines – the day-to-day operations of the SSA are determined by internally derived policies and guidelines. As noted above, a central thesis of this chapter is that in order to carry out disability evaluations intelligently on your patients, you need to have at least rudimentary knowledge about the workings of the agencies that administer disability programs.

Types of disability and disability agencies

Medical problems can interfere with a person's ability to carry out activities in many different arenas. Correspondingly, there are many types of support given to people with disabilities, and many agencies to administer benefit programs. Table 4.2 shows some of the common forms

Table 4.2 *Types of disability*

Nature of disability	Type of assurance sought	Organization involved
Limited walking ability	Disabled parking sticker	Department of Motor Vehicles
Diminished ability to perform household chores	Chore worker service	Private insurance company; workers' compensation carrier; Medicare; Medicaid
Diminished ability to perform self-care	Personal attendant	Private insurance company; workers' compensation carrier; Medicare; Medicaid
Limited ability to work	Job accommodations	Equal Employment Opportunity Commission
Limited ability to work	Time off work, with protection from being fired	US Department of Labor (Family and Medical Leave Act)
Inability to work	Wage replacement payments	Workers' compensation; Social Security Disability Insurance; Supplemental Security Income; private insurance

of disability, the benefits that are available for individuals with these disabilities, and the organizations that evaluate disability requests and/or administer benefits in the USA. These organizations include private insurance companies and a variety of state or federal governmental agencies. In the discussion below, the term "disability agency" will be used to refer to any organization that evaluates disability applications or dispenses disability benefits.

For simplicity, the present chapter will focus on work disability. Work disability can be subcategorized in several ways. The most important distinctions are between total and partial disability, and between temporary and permanent disability. Various disability agencies have programs tailored to these different categories of work disability. For example, the SSA programs are designed for individuals who are permanently and totally disabled; workers' compensation time-loss benefits are paid to individuals who are totally, temporarily disabled; and many private disability insurance policies provide benefits when an individual's disability prevents them from performing their usual work, even if they are not totally disabled.

Definitions: disability and impairment

"Disability" and "impairment" are fundamental concepts that provide the conceptual cornerstones for disability programs. As noted above, disability can be informally defined as the inability to carry out certain activities because of a medical problem. Unfortunately, there is no unique formal definition of disability, since various agencies that administer disability programs define the term slightly differently. These differences reflect a fundamental reality about disability agencies. It is that an agency does not develop definitions to satisfy people's intellectual needs for conceptual clarity. Definitions serve the much more practical function of identifying the criteria that applicants must meet in order to be eligible for benefits.

Thus, agencies have different definitions because they have different mandates and different eligibility criteria. For example, the SSA defines disability as: "the inability to engage in any substantial gainful activity by reason of any medically determinable physical or mental impairment that can be expected to result in death or that has lasted or can be expected to last for a continuous period of not less than 12 months" (reference 13, p. 2). This definition reflects three facts about eligibility criteria for the SSD and SSI programs:

1 applicants must be totally disabled from work;
2 the work disability must be "permanent" (or at least long term);
3 causation is irrelevant, i.e. an individual is eligible for benefits regardless of how or why they became disabled.

In contrast, the AMA Guides defines disability as "an alteration of an individual's capacity to meet personal, social, or occupational demands or statutory or regulatory requirements because of an impairment" (reference 7, p. 8). This very broad definition reflects the fact that the Guides describes an evaluation system that is relevant to many kinds of disability (rather than just work disability) and that permits gradations in disability to be identified (rather than just the two categories of totally disabled and nondisabled).

An impairment can best be understood as a deficiency in the functioning of an organ or body part that leads to incapacitation or disadvantage in various arenas (such as inability to work, or inability to carry out routine activities at home). The formal definition of impairment given in the AMA Guides is: "a loss, loss of use, or derangement of any body part, organ system, or organ function" (reference 7, p. 2). Impairment is conceptualized as existing at the level of organs or body parts. Thus, one might say: "Mr Jones' heart has been impaired since he suffered a myocardial infarction" or "Mrs Brown's right hand is impaired because of her carpal tunnel syndrome."

Disability agencies assume significant linkages

between impairment and disability. First, they construe impairment as a necessary condition for disability. The logic underlying this requirement is simple. Disability programs are designed to assist individuals who are unable to compete in the workplace because of a medical condition. In essence, disability programs attempt to partition individuals who fail in the workplace into two large groups: those who fail because of a medical condition and those who fail for other reasons (e.g. lack of demand for their skills). Therefore, disability programs require evidence that an applicant has a medical problem underlying their workplace failure. Impairment provides the required evidence because it can be viewed as a marker that an individual has a medical problem which diminishes their capability. Conversely, if an individual has no impairment, this means that they do not have limitations due to a medical condition. Second, disability agencies typically assume that the severity of a patient's impairment correlates with the severity (or probability) of their being disabled from work. Thus, even when an agency grants awards only on the basis of work disability, the agency will often seek information about a patient's impairment in order to rationalize its decision about whether or not to award disability benefits.

As a practical matter, disability agencies typically ask physicians to make judgments about both impairment and disability in patients whom they evaluate. In some instances, the agency operates under a mandate to compensate patients for impairment. In that setting, the physician's impairment rating has a direct bearing on the award that a patient receives, as the size of the award is linked to the severity of the patient's impairment. In other instances, the agency makes payments only if a patient is judged to be disabled from work. In the latter setting, an impairment rating may well be performed, but it serves only as an intervening step in the broader task of determining whether or not the patient warrants a disability award.

A note of caution is needed here. Although it is possible to distinguish conceptually between impairment (meaning dysfunction of an organ or body part) and disability (meaning an activity limitation secondary to an impairment), in many practical situations the distinction is unclear. For example, the notion of a dysfunctional organ does not readily apply to psychiatric impairments. In essence, the distinction between impairment and disability is easy to make in some medical conditions, and difficult to make in others. The inherent difficulty in distinguishing between impairment and disability is greatly aggravated by the lack of precision that abounds in discussions of the two concepts. For example, consider the following statement from the Medical Aid Rules of the Washington State Department of Labor and Industries (DLI): "The Department of Labor and Industries has promulgated the following rules and categories to provide a comprehensive system of classifying unspecified permanent partial disabilities in the proportion they rea-

sonably bear to total bodily impairment" (reference 14, p. 37). This statement is semantically opaque, and adds confusion rather than clarity to the distinction between impairment and disability.

The mechanics of disability evaluations

Figure 4.1 shows the participants who are typically involved in a determination about whether or not an applicant warrants work disability benefits.

1   The application process typically has to be initiated by the patient who alleges that they is unable to work.
2   The central person in the communication loop is the adjudicator or claims manager who works for the insurance company or disability agency to which the patient applies.
3   The adjudicator gathers information from the applicant, and then contacts the applicant's treating physician. Frequently, the contact is indirect – the applicant is given an information form and told that his/her treating physician needs to fill it out. An example of the physician's portion of a disability form is given in Fig. 4.2.

   Depending on the disability agency involved, the adjudicator may have only a single interaction with a treating physician, or may have multiple interactions over time. For example, when the SSA processes an application for SSDI, the treating physician is asked to provide information only once. At the opposite extreme, claims managers for workers' compensation claimants typically have multiple interactions with treating physicians.
4   The adjudicator can turn to various consultants within his/her agency for help with claims. These include vocational consultants, legal consultants, and medical consultants.
5   The adjudicator frequently will request information from a physician who is not involved in the applicant's care. Large agencies such as the SSA hire physicians to review information on applicants. Another option is to have an applicant undergo an independent medical examination. Typically, these examinations are performed by physicians who are not regular employees of the disability agency, but are commissioned to perform examinations on disability applicants.

   Adjudicators for some agencies will ask the treating physician to review an independent medical examination report and express agreement or disagreement with its conclusions. In other agencies, for example the SSA, the adjudicator collates information from various sources, but does not ask the treating physician to comment on the reports of others.
6   The adjudicator may interact with a variety of other individuals. Examples include a vocational rehabilita-

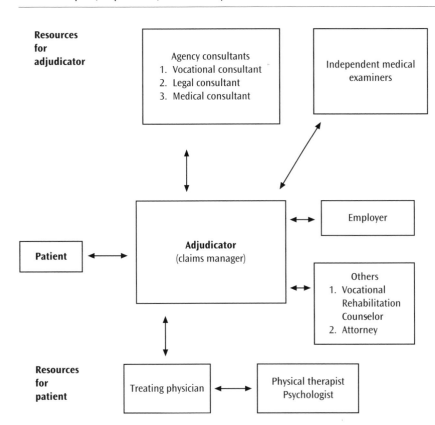

Figure 4.1 *Typical participants in a disability claim.*

tion counselor, an attorney who represents an applicant, and the applicant's former employer.

7 The adjudicator is the individual who ultimately makes the determination of whether the applicant meets eligibility criteria for disability benefits.

Conceptual models of disability

Agencies that administer disability programs develop procedures to facilitate efficient decision-making. These procedures embody a conceptual model of the manner in which disability can be assessed. Unfortunately, most disability agencies do not make their policies and conceptual models available to the public. Thus, a discussion of them is of necessity speculative. The only exception to this generalization is the SSA, which runs the two biggest disability programs in the world – SSDI and SSI. Several monographs have been written about the SSA.[12,15,16] They emphasize that the SSA strives to use disability evaluation procedures that are inexpensive, uniform across the USA, and based on objective findings of incapacitation. These administrative objectives seem innocuous enough. However, they have profound implications. In essence, the SSA has to make significant simplifying assumptions about disability in order to achieve its administrative goals.

The most fundamental simplifying assumption made by disability agencies is that impairment and disability should be "transparent" to an experienced physician, i.e.

that activity limitations described or demonstrated by patients should be highly correlated with evidence of tissue damage or organ dysfunction that can be objectively assessed by a physician. This assumption underlies the routine demand that disability adjudicators make for the "objective findings" on which physicians rely when they make conclusions about activity limitations of patients.

The assumption that impairment and disability can be objectively assessed is so pervasive that most physicians – and essentially all disability adjudicators – accept it without question. It is thus surprising to discover that physicians have not always made this assumption. In fact, when the SSDI program was being considered by Congress during the 1950s, physician groups almost uniformly protested that they would not be able to carry out the assessments that were envisaged in the SSDI-enabling legislation.[16]

Some impairments can be assessed accurately by objective means. For example, physicians have tools to quantify impairment stemming from amputations or complete spinal cord injuries. However, in many medical conditions – including most chronic pain syndromes – physicians cannot objectively identify impairments that rationalize the activity limitations that patients report. In a monograph on the SSDI and SSI programs, Osterweis *et al.* summarize the problem as follows: "The notion that all impairments should be verifiable by objective evidence is administratively necessary for an entitlement program. Yet this notion is fundamentally at odds with a realistic understanding of how disease and injury operate to inca-

Physician name: _____ Phone number: _____ ID no.:
_____

Specialty: _____ Patient's Account Number:
_____

Address:
_____

1. Diagnosis: _____ 2. Diagnosis code:
_____

3. Was condition due to an accidental injury?   Yes   No 4. Date accident occurred _____ Nature of injury
_____

5. Where did injury happen?   At work   At home   Other
(Specify) _____

3. When did patient first consult you for this condition? Date: _____ Date of most recent examination:
_____

7. Has patient ever had same or similar condition: Yes   No   If yes, when?
_____

8. Describe any other disease or infirmity affecting present condition:
_____

9. Please give patient's last known weight: _____ height:
_____

10. Referring physician's name and address:
_____

11. Was patient under the influence of any intoxicant or narcotic at time of accident?   Yes   No Did it
contribute to the injury? _____
     If yes, under the direction of a physician? _____

12. Was patient hospitalized solely due to this condition?   Yes   No Where?
_____

13. Was patient disabled?   Yes   No   Total or partial?
_____

14. On what dates: From _____   To _____   Return to work:
_____

15. *Please list any procedure codes: A) _____ B) _____ C)
_____

16. **Please list the objectives disability factors (disabling signs and symptoms):
_____
_____
_____

*   Please attach a copy of the bill for services you rendered to this patient.
**   If length of this disability period exceeds normal duration for this diagnosis, please attach copies of all supporting
documentation.

Completed by (print): _____ Position:
_____

Physician's signature: _____ Date:
_____

Figure 4.2 *Physician's portion of a disability form (from a private insurance company).*

pacitate people. Except for a very few conditions, such as the loss of a limb, blindness, deafness, paralysis, or coma, most diseases and injuries do not prevent people from working by mechanical failure. Rather, people are incapacitated by a variety of unbearable sensations when they try to work" (reference 16, p. 28).

This statement by Osterweis *et al.* succinctly captures the dilemma that arises when a physician attempts to determine whether one of his/her chronic pain patients is disabled. The disability agency to which the patient is applying indicates that it will award benefits only if there is objective evidence that the patient is incapacitated. The patient reports "unbearable sensations" that preclude work. The physician often cannot identify evidence of organ damage that makes the pain complaints seem inevitable or even plausible. He/she has the difficult task of reconciling the subjective assessment of the patient with the demands of the disability agency for objectivity.

STRATEGIES FOR DISABILITY EVALUATIONS

Preparation

The discussion above explains the context within which physicians operate when they carry out disability evaluations on their patients, and describes some of the reasons why disability evaluations are difficult. But the practical question still remains: what should you do when you are asked to fill out a disability form?

The answer to this question is do not wait for the form to cross your desk – do some homework up front. At the very least, you should consider two issues prior to the time when you might be asked to fill out a disability form:

1 What are your attitudes toward disability?
2 How do you integrate disability *evaluation* into an overall strategy of disability *management*?

What are your attitudes toward disability?

Some physicians experience a lot of empathy for patients who are applying for disability awards. They believe that the patients are likely to experience severe emotional and physical stress if economic circumstances force them to remain in the work force. At the opposite extreme, some physicians perceive disability applicants as con artists who are trying to manipulate "the system" and get benefits that they do not deserve. The available evidence suggests that both of these perspectives are oversimplified.

For most workers, the work place provides many benefits. In addition to financial rewards, work provides individuals with social contacts and binds them to the community. The psychosocial benefits of work can best be appreciated by the extensive research on unemployment among people who are not disabled. The general thrust of this research is that when individuals are separated from the work place – for example, by being laid off during an economic recession – they and their families are at increased risk for a number of adverse outcomes, including depression, anxiety, substance abuse, social isolation, family dissolution, and suicide.[17-21] The implication of this research is clear: the mental health of most people – even those with significant medical problems – is better served by staying in the work force than by leaving it.

In addition to the psychological losses associated with separation from the work place, injured workers suffer severe economic losses when they become disabled.[22] Thus, the notion that disabled people are "milking the system" is almost certainly wrong. In fact, one of the tragedies of disability is that everyone seems to lose – the injured workers, their families, the people who pay disability insurance premiums, and society at large.

Many observers of disability systems have speculated that the process of interacting with disability agencies has detrimental effects on patients.[23] For example, Hadler[24] has argued that as patients try to prove their incapacitation to disability adjudicators, they become more and more convinced that they really are disabled. Some observers have suggested the term "disability syndrome" to describe the set of dysfunctional attitudes and beliefs that develops over time as an individual adapts to the role of being a disabled person. Thus, patients who seem straightforward and highly motivated just after an injury often become more resistant to rehabilitation later on.

A related point is that disability seems to act like quicksand for many people, i.e. once they enter the disability system, they tend to get "stuck" there and to sink into protracted disability. The most striking evidence for this conclusion comes from long-term outcome studies on SSDI beneficiaries. These studies indicate that, after an individual has been accepted for SSDI, the probability is only about 3% that they will ever return to the work force.[25] Also, numerous studies on disabled workers with industrial compensation claims have shown that, although the vast majority of them return to work within a few weeks after injury, those who are still disabled at 6 months after injury have a high probability of very protracted disability.[26,27]

How do you integrate disability evaluation into an overall strategy of disability management?

This chapter focuses on disability evaluation. In practical situations, however, treating physicians do not perform disability evaluations in isolation. Broadly speaking, treating physicians need to develop strategies for disability *management* for the patients they are treating. Disability management encompasses at least four areas: assessment of disability risk, establishment of a treatment contract with a patient, prevention of disability, and evaluation of disability. These areas are linked, e.g. if a physician fails to assess disability risk adequately or to develop reasonable disability prevention strategies, they will probably find disability evaluation particularly difficult.

It is beyond the scope of this chapter to discuss assessment of disability risk, treatment contracts, or disability prevention. However, a few examples are given below to convey an idea of what these areas entail.

Disability management starts with an assessment of a patient's risk of sliding into long-term disability. Experts in disability have asserted that there are "red flags" which signify that a patient is at risk for protracted disability.[28,29] Although these lists have not been empirically validated, they highlight the general point that the treating physician should be thinking about a patient's risk for long-term disability before the patient brings in disability forms to be signed.

The second crucial aspect of disability management involves contracting with a patient. If you anticipate that a patient is likely to seek disability benefits, what ground rules do you establish with him/her? One strategy is to agree to treat patients only if they express a commitment to return to work.

Disability prevention refers to interventions by a physician to help prevent a patient from sliding into long-term disability. For example, a treating physician might refer a patient to a work-hardening program, or recommend that the patient return to work rapidly after injury, but in a light-duty capacity. A variety of disability prevention strategies have been proposed.[30–32]

The key issues in a disability evaluation

When a physician – either an independent medical examiner or a treating physician – carries out a disability evaluation, they are expected to perform the kind of thorough history and physical examination that would be carried out in a clinical setting. In addition, disability adjudicators ask the physician to address issues that permit the disability agency to determine whether an applicant is eligible for benefits.[3] These typically include:

1 diagnosis;
2 causation;
3 need for further treatment;
4 impairment;
5 ability to work.

Examples of the questions posed by disability agencies are given in Table 4.3. The second column of this table lists questions that were addressed to an independent medical examiner by a workers' compensation board. The patient was a woman who had sustained a noncatastrophic neck injury in the course of her work. The third column lists questions that were addressed to a physician who was treating a man for a nonwork-related median neuropathy. The patient had a disability policy through a private insurance company. The questions were written by the company. Table 4.3 is organized to show how questions were worded by the two agencies, and which of the key issues the questions addressed. Note that the questions from the workers' compensation board addressed all five of the issues listed above, whereas the questions from the private insurance company addressed only three of them. This presumably reflects the different mandates of the two agencies, e.g. workers' compensation programs are responsible only for injuries that occur at work, whereas many private disability programs provide benefits regardless of how a policy-holder became disabled.

Each of the key areas is discussed further below.

Diagnosis

Physicians are familiar with making diagnoses – in fact, diagnosis is a central component of any clinical evaluation. However, most physicians are not familiar with

Table 4.3 *Typical issues addressed and specific questions asked in disability evaluations*

Issue addressed	Specific questions asked	
	Workers' compensation system[a]	Private insurance company[b]
Diagnosis	What are the diagnoses based on objective findings?	Diagnoses ――― Subjective symptoms ――― Objective findings ―――
Causation	Please state which, if any, of the diagnosed conditions are work related	
Maximal medical improvement	Is the patient medically stable or have they reached preinjury status? What treatment would you recommend?	Has the patient reached maximal medical improvement? Would any further therapy be reasonably expected to result in full or partial recovery?
Impairment rating	If the patient is medically stable, do they have a ratable permanent partial impairment according to the AMA *Guidelines*, 5th edition?	
Ability to work	Can the patient return to their job of injury? (The job description is attached)	1. Rate the patient's physical impairment: Class 1 – no limitation Class 2 – capable of medium work Class 3 – capable of light work Class 4 – capable of sedentary work Class 5 – incapable of minimal activity or sedentary work 2. Please describe fully how the patient's symptoms/limitations affect their ability to work 3. Would job modification enable the patient to work with impairment? 4. Would vocational counseling and/or retraining be recommended?

a. Questions to an independent medical examiner.
b. Questions to a treating physician.

the need to justify diagnoses on the basis of objective findings. The term "objective findings" is not precisely defined, but in general it refers to laboratory or physical findings that are not subject to voluntary control or manipulation by a patient. In clinical practice, physicians diagnose patients on the basis of recognizable patterns of symptoms and clinical signs. They generally make informal attempts to assess the credibility of patients, and they may discount a patient's symptoms if he/she does not appear to be credible. But they do not make the sharp distinction between objective and subjective findings that disability agencies demand.[33]

Causation

Causation is crucial for agencies that are responsible only for injuries that occurred as a result of a specific type of exposure. For example, workers' compensation systems are responsible only for injuries that occurred in the work place; motor vehicle insurance companies are responsible only for injuries that occurred in automobile accidents. The concept of causation is a legal one – it identifies who is legally and financially responsible for a patient's medical condition.

In catastrophic injuries, such as spinal cord injuries, there is usually no problem in establishing the time and place where the problem began. However, the situation is very different for common musculoskeletal problems such as low back pain. First, episodes of low back pain can start in the absence of any obviously injurious stimulus. Second, an individual is not necessarily incapacitated by low back pain, thus it is possible for them to be injured in one setting but to attribute the onset of symptoms to something else. Third, most episodes of low back pain are not accompanied by unambiguous biological markers.[34,35] Thus, a physician cannot count on a test to determine whether or not a patient has a low back problem or to determine when and how the problem began. Finally, low back pain tends to follow a waxing and waning course, with multiple exacerbations and remissions. Thus, a patient's symptoms at any given time are most plausibly construed as a complex result of multiple causes. The significance of any single putative cause is difficult to assess. For all these reasons, physicians have difficulty determining the legal cause of symptoms in a patient with low back pain.

The inherent difficulty in making causal statements regarding such conditions is aggravated by the fact that most physicians do not have much training in the niceties of causal assessment in forensic settings.[36]

Need for further treatment

Disability agencies generally adopt an idealized model of the course of recovery following an injury. The model is shown in Fig. 4.3. It embodies the assumption that people show rapid improvement following injury, but then level off and reach a plateau. When they reach the plateau,

they are considered to have achieved maximal medical improvement. From an administrative perspective, the model is convenient because it provides guidelines for intervention and decision-making. For example, when a patient has reached point X on the graph (Fig. 4.3), curative treatment should be abandoned, and a permanent partial impairment rating should be made.

Unfortunately, patients frequently present with clinical problems that are hard to conceptualize in terms of the idealized recovery shown in Fig. 4.3.[37] The difficulties in this area are myriad. For example, it is not at all clear that patients with repetitive strain injuries should be expected to follow the trajectory shown in this figure. Another problem is that patients may have comorbidities that complicate recovery and make it difficult to determine when they have reached maximal medical improvement, e.g. a diabetic who has a work-related carpal tunnel syndrome.

A final complication of the maximal medical improvement concept is that a patient who has reached maximal benefit from a particular kind of treatment may not have reached maximal benefit from treatment in general. For example, consider a patient who is examined 6 months after a low back injury. Assume that the patient's treatment has consisted entirely of chiropractic care during the 6-month interval and that they have not shown any measurable improvement during the past 2 months. This patient might be judged to have reached maximal medical benefit from chiropractic care, but an examining physician would understandably be uncertain about whether the patient could benefit from physical therapy, epidural steroids, lumbar surgery, aggressive use of various medications, or other therapies not provided by the chiropractor. This problem is not just a hypothetical one, since examiners routinely find that even very chronic patients have not had exposure to all the plausible treatment approaches for their condition.

Impairment

The concept of impairment has been discussed above. Although most physicians are somewhat familiar with the concept, they often do not have expertise in the techniques required to carry out impairment ratings. The complexity of these techniques is apparent when we consider that the fifth edition of the AMA *Guides to the Evaluation of Permanent Impairment*[7] is 613 pages long.

Impairment ratings are essentially always performed by physicians, typically in the context of an overall evaluation of a patient's medical condition. The ratings are usually made only after a patient has reached maximal medical improvement from treatment, i.e. when his/her recovery following an injury or illness appears to have reached a plateau. In this setting, the task of the examining physician is to ascertain how much permanent partial impairment a patient has sustained.

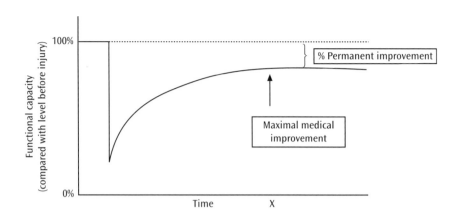

Figure 4.3 *Hypothetical recovery curve following an injury.*

When a physician assesses a patient's impairment, he/she potentially asks three questions:

1 Is there a diagnosis? That is to say, does the patient have a recognizable medical condition that reasonably accounts for the clinical findings?
2 Is there any impairment associated with the patient's medical condition?
3 If so, how severe is the impairment?

A diagnosis is a necessary condition for a determination that a patient has impairment. However, it is not a sufficient condition, i.e. a patient could have a recognizable disorder but no associated permanent impairment of the affected organ. For example, some patients receive a diagnosis of lumbar strain on the basis of their reports of back pain, but have no ratable impairment in the lumbar spine.

Some conceptual problems arise about whether impairment can be localized to an organ or body part, and about whether impairment and disability can be distinguished. But these pale compared with the two really difficult issues in impairment: determining the severity of impairment and assessing impairment caused by pain.

The quantification of impairment: general problems

The AMA impairment system represents an ambitious attempt to quantify impairment affecting essentially all organ systems and body parts. Whole-person impairment is a key unifying concept in the AMA system. It is conceptualized as a unidimensional scale running from 0% (for an individual with no measurable deficit) to 100% whole-person impairment (for a person who is comatose or has some other type of problem that is totally incapacitating).

For some conditions – such as renal impairment – the AMA *Guides* specifies impairment only in terms of whole-person impairment. For other conditions – especially ones involving the extremities – the *Guides* has physicians go through a series of abstractions to reach a whole-person impairment rating. For example, consider a man who sustains a traumatic amputation of the thumb of the right hand at the metacarpophalangeal joint. This corresponds to a 100% impairment of the right thumb.

According to Tables 16-1, 16-2, and 16-3 of the *Guides* (reference 7, pp. 438–9), a 100% impairment of the thumb corresponds to a 40% impairment of the hand. A 40% impairment of the hand, in turn, corresponds to a 36% impairment of the upper extremity. Finally, a 36% impairment of the upper extremity corresponds to a whole-person impairment of 22%. Thus, the man would receive a whole-person impairment of 22%.

Regardless of whether or not there are intermediate steps, the endpoint of impairment ratings in the AMA system is whole-person impairment. The whole-person impairment construct has two essential features: it measures the severity of impairment (with a range of 0–100%), and it permits direct comparisons to be made among impairments involving different organs and different body parts.

The AMA system has several flaws. Most fundamentally, impairment is extremely difficult to quantify for some kinds of medical conditions, especially psychiatric conditions and chronic pain syndromes. Second, although the "whole-person impairment" construct seems to integrate impairment ratings, this integration comes at a cost. Most importantly, whole-person impairment is a very abstract construct that obscures crucial differences among patients. For example, imagine a patient who has a 50% whole-person impairment because of renal insufficiency, and another one who has a 50% whole-person impairment because of a spinal cord injury. Although these two individuals would be judged as equivalent by the AMA system, they would have completely different types of activity limitations.

It is important to note that some disability agencies, for example the SSA, do not use quantitative measures of impairment. The SSA relies on "listings" to determine whether an applicant has severe enough impairment to be considered totally disabled from work. A listing essentially consists of a diagnosis along with some markers of severity. For example, one listing is for "Other vertebrogenic disorders (e.g. herniated nucleus pulposus, spinal stenosis) with the following persisting for at least 3 months despite prescribed therapy and expected to last 12 months. With both 1 and 2: (1) Pain, muscle spasm, and significant limitation of motion in the spine; and (2) Appropriate radicular distribution of significant motor loss with muscle weakness and sensory and reflex loss" (reference 13, p. 19). Thus, the SSA uses a few crude markers of severity of impairment, but does not ask evaluators to quantify impairment precisely.

Impairment caused by pain

Several reviewers have concluded that impairment assessment in painful conditions is extremely difficult, and that no completely satisfactory system for making such assessments exists.[7,16,33,38] Disability agencies have largely ignored the problem, presumably because they are committed to the model that impairments should be objectively measurable. For example, the Washington State DLI provides the following guidelines for the assessment of permanent impairment in patients with dorsolumbar or lumbosacral problems: "Gradations of clinical findings of low back impairments in terms of 'mild', 'moderate' or 'marked' shall be based on objective medical tests. All of the low back categories include the presence of complaints of whatever degree" (reference 14, p. 42). In essence, this statement means that patients' complaints of pain are to be ignored in the impairment assessment process.

As Osterweis *et al.* noted (see quote above), disability agencies conceptualize impairment in terms of measurable "mechanical failure" of a body part or organ. This conceptual system is most applicable to dramatic injuries such as amputations or nerve injuries that render a body part functionless because of paralysis. The mechanical failure model implicitly assumes that an individual will use all of their body parts optimally unless they mechanically fail, i.e., that they will not limit activities on the basis of subjective factors such as pain, discouragement, fear of reinjury, etc.

The model is thus a caricature that describes robots more than people. For example, one of the most memorable examples of an individual whose goal-oriented behavior was limited only by objective bodily damage was Arnold Schwarzenegger in the movie *The Terminator*. Reese (the Terminator's human adversary) described the Terminator to Sarah Conner as follows: "That terminator is out there .... It doesn't feel pity or remorse or fear. And it absolutely will not stop – ever ..." As the movie unfolds, it becomes abundantly clear that the Terminator was relentless in its pursuit of Sarah Conner – it could be stopped only by fires, explosions, etc. that tore off body parts.

In contrast to robots or Terminators, human beings do not persist in activities until their bodies fail mechanically. As described by Osterweis *et al.* (reference 16, p. 28), they experience "unbearable sensations" that lead them to discontinue activities even though their bodies are (or appear to be) mechanically intact.

The distinction between mechanical failure and unbearable sensations as a cause of incapacitation has profound ramifications. The central dilemma is that mechanical failure is publicly observable, whereas unbearable sensations (such as pain) are directly observable only by the individual experiencing them. Physicians face this dilemma repeatedly as they evaluate impairment in patients with chronic pain. The patients communicate the sense that they are severely incapacitated by pain, and ask their physicians to support these claims. Typically, a physician who evaluates such a patient cannot identify tissue damage/organ pathology that make the limitations communicated by the patient seem inevitable or even plausible. The physician then has the dilemma of integrating the subjective reports of the patient with the objective evidence of tissue damage/organ pathology/mechanical failure to come up with some final judgment about the extent to which the patient really is incapacitated. At one extreme, a physician might simply ignore the patient's self-assessments, and make a disability determination based strictly on objective findings of tissue damage/ organ pathology. At the opposite extreme, the physician might accept the patient's definition of the situation, and give a disability rating that is congruent with the patient's self-assessment. Most physicians feel uncomfortable with either extreme, but it has proved extremely difficult to find some middle ground in which both objective evidence and self-assessments by patients can be incorporated into disability evaluations.

Systems for measuring impairment caused by pain

Probably the most widely used system for incorporating pain into impairment assessments is the one developed by the SSA.[33,39] As noted above, the SSA does not have a formal process for quantifying impairment. However, it does require evaluators to do something similar, i.e. to make a qualitative determination of whether an applicant's illness or injury is so severe that it precludes gainful employment. SSA evaluations in the context of painful conditions proceed in accordance with the following principles:

1 A physician evaluation is needed:
   a to make the qualitative determination of whether or not there is any impairment;
   b to determine whether an applicant's impairment is likely to produce the types of symptoms (including pain) of which he/she complains.
2 A physician cannot reliably determine the amount of pain that a person with a certain impairment has or the extent to which the pain interferes with activities.
3 The severity of activity limitations imposed by impairment should be assessed largely on the basis of restrictions that the applicant actually demonstrates in his/her day-to-day life, as indicated in interviews with the patient, family members, coworkers, etc.
4 The adjudicator who processes an SSD application should assess the credibility of the applicant, and consider this in reaching a conclusion about the severity of the applicant's activity limitations.

The 5th edition of the American Medical Association's *Guides to the Evaluation of Permanent and Impairment* describes a new system for assessing pain-related impairment. The system has been elaborated and modified in the companion volume *Mastering the Guides*.[40]

Key elements of this system are:

1 It provides a systematic algorithm for physicians to follow when they rate impairment associated with pain. This increases the likelihood that ratings will have acceptable reliability.
2 It follows the general approach of the *Guides* in that judgments about the severity of pain-related impairment are made by physicians.
3 It recognizes that pain is subjective, so that an evaluator must consider self-report data in the assessment of pain-related impairment. It also recognizes that the significance of pain for an individual is related to the extent to which his or her daily activities are restricted because of pain. The assessment algorithm includes a self-report measure in which patients describe the impact of their pain on their ability to perform activities of daily living.
4 However, the system also recognizes that patients might embellish their presentations. It instructs examiners to temper patients' self-reports by assessing their credibility and their pain behaviors (observable expressions of pain, distress, and suffering). The physician evaluator is asked to balance self-reports by a patient with clinical judgment based on his or her experience and observation of the patient throughout the evaluation process.
5 The system acknowledges that chronic pain is sometimes independent of any well-established medical condition. In this setting, examiners can use the system to assess the magnitude of pain-related impairment, but they are instructed to designate the impairment they identify as unratable.

At this point, there are no validity data on either of the above two systems. Thus, in principle, you could use concepts from either of them, or some entirely different system, to make judgments about pain-related impairment in your patients. As a practical matter, however, you will be discouraged from using any system that factors pain into impairment ratings. Most disability agencies discourage physicians from factoring pain into impairment ratings by demanding that conclusions be based on objective findings, and by requiring rating physicians to use assessment procedures that de-emphasize pain.

Ability to work

As discussed above, a physician evaluation is needed to provide a diagnosis for a disability applicant and to assess (either qualitatively or quantitatively) impairment associated with the diagnosed medical condition. In theory, a nonmedical adjudicator could use this medical information to determine whether or not the applicant was actually incapacitated from work. In practical situations, however, physicians are almost always asked not only about a disability applicant's diagnosis and impairment, but also about his/her ability to work. In theory, the examining physician could make some inference about the ability of an applicant to work on the basis of his/her diagnosis and rated impairment. In practice, physicians face enormous obstacles when they try to do this. Problems include the following:

1 The severity of impairment is often difficult to assess, especially for conditions in which pain plays a major role.
2 The linkages between impairment and work disability are highly variable, and are often job specific.
   For example, a person with a spinal cord injury might be able to work as a research scientist, but would be unable to do heavy manual labor. A person with impairment from a traumatic brain injury might show the opposite pattern.
3 The examinations that physicians carry out in their offices typically do not provide detailed information about the ability of patients to carry out various tasks. For example, a physician rarely gets detailed information regarding a patient's tolerances for lifting, walking, or sitting from an office evaluation.
4 Physicians often do not have details about the demands imposed by various jobs.
5 The vocational implications of a patient's activity restrictions depend to a substantial degree on the availability of accommodations in his/her work place. As a simple example, a paraplegic would be unable to perform work in a third floor office of a building that had no elevator, but might be completely capable of working in a building that was wheel chair accessible.

General principles for disability evaluation

Disability evaluation requires flexibility on your part, because there is significant variation from one evaluation to another. One factor underlying this variation is that different disability agencies require you to address different questions. Second, there is enormous variation in the medical, psychological, and social problems with which patients present. Because of the heterogeneity of disability evaluations, no specific guidelines for performing them can be outlined. Some general principles are given below:

1 *Understand the context.* You should know something about the disability agency to which your patient is applying, and the implications of the opinions you state on a disability form. For example, is the patient seeking wage-replacement benefits (as provided, for example, by SSA or workers' compensation), or simply time off work without pay (as provided by the

Family and Medical Leave Act)? Is he/she applying for permanent disability or temporary disability? Does the agency to which the patient is applying provide benefits for individuals with partial disability (e.g. an inability to perform a specific kind of work), or must the individual be totally disabled in order to be eligible? Does it provide any kind of vocational rehabilitation benefits?

2 *Consider the five key issues that you will probably be asked to address.* Most disability forms require you to address the issues discussed above, i.e. diagnosis, causation, need for further treatment, impairment, and ability to work. You will be able to fill out a form more coherently if you have considered how these issues apply to your patient before you work on the form.

3 *Read the questions in a disability form carefully.* Your disability evaluation needs to be directed toward the questions raised by the disability agency to which your patient is applying. The specific questions addressed to you will vary from one disability agency to another. Basically, disability agencies ask physicians different questions because they have different kinds of obligations to their beneficiaries, and different methods for processing disability applications. Consider, for example, the kinds of questions that you might face regarding a patient's activity restrictions and/or work capacity. Sometimes, you will be asked to state the physical limitations of a patient, e.g. to state how many hours the patient can sit during a day, how many pounds he/she can lift, etc. In other situations, you will be given detailed information about specific jobs, and asked whether your patient can perform the essential functions of the jobs. These job analyses typically request much more than a simple yes–no answer. For example, they often ask whether the worker can do the job on a full-time rather than a part-time basis, whether modifications in the job would help, what these modifications should be, etc. Other agencies will ask you to state in very broad terms the category of work in which a patient can engage – from sedentary to very heavy. In still other situations, you will be asked whether your patient can go back to his/her usual line of work, and, if not, whether he/she can do any kind of work. In essence, even if you have given careful thought to key issues related to your patient's disability, you will also need to give careful attention to the issue of communicating this information within the framework provided by a disability evaluation form.

If you feel that a disability form constrains you so much that you cannot communicate crucial information regarding your patient, you should write a letter to supplement the form.

4 *Discuss the disability form with your patient.* This is time-consuming and may complicate your evaluation task. But it is important to know the patient's assessment of their physical capacities, and their ability to perform various kinds of work. One reason for this is that patients' self-assessments are important predictors of whether they actually will remain on disability benefits.[40] Second, patients can provide information about the demands of their prior jobs. This information sometimes conflicts sharply with the information supplied by disability agencies.

5 *Distinguish between short-term and long-term disability.* It is often reasonable for treating physicians to support requests for temporary disability by their patients. Patients who are certified as temporarily disabled typically receive time-limited wage replacement payments. These protect the patients from financial devastation while they are going through medical treatment. But physicians should be much more cautious in responding to requests for permanent disability, e.g. SSDI, or pensions through the workers' compensation system.

6 *Ask for help.* When physicians treat complex patients, they frequently seek consultations from specialists regarding medical issues. When a physician treats a patient who is applying for disability benefits, a consultation from a physician familiar with disability evaluations can be just as important as a consultation that focuses on the pathophysiology of the patient's medical condition. Also, treating physicians often need objective data to help them determine a patient's physical limitations and work potential. It is appropriate to indicate the kinds of information you need in order to answer questions raised by a disability agency. For example, you might request a formal functional capacities evaluation[30–32,42] or an evaluation by a vocational rehabilitation counselor.

7 *Recognize that your opinions count.* You may feel on the defensive because of the wording of questions on disability forms. For example, they typically insist that you reach conclusions based strictly on objective findings. Thus, you may feel that there is no room for you to express your clinical impressions about the ability of a patient to perform various activities. You may also feel overwhelmed when a panel of independent medical examiners makes flat statements, such as "There are no objective findings that preclude this patient from working on a full-time basis." In these settings, it is important to realize a few things. First, the concept that activity restrictions should be closely linked to objective findings embodies the "mechanical failure" model of disability. The relevance of this model to patients with chronic pain is questionable. Second, if patients' subjective assessments are to be considered in disability evaluations, the credibility of the patients becomes crucial. In general, a treating physician who sees a patient over time is in a better position than an independent medical examiner to evaluate the credibility of a patient's symptoms. Finally, the courts have generally supported the position that the opinions of a treating physician should

be given special weight in any decision that an agency makes regarding a disability application.[11,43]

CASE HISTORIES

Two hypothetical case histories are presented below in some detail. They illustrate the kinds of issues that treating physicians face in the arena of disability evaluation, and suggest solutions to them. One involves a patient seeking SSDI, the other involves an injured worker with a workers' compensation claim.

Case history 1

Ms Smith is a 42-year-old right-handed woman whom you evaluate for the first time on 4/20/00. She has a history of a Colles fracture of the right wrist from a fall during a hike on 6/24/99. Her fracture healed uneventfully, but, while she was in a cast, she developed swelling and paresthesiae in the right hand. She was eventually found to have carpal tunnel syndrome. But after a carpal tunnel release, she continued to have swelling and paresthesiae in the right hand, along with diffuse pain involving the entire right upper extremity. On 11/6/99, she was diagnosed with complex regional pain syndrome, type II. She failed to improve from a series of stellate ganglion blocks, and courses of prednisone, terazosin, gabapentin, mexiletine, and amitriptyline. She is now is on oxycontin 20 mg t.i.d. plus up to four 5-mg short-acting oxycodone tablets per day for breakthrough pain.

Her other medication is sertraline 100 mg q.d. for depression. She continues to complain of pain running the length of her right arm and paresthesiae into the right hand. She also reports that her hand frequently swells, and that it is cool, discolored, and sweaty. When asked about strength in her right upper extremity, she says that it feels diffusely weak, but acknowledges that pain is the main thing that limits her use of the extremity.

Past medical history is noncontributory – the patient has no general medical problems and no history of injuries or dysfunction involving the right upper extremity.

Social history is noteworthy in that the patient worked as a receptionist in a medical office between the ages of 18 and 30. For the next 11 years, she did medical transcription work. She denies any history of prolonged time away from work for any reason except childbirth. However, she says that she has not been able to do any kind of work since her injury on 6/24/99. Physical examination reveals findings consistent with complex regional pain syndrome. There is no clinically apparent loss of function in the right median nerve.

You refer the patient to a multidisciplinary pain management center. The patient enters a 4-week functional restoration program at the center on 6/14/00.

- 9/15/00. The patient returns to your care after completing the multidisciplinary functional restoration program and a 6-week follow-up program. She is now off opiates. She reports that her mood improved dramatically and her activity tolerances increased somewhat during her multidisciplinary treatment program. Progress notes from the center generally support this assessment. However, the patient maintains that she is still unable to work.
- 10/15/00. The patient indicates that she has applied for Social Security Disability benefits. She brings in a letter from the SSA requesting medical information. The content of the letter is shown in Fig. 4.4. To address items 1 and 7, you enclose a copy of your initial evaluation and all progress notes. You indicate that items 2–6 should be answered by other physicians who have treated the patient. Your progress notes include an updated physical examination that addresses the information requested in items 8–12.
- 6/10/01. The patient is still under your care. She is not working. She is back on opiates, although in low doses. Her symptoms have not changed much during the past 8 months. She tells you that her application for SSDI has been denied. She indicates that she plans to appeal the denial.

General comments

SSDI applications are very simple in terms of the demands made upon physicians. A treating physician is asked to render an opinion about a patient only once. As Fig. 4.4 shows, the information requested is factual in nature. Note that the physician is not asked to give an opinion about causation of the patient's condition. This reflects the fact that SSDI provides benefits for disabled individuals regardless of how or why they became disabled. Also, none of the questions asks you to provide a diagnosis, or to render opinions about further treatment, impairment, or ability to work. This reflects the SSA philosophy that treating physicians should provide data rather than opinions. These data are reviewed by a team consisting of an adjudicator and a physician. The SSA takes the position that they are the ones who should make judgments about the severity of an applicant's impairment, his/her ability to work, etc.

The present case history ends with Ms Jones saying she will appeal the denial of her SSDI application. Although accurate statistics are not available, many experts believe that patients with painful conditions routinely have their initial SSDI applications denied.[16] After initial denial, applicants have the right to go through a series of appeals.[39] These appeals are often successful. In fact, about 25% of all SSDI awards are granted on appeal rather than at the point of initial evaluation.[15]

It is worth noting that a treating physician can play a more active role than the one described in this example. The teams who evaluate applicants are supposed to fol-

Your patient has applied for disability under the Social Security Act. We would appreciate information from your records for the following problems:

ALLEGATION: right arm condition

The following items are especially important! If you do not have information on a particular item, please tell us.

1. History and physical examination findings
2. Consultative examination reports
3. Psychological and/or psychiatric reports
4. Operative and pathology reports
5. X-ray reports of involved area(s)
6. CAT scan, myelogram, ultrasound, bone scan, or MRI scan reports
7. Outpatient progress notes
8. Height and weight
9. Description of gait and station
10. Clinical description of involved joints
11. Range of motion in degrees
12. Neurological findings

Figure 4.4 *Information requested by the social security administration for a disability applicant. Letters like this do not actually come directly from the Social Security Administration. the Social Security Administration contracts with state agencies called Disability Determination Services. Medical information regarding a disability applicant is evaluated by a disability Determination Service, and a final report with recommendations is forwarded to the local office of the Social Security Administration.*

low explicit rules when they perform their evaluations. In particular, they match the medical data they gather with a set of "listings" that the SSA has developed. A listing is a set of clinical indicators (typically a diagnosis along with certain markers of disease severity) that are considered prima facie evidence that an individual is totally disabled. The listings used by the SSA are available in *Disability Evaluation Under Social Security*.[13] A physician who believes that a patient is disabled can quote from this publication to buttress his/her opinion. In the present example, the treating physician might note that Ms Jones shows evidence of "persistent disorganization of motor function," as described in Section 11.00, Part C of this publication (reference 13, p. 63).

Case history 2

January 10, 2000

Mr Smith, a 40-year-old auto mechanic who works in Washington State and is eligible for workers' compensation benefits through the Department of Labor and Industries (DLI), sees you on an urgent basis. He indicates that he sustained a low back injury earlier in the day in the course of his work. He was bent over the hood of a car and was lifting out a carburetor when he felt a "pop" in his low back, and abrupt onset of severe low back pain (LBP). He denies pain, sensory loss, or motor loss in the lower extremities. He has not noticed any problems with bowel or bladder control.

Past medical history is noteworthy in that the patient had a workers' compensation claim from age 37 to age 39 because of a low back injury that he sustained at work. During that time, he underwent L4–5 and L5–S1 diskectomies for right lower extremity sciatica, followed by an L4–S1 fusion with Steffee plates. His radicular symptoms resolved, but he has had ongoing LBP. His claim was closed after his last surgery, and he returned to the work force 6 months ago. His employer now is different from the one he had when he was injured 3 years ago. The rest of his past medical history is unremarkable.

Social history indicates that the patient is a high-school graduate. All of his work experience has been in the area of automobile repair. He is married, and has two children aged 10 and 7.

Physical examination is noteworthy in that he stands leaning forward, with complete flattening of the lumbar lordotic curve. He walks very slowly. Palpation reveals diffuse spasms in the lumbar paraspinal muscles, along with significant soft-tissue tenderness. The patient demonstrates virtually zero range motion of the lumbar spine in all planes. Straight leg raising is limited by back pain rather than radicular symptoms. Neurologic examination reveals diffuse, bilateral lower extremity weakness that appears to reflect pain inhibition. The only focal sign is a diminished right ankle jerk, which the patient says has been present since his original back injury. He is positive on three of the five Waddell signs.

He says he is in too much pain to work.

The patient asks you to fill out a Labor and Industries Accident Form. You indicate the following:

- 41 – Diagnosis = lumbosacral strain (847.2).
- 45 – Objective findings = muscle spasms, severely restricted lumbar range of motion in all planes, diminished right ankle jerk
- 47 – Was the diagnosed condition caused by this injury or exposure? Probably.
- 48 – Will the condition cause the patient to miss work? Yes, for 10 days.
- 49 – Is there any preexisting impairment of the injured area? Yes.
- 50 – Has the patient ever been treated for the same or similar condition? Yes.

Comments

1 The patient's presentation is a typical one – acute onset of nonradicular low back pain.

2 In filling out the required accident report, you are forced to make several judgments about the patient's disability:

   a You have to decide whether to conceptualize the patient's problem as a new injury, or as an aggravation of the lumbar spine problem he developed at age 37. If the problem is conceptualized as a new injury, claim opening is fairly easy. If it is conceptualized as an aggravation, DLI will ask you to review past records on the patient and indicate whether there is objective evidence that his condition has worsened.

      i The diagnosis of lumbosacral strain embodies the concept that you are conceptualizing the patient's problem as a new injury.

   b Administrative agencies always demand that a physician buttress his/her conclusions with objective findings. This embodies the administrative myth that reports of incapacitation by patients should be closely correlated with objectively measurable signs of tissue injury or organ dysfunction. Despite the aura of objectivity connoted by the demand for objective findings, the objectivity is somewhat illusory because there is no clear definition of "objective findings."

      i Most physicians would accept the objectivity of a depressed ankle jerk reflex. In this patient, it is quite likely that the depressed right ankle jerk reflex stems from the back injury 3 years ago. But since the Department of Labor and Industries insists on objective findings, you should strongly consider listing the abnormal reflex in answer to item 45.

      ii The status of muscle spasms and restricted lumbar range of motion is less clear. They are not completely objective, since patients have some control over the tightness of muscles in their backs and over how much they move when a physician assesses active range of motion.

      iii What *is* clear is that you need to answer item 45 in some way. As a practical matter, the claims

managers who review accident reports are likely to accept virtually any answer you give.

   c When a physician gives a diagnosis (item 41), states objective findings that support the diagnosis (item 45), and says that the diagnosed condition was probably caused by the patient's work (item 47), he/she is in effect urging the DLI to accept the patient's problem as a work injury. This is a necessary step on the way to medical or disability benefits, i.e. a worker must have a valid workers' compensation claim before he/she can obtain benefits from the DLI.

   d When you indicate that Mr Smith's condition will cause him to lose 10 days of work (item 48), you are supporting the idea that he is work disabled, and therefore entitled to disability benefits. In the language of workers' compensation law, Mr Smith deserves benefits if he is judged to be temporarily, totally disabled from work.

   e Items 49 and 50 address the issue of previous problems that Mr Smith has had with his lumbar spine. As noted above, his new symptoms can be construed as either an aggravation of an old lumbar spine condition or as a new injury.

   f In a general way, it is important to note that, in filling out the required accident report, you have made important disability judgments regarding Mr Smith. You have indicated that he has a legitimate musculoskeletal injury, that the injury was probably caused by his work, and that he will be disabled from work because of the injury. These judgments are typically made primarily on the basis of what the patient says – you rarely have completely objective indices of the severity of a patient's incapacitation from low back pain, and you often do not have independent confirmation that the patient became symptomatic because of his work.

   g The DLI system tends to be permissive when it processes accident reports, i.e. the accuracy of the physicians statements is rarely questioned.

February 10, 2000

Mr Smith has undergone evaluation by a spine surgeon. He is felt not to be a candidate for further surgery. He is getting conservative therapy consisting of physical therapy and medications. He appears to have improved modestly, but continues to complain of persistent, localized low back pain that precludes employment. His employer contacts you and requests a conference to discuss Mr Smith's ongoing symptoms and prospects for return to work.

Comments

1 Many experts in workers' compensation emphasize that treating physicians can do a better job if they talk with employers, or even visit work sites. Aside from

the time required for this, you have to be aware of the possibility of an employer presenting a distorted picture of a worker or of the job to which the worker might return. Probably the best way to deal with this is to have a conference that includes both the injured worker and a representative of the employer.

March 10, 2000

You receive a letter from the DLI. It asks whether Mr Smith has reached maximal medical improvement, and whether he continues to have impairments that prevent him from working. It insists that you present the objective findings on which your conclusions are based. You respond that Mr Smith's functional capacities as measured by his physical therapist continue to increase, so that he is not yet at maximal medical improvement. You express the view that he is not currently able to return to his job as an auto mechanic. You cite his limited lumbar range of motion and his diminished right ankle jerk reflex as objective findings supporting your conclusion.

Comments

1 The issue of maximal medical improvement is closely linked to disability issues for an individual with a workers' compensation claim. Typically, compensation systems accept the judgments of treating physicians more or less at face value while a worker is recovering from an injury. But when an injured worker has reached maximal medical improvement, compensation law generally requires that some permanent decision be made about the worker's employment capabilities. As a result, claims managers are more likely to challenge the opinions of the attending physician, e.g. by commissioning an independent medical examination.

2 The demand for "objective findings" reflects the myth that work incapacitation can be objectively assessed by a physician. In fact, your conclusion that Mr Smith cannot work as an auto mechanic is based largely on the following considerations: (1) he has a complex lumbar spine problem that can produce intolerance of physically demanding work; (2) he has repeatedly stated that he cannot handle the physical demands of work as an auto mechanic; (3) having treated him for 2 months, you have formed the clinical judgment that his reports regarding his physical capacities are credible. This is an example of the fundamental dilemma of assessing disability based on pain. The patient reports severe activity restrictions because of his pain, but there is nothing you can do in your office to confirm or discount his statements about his activity restrictions. To a large extent, your decision about whether to support his assertions rests on whether you find the assertions credible. But the compensation system insists that you rationalize your disability determination on the basis of objective findings. As

suggested in the case history, probably the best way to address this mismatch is simply to state the patient's physical findings, and disregard the fact that the physical findings do not lead inevitably to a conclusion about the patient's work capacity.

April 10, 2000

Mr Smith has now been assigned a vocational rehabilitation counselor by the DLI. The vocational rehabilitation counselor has filled out a job analysis for the position that Mr Smith held at the time of his injury. You review the job analysis with Mr Smith at his next scheduled visit. He complains that it is grossly inaccurate. For example, while the job analysis says that his job requires lifting objects weighing no more than 35 pounds, Mr Smith insists that prior to his injury he had to lift objects weighing up to 100 pounds. He also asserts that he is unable to spend long periods of time bent over the hood of a car. You request a formal physical capacities evaluation to determine his lifting capacity and his ability to work in the postures required by his auto mechanic job. Based on Mr Smith's statements, your physical examination findings, and the results of the physical capacities evaluation, you indicate that Mr. Smith is not able to do the work described in the job analysis.

Comments

1 It is common for injured workers to complain that job analyses provide a distorted picture of what their work actually requires. It is important for you to discuss a job analysis with an injured worker so that you learn whether there is a significant difference between the job as it is described in the job analysis and the worker's perception of what the job requires.

2 Physical capacities evaluations are usually performed by physical therapists. The purpose of such an evaluation is to provide objective data about what an injured worker actually does in a test situation, e.g. how much he/she lifts, how long he/she sits continuously, etc. A physical capacities evaluation is by no means a foolproof solution to the problem of determining activity limitations in a patient with a chronic pain problem. In fact, a recent review concludes that there is no firm evidence that such evaluations predict work performance.[44] But at least they provide some performance data, which is more than a physician can glean simply by carrying out an office examination on a patient.

May 10, 2000

Mr Smith brings two forms to his scheduled office visit. The first is from a company that has financed the purchase of the car he owns. When he arranged financing, he purchased an insurance option – it stipulates that his car payments will be deferred if his treating physician asserts that he is totally disabled from any kind of work, and that the disability is likely to continue for more than a year. You agree to support his request for deferment. The second form is from the Department of Motor Vehicles. It is an application for a disabled parking sticker. The patient says he needs to have a disabled parking sticker because his back pain becomes intolerable if he has to walk more than a quarter of a mile. You tell him that you will not support his application for a disabled parking sticker.

Comments

1 These two requests have no inherent relation to Mr Smith's DLI claim. But they give a flavor of the types of disability decisions a treating physician is called upon to make. These "extraneous" disability requests can create stress for the treating physician, and may well have an impact on a patient's perceptions regarding his work disability. The car insurance form is a problem because it requires you to characterize Mr Smith as having long-term, total disability. This message is likely to be incongruent with messages that you expect to give Mr Smith in relation to his DLI claim. A disabled parking sticker may also affect Mr Smith's perception of himself as an able-bodied rather than a disabled person. Although there is no logical incompatibility between Mr Smith's having a disabled parking sticker and his returning to work, there may well be a psychological inconsistency.

June 10, 2000

Mr Smith indicates that his DLI claims manager has strongly urged him to apply for Social Security Disability. He indicates that he has started the SSDI application process, and has been told that disability adjudicators for the SSA will soon be asking you to provide information about his medical condition. You urge him to delay the SSDI application process until he has received definitive information about whether the DLI will provide vocational rehabilitation services for him.

Comments

1 You may well be surprised that a workers' compensation agency, which is nominally devoted to helping individuals return to work, would urge an injured worker to apply for SSDI, a program established for individuals who are totally and permanently disabled. Yet, clinicians who treat injured workers see this pattern frequently.

2 In terms of perceptions of disability by an injured worker, an SSDI application represents a "kiss of death." An individual can obtain an SSDI award only if they can convince adjudicators that they are totally and permanently disabled. Long-term studies show that only about 3% of individuals who are awarded SSDI benefits ever return to the work force on a sustained basis. Although it is theoretically possible for a person to continue to seek employment while they

are applying for SSDI, informal observation and the limited data available[45] strongly suggest that an individual's probability of vocational rehabilitation is low once they start the SSDI application process.

3 The treating physician is often in an uncomfortable position when an individual on workers' compensation starts an SSDI application. On the one hand, the physician will appropriately anticipate that the worker will be more refractory to vocational rehabilitation once he starts the SSDI application process. On the other hand, they may well be concerned about time lines and back-up plans for the worker. One issue is that individuals who apply for SSDI on the basis of painful conditions such as low back pain often have their initial claims denied.[16] Their claims may be accepted upon appeal, but the process of going through multiple levels of the SSA appeals process can easily take more than a year. In the meantime, the worker faces the risk of having his time loss benefits abruptly terminated by the DLI. From this perspective, an early application for SSDI might be viewed as an "insurance policy" for a worker who is having difficulty returning to work, even if they have not totally given up this goal. In an ideal world, workers' compensation agencies would work cooperatively with other agencies to make sure that injured workers do not get caught in the middle between different benefit programs. In fact, this kind of cooperation rarely occurs.

July 10, 2000

Mr Smith's claims manager schedules him for an independent medical examination. The examination is performed by an orthopedist, a physiatrist, and a psychiatrist. The orthopedist and physiatrist collaborate to generate a medical/surgical report; the psychiatrist submits a separate report. The medical/surgical report states that the patient has reached maximal medical improvement from his lumbar strain of 1/10/00. He is felt to have no permanent partial impairment over and above the 10% impairment that was awarded when his earlier lumbar spine claim was closed. The report states: "There are no objective findings that would prevent Mr Smith from working on a full-time basis in a job with medium physical requirements." The psychiatrist diagnoses "pain disorder associated with both psychological factors and a general medical condition" [*Diagnostic and Statistical Manual of Mental Disorders*, 4th edn (DSM-IV) 307.89] (reference 46, p. 458). Both the medical/surgical and the psychiatric reports indicate that Mr Smith's claim is ready for closure. A copy of the independent medical examination report is sent to you, and you are asked: (1) to indicate your agreement or disagreement with it; and (2) to state the objective findings on which your opinions are based. You respond that Mr Smith probably has reached maximal medical improvement, but that you are concerned about his ability to work on a full-time basis. You note that he has shown consistent activity limitations, and that his reported activity limitations are credible. You indicate that he needs a careful vocational assessment and identification of specific job options before his claim is closed.

Comments

1 Independent medical examinations routinely perpetuate the myth that impairments and associated work restrictions can be objectively measured by physicians. The statement: "There are no objective findings that would prevent Mr Smith from working on a full-time basis in a job with medium physical requirements" could be made about virtually every patient with low back pain. But the reality is that back pain is the most common cause of disability in working aged people.[27,47,48] To paraphrase Osterweis et al.,[16] back pain disables people not because their backs fail mechanically, but because back problems can create unbearable sensations that limit activities. Treating physicians need to avoid falling into the conceptual trap of concluding that disability can be supported only if there are objective findings that make the disability inevitable.

2 Nonpsychiatric physicians may well feel intimidated by psychiatric evaluations that purport to say what is "really" underlying an injured worker's pain complaints. It is important to realize that, although psychiatric disorders may well be major factors underlying the pain complaints of some patients, this is by no means universal. Even if a chronic low back pain patient has a psychiatric condition, the role that this plays in his ongoing pain complaints is often uncertain. Also, while diagnostic criteria for some psychiatric disorders – such as major depressive disorder – are well established, the diagnoses given to many chronic pain patients are much less well validated. In particular, you should look with some skepticism on a diagnosis of pain disorder with both psychological factors and a general medical condition.[49,50]

3 An attending physician might well feel overwhelmed by a strongly worded independent medical examination report signed by three physicians. It is thus important to recall that courts have generally taken the position that the opinions of treating physicians should be given great weight.[11,43] The important practical point is that, if you disagree with the conclusions of an independent medical examination, you should feel free to state your objections.

August 10, 2000

The DLI claims manager retains a vocational rehabilitation counselor to carry out an employability assessment on Mr Smith, i.e. to see whether Mr Smith's physical capabilities and past work history permit him to work in any field other than auto repair. The vocational rehabilitation

counselor notes that, at the age of 18, Mr Smith worked for 3 months as a dishwasher, and asks you to sign a job analysis for this kind of work. You meet with Mr Smith to discuss the job analysis. He protests that dishwashing requires more bending, lifting, and standing than he can do. He also notes that he and his family will be impoverished if he is left with no choice other than doing entry level work. You refuse to sign the job analysis on the grounds that the physical demands of dishwashing exceed Mr Smith's capabilities.

Comments

1 The DLI system requires that, if an injured worker is unable to return to the job he had at the time of injury, a vocational rehabilitation counselor is assigned to review his entire work history, and to determine whether, based on his skills and physical capabilities, the worker can perform any kind of work. Most workers who go through this kind of vocational assessment are placed into one of three categories:

   a They are judged to be employable based on the types of work they have performed at some earlier time in their lives (workers in this category typically have their time loss benefits terminated).

   b They are judged to need vocational retraining in order to be employable (workers in this category are typically authorized for vocational rehabilitation services).

   c They are judged to be unemployable under any circumstances (workers in this category typically receive a pension).

2 Injured workers and treating physicians often look at category 1 with some skepticism. One issue is that workers may be judged employable on the basis of entry level work that they did when they first entered the labor force. Even if a worker is physically able to do such entry level work (e.g. a job at a fast food restaurant), the remuneration from the work is often very low. Also, some of the jobs that are proposed by vocational rehabilitation counselors seem contrived. For example, a person with a severe lumbar spine condition might be judged to be employable as a telephone solicitor.

October 10, 2000

Mr Smith is accepted for vocational rehabilitation services. He and his vocational rehabilitation counselor develop a plan for him to work in an auto parts store. It is determined that Mr Smith will need 6 months of training in order to have the skills needed for this kind of work. The DLI insists that you review the physical requirements of a salesman in an auto parts store. You review the appropriate job analysis with Mr Smith, and sign it. Mr Smith goes through the 6-month training program, and shortly thereafter is hired for a full-time position as a salesman in an auto parts store. Although he continues to complain of back pain, he is able to carry out his job responsibilities consistently, with no time lost from work because of back pain. His DLI claim is closed 4 months after his successful return to work.

Comments

1 A formal vocational rehabilitation plan represents the last step in the DLI's procedures for assisting injured workers return to the work force. A vocational rehabilitation counselor assigned by the DLI first works with an injured worker to develop a vocational rehabilitation plan. The DLI provides only modest funding (about $3,000) for retraining, and generally insists that the attending physician indicate that the job for which the patient will be trained is within his physical capacities.

2 This case history has a happy ending. Mr Smith makes a successful reentry into the work force, and his claim is closed. In real-life situations, the likelihood of the outcome described in the example is low for a person who has had multiple spine surgeries and has been disabled for 3 of the past 4 years. Moreover, an outcome that is successful from the standpoint of an individual claim may not be successful from the standpoint of the person with a chronic low back problem.[26,51,52] Long-term follow-up data indicate that an individual such as Mr Smith is at high risk of having yet another back injury and filing another compensation claim prior to the time when he reaches retirement age.

General comments

The disability issues involved in case history 2 are much more complex than those in case history 1. To a large extent, this reflects the fact that the SSA and workers' compensation systems have different mandates, and use different procedures. A few points are worth emphasizing:

1 The treating physician in this example included Mr Smith in crucial decisions, and generally paid a great deal of attention to Mr Smith's concerns. Some physicians might take a very different approach to this kind of patient. For example, a physician might focus on the fact that Mr Smith lacked unequivocally objective findings, and support early closure of the claim.

2 Judgments about disability in the workers' compensation system are multilayered and interwoven. It is rarely the case that a treating physician renders a single judgment about the ability of a patient to work. Instead, as the example shows, the physician is repeatedly asked or required to make judgments that bear on the disability status of his/her patient.

3 The questions posed to the physician in the above example were not explicitly about pain. Pain was central to the entire problem because Mr Smith's medical condition was one in which activity limitations are created primarily by pain. But the role of pain was constantly obscured by the demand of the DLI system to have decisions rationalized in terms of objective findings. In essence, questions were posed to the treating physician in a manner that pressured him or her to construe Mr Smith's limitations in terms of an objective "mechanical failure" model of incapacity. The challenge for a treating physician is to continue to consider how pain is affecting his or her patient in the face of ongoing pressure to be "objective".

4 In the example, the physician ended up interfacing between the patient and several organizations, i.e. the DLI, the SSA, the Department of Motor Vehicles, and Mr Smith's automobile credit company. It is not unusual for a treating physician to make disability determinations for two or more agencies at the same time. As the example shows, the contradictory needs of different agencies make the difficult task of disability evaluation even more taxing.

CONCLUDING REMARKS

This chapter can only point out some of the problems associated with disability evaluation. It by no means gives you all the information you need to conduct disability evaluations on your patients effortlessly. Unfortunately, there is no cookbook for performing disability evaluations. One reason for this is that there is enormous variation from one disability evaluation to another. Busy physicians may want a simple answer to the question "How should I fill out Mr Smith's disability form?" but in reality this is no simpler than the question "What medical or surgical treatment should I provide for Mr Smith's pain?" In both instances, it is necessary to answer the question on the basis of factors that are specific to Mr Smith.

Another complicating factor is that there is strikingly little published information on the subject of disability evaluation, given that millions of evaluations are carried out each year in the USA. At a very basic level, we have very little evidence about whether the decisions made by large agencies such as the SSA are, on the whole, good or bad, i.e. whether the SSA is awarding benefits to individuals who are truly disabled, but withholding them from individuals who are actually able to work.[33,39] In the face of this large-scale uncertainty, it is difficult for an individual physician to know whether he/she is rendering appropriate judgments regarding his/her patients.

But this chapter should help you understand that you are not alone, i.e. that disability evaluation is difficult for everyone. This is particularly the case for disability evaluation in the context of chronic pain. As noted earlier, chronic pain fundamentally challenges the assumption of administrative agencies that impairments should be objectively observable. At this point, no disability agency has resolved this challenge.

Some of you will understandably be tempted to say "Why bother?" That is to say, why should a physician take the extra time to learn about disability agencies, disability evaluation methods, the ethics of disability evaluation, etc? To some extent, the answer to this question is: "Because you have no choice." Society forces physicians to make judgments about the capacities of their patients. Physicians may perform disability evaluations thoughtfully or thoughtlessly, but they don't have the option of simply not doing them.

Another answer to the "Why bother" question is that disability evaluation and disability management generally are important. In an ideal world, we would cure all our patients completely, and would not have to worry about disability because there would be none. In the real world, our interventions are only partially effective in ameliorating conditions that compromise the ability of patients to work. In that imperfect world, we have to be concerned about residual impairment and workplace disadvantage of our patients after treatment has been optimized. We need to do whatever we can to help them return to economic productivity, and we need to recognize that we do them a disservice if we either grossly overstate or grossly understate their capacities to disability adjudicators.

REFERENCES

1. US Department of Labor Employment and Training Administration. *Dictionary of Occupational Titles*, 4th edn revised. Washington, DC: US Government Printing Office, 1991.
2. Nachemson A. Chronic pain – the end of the welfare state? *Q Life Res* 1994; **3** (Suppl. 1): S11–17.
3. Peterson KW, Babitsky S, Beller TA, *et al*. The American Board of Independent Medical Examiners. *J Occup Environ Med* 1997; **39**: 509–14.
4. Holleman WL, Holleman MC. School and work release evaluations. *JAMA* 1988; **260**: 3629–34.
5. Ziporyn T. Disability evaluation: a fledgling science? *JAMA* 1983; **250**: 873–80.
◆ 6. Sullivan MD, Loeser JD. The diagnosis of disability. *Arch Intern Med* 1992; **152**: 1829–35.
7. Cocchiarella L, Andersson GBJ eds. *Guides to the Evaluation of Permanent Impairment*, 5th edn. Chicago, IL: American Medical Association, 2001.
8. Demeter SL, Andersson GBJ, Smith GM. Disability Evaluation. Chicago, IL: American Medical Association, 1996.
9. Rondinelli RD, Katz RT eds. *Impairment Rating and Disability Evaluation*. Philadelphia, PA: Saunders, 2000.
10. Williams CA. *An International Comparison of Workers' Compensation*. Boston, MA: Kluwer Academic Publishers, 1991.
11. Wolfe F, Potter J. Fibromyalgia and work disability. *Rheum Dis Clin North Am* 1996; **22**: 369–91.
12. Derthick M. *Agency Under Stress*. Washington, DC: The Brookings Institution, 1990.
13. US Government. *Disability Evaluation under Social Security*. SSA Publication no. 64-039. Washington, DC: US Government Printing Office, 1994.
14. DLI. *Medical Aid Rules and Fee Schedules*. Olympia, WA: State of Washington, Department of Labor and Industries, 1999.
15. Committee on Ways and Means, US House of Representatives. *1996 Green Book*. Washington, DC: US Government Printing Office, 1996.
◆ 16. Osterweis M, Kleinman A, Mechanic D, eds. *Pain and Disability*. Washington, DC: National Academy Press, 1987.
17. Atkinson T, Liem R, Liem J. The social cost of unemployment: implications for social support. *J Health Soc Behav* 1986; **54**: 454–60.
18. Mrazek PI, Haggerty RJ eds. *Reducing Risks for Mental Disorder*. Washington, DC: National Academy Press, 1994.
19. Kaplan GA, Roberts RE, Camacho TC, *et al*. Psychosocial predictors of depression. *Am J Epidemiol* 1987; **125**: 206–20.
20. Hamrnarstrom A, Janlert U. Nervous and depressive symptoms in a longitudinal study of youth unemployment – selection or exposure? *J Adolesc* 1997; **20**: 293–305.
21. Rahmqvist M, Carstensen J. Trend of psychological distress in a Swedish population from 1989 to 1995. *Scand J Soc Med* 1998; **3**: 214–22.
22. Reno VP, Mashaw JL, Gradison B eds. *Disability*. Washington, DC: National Academy of Social Insurance, 1997.
23. Robinson JP, Rondinelli RD, Scheer, SJ. Industrial rehabilitation medicine. 1. Why is industrial rehabilitation medicine unique? *Arch Phys Med Rehabil* 1997; **78** (Suppl. 3): S3–9.
24. Hadler NM. If you have to prove you are ill, you can't get well. the object lesson of fibromyalgia. *Spine* 1996; **21**: 2397–400.
25. Muller LS. Disability beneficiaries who work and their experience under program work incentives. *Soc Security Bull* 1992; **55** (2): 2–19.
26. Robinson JP. Disability in low back pain: what do the numbers mean? *Am Pain Soc Bull* 1998; **8** (2): 9–13.
27. Cheadle A, Franklin G, Wolfuagen C, *et al*. Factors influencing the duration of work-related disability: a population-based study of Washington State workers' compensation. *Am J Public Health* 1994; **84** (2): 190–6.
28. Frymoyer JW, Cats-Baril W. Predictors of low back pain disability. *Clin Orthop Rel Res* 1987; **221**: 89–98.
29. DLI. *Attending Doctor's Handbook*, revised edn. Olympia, WA: State of Washington, Department of Labor and Industries, 1999.
30. Rondinelli RD, Robinson JP, Scheer SJ. Industrial rehabilitation medicine. 4. Strategies for disability man-

agement. *Arch Phys Med Rehabil* 1997; **78** (Suppl. 3): S21–8.

31. King PM ed. *Sourcebook of Occupational Rehabilitation*. New York, NY: Plenum Press, 1998.

32. Scheer SJ ed. *Medical Perspectives in Vocational Assessment of Impaired Workers*. Gaithersburg, MD: Aspen, 1991.

◆ 33. Robinson JP. Evaluation of function and disability. In: Loeser JD ed. *Bonica's Management of Pain*, 3rd edn. Philadelphia, PA: Lippincott, Williams and Wilkins, 2001.

34. Jensen MC, Brant-Zawadzki MN, Obuchowski N, *et al*. Magnetic resonance imaging of the lumbar spine in people without back pain. *N Engl J Med* 1994; **331** (2): 69–73.

35. Deyo RA. Magnetic resonance imaging of the lumbar spine. Terrific test or tar baby? *N Engl J Med* 1994; **331** (2): 115–16.

36. Kramer MS, Lane DA. Causal propositions in clinical research and practice. *J Clin Epidemiol* 1992; **45:** 639–49.

37. Subcommittee Report on "Fixed and Stable." Meeting of the Washington State Medical Association Industrial Relations/Rehabilitation Committee. Unpublished, December, 1996.

38. US Government. *Report of the Commission on the Evaluation of Pain*. SSA Publication no. 64-031. Washington, DC: US Government Printing Office, 1987.

39. Robinson JP, Wolfe C. Social Security disability insurance and supplemental security income. In: Rondinelli RD, Katz RT eds. *Impairment Rating and Disability Evaluation*. Philadelphia, PA: Saunders, 2000.

40. Cocchiarella L, Lord SJ. *Master the AMA Guides*, 5th edn. Chicago, IL: AMA Press, 2001.

41. Hildebrandt J, Pfingsten M, Saur P, *et al*. Prediction of success from a multidisciplinary treatment program for chronic low back pain. *Spine* 1997; **22:** 990–1001.

42. Rondinelli RD, Robinson JP, Scheer SJ, Weinstein SM. Occupational rehabilitation and disability determination. In: DeLisa JA, Gans BM eds. *Rehabilitation Medicine: Principles and Practice*, 3rd edn. Philadelphia, PA: Lippincott-Raven, 1998.

43. Ruskell RC. *Social Security Disability Claims*, 3rd edn. Norcross, GA: The Harrison Company, 1993.

● 44. King PM, Tuckwell N, Barrett TE. A critical review of functional capacity evaluations. *Phys Ther* 1998; **78:** 852–66.

45. Rucker KS, Metzler HM. Predicting subsequent employment status of SSA disability applicants with chronic pain. *Clin J Pain* 1995; **11:** 22–35.

46. American Psychiatric Association. *Diagnostic and Statistical Manual of Mental Disorders*, 4th edn. Washington, DC: American Psychiatric Association, 1994.

47. Lawrence R, Helmick C, Arnett F, *et al*. Estimates of the prevalence of arthritis and selected musculoskeletal disorders in the United States. *Arthritis Rheum* 1998; **41:** 778–99.

48. Dionne CE Low back pain. In: Crombie IK, Croft PR, Linton SJ, *et al*. eds. *Epidemiology of Pain*. Seattle, WA: IASP Press, 1999.

49. King SA. Review: DSM-IV and pain. *Clin J Pain* 1995; **11:** 171–6.

50. Sullivan MD. DSM-IV pain disorder: a case against the diagnosis. *Int Rev Psychiatry* 2000; **12:** 91–8.

51. Butler RJ, Johnson WG, Baldwin ML. Managing work disability: why first return to work is not a measure of success. *Ind Labor Relations Rev* 1995; **48:** 452–69.

52. Johnson WG, Baldwin M. *Returns to Work by Ontario Workers with Permanent Partial Disabilities*. Report to the Workers' Compensation Board of Ontario. Ottawa: Workers' Compensation Board of Ontario, 1993.

5

Aspects of the chronic pain history and its application to treatment decisions

DAVID A FISHBAIN

The purpose of this chapter is to outline the important aspects of the office chronic pain history and examination. Issues determined to be important by previous research will be presented in a practical format with suggested measurement instruments.

This chapter is also written as a procedural guide to the chronic pain history and examination process. Therefore, it has been written around a number of algorithms, which will be referred to and discussed. These algorithms are based on a number of basic questions:

1 Does the patient have nonspecific low back pain (LBP) and/or neck pain or total body pain?
2 Does the patient have chronic pain (CP)?
3 Does the patient suffer from fibromyalgia syndrome (FMS) or myofascial pain syndrome (MFPS)?
4 Does the chronic pain patient (CPP) have psychiatric comorbidities and do they require psychiatric treatment?
5 Does the CPP have behavioral comorbidities not otherwise designated as psychiatric diagnoses?
6 Does the CPP have the other "usual" CP comorbidities?
7 Does the CPP require referral to a pain facility?
8 Does the CPP have a neuropathic pain component?
9 What is the extent of functional impairment and perceived disability secondary to the CP?

10 At what point should the CPP receive neural blockade and neuroaugmentation/neurosurgical pain relief techniques?
11 Is the CPP a candidate for opioid treatment?

The suggested chronic pain history and examination will be organized in such a way as to generate information to answer these questions. Therefore, this chapter will not be presented in the usual format; instead, discussion will relate to the algorithms outlined. It is intended that this chapter will integrate the other chapters in this textbook into this framework. It will primarily deal with the CP history and examination as it pertains to low back pain (LBP), neck pain, and total body pain.

THE PAIN HISTORY

The algorithm in Fig. 5.1 defines the pain physician's tasks in the evaluation of a patient complaining of pain.

The style for a single universal medical pain history is still being developed.[1] One issue makes the pain history different from the traditional medical history: pain patients rarely have one chief complaint – usually, there are associated complaints or symptoms. Pain history questions should have practical value in developing clues which will eventually help with treatment decisions about the pain These questions are presented in Table 5.5.

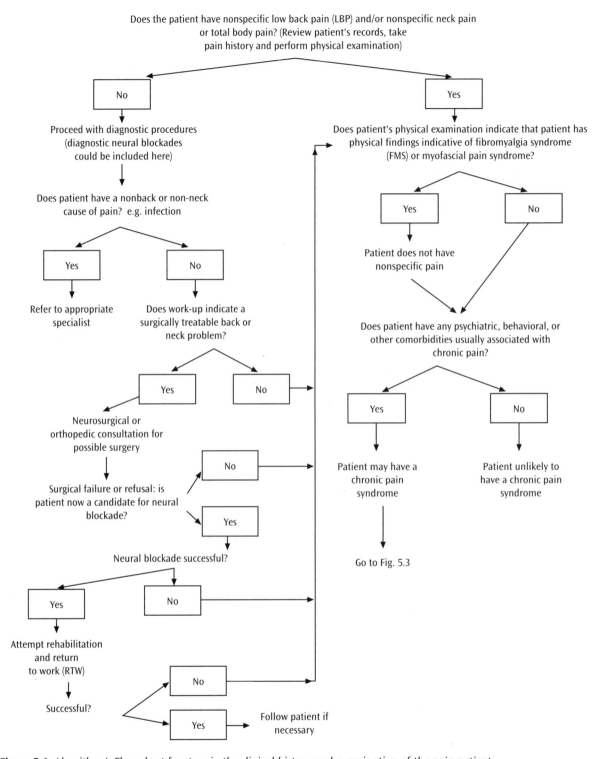

Figure 5.1 *Algorithm I. Flow chart for steps in the clinical history and examination of the pain patient.*

Table 5.1 is organized around a series of 24 topics and their clinical and diagnostic significance. The questions relate to a specific set of issues commonly found in pain patients. These issues are:

1 Does the pain patient have a disk problem, spinal stenosis, or myofascial pain syndrome, or fibromyalgia, osteoarthritis, or low back decompensation[2] syndrome?

2 Is the pain pattern unusual?
3 Is the pain intermittent?
4 Is the pain chronic?
5 Is the pain of significant severity?
6 Does the pain have a neuropathic component or elements of complex regional pain syndrome?
7 Are there psychophysiological responses to the pain?
8 Are there alleged conversion symptoms which are really pain-dependent phenomena?

The next part of the pain history is an attempt to measure the patient's pain. This is important for the documentation of the effects of treatment and for treatment outcome. It is important to remember that pain defies objective measurement and its intensity can only be measured indirectly.[5] Patients respond to pain measurement tools according to their own internal pain scale (i.e. they place their own values on the pain measurement scales). Thus, a certain pain level for one patient is not necessarily equivalent to the same pain level on the same tool for another patient. Pain measurements are, therefore, meaningless in terms of patient comparisons, but they are important within the same patient.

There are essentially two types of pain scales currently being utilized to measure pain: single-dimension rating scales and multiple-dimension scales. Single-dimension rating scales, include the verbal descriptor scale, behavioral rating scale, simple numerical rating scale (0–10), point box scale (0–10), visual analog scale (10 cm), numerical rating scale (0–100), pain relief scale, and the 21-point box scale.[6–8] The visual analog scale (VAS) is the most researched and accepted method, and is the most widely utilized in measuring clinical pain.[5,8,9] The VAS consists of a 10-cm line anchored by two extremes of pain: "no pain" and "pain as bad as it could be." Patients are asked to make a mark on the line that represents their level of perceived pain intensity.

Although the VAS is subject to response biases,[5] it has been shown to be internally consistent in both experimentally induced pain and chronic clinical pain, thereby demonstrating validity.[5] The VAS has been shown to be more sensitive than verbal rating scales,[10] and may be more reliable.[5] Also, VAS scores appear to predict chronic pain patient status at 6 months.[11] Of the rating scale methods, the VAS is preferable for clinical application. However, even the VAS may have poor sensitivity to treatment effects.[5,12]

The VAS scale can also be utilized in other ways. The patient can be asked to rate his/her pain at "this point in time" or as "average pain level over the last 24 h" or "average pain over the last month" (Fig. 5.2). By combining visual analog scales based on different directions, the intensity, frequency, and duration of clinical pain can be indirectly assessed.[5]

There are also any number of multiple-dimension scales. These include the Dallas Pain Questionnaire, West Haven–Yale Multidimensional Pain Inventory, Western Ontario and McMaster Osteoarthritis Index, Descriptor/ differential scale, Wisconsin Brief Pain Questionnaire, Millon Scale, and the McGill Pain Questionnaire.[6,13] In the author's opinion, none of these tools possesses the simplicity and utility of various forms of the VAS. In addition, many of these tools measure constructs which are not usually the focus of treatment or treatment outcome. This author would not recommend their routine use unless there is interest in the treatment outcome in a specific construct of one of these tools.

THE "NONSPECIFIC" PAIN PROBLEM

The algorithm in Fig. 5.1 revolves around the central question of whether the pain is "specific" or "nonspecific." "Specific pain" is defined as pain for which an underlying cause can be identified.[14] It is claimed that a definite somatic cause for the pain can be identified in 10–20% of cases.[15,16] Thus, the "nonspecific" pain diagnosis is determined or defined by the process of excluding "specific" pain.[16] If the pain physician is not convinced of the specificity of the pain after the record review, pain history, and physical, he/she should proceed with further diagnostic procedures including laboratory investigation[17] (Fig. 5.1). This process could in theory lead to consideration for surgery. Finally, this part of the algorithm also allows for the possibility of neural blockade[18] for diagnosis or treatment.

THE FIBROMYALGIA SYNDROME AND MYOFASCIAL PAIN SYNDROME ISSUE

The second question in the evaluation of pain after "specific" pain has been ruled out is related to whether the pain patient has physical findings indicative of fibromyalgia syndrome (FMS) or myofascial pain syndrome (MFPS). These are a group of soft-tissue pain syndromes characterized by widespread pain and tender points in FMS[19] and regional pain and trigger points in MFPS.[20] These syndromes are commonly found in patients with intractable pain of other causes.[23] For example, the proportion of new patients with FMS presenting in rheumatology clinics has been reported to be 10–20%,[21] with other pain facilities reporting 30–100%.[22,24] In an early study, our group[25] had reported that of LBP patients with chronic intractable benign pain (CIBP) 96.7% had one or more trigger points. Of the neck pain patients with CIBP, 100% had one or more trigger points.[25] It was concluded that the vast majority of CIBP patients demonstrate physical findings indicative of musculoskeletal disease.[25] Thus, it is unlikely that a significant number of pain patients presenting to a pain facility will have true "nonspecific" pain if an adequate soft-tissue examination is performed.[25]

The issue of whether the pain patient has "nonspecific" pain or a defined soft-tissue syndrome such as FMS or MFPS is important behaviorally. The pain patient needs and awaits an explanation for the pain to legitimize the symptoms.[14] In addition, there may be legal and financial reasons as to why the pain patient requires a formal diagnosis. Borkan et al.[26] demonstrated that pain patients considered "delegitimation," referring to the reputation of the patient's experience of pain and suffering, as one of the major perceived difficulties of the pain experience. In another study, addressing this issue in a different way,

Table 5.1 *Pain history questions and diagnostic significance*

	Pain question	Clinical and diagnostic significance
1	Pain onset related to trauma or insidious	Trauma-related pain more likely to be disk or muscular problems; insidious pain more likely to be spinal stenosis or arthritic
2	Duration of pain?	Longer than 6 months – likely to be chronic; longer than 2 years – more likely not to respond to treatment
3	Exact details of how the injury occurred and why it occurred	Will help to determine whether mechanical displacement occurred
		Will help to determine whether the patient perceives the injury as being caused by someone else's negligence or as purely an accidental event
4	Location of all pains	Generally, a CPP has either LBP that may radiate to the lower extremities, neck pain that may radiate to the upper extremities, headache that may or may not be associated with neck pain, or any combination of the three syndromes
		Any deviation from these patterns is unusual
5	Pain referral patterns?	Generally, pain is referred proximally to distally; anything else is unusual
6	Is the CPP *pain free* under any circumstances, e.g. lying down, sitting, etc.?	If the CPP has pain-free periods, the pain syndrome could be a variant of intermittent pain with a much better prognosis
		If the CPP is pain-free sitting, he/she is likely to have a spinal stenosis pain pattern
7	Is the CPP never pain free under any circumstances?	This is the true CPP pain pattern
8	What particular movements accentuate the pain, e.g. standing, walking, sitting, bending, lifting?	Disk syndromes are typically made worse by sitting; these patients are most comfortable shifting positions
		Spinal stenosis pain pattern typically precipitated by standing and walking with relief when sitting
9	Any particular weather makes pain worse?	CPP's pain typically made worse by wet/cold weather
10	What relieves pain?	Usually CPP's pain relieved by rest/lying down and often heat
11	What is the pain pattern when getting up in the morning?	Patient who describes significant pain in the morning in association with stiffness which improves as day goes on usually has osteoarthritic problems
12	Does pain increase as the day goes on?	This could be a low back decompensation syndrome[a]
13	How do medications (narcotics) affect the pain?	Generally, most CPPs will complain that narcotics never alleviate the pain entirely
14	Does the pain awaken the patient?	Most CPPs with significant pain will complain of being awakened by pain
15	Are there psychophysiological responses that follow severe pain?	Some CPPs will complain of dizziness, nausea, vomiting, passing out, increased blood pressure, and headaches in relationship to increases in pain
16	Are there alleged conversion symptoms which are precipitated by increases in pain?	Some CPPs will complain of muscle weakness or numbness with increased pain;[b] as these symptoms are often alleged to be conversion symptoms, it is important to realize that in most CPPs these symptoms are pain dependent
17	How does the CPP describe his/her pain?	Pain described as shooting, burning, or like lightening indicates a neuropathic pain component
18	Does CPP complain of sensory changes in areas of decreased hypoalgesia, increased hyperalgesia, hyperpathic response to normal stimuli, abnormal paresthesiae, and unpleasant dysesthesiae	CPP may have a neuropathic pain component

disorders of the back." However, "nonspecific" pain is not the same and does not necessarily equal chronic pain (CP).[14] As such, the last major question in the algorithm in Fig. 5.1 relates to whether the referred pain patient has chronic pain and can he/she then be labeled a chronic pain patient (CPP)? This decision is important as the chronic pain patient (CPP) is a candidate for treatments which would otherwise not be available to the non-CPP.

Although the above decision appears simple, there is little information in the literature as to how this decision is to be made.[170] The problem begins with the lack of a definition for chronic pain. For example, the International Association for the Study of Pain Task Force on Taxonomy, in the classification of chronic pain, has chosen not to define chronic pain.[171] In addition, the task force has decided not to adopt chronic pain syndrome as a diagnosis to be utilized for billing purposes because

such a category evades the requirement for accurate physical and psychiatric diagnoses.[171]

The second algorithm is presented in Fig. 5.3. The purpose of this algorithm is to utilize comorbidities usually associated with chronic pain in order to make treatment decisions. This algorithm revolves around the issue of whether the CPP has some associated comorbidities and, thus, according to Table 5.9, may fulfill the criteria for chronic pain syndrome. The next issue is then whether these comorbidities indicate a need for referral for treatment to a pain facility.

As a tentative guide for making the decision for referral, the author recently published a set of criteria,[172] which are presented in Table 5.10. A closer inspection of these criteria indicates that a patient first has to be diagnosed as suffering from chronic pain (major inclusion criteria). For consideration for referral, the patient then requires

Table 5.11 *Possible inclusion and exclusion criteria for potential chronic narcotic treatment*

I Inclusion criteria (1 or 2 and 3 required)
1 CPPs who are depressed and suicidal because of their pain, especially if they have failed antidepressant treatment
2 CPPs whose quality of life is extremely poor and intolerable because of pain
3 Failure of all forms of pain treatment, including blocks and pain facility treatment which includes detoxification

II Exclusion criteria (any one of 1–5 required)
1 A history of alcohol abuse and/or dependence
2 Any history of illicit drug use (cannabinoids, cocaine, etc.)
3 Any history of unauthorized escalation of therapeutic drugs such as benzodiazepines
4 Any history of other addictive behaviors[a]
5 Heavy smokers with inability to quit

From Fishbain.[174]
a. See Portenoy.[173]

Table 5.12 *Spectrum of aberrant drug-related behaviors that raise concern about the potential for addiction*

More suggestive of addiction
Selling prescription drugs
Prescription forgery
Stealing of drugs from others
Injecting oral formulations
Obtaining prescription drugs from nonmedical sources
Concurrent abuse of alcohol or illicit drugs
Repeated dose escalation or similar noncompliance despite multiple warnings
Repeated visits to other clinicians or emergency rooms without informing prescriber
Drug-related deterioration in function at work, in the family, or socially
Repeated resistance to changes in therapy despite evidence of adverse drug effects

Less suggestive of addiction
Aggressive complaining
Drug hoarding during periods of reduced symptoms as patient needs more drugs when symptoms increase
Requesting specific drugs
Openly acquiring similar drugs from other medical sources
Occasional unsanctioned dose escalation or other noncompliance
Unapproved use of the drug to treat another symptom
Reporting psychic effects not intended by the clinician
Resistance to a change in therapy associated with tolerable adverse effects
Intense expressions of anxiety about recurrent symptom

From Portenoy.[173]

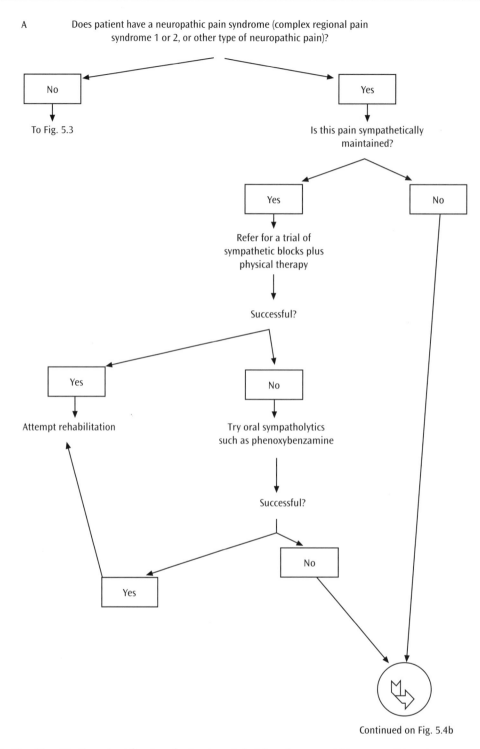

Figure 5.4 *Algorithm III. Flow chart for steps for treatment decisions for comorbid neuropathic pain.*

one minor inclusion criterion. The minor inclusion criteria are essentially the list of comorbidities (discussed above) plus the criteria of failure of "conservative" management and failure of one isolated mode of treatment.

Failure of pain facility treatment (next step in the second algorithm, Fig. 5.3) makes the CPP a candidate for neural blockade. Failure of neural blockade makes the CPP a candidate for oral chronic opioid analgesic treatment. To help with this last decision, the author has published a set of criteria[174] that allow the pain physician to decide whether the CPP is a candidate for this type of treatment. These criteria are presented in Table 5.11. The exclusion criteria in this table are heavily dependent on the psychiatric comorbidities being recognizable. These relate mainly to a history of alcohol abuse and illicit drug use. In addition, CPPs with psychiatric comorbidities I (substance abuse/dependence), V, and VI in Table 5.2 would also fulfill these exclusion criteria. Two other

B

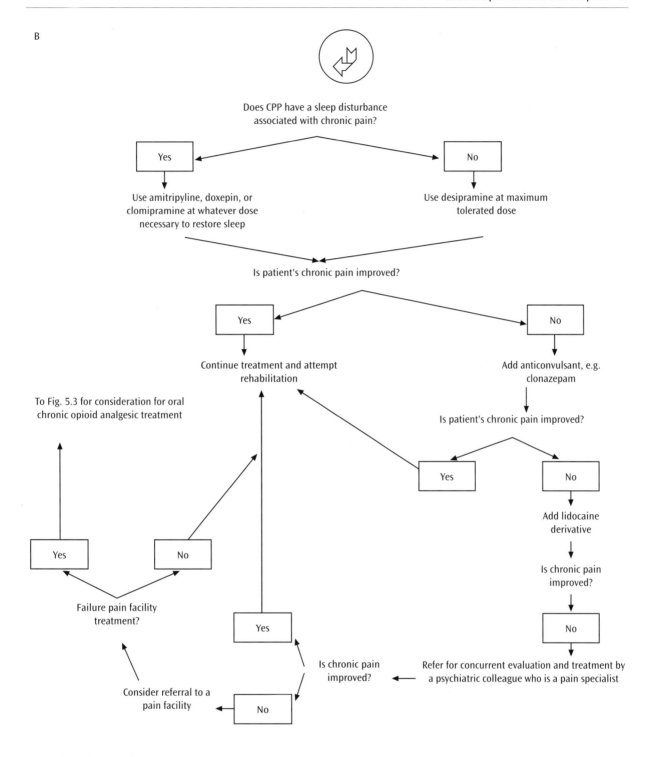

Figure 5.4 *Continued.*

exclusion criteria (3 and 4) in Table 5.11 relate to what has been termed by Portenoy[173] to be addictive behaviors. A full list of addictive behaviors is presented in Table 5.12. As pointed out above, a history of addiction behaviors can be utilized as exclusion criteria for a decision about narcotic pain treatment (Table 5.11). In addition, addictive behaviors can also be used to monitor oral chronic opioid analgesic treatment. Demonstration of these behaviors during oral chronic opioid analgesic treatment

should lead one to suspect that there may be underlying addictive problems.

Failure of chronic narcotic pain treatment or recognition of CPP addictive problems would make the CPP a candidate for consideration for neuroaugmentation techniques or other neurosurgical techniques (algorithm II in Fig. 5.3).

Algorithm III is presented in Fig. 5.4. The purpose of this algorithm is to outline a method for utilizing the

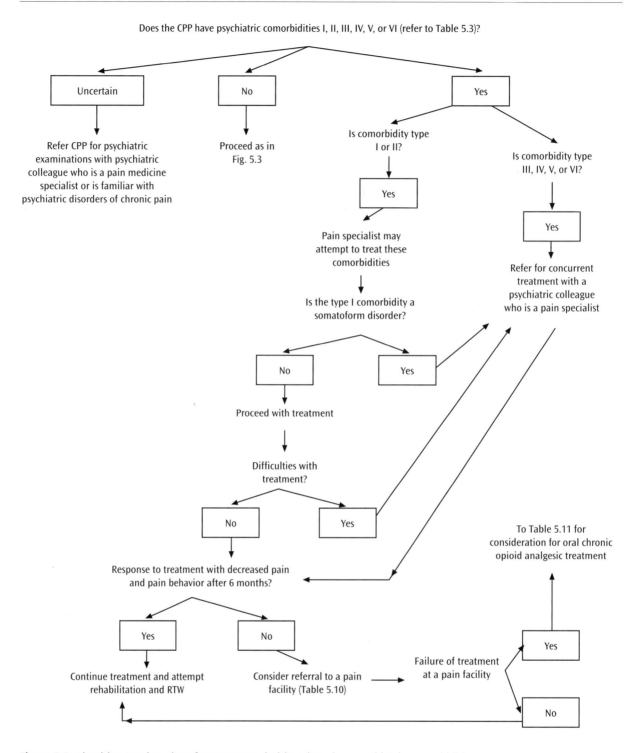

Figure 5.5 *Algorithm IV. Flow chart for treatment decisions based on psychiatric comorbidities.*

neuropathic pain comorbidity in making psychopharmacologic and other treatment decisions. This type of approach has been advocated by Fields and Liebeskind.[175]

Algorithm IV is presented in Fig. 5.5. The purpose of this algorithm is to utilize the CPP's psychiatric comorbidities in making treatment decisions. This algorithm is based around the questions of whether the CPP has any

category of psychiatric comorbidity. If the answer is no (refer to algorithm IV, Fig. 5.5), the pain physician may proceed as in algorithm II (Fig. 5.3). However, if the pain physician is uncertain about the presence of any psychiatric comorbidities, a consultation should be sought with a psychiatrist familiar with chronic pain or who is a pain specialist. CPPs who demonstrate psychiatric comorbidities III–VI should be treated in collaboration with a psychiatric colleague. This is because these comorbidities relate to either psychoactive drug misuse or to a number of concurrent psychiatric comorbidities. As pointed out, the presence of more than one psychiatric comorbidity or a psychoactive drug misuse comorbidity makes that CPP a difficult treatment problem.

As seen in algorithm IV (Fig. 5.5), the pain physician may attempt to treat type I and type II psychiatric comorbidities except if the type I comorbidity is a somatoform disorder. Under these circumstances concurrent treatment with a psychiatric colleague is recommended. Difficulties after 6 months of treatment for CPPs with type I or II psychiatric comorbidities should lead to consideration for referral to a pain facility (algorithm IV). Failure of pain facility treatment should lead to consideration for chronic opioid analgesic therapy as in algorithm II.

CONCLUSIONS

Psychiatric, behavioral, and other comorbidities are extremely important in the proper management of chronic pain. As such, decisions about chronic pain treatment should be based on an understanding of the comorbidities associated with chronic pain.

Acknowledgment We thank Ms Sandy Vassilatos for typing the manuscript.

REFERENCES

1. Longmire DR. Evaluation of the pain patient. In: Raj PP ed. *Pain Medicine a Comprehensive Review*. St Louis, MO: Mosby, 1996: 26–35.

● 2. Braddom L. Perils and pointers in the evaluation and management of back pain. *Semin Neurol* 1998; **18:** 197–210.

◆ 3. Fishbain DA, Goldberg M, Steele-Rosomoff R, Rosomoff HL. Chronic pain patients and the non-organic physical sign of nondermatomal sensory abnormalities (NDSA). *Psychosomatics* 1991; **32:** 294–303.

4. Patt RB, Ellison N. Breakthrough pain. In: Aronoff G ed. *Evaluation and Treatment of Chronic Pain*, 3rd edn. Philadelphia, PA: Williams and Wilkins, 1998: 377–87.

● 5. Chapman CR, Casey KL, Dubner R, *et al*. Pain measurement: an overview. *Pain* 1985; **22:** 1–31.

6. Valley MA. Pain measurement. In: Raj PP ed. *Pain Medicine a Comprehensive Review*. St Louis, MO: Mosby, 1996: 36–44.

7. Jensen MP, Miller L, Fisher LD. Assessment of pain during medical procedures: a comparison of three scales. *Clin J Pain* 1998; **14:** 343–9.

● 8. Sriwatanakul K, Kelvie W, Lasagna L. Studies with different types of visual analog scales for measurement of pain. *Clin Pharmacol Ther* 1983; **34:** 234–9.

◆ 9. Price DDR, McGrath PA, Rafi A, Buckingham B. The validity of visual analogue scales as ration scale measures for chronic and experimental pain. *Pain* 1983; **17:** 45–56.

◆ 10. Jensen MP, Karoly P, Braver S. Measurement of clinical pain intensity: a comparison of six methods. *Pain* 1986; **27:** 117–26.

11. Yang JC, Clark WC, Janal MN. Sensory decision theory and visual analogue scale indices predict status of chronic pain patients six months later. *J Pain Symptom Manage* 1991; **6:** 58–64.

12. Huskisson EC. Measurement of pain. *Lancet* 1974; **82:** 1127–32.

13. Deyo RA. Measuring the functional status of patients with low back pain. *Arch Phys Med Rehabil* 1988; **69:** 1044–53.

● 14. Cedraschi C, Nordin M, Nachemson AL, Vischer TL. Health care providers should use a common language in relation to low back pain patients. *Baillière's Clin Rheumatol* 1998; **12:** 1–13.

◆ 15. Haldeman S. Failure of the pathology model to predict back pain. *Spine* 1990; **15:** 718–24.

16. Deyo RA, Fihillips WR. Low back pain: a primary care challenge. *Spine* 1996; **21:** 2826–32.

17. Kennedy LD. Laboratory investigation. In: Raj PP ed. *Pain Medicine: a Comprehensive Review*. St Louis, MO: Mosby, 1996: 47–54.

18. Raj PP. Diagnostic nerve block. In: Raj PP ed. *Pain Medicine a Comprehensive Review*. St Louis, MO: Mosby, 1996: 83–90.

◆ 19. Wolfe F, Smythe HA, Yunus MB. The American College of Rheumatology 1990 criteria for the classification of fibromyalgia: report of the Multicenter Criteria Committee. *Arthritis Rheum* 1990; **33:** 160–72.

20. Simons DG. Referred phenomena of myofascial trigger points. In: Vechiet L, Albe-Fessard D, Lindblom U eds. *New Trends in Referred Pain and Hyperalgesia*. Amsterdam: Elsevier, 1993: 341.

21. Wolfe F, Ross K, Anderson J, *et al*. The prevalence and characteristics of fibromyalgia in the general population. *Arthritis Rheum* 1995; **38:** 19–28.

22. Han SC, Harrison P. Myofascial pain syndrome and trigger-point management. *Reg Anesth* 1997; **22:** 89–101.

23. Gerwin R. A study of 96 subjects examined both for fibromyalgia and myofascial pain. *J Musculoskeletal Pain* 1995; **3:** 121.

24. Hubbard Jr DR. Chronic and recurrent muscle pain: pathophysiology and treatment, and review of pharmacologic studies. *J Musculoskeletal Pain* 1996; **4:** 123–43.

◆ 25. Rosomoff HL, Fishbain DA, Goldberg M, *et al*. Physical findings in patients with chronic intractable benign pain of the neck and/or back. *Pain* 1989; **37:** 279–87.

26. Borkan JM, Reis S, Hermoni D, Biderman A. Talking about the pain: a patient-centered study of low back pain in primary care. *Soc Sci Med* 1995; **40:** 977–88.

◆ 27. Deyo RA, Diehl AK. Patient satisfaction with medical care for low-back pain. *Spine* 1986; **11:** 28–30.

◆ 28. Abenhaim L, Rossignol M, Gobeille D. The prognostic consequences in the making of the initial medical diagnosis of work-related injuries. *Spine* 1995; **20:** 791–5.

29. Bohr T. Problems with myofascial pain syndrome and fibromyalgia. *Neurology* 1996; **46:** 593–7.

30. Cathey MA, Wolfe K, Dleinhekss SM, Hawley DJ. Socioeconomic impact of fibrositis: a study of 81 patients with primary fibrositis. *Am J Med* 1986; **81:** 78–84.

31. Feinstein A. The pre-therapeutic classification of comorbidity in chronic disease. *J Chronic Dis* 1970; **23:** 455.

32. Merikangas KR, Gelernter CS. Comorbidity for alcoholism and depression. *Psychiatr Clin North Am* 1990; **13:** 613–31.

● 33. Fishbain DA, Cutler RB, Steele-Rosomoff R, Rosomoff HL. The problem oriented psychiatric examination of the chronic pain patient and its application to the litigation consultation. *Clin J Pain* 1994; **10:** 38–51.

● 34. Fishbain DA, Cutler RB, Rosomoff HL, Rosomoff RS. Comorbidity between psychiatric disorders and chronic pain. *Curr Rev Pain* 1998; **2:** 1–10.

35. American Psychiatric Association. *Diagnostic and Statistical Manual of Mental Disorders*, 4th edn. Washington, DC: American Psychiatric Association 1994;

◆ 36. Fishbain DA, Goldberg M, Meagher BR, Rosomoff H. Male and female chronic pain patients categorized by DSM-III psychiatric diagnostic criteria. *Pain* 1986; **26:** 181–97.

● 37. Romano JM, Turner JA. Chronic pain and depression: does the evidence support a relationship. *Psychol Bull* 1985; **97:** 18–34.

● 38. Fishbain DA, Cutler R, Rosomoff HL, Rosomoff RS. Chronic pain-associated depression: antecedent or consequence of chronic pain: a review. *Clin J Pain* 1997; **13:** 116–37.

● 39. Fishbain DA, Steele-Rosomoff R, Rosomoff HL. Drug abuse dependence, and addiction in chronic pain patients. *Clin J Pain* 1992; **8:** 77–85.

● 40. Fishbain DA. DSM-IV: implications and issues for the pain clinician. *Am Pain Soc Bull* 1995; 6–18.

● 41. Katon W. Panic disorder and somatization: review of 55 cases. *Am J Med* 1984; **77:** 101–6.

42. Gilcrist JC. Psychiatric and social factors related to low-back pain in general practice. *Rheumatol Rehabil* 1976; **18:** 10?-107.

43. Asmudson GJ, Norton GR, Jacobson SJ. Social, blood/injury, and agoraphobic fears in patients with physically unexplained chronic pain: are they clinically significant. *Anxiety* 1988; **2:** 87–95.

44. Gureje O, VonKorff M, Sim GE, Gater R. Persistent pain and well-being: a World Health Organization study in primary care. *J Am Med Assoc* 1998; **280:** 147–51.

● 45. Weisberg JN, Keefe FJ. Personality disorders in the chronic pain population: basic concepts, empirical findings, and clinical implications. *Pain Forum* 1997; **6:** 19.

● 46. Fishbain DA. Can personality disorders in chronic pain patients be accurately measured. *Pain Forum* 1997; **6:** 16–19.

47. Fishbain DA, Cutler RB, Rosomoff HL, Steele-Rosomoff R. Comorbid psychiatric disorders in chronic pain patients with psychoactive substance use disorders. *Pain Clin* 1998; **11:** 79–87.

48. Fishbain DA, Cutler RB, Rosomoff HL, Steele-Rosomoff R. False information on chronic pain patient illicit drug use as determined by urine toxicology. *Clin J Pain* 1999; **15** (2): 102–10.

49. Beck AT, Ward CH, Mendelson M, *et al*. An inventory for measuring depression. *Arch Gen Psychol* 1961; **4:** 561–71.

◆ 50. Berndt S, Maier C, Schutz HW. Polymedication and medication compliance in patients with chronic non-malignant pain. *Pain* 1993; **52:** 331–9.

● 51. Hedlund JL, Vieweg BW. The Michigan alcoholism screening test (MAST): a comprehensive review. *J Operational Psychol* 1984; **15:** 55–65.

◆ 52. Pokorny AD, Miller BA, Kaplan HB. Testing for alcoholics. The brief mast: a shortened version of the Michigan Alcoholism Test. *Am J Psychiatry* 1972; **129:** 342–5.

◆ 53. Steinweg DL, Worth H. Alcoholism: keys to the CAGE. *Addict Behav* 1993;**18:** 520–3.

54. Bush K, *et al*. The AUDIT alcohol consumption questions (AUDIT-C): an effective, brief screening test for problem drinking. *Arch Intern Med* 1998; **158:** 1789–95.

55. Baillie AJ, Mattick RP. The benzodiazepine dependence questionnaire: development, reliability and validity. *Br J Psychol* 1996; **196:** 276–81.

56. Skinner HA. The drug abuse screening test. *Addict Behav* 1982; **7:** 363–71.

57. Ling W, McLellan T, Woody GE. Assessing pathological detoxification fear among methadone maintenance patients: the DFSS. *J Clin Psychol* 1987; **43:** 528–39.

58. Spielberger CD, Gorsuch RL, Lusheme RR. *Manual for the State–Trait Anxiety Inventory*. Palo Alto, CA: Consulting Psychologists Press 1970;

59. Muse M, Frigola G. Development of a quick screening instrument for detecting posttraumatic stress disorder in the chronic pain patient: construction of the posttraumatic chronic pain test (PCPT). *Clin J Pain* 1987; **2:** 151–3.

60. Sher KJ, Frost RO, Kushner M, *et al*. Memory deficits in compulsive checkers: replication and extension in a clinical sample. *Behav Res Ther* 1989; **27:** 65–9.

61. Davidson JRT. Biological therapies for posttraumatic stress disorder: an overview. *J Clin Psychiatry* 1997; **58** (9): 29–32.

◆ 62. Fishbain DA, Trescott J, Cutler B, *et al*. Do some chronic pain patients with atypical facial pain overvalue and obsess about their pain? *Psychosomatics* 1993; **34:** 355–9.

63. Kremer E, Atkinson JH, Fagnelzi RM. Measurement of pain: patient preference does not confound pain measurement. *Pain* 1981; **51:** 281–7.

64. Cornwal A, Doncleri DC. The effect of experimentally induced anxiety on the experience of pressure pain. *Pain* 1988; **35:** 105–13.

65. Weisberg JN, Gorin A, Drozd K, Gallagher RM. The relationship between depression and psychophysiological reactivity in chronic pain patients. In: *Proceedings of the International Association for the Study of Pain, 8th World Congress on Pain*. Vancouver: IASP Press, 1996: 71.

66. Krass S, Gallagher RM, Myers P, Friedman R. The effect of chronic pain and depression on pain perception in chronic pain patients. In: *Proceedings of the American Pain Society 15th Annual Meeting*. Washington, DC: APS 1996; A-684, A-71.

67. Katon WJ. Depression in patients with inflammatory bowel disease. *J Clin Psychiatry* 1997; **58:** 20–3.

68. Angst J. Depression and anxiety: implications for nosology, course, and treatment. *J Clin Psychiatry* 1997; **58:** 3–5.

69. Fava M, Alpert JE, Borus JS. Patterns of personality disorder comorbidity in early-onset versus late-onset major depression. *Am J Psychiatry* 1996; **153:** 1308–12.

70. Williams DA, Thron BE. An empirical assessment of pain beliefs. *Pain* 1989; **36:** 351–8.

71. Waddell G, Newton M, Henderson I, *et al*. A fear-avoidance beliefs questionnaire (FABQ) and the role of fear-avoidance beliefs in chronic low back pain and disability. *Pain* 1993; **52:** 157–68.

72. Rosenstiel AK, Keefe FJ. The use of coping strategies in chronic low back pain patients: relationship to patient characteristics and current adjustment. *Pain* 1983; **17:** 33–44.

73. Spielberger CD, Jacobs GA, Russell S, Crane RS. Assessment of anger: the state–trait anger scale. *Adv Pers Assess* 1983; **2:** 112–34.

74. Bernstein IH, Matthew E, Jaremko, Hinkley BS. On the utility of the West Haven–Yale multidimensional pain inventory. *Spine* 1995; **20:** 956–63.

75. Asmundson GJG, Norton GR, Allerdings MD. Fear and avoidance in dysfunctional chronic back pain patients. *Pain* 1997; **69:** 231–6.

76. Vlaeyen JWS, Kole-Snijders AMJ, Boeren RGB, van Eeek H. Fear of movement/(re)injury in chronic low back pain and its relation to behavioral performance. *Pain* 1995; **62:** 363–72.

77. Lorig K, Chastain RI, Ung E, Large P. Development and evaluation of a scale to measure perceived self-efficacy in people with arthritis. *Arthritis Rheum* 1989; **32:** 37–44.

78. Buysse DJ, Reynolds III CF, Monk TH, *et al*. The Pittsburgh sleep quality index: a new instrument for psychiatric practice and research. *Psychiatry Res* 1989; **28:** 193–213.

79. Frank E, Anderson MSW, Rubinstein D. Frequency of sexual dysfunction in "normal" couples. *New Engl J Med* 1978; **299:** 111–115.

80. Schneider RA. Concurrent validity of the beck depression inventory and multidimensional fatigue inventory-20 in assessing fatigue among cancer patients. *Psychol Rep* 1998; **82:** 883–6.

81. Derogatis LR. *The SCL-90-R Manual II: Administration, Scoring and Procedures*. Towson, MD: Clinical Psychometric Research 1983;

82. Korbon GA, DeGood DE, Schroeder ME. The development of a somatic amplification rating scale for low back pain. *Spine* 1987; **12:** 787–91.

83. Riley JF, Ahern DK, Follick MJ. Chronic low back pain and functional improvement: assessing beliefs about the relationship. *Arch Phys Med Rehabil* 1988; **69:** 579–82.

84. Guck TP, Fleischer TD, Willcockson JC, *et al*. Predictive validity of the pain and impairment relationship scale in a chronic nonmalignant pain population. *Arch Phys Med Rehabil* 1999; **80:** 91–5.

85. Tait RC, Pollard CA, Margolis RB. The pain disability index: psychometric and validity data. *Arch Phys Med Rehabil* 1987; **68:** 438–41.

◆ 86. Richards JS, Nepomuceno C, Riles R, Suer Z. Assessing pain behavior: the UAB pain behavior scale. *Pain* 1982; **14:** 393–8.

◆ 87. Galer BS, Jensen MP. Development and preliminary validation of a pain measure specific to neuropathic pain: the neuropathic pain scale. *Neurology* 1997; **48:** 332–8.

88. Sandroni P, Low PA, Ferrer T, *et al*. Complex regional pain syndrome I (CRPS I): prospective study and laboratory evaluation. *Clin J Pain* 1998; **14:** 282–9.

◆ 89. Follick MJ, Smith TW, Ahern DK. The sickness impact profile: a global measure of disability in chronic low back pain. *Pain* 1985; **21:** 67–76.

90. Millard RW. The functional assessment screening questionnaire application for evaluating pain related disability. *Arch Phys Med Rehabil* 1989; **70:** 303–7.

91. Herda CA, Siegeris K, Basler HD. The pain beliefs and perceptions inventory: further evidence for a 4-factor structure. *Pain* 1994; **57:** 85–90.

92. Williams DA, Robinson ME, Geisser ME. Pain beliefs: assessment and utility. *Pain* 1994; **59:** 71–8.

93. Williams DA, Keefe FJ. Pain beliefs and the use of cognitive–behavioral coping strategies. *Pain* 1991; **46:** 185–90.

94. Panzarella JP. The nature of work, job loss, and the diagnostic complexities of the psychologically injured worker. *Psychiatr Ann* 1991; **21:** 10–15.

95. Fagin L. Stress and unemployment. *Stress Med* 1984; **1:** 27–36.

◆ 96. Fishbain DA, Rosomoff HL, Cutler R, Rosomoff RS. Do chronic pain patients' perceptions about their preinjury jobs determine their intent to return to the same type of job post-pain facility treatment? *Clin J Pain* 1995; **11:** 267–78.

97. Rosomoff HL, Fishbain DA, Cutler R, Steele Rosomoff R. Do chronic pain patients' perceptions about their pre-

injury jobs differ as a function of workers' compensation and non-worker compensation status? *Clin J Pain* 1995; **11:** 279–86.

◆ 98. Fishbain DA, Cutler R, Rosomoff HL, *et al.* Impact of chronic pain patients' job perception variables on actual return to work. *Clin J Pain* 1997; **13:** 197–205.

99. Fishbain DA, Cutler R, Rosomoff HL, *et al.* The prediction of chronic pain patient "intent," discrepancy with intent" and "discrepancy with non-intent" for return to work post pain facility treatment. *Clin J Pain* 1999; **15** (2): 141–50.

100. Fernandez E, Turk DC. The scope and significance of anger in the experience of chronic pain. *Pain* 1995; **61:** 165–75.

101. Fernandez E. Milburn TW. Sensory and affective predictors of overall pain and emotions associated with affective pain. *Clin J Pain* 1994; **10:** 3–9.

102. Kerns RD, Rosenberg R, Jacob MC. Anger expression and chronic pain. *J Behav Med* 1994; **17:** 57.

103. Burns JW, Johnson BJ, Devine J, *et al.* Anger management style and the prediction of treatment outcome among male and female chronic pain patients. *Behav Res Ther* 1998; **36:** 1051–62.

104. Deffenbacher JL, Demm PM, Brandon AD. High general anger: correlates and treatment. *Behav Res Ther* 1986; **24:** 481–9.

105. Nordin M, Cedraschi C, Skovron ML. Patient–health care provider relationship in patients with non-specific low back pain: a review of some problem situations. *Baillière's Clin Rheum* 1998; **12:** 75–91.

106. Cherkin DC, Deyo RA, Street JH, Barlow W. Predicting poor outcome for back pain seen in primary care using patients' own criteria. *Spine* 1996; **21:** 2900–7.

107. Main CJ, Spanswich CC. Personality assessment and the Minnesota Multiphasic personality inventory. *Pain Forum* 1995; **4:** 90–6.

◆108. Fishbain DA. Some difficulties with predictive validity of the Minnesota Multiphasic Personal inventory. *Pain Forum* 1996; **5:** 81–2.

109. DeGood DE, Shutty Jr MS. Assessment of pain beliefs, coping and self-efficacy. In: Turk DC, Melzak R eds. *Handbook of Pain Assessment*. New York, NY: Guilford Press 1993.

110. Williams DA, Thorn BE. An empirical assessment of pain beliefs. *Pain* 1989; **36:** 351–8.

●111. Tan SY. Cognitive and cognitive behavioral methods for pain control: a selective review. *Pain* 1982; **12:** 201–28.

●112. Jensen MP, Turner JA, Romano JM, Karoly P. Coping with chronic pain: a critical review of the literature. *Pain* 1991; **47:** 249–83.

113. Turner JA, Romano JM. Behavioral and psychological assessment of chronic pain patients. In: Loeser JD, Egan KJ eds. *Managing the Chronic Pain Patient*. New York, NY: Raven Press, 1989: 165–79.

114. Gill KM, Keefe FJ, Crisson JE, Van Dalfsen PJ. Social support and pain behavior. *Pain* 1987; **29:** 209–17.

115. Kerns RD, Southwick S, Giller EL, *et al.* The relationship between reports of pain related social interactions and expressions of pain and affective distress. *Behav Ther* 1991; **22:** 101–11.

116. Lousberg R, Schmidt Anton JM, Groenman NH. The relationship between spouse solicitousness and pain behavior: searching for more experimental evidence. *Pain* 1992; **51:** 75–9.

117. Romano JM, Turner H, Jensen MP, *et al.* Chronic pain patient–spouse behavioral interactions predict patient disability. *Pain* 1995; **63:** 353–60.

118. Schwartz L, Slater MA, Birchler GR, Atkinson JH. Depression in spouses of chronic pain patients: the role of patient pain and anger, and marital satisfaction. *Pain* 1991; **44:** 61–7.

119. Hughes AM, Medley I, Turner GN, Bond MR. Psychogenic pain: a study of marital adjustment. *Acta Psychiatr Scand* 1987; **75:** 166–70.

120. Pawlicki RE. A neglected issue: the family of the chronic pain patient. *Am Pain Soc Bull* 1992; **Oct/Nov:** 5–6.

121. Faucett JA, Levine JD. The contributions of interpersonal conflict to chronic pain in the presence or absence of organic pathology. *Pain* 1991; **44:** 35–43.

122. Pilowsky I, Creltenden I, Townley M. Sleep disturbance in pain clinic patients. *Pain* 1985; **23:** 27–33.

123. Wittig RM, Zorck FJ, Blumer D, *et al.* Disturbed sleep in patients complaining of chronic pain. *J Nerv Ment Dis* 1982; **170:** 429–35.

◆124. Atkinson JH, Ancoli-Israel S, Slater MA, *et al.* Subjective sleep disturbance in chronic back pain. *Clin J Pain* 1988; **4:** 225–32.

125. Hemmeter U, Kocher R, Ladewig M, *et al.* Sleep disorders in chronic pain and fibromyalgia syndrome. *Schweiz Med Wochenschr* 1995; **125:** 2391–7.

126. Morin CM, Gibson D, Wade J. Self-reported sleep and mood disturbance in chronic pain patients. *Clin J Pain* 1998; **14:** 311–14.

●127. Labbe EE. Sexual dysfunction in chronic back pain patients, implications for clinical research and practice. *Clin J Pain* 1988; **4:** 143–9.

128. Maruta T, Osborne D. Sexual activity in chronic pain patients. *Psychosomatics* 1978; **19:** 531–537.

129. LaBan MM, Burk RD, Johnson EW. Sexual impotence in men having low-back syndrome. *Arch Phys Med Rehabil* 1966; **49:** 715–23.

130. Feuerstein M, Carter RL, Papciak AS. A prospective analysis of stress and fatigue in recurrent low back pain. *Pain* 1987; **31:** 333–44.

131. Wendt JK, Wang S, Mendoza T. The impact of pain on fatigue levels in a non-patient community-dwelling population. In: *Proceedings of the 17th Annual Meeting American Pain Society*. Seattle, WA: American Pain Society 1998: 204.

●132. Lipowski ZJ. Somatization: the concept and its clinical application. *Am J Psychiatry* 1988; **145:** 1358–66.

●133. Sullivan M, Katon W. The path between distress and somatic symptoms. *Am Pain Soc J* 1993; **2:** 141–9.

of each of these elements will lead to a more complete understanding of the patient's experience of pain.

Pain behaviors

Pain behaviors are overt expressions that communicate pain and distress to others. They include verbal or motor behaviors that are almost automatic, such as limping and wincing, or they can be higher order behavioral patterns such as taking medication or help-seeking. Pain behaviors may result from reflexive avoidance of aversive experience or defense response to protect oneself. This is particularly evident in the case of acute pain. For example, we have all seen a person with a sprained ankle limp in an attempt to protect the injured area. In this case, pain behaviors serve to protect a person from exacerbating the pathology and exacerbating the pain. However, there are cases where some patients acquire and maintain pain behaviors because of environmental contingencies that provide reinforcement for the behaviors.[8] For example, if pain leads to limping and limping elicits attention from family members, a contingency pattern of limping – positive reinforcement – may become established. Once such a contingency is established, pain may no longer be necessary to maintain limping behavior. Pain behaviors cease to serve as a protective mechanism, rather their functions become a way of ensuring the reinforcements.

It is important to assess the functions that observed pain behaviors serve. Since patients' behaviors affect how people, including health care providers, respond, maintenance of maladaptive pain behaviors will contribute to disability. Consequently, pain assessment, particularly for chronic pain, must include pain behaviors and the relevant reinforcement contingencies along with the assessment of physical pathology.

Suffering

Another direction from nociception through pain experience is more phenomenologic than pain behaviors – suffering. Suffering is loosely defined as "a state of severe distress associated with events that threaten the intactness of person."[14] Patients with chronic or recurring acute pain are at risk to experience suffering because the impact of pain puts their physical, psychologic, occupational, and social integrity in jeopardy owing to pain and related functional limitations. Social and occupational rewards that the patient used to enjoy may no longer be available. Moreover, pessimism about obtaining relief may leave a person with little hope for the future – pain is interminable, uncontrollable, and there is no end in sight. Suffering is an internally processed state; thus it, unlike pain behaviors, cannot be observed by others.

It is often assumed that pain behaviors and suffering are opposite sides of the same coin and that both must be present for persons with substantial pain experience. It is important to remember, however, that they are distinct categories of human experience; the absence of pain behaviors does not mean that the person is free from suffering, or vice versa.

ASSESSMENT OF THE PERSON WITH CHRONIC PAIN

It should be apparent from the above that all types of pain – chronic or acute recurrent pain syndromes – represent a complex combination of contributing components in which both physical and psychologic influences are represented. The fact that significant psychologic factors contributing to pain problems can be identified does not preclude the existence of physical pathology, nor do abnormal physical findings necessarily imply the absence of significant psychologic or behavioral contributors to pain and subsequent disability.

Purposes of assessment

There are a number of purposes of assessment, including:

- diagnosis;
- decision-making and treatment planning;
- evaluation of change in symptoms and impact of treatment;
- prediction of response to treatment; and
- program evaluation.

These purposes are not mutually exclusive. The purposes of the assessment, however, should guide the nature and content of the assessment process. For example, when a patient with chronic pain is being evaluated to make decisions regarding treatment, a comprehensive assessment of multiple areas – physical, psychosocial, and behavioral – may be indicated. Assessment of response to a pharmacological intervention may not require such an extensive evaluation but may focus on changes in symptoms. Program evaluation may focus more on objective instruments and procedures, whereas individual assessment may include open-ended interviews. The comprehensiveness of the assessment should also be related to patients' capacity to respond. It would be inappropriate to ask a patient with end-stage cancer to complete lengthy self-report questionnaires. For these individuals, several simple questions regarding pain severity and related symptoms may be all that are used.

Evaluative questions for pain assessment

Our conceptualization of the multiple levels of the pain experience leads to three central questions that can guide assessment of people who report pain:[15]

1 What is the extent of the patient's disease or injury? (nociception, physical impairment)

2 What is the magnitude of the illness? That is to say, to what extent is the patient suffering, disabled, and unable to enjoy usual activities? (pain and suffering)

3 Does the patient's behavior during his or her interactions with the physician seem reasonable given the nature and extent of the disease or injury? Is there any evidence that symptoms are amplified for psychologic or social reasons or purposes? (pain behaviors)

In this chapter, we will focus on questions 2 and 3 – the impact of pain on the adult patient's life and his or her behavioral response to pain. (For discussion of the assessment of physical factors associated with pain and pain assessment in children, see Turk and Melzack.[16])

ASSESSMENT FORMATS

Assessment of the person with chronic or acute recurrent pain may be accomplished by unstructured or semistructured clinical interviews, self-report instruments, and direct observation or observation by significant others such as family members. Multimethod assessment has a distinct advantage. Interviews have a great deal of flexibility but do not provide normative data and are difficult to quantify. The advantages of the self-report measures are that they are efficient, standardized, and permit assessment of important areas such as attitudes, beliefs, and mood states that may not be directly observable. The advantages of observation methods are that they can be unobtrusive and that they are less reactive and more objective than self-report measures and interviews.

Clinical interviews

Clinical interviews provide the opportunity to gather a wide range of information from patients and their significant others. When conducting an interview with a pain patient, clinicians should focus not simply on factual information but also on the patient's and significant other's specific thoughts (i.e. appraisals, interpretations, meaning of symptoms, expectations) and feelings and they should observe specific behaviors. Some of the areas that should be assessed during a clinical interview are outlined in Table 6.1.

It is increasingly recognized that a patient's interpretation of the meaning of pain and the extent to which pain forms a focus of attention can have profound effects on the patient's response to pain. In light of this, it is important to gather information on patients' appraisals of the pain problems, their thoughts and images of what is happening in their bodies when they are experiencing pain, and, similarly, their significant others' explanatory model

Table 6.1 *Targets covered in interview*

The history of the problem from the point of view of the patient
Patient's concerns about problem (e.g. degeneration, reinjury, paralysis)
How the patient thinks about his or her problem and the health care system
Cognitive and behavioral antecedents that are consistently associated with fluctuations in pain (e.g. when certain topics are discussed)
Thoughts and feelings that precede, accompany, and follow exacerbation of pain
Problems that have arisen because of pain
How the patient expresses pain
How others react to the patient's pain and disability
What effect the patient believes the problem is having on others
Activity patterns
Learning history (prior history of pain or chronic illness)
Marital relationship including sexual functioning
Current or recent life stresses
Vocational history and goals for return to work
Job satisfaction (employers, coworkers, job conditions)
Compensation–litigation status
Benefits from having pain and disability
Patterns of alcohol and medication use
Mental status examination including anxiety and depression
What the patient has tried to do to alleviate the pain
Inconsistencies and incongruities between patient's report and behavior or between patient's and significant other's reports
Patient's and significant other's goals for treatment

for the cause and implication of pain.

During the clinical interview, the assessor should attend to the temporal association of these cognitive, affective, and behavioral events – their specificity versus generality across situations, the frequency of their occurrence, and so forth – in order to elucidate the topography of the target behaviors, including the controlling variables. The patient's reports of specific thoughts, behaviors, emotions, and physiologic responses that precede, accompany, and follow pain episodes or exacerbation, as well as the environmental conditions and consequences associated with cognitive, emotional, and behavioral responses in these situations, all need to be attended to by the clinicians. The interviewer should seek information that will assist in the development of appropriate goals for the patient, and possible reinforcers for the successful attainment of these goals.

It is important for the health care professional to adopt the patient's perspective (see Table 6.2). Patients' beliefs about the causes of their pain, its trajectory, and what treatments will benefit them appear to have an important influence on their emotional adjustment and compliance with therapeutic interventions. A habitual pattern of maladaptive thought may contribute to a sense of hopelessness, dysphoria, and unwillingness to engage in activity. During the interview, attempts should be made to determine both patients' and spouses' expectancies and goals for treatment.

In many cases, patients have fears based on misinformation or faulty concepts of anatomy and medicine. Thus, the patient who has been told that he or she has "degenerative disk disease" may believe that his spine is fragile and unstable, and that movement will hasten the process of degeneration and disability. Patients told that they have a pinched nerve or "slipped disk" compressing a nerve may fear that they may damage their spinal cord and become paralyzed if they increase activity. If patients interpret their persistent pain as a signal of ongoing and progressive tissue damage, it is understandable that they avoid any activities that increase pain. If spouses have such fears, they are likely to reinforce pain behaviors by overprotecting the patient, and may even sabotage treatment aimed at increasing physical activity. The evaluator should seek information that will assist in the development of potential alternative behaviors, appropriate goals for the patient, and possible reinforcers for these alternatives.

The marital relationship is particularly important as a spouse can be a major source of support but can also be an impediment to rehabilitation. It is important to examine the quality of marital relationship and the manner of marital interaction (e.g. enabling, reinforcing). What would happen to the marriage if pain were alleviated? One component of the marital relationship frequently affected by pain is sexual activity. The assessor should examine this aspect of the marital relationship to determine whether the pain has led to any significant dysfunction.

Many chronic pain patients seen in pain treatment facilities have problems with excessive alcohol, opioid, or sedative–hypnotic medication use, even if not abuse.

Such use complicates the assessment of the pain problem for a number of reasons. Patients may use their pain to legitimize alcohol or substance abuse. Patients may mislabel withdrawal symptoms as an increase in "pain." Chronic use of opioid, barbiturate, and anxiolytic drugs can produce dysphoria and other symptoms that mimic depression, such as decreased energy, sleep disturbance, and appetite and weight changes. It is important to examine prior history of alcohol and illicit substance use and to identify changes in the usual pattern that have evolved since the pain onset.

The evaluator should inquire about vocational history and identify factors that might impede return to work. The patient's satisfactions with jobs, employers, and coworkers prior to pain onset are assessed. Patients should be asked directly about their specific plans, if any, for return to work and about potential barriers other than pain to returning to work.

Patients may fear losing the financial support, particularly if the former job is unpleasant or no longer available, if vocational options appear limited, or if the patient fears reinjury or increased pain upon return to work. These concerns may serve as disincentives to rehabilitation.

If litigation is pending, the implications of improvement in pain and disability for the case should be explored prior to making decisions about treatment. It has been suggested that pending litigation should constitute grounds for exclusion from a rehabilitation program if the law appears to be an important factor in the promotion of continued disability. In some studies, however, litigation has not emerged as a significant predictor of outcome.

Measurement of pain by self-report

There is no "pain thermometer." Measurement of pain is dependent on patients' self-reports, or the inferences we make based on the behavior we observe. Patients can quantify their pain by providing a single, general rating of pain: "Is your usual pain 'mild,' 'moderate,' or 'severe'?" or "Rate your typical ('at its worst,' 'at its least') pain from 0 (no pain) to 10 (the worst pain you can imagine)." In these instances, the patient must quantify and average his or her pain retrospectively. Pain, however, is likely to vary over time and with different activities. In addition, ratings of "usual" pain tend to use current pain as their reference point. Thus, asking about usual or typical pain may not accurately reflect pain severity over time. More valid information may be obtained by asking about the current level of pain ("severity of pain right now"). Several simple methods can be used to evaluate current pain intensity: numeric scales, descriptive rating scales, visual analog scales, and box scales (Fig. 6.1).[17]

Pain diaries may be useful to assess the severity of pain on a regular basis rather than depending upon ret-

Table 6.2 *Entering the patient's perspective*

What do you think is wrong with you?

Why do you think your pain started when it did?

What do you think is happening to your body?

What do you think of the explanations given to you by others you have consulted?

Do you understand the explanation(s) and find it acceptable?

Do you have any fears about your pain?

What are the main problems that your pain has caused you?

What do your family, friends, and coworkers think about your pain?

Do you have any ideas or opinions on how this type of pain is treated?

What do you hope to gain from treatment?

If your pain is not entirely relieved by the treatment, what will you do?

rospective recall. For example, patients may be asked to rate their pain at the end of the day or several times a day for a period of a week or more. These diaries can also ask about other factors such as use of medication, activities, mood, and thoughts. Sophisticated technology using computers to "interview" patients about pain and related factors have recently been used.[18,19] There are advantages to computerized diaries such as reminding patients to provide measurements and preventing patients from completing "daily" diaries after a number of days. There are also disadvantages of such technology, including cost, intrusiveness, and sensitization to pain.[20,21] Daily diary ratings, whether hand written or computerized, will provide more precise information about pain severity and also about the relationship of pain to important mediators and responses to the presence of pain.

Pain has three components: sensory–discriminative, motivational–affective, and cognitive–evaluative.[22] The scales in Fig. 6.1 address only the sensory intensity component. Similar tools can be used to evaluate the motivational–affective components of pain, given that they have suitable anchors and one modifies the instructions appropriately. For example, the endpoints on the scales contained in Fig. 6.1 can be modified so that 0 indicates no distress or no unpleasantness and 10 refers to extreme or severe distress, or extreme unpleasantness.

One of the most frequently used pain assessment instruments is the McGill Pain Questionnaire (MPQ).[23] This instrument has three parts, including a descriptive scale (present pain intensity) with numbers assigned to each of five adjectives: 1 (mild), 2 (discomforting), 3 (distressing), 4 (horrible), and 5 (excruciating). The second part includes the ventral and dorsal views of a human figure upon which patients can mark the location of their pain. The third part is a pain rating index based on patient selection of adjectives from 20 categories reflecting sensory, affective, and cognitive components of pain. The MPQ provides a great deal of information but takes much longer to complete than the scales presented in Fig. 6.1. A short form of the MPQ consisting of 15 adjectives that represent sensory and affective dimensions of pain, each of which is rated from 0 (none) to 3 (severe), has been developed.[24]

Self-report of functional activities

Traditional physical and laboratory measures do not provide direct assessment of symptoms (i.e. subjective interpretations) or functional activities in everyday life, but they can be proxies. Commonly used physical tests of muscle strength and range of motion correlate poorly with actual patient behavior.[25] Similarly, radiographic indicators are only weak predictors of long-term functional capacity.[26] In contrast, self-report functional status instruments quantify symptoms, function, and behavior more directly.[27]

Several self-report measures assess a patient's ability to engage in functional activities such as walking up stairs, sitting for a specific time, lifting specific weights, performing activities of daily living, and the severity of pain during these activities. Although the validity of self-reports of ability to perform activities is questionable, studies have found good correspondence among self-reports, disease characteristics, physicians' or physical therapists' ratings of functional abilities, and objective functional performance.[28,29] Moreover, self-report instruments are economical and efficient. They enable the assessment of a wide range of relevant behaviors and permit social and mental functions to be evaluated. There are a number of brief functional assessment scales such as the Roland–Morris Disability Scale,[30] Functional Status Index,[29] and Oswestry Disability Scale.[31] The measures require no more than 5–10 min to complete. A more extensive instrument, the Sickness Impact Profile, includes over 120 questions to examine a range of physical activities and psychologic features.[32]

PSYCHOLOGIC ASSESSMENT OF PAIN PATIENTS

A number of studies have reported on the role of individual differences or personality factors in pain assessment. These factors have been shown to be of particular importance is predicting response to surgery[33] and the development of disability.[34]

A
Draw a vertical line to indicate your current level of pain:

None   Severe

B
Place an X through the box below to indicate your current level of pain:

No pain	0	1	2	3	4	5	6	7	8	9	10	Pain as bad as it can be

Figure 6.1 *Examples of pain intensity rating scales. (A) Visual analog scale; (B) box intensity scale.*

avoidance of movement, resulting in further physical deconditioning and a worsening of the pain problem, has been termed fear avoidance.[11,12] Recently, Crombez and colleagues[7] have extended the model to include specific anxiety-related beliefs about reinjury.

Figure 7.1 suggests a number of other mechanisms by which chronic pain might disrupt psychological functioning and cause further difficulties. These include the well-documented association between pain and depression[13,14] (see below), family influences on the development and maintenance of disability,[15,16] and the role of anger and frustration in the experience of chronic pain.[17] None of these factors are mutually exclusive, and a combination of several or all variables may be relevant within the one presentation.

Having set out these principal areas, we can now turn to the methods by which they are assessed. Table 7.1 lists the major assessment formats, and includes a brief description of the advantages and disadvantages associated with each method. Self-report questionnaires are the most common means of gathering information about the experience of chronic pain, and it is appropriate to reflect upon the issues of demand characteristics and response bias before reviewing the methods themselves. As noted by Williams,[18] it should not come as any surprise if a chronic pain patient, when asked to complete a number of questionnaires prior to receiving much sought-after treatment in a pain clinic, is influenced by social desirability response biases. The context in which assessment takes place should always be considered when interpreting the findings; however, it is not always clear how

that context may influence responding. For example, is a chronic pain patient who presents as a stoical "good coper" to be preferred to a patient who clearly expresses distress and the desire for help from those empowered to provide it? Following treatment, would the patient be considered "ungrateful" or "not trying hard enough" if he or she did not report improvements – irrespective of the actual outcome of the intervention? Or would the report of significant benefits prompt the patient's discharge from the clinic, leaving no hope for future treatment?

Issues such as these are of greater complexity than simply "faking good" or "faking bad," yet they are rarely addressed in the pain literature.[4] However, as clinicians, we need to be wary of overinterpreting the meaning of questionnaire scores when making judgments about patient function or experience. After all, a score on a questionnaire is nothing more than a subjective label given to an hypothetical construct – it is not a property of the individual tested.

Bearing these issues in mind, we can now examine the essential components of a comprehensive assessment battery for use in the pain clinic. As shown in Table 7.2, these assessment components can be divided into several domains, each to be considered in turn: pain quality, mood, personality, coping, pain beliefs, physical disability, family response, and health care usage. There are several "multiaxial" pain questionnaires, such as the Sickness Impact Profile,[19] the Arthritis Impact Measurement Scale,[20] and the Multidimensional Pain Inventory,[21] which assess physical, psychological, and social dimensions of pain within the one instrument. Equally, non-

Table 7.1 *Formats of assessment in chronic pain*

Method	Advantages	Disadvantages
Clinical interview (structured or semistructured)	Rich source of information; adaptable to needs/presentation of individual; multiple domains of assessment possible simultaneously (e.g. pain behaviors, communication skills)	Time-consuming; requires considerable interviewer skill in order to obtain optimal information
Self-report questionnaire	Easily and rapidly administered to large numbers; multiple measures for cross-validation possible	Potential for response bias; forced choice formats not suitable for all patients
Significant other report	Provides collaborative information about patient's physical ability and psychological status; may provide information not otherwise obtained	Potential for response bias; information will not be available for all patients
Measures of health services usage, e.g. number of GP and/or hospital visits, medication usage, receipt of disability-related income support	Objective indices of health status	Information can be time-consuming to collect; questionable applicability of information in certain cases (e.g. patients with multiple health problems)
Structured observer rating scales	Provides direct measure of patient's function; can generate clinically useful information as well as provide an index to compare post-treatment changes	Assessment must be standardized; requires training of coders and regular reviewing to prevent "observer drift"

Table 7.2 *Primary domains of psychosocial assessment in chronic pain*

Pain quality	Intensity, duration, frequency, distress, interference
Mood/affect	Depression, anxiety, anger
Personality	Stable traits associated with chronic pain
Coping skills	Cognitive and behavioral pain management strategies
Pain beliefs	Self-efficacy, catastrophizing, future health status
Physical disability	Self-reported disability, objectively tested
Family factors	Spouse responses to pain behaviors, marital satisfaction
Health care usage	Medication, clinical attendances

pain-specific general health measures, such as the SF-36[22] and the WHOQoL,[23] are becoming more commonly used with pain patients because of their potential for cross-study comparisons with other patient groups. However, these compound measures are unavoidably restricted in the domains that they can cover – and as will be seen, there are many alternative assessment options for the enthusiastic practitioner to explore.

Assessment of pain: intensity, frequency, duration

The most common methods for measuring the severity of pain are via numerical rating scales (e.g. 0–10 scale or 0–100 scale, where 0 = *no pain*, 10/100 = *pain as bad as it could be*), or visual analog scales (e.g. 10-cm line, anchored at either end by the descriptors listed above; see Chapter Ch6). These are simple to administer, readily comprehensible even for those with poor language skills, and have been shown to be sensitive to change following treatment.[24] Psychometric support for the use of visual analog scales has been demonstrated,[25] although it appears that individuals vary considerably in the processes by which they arrive at a given pain rating.[26] Verbal rating scales, in which the respondent selects an adjective to describe the intensity of his or her pain from among a set list (e.g. none–mild–moderate–severe) are not generally recommended.[25] These rating scales require a level of literacy which will exclude a proportion of patients, assume equal distance between points (words) on the scale which may be unwarranted, and force the respondent to choose from a list which may not accurately describe his or her personal experience of pain.

However, even among the more reliable and valid rating scale options, there are a number of caveats to be considered. First, as pain is not a unidimensional phenomenon, the affective component must be included in any assessment.[18] It is therefore advisable to separate the assessment of pain intensity from the assessment of pain distress. Pain effect can be measured using the visual analog or numerical rating scales described above. Second, the estimation of average pain levels is influenced by the level of pain being experienced at the time of evaluation: obtaining an estimate of present pain before rating average pain levels provides an anchor for the general estimate.[24]

Numerical rating scales and visual analog scales have the attraction of being brief and simple to complete and score. More demanding of the patient in terms of time and effort, but overcoming several of the shortcomings of these "one-off" recordings, is the use of a pain diary for example.[27] In addition to its usefulness as a more accurate representation of daily pain levels, diary monitoring can reveal relationships between pain and other variables (e.g. medication use and activity levels) which the patient may not have been aware of. Equally, the patient who rates his or her pain as "10 out of 10 at all times" when providing a "snapshot" estimation of pain may begin to see some variation when asked to perform the diary exercise over time. Twelve ratings over 4 days is sufficient to ensure that reliability in the measurement has been achieved.[24] Computerized diary formats now exist, which have the added advantage of randomly prompting for pain ratings over the course of the day.

Finally, the McGill Pain Questionnaire[28,29] is a widely used self-report measure of pain intensity which quantifies three components of pain: sensory–discriminative, motivational–affective, and cognitive–evaluative. Although it has been used in a large number of studies,[30] making cross-study comparisons possible, the three-factor structure of the questionnaire is open to debate.[5,18] The McGill Pain Questionnaire also takes longer to complete than the other scales mentioned and requires reasonably sophisticated language skills (e.g. capable of discriminating between "taut" and "rasping" descriptors). However, it has been translated into several different languages, and there is clinical utility in identifying a patient who describes his or her pain as "terrifying" or "torturing."

Ultimately, the choice of pain measure must be determined in part by the type of question that is being asked. For example, most cognitive behavioral pain management programs include a measure of average pain intensity among their outcome measures.[31] However, given that obtaining pain relief is de-emphasized as a goal in pain management programs, it is questionable whether such measures are of most value. Perhaps more useful information would be obtained from questions concerning the frequency of painful episodes (e.g. "number of flare-ups in the past 2 weeks"), the duration of the flare-ups (in hours/minutes), or an estimate of the perceived intensity of these pain increases. These outcome measures may better reflect the effective use of the coping skills taught on a self-management program.

requirements of reliability (stability over time, reproducibility by others, internal consistency) and validity (true measurement of the construct that it purports to measure). Beware the seduction of the title of the questionnaire: this confers no psychometric advantage or guarantee of validity.

- Respondent fatigue. Completing lengthy questionnaires can be laborious, particularly for pain patients whose concentration may be poor and who may have limited tolerances for sitting and/or writing. The practitioner needs to balance the desire for a comprehensive assessment with the risk of overextending patients and introducing error (missing responses, completing items semirandomly in order to finish the assessment more quickly) into the assessment.

Bearing these issues in mind, there is clearly a wealth of material to draw upon when assessing the psychosocial status of chronic pain patients. Ultimately, the clinical care that we provide to these patients is largely dependent upon an accurate, sensitive assessment of the various difficulties with which they present. As research progresses, we can look forward to even more reliable, valid, and economical methods of understanding this complex patient group.

REFERENCES

1. Skevington SM. *Psychology of Pain.* Chichester: John Wiley and Sons, 1995.
2. Williams ACdeC, Erskine A. Chronic pain. In: Broome A, Llewelyn S eds. *Health Psychology: Processes and Applications.* London: Chapman and Hall, 1995.
3. Williams ACdeC. Measures of function and psychology. In: Wall PD, Melzack R eds. *Textbook of Pain*, 4th edn. Edinburgh: Churchill Livingstone, 1999.
4. Turk DC, Melzack R. *Handbook of Pain Assessment,* 2nd edn. New York, NY: Guilford Press, 2001.
5. Karoly P, Jensen MP. *Multimethod Assessment of Chronic Pain.* New York, NY: Pergamon Press, 1987.
6. Eccleston C, Crombez G. Pain demands attention: a cognitive–affective model of the interruptive function of pain. *Psychol Bull* 1999; **125:** 356–66.
7. Crombez, G, Vlaeyen JW, Heuts PH, Lysens R. Pain-related fear is more disabling than pain itself: evidence on the role of pain-related fear in chronic back pain disability. *Pain* 1999; **80:** 329–39.
8. Morin CM, Gibson D, Wade J. Self-reported sleep and mood disturbance in chronic pain patients. *Clin J Pain* 1998; **14:** 311–14.
9. Harding VH, Williams ACdeC, Richardson PH. The development of a battery of measures for assessing physical functioning of chronic pain patients. *Pain* 1994; **58:** 367–75.
10. Bortz, WM. The disuse syndrome: a commentary. *West J Med* 1984; **141:** 691–4.
11. Letham J, Slade PD, Troup JDG, Bentley G. Outline of a fear-avoidance model of exaggerated pain perception. *Behav Res Ther* 1983; **21:** 401–8.
12. Waddell G, Newton M, Henderson I, *et al.* A Fear-Avoidance Beliefs Questionnaire (FABQ) and the role of fear-avoidance beliefs in chronic low back pain and disability. *Pain* 1993; **52:** 157–68.
13. Von Korff M, Le Resche L, Dworkin S. First onset of common pain symptoms: a prospective study of depression as a risk factor. *Pain* 1993; **55:** 251–8.
14. Turk DC, Salovey P. Chronic pain as a variant of depressive disease: a critical reappraisal. *J Nerv Ment Dis* 1984; **172:** 398–404.
15. Fordyce WE. *Behavioral Methods in Chronic Pain and Illness.* St Louis, MO: Mosby, 1976.
16. Payne B, Norfleet MA. Chronic pain and the family: a review. *Pain* 1985; **26:** 1–22.
17. Fernandez E, Turk DC. The scope and significance of anger in the experience of chronic pain. *Pain* 1995; **61:** 165–75.
18. Williams, ACdeC. Pain measurement in chronic pain management. *Pain Rev* 1995; **2:** 39–63.
19. Bergner M, Bobbitt RA, Carter WB, Gilson BS. The Sickness Impact Profile: development and final revision of a health status measure. *Med Care* 1981; **19:** 787–805.
20. Meenan RF, Gertman PM, Mason JH, Dunaif R. The Arthritis Impact Measurement Scales: further investigation of a health status measure. *Arthritis Rheum* 1982; **25:** 1048–53.
21. Kerns RD, Turk DC, Rudy TE. The West Haven–Yale Multidimensional Pain Inventory (WHYMPI). *Pain* 1985; **23:** 345–56.
22. Ware JE, Sherbourne CD. The MOS 36-item shortform health survey (SF-36). I. Conceptual framework and item selection. *Med Care* 1992; **30:** 473–83.
23. Anderson RT, Aaronson NK, Wilkin D. Critical review of the international assessments of health-related quality of life. *Quality Life Res* 1993; **2:** 369–95.
24. Jensen MP, McFarland CA. Increasing the reliability and validity of pain intensity measurement in chronic pain patients. *Pain* 1993; **55:** 195–203.
25. Jensen MP, Karoly P. Self-report scales and procedures for assessing pain in adults. In: Turk DC, Melzack R eds. *Handbook of Pain Assessment*, 2nd edn. New York, NY: Guilford Press, 2001.
26. Williams ACdeC, Davies HTO, Chadury Y. Simple pain rating scales hide complex idiosyncratic meaning. Pain 2000; **85:** 457–63.
27. Spence SH, Sharpe L, Newton-John TRO, Champion D. Effect of EMG biofeedback compared to applied relaxation training with chronic, upper extremity cumulative trauma disorders. *Pain* 1995; **63:** 199–206.
28. Melzack R. The McGill Pain Questionnaire: major properties and scoring methods. *Pain* 1975; **1:** 277–99.
29. Melzack R. The short-form McGill Pain Questionnaire. *Pain* 1987; **30:** 191–7.
30. Melzack R, Katz J. The McGill Pain Questionnaire:

appraisal and current status. In: Turk DC, Melzack R eds. *Handbook of Pain Assessment*, 2nd edn. New York, NY: Guilford Press, 2001.

31. Morley S, Eccleston C, Williams ACdeC. Systematic review and meta-analysis of randomized controlled trials of cognitive behaviour therapy and behaviour therapy for chronic pain in adults, excluding headache. *Pain* 1999; **80:** 1–13.

● 32. Gamsa A. The role of psychological factors in chronic pain. I. A half century of study. *Pain* 1994; **57:** 5–15.

33. Beck AT, Ward CH, Mendelson M, *et al*. An inventory for measuring depression. *Arch Gen Psychiatry* 1961; **4:** 561–71.

34. Beck AT, Steer RA, Garbin MG. Psychometric properties of the Beck Depression Inventory: twenty-five years of evaluation. *Clin Psychol Rev* 1988; **8:** 77–100.

35. Geisser ME, Roth RS, Robinson ME. Assessing depression among persons with chronic pain using the Center for Epidemiological Studies Depression Scale and the Beck Depression Inventory: a comparative analysis. *Clin J Pain* 1997; **13:** 163–70.

36. Zigmond AS, Snaith RP. The Hospital Anxiety and Depression Scale. *Acta Psychiatry Scand* 1983; **67:** 361–70.

37. Main CJ, Waddell G. The detection of psychological abnormality using four simple scales. *Curr Concepts Pain* 1984; **2:** 10–15.

38. Spielberger CD. *Manual for the State–Trait Anxiety Inventory (Form 1)*. Palo Alto, CA: Consulting Psychologists Press, 1983.

39. McCraken LM, Zayfert C, Gross RT. The Pain Anxiety Symptoms Scale: development and validation of a scale to measure fear of pain. *Pain* 1992; **50:** 67–73.

40. McNeil DW, Rainwater AJ. Development of the Fear of Pain Questionnaire – III. *J Behav Med* 1998; **21:** 389–410.

41. Zvolensky MJ, Goodie JL, McNeil DW, *et al*. Anxiety sensitivity in the prediction of pain-related fear and anxiety in a heterogeneous chronic pain population. *Behav Res Ther* 2001; **39:** 683–96.

42. Vlaeyen JW, Kole-Snijders AMJ, Boeren RGB, van Eek H. Fear of movement/(re)injury in chronic low back pain and its relation to behavioral performance. *Pain* 1995; **62:** 363–72.

43. Jensen MP, Karoly P, Huger R. The development and preliminary validation of an instrument to assess patients' attitudes towards pain. *J Psychosom Res* 1987; **31:** 393–400.

44. Tait RC, Chibnall JT. Development of a brief version of the Survey of Pain Attitudes. *Pain* 1997; **70:** 229–35.

45. Burns JW, Johnson BJ, Devine J, *et al*. Anger management style and the prediction of treatment outcome among male and female chronic pain patients. *Behav Res Ther* 1998; **36:** 1051–62.

46. Spielberger CD. *State–Trait Anger Expression Inventory Professional Manual*. Odessa, FL: Psychological Assessment Resources, 1988.

47. Siegel JM. The Multidimensional Anger Inventory. *J Pers Soc Psychol* 1986; **51:** 191–200.

48. Watson D. Neurotic tendencies among chronic pain patients: an MMPI item analysis. *Pain* 1982; **14:** 365–85.

49. Derogatis LR. *SCL-R90*. Towson, MD: Clinical Psychometric Research, 1977.

50. Hampson S. State of the art: personality. *Psychologist* 1999; **12:** 284–88.

51. Block J. A contrarian view of the five-factor approach to personality description. *Psychol Bull* 1995; **117:** 187–215.

● 52. Jensen MP, Turner JA, Romano JM, Karoly P. Coping with chronic pain: a critical review of the literature. *Pain* 1991; **47:** 249–83.

53. Lazarus RA, Folkman S. *Stress, Appraisal and Coping*. New York, NY: Springer Press, 1984.

54. Brown GK, Nicassio PM. Development of a questionnaire for the assessment of active and passive coping strategies in chronic pain patients. *Pain* 1987; **31:** 53–64.

55. Rotter JB. Generalised expectancies for internal versus external locus of control. *Psychol Monogr* 1966; **80:** 1–28.

56. Rosensteil AK, Keefe FJ. The use of coping strategies in low back pain patients: relationship to patient characteristics and current adjustment. *Pain* 1983; **17:** 33–40.

57. Vitaliano PP, Russo J, Carr JE, *et al*. The Ways of Coping Checklist: revision and psychometric properties. *Multivariate Behav Res* 1985; **20:** 3–26.

58. Coughlan GM, Ridout KL, Williams AC de C, Richardson PH. Attrition from a pain management programme. *Br J Clin Psychol* 1995; **34:** 471–9.

59. Nicholas MK. The Pain Self-Efficacy Questionnaire: self-efficacy in relation to chronic pain. In: *Proceedings of the British Psychological Society Annual Conference*, April 1989, St Andrews. Leicester: British Psychological Society.

60. Kerns RD, Rosenberg R, Jamison RN, *et al*. Readiness to adopt a self-management approach to chronic pain: the Pain Stages of Change Questionnaire. *Pain* 1997; **72:** 227–34.

61. Jensen MP, Nielsen WR, Romano JM, *et al*. Further evaluation of the pain stages of change questionnaire: is the transtheoretical model of change useful for patients with chronic pain? *Pain* 2000; **86:** 255–64.

62. Waddell G, Somerville D, Henderson I, Newton M. Objective clinical evaluation of physical impairment in chronic low back pain. *Spine* 1992; **17:** 617–28.

63. Pollard CA. Preliminary validation study of the Pain Disability Index. *Percept Motor Skills* 1984; **59:** 974.

64. Tait RC, Chibnall JT, Krause S. The Pain Disability Index: psychometric properties. *Pain* 1990; **40:** 171–82.

65. Fairbanks JCT, Davies JB, Couper J, O'Brien JP. The Oswestry low back pain disability questionnaire. *Physiotherapy* 1980; **66:** 271–3.

66. Roland M, Morris R. A study of the natural history of back pain. Part I. Development of a reliable and sensitive measure of disability in low back pain. *Spine* 1983; **8:** 141–4.

67. Lousberg R, Schmidt AJM, Groenman NH. The relationship between spouse solicitousness and pain behavior: searching for more experimental evidence. *Pain* 1992; **51:** 75–9.

◆ 68. Romano JM, Turner JA, Jensen MP, *et al.* Chronic pain patient–spouse behavioral interactions predict patient disability. *Pain* 1995; **63:** 353–60.

69. Newton-John TRO. Responding to pain behaviours: when helping does not help. In: Gifford L ed. *Topical Issues in Pain*. Cornwall: CNS Press, 2000: 165–75.

70. Kerns RD, Rosenberg R. Pain-relevant responses from significant others: development of a significant-other version of the WHYMPI scales. *Pain* 1995; **61:** 245–9.

71. Roy R. The interactional perspective of pain behavior in marriage. *Int J Fam Ther* 1985; **7:** 271–83.

72. Romano JM, Turner JA, Friedman LS, *et al.* Observational assessment of chronic pain patient–spouse behavioral interactions. *Behav Ther* 1991; **22:** 549–67.

73. Locke HJ, Wallace KM. Short marital adjustment and prediction tests: their reliability and validity. *Marriage Fam Living* 1959; **21:** 251–5.

74. Spanier GB. Measuring dyadic adjustment: new scales for assessing the quality of marriage and similar dyads. *J Marriage Fam* 1976; **38:** 15–28.

75. Moos R, Moos B. *Family Environment Scale Manual*. Palo Alto, CA: Consulting Psychologists Press, 1981.

8

Assessment of neuropathic pain

TROELS S JENSEN AND HANNE GOTTRUP

Normally, the pain system has an important protective role by alerting the individual to the threat of tissue damage. Following disruption of the somatosensory system the expected result is loss of sensation and analgesia in the involved area.[1-5] On rare occasions, however, this loss of sensation presents itself with a paradox: pain in the hypoesthetic area. This type of pain, termed neuropathic pain, is important for several reasons: the pain is severe, it is long-lasting, and it is often resistant to treatment with current analgesics. In addition – as discussed in more detail below – neuropathic pains may be difficult to diagnose, with a risk of both false-positive and false-negative diagnoses.

Neuropathic pain is not a single entity; it includes heterogeneous conditions that differ not only in etiology but also in location.[6-8] Disorders such as diabetes, immune deficiencies, and malignant, traumatic and ischemic conditions may all give rise to the same type of pain. The anatomical sites of lesions causing neuropathic pain are multiple: they can be located at any level from the peripheral receptor to the highest cortical centers, the most common being peripheral nerves, major nerve plexuses, dorsal nerve roots, spinal cord, and the thalamus.[1,3,4] In spite of the diverse etiology and topography, the clinical picture is in many cases surprisingly similar, suggesting that these disorders share common mechanisms.[3,9]

Recent studies have shown a cascade of temporally related biological changes following damage to the nervous system, which eventually results in a sensitization of neural elements involved in the processing of noxious information.[5,8-13] Although the significance of these molecular changes following nerve damage is still being explored, they may represent a link between different neuropathic conditions. Hence, understanding of the dynamic events following nerve damage may be key to understanding this hyperexcitability and how to treat it.

A major contribution to this new information has been the demonstration of changes in the nervous system following sustained noxious input, which is different from the normal processing of noxious information. This plasticity of the nervous system is displayed at many levels of the neuraxis from the peripheral nociceptor to the spinal cord and even to the cortex of the brain.[5,8,15,16] This chapter reviews the etiology of the symptoms of neuropathic pain conditions and examines how these conditions can be diagnosed both at the bedside and in the laboratory using more sophisticated experimental techniques.

In the evaluation of a patient with a suspected neuropathic pain disorder it is important to assess and classify the condition on the basis of the underlying disorder, the anatomical location, the characteristics of the pain, the pain intensity, the associated features, and the possible mechanisms involved. It is important to emphasize that the evaluation of neuropathic pain is often complicated, time-consuming, and may require the use of laboratory techniques.[17-19]

CLASSIFICATION OF NEUROPATHIC PAIN

Neuropathic pain has usually been classified on the basis of the underlying etiology, e.g. peripheral diabetic neuropathy, nerve damage due to injury, spinal or brain lesions following infarction, or multiple sclerotic plaques. At other times, the pain is defined on the basis of the location of the lesion: is the lesion in the peripheral nerves, in the spinal roots, in the spinal cord, or in the brain? Table 8.1 presents a commonly used scheme for classifying neuropathic pain on the basis of either etiology or anatomy. More recently, a mechanism-based classification has been suggested by Woolf *et al.*[8] In this latter case an attempt has been made to elucidate the various mechanisms that may be involved in the particular pain felt by a patient and link such a mechanism to a rational type of treatment. It is beyond the scope of this chapter to present a detailed description of current mechanisms, some of which are still hypothetical.[5,11–13] Briefly, however, these mechanisms include:

a   Pathological activity or sensitized nociceptors with recruitment of silent nociceptors and ectopic activity in spinal ganglion cells. The increased afferent neuronal barrage causes sensitization of the dorsal horn neurons.
b   A severe loss of small fiber input may also give rise to central sensitization due to a spinal reorganization from sprouting of large myelinated fibers into superficial "nociceptive" laminae in the dorsal horn.
c   Inflammation along nerve trunks, producing ectopic activity and therefore representing a source for central sensitization.
d   Increased sympathetic activity, producing further sensitization of nociceptors.
e   Altered brain processing due to plastic changes with recruitment of new brain areas not usually involved in pain. This may lead to changed modulation of input.

Because of the intimate connection between the periphery and the central parts, and because of the considerable plasticity in the nociceptive system, different mechanisms may be involved in each patient and one mechanism may account for several etiologically different conditions and be the source of different symptoms. For example, a diabetic patient may have steady pain, touch-evoked pain, paroxysms, and nonpainful paresthesiae. In these cases several mechanisms can be involved, such as tissue injury due to ischemia, sensitization of peripheral receptors, ectopic activity in sprouting regenerating fibers, phenotypic changes in dorsal root ganglion (DRG) cells, and spinal reorganization.[1–5,10,14,17–21] An additional approach to classifying pain involves the use of specific pharmacological agents.[6–7,19] Although a mechanism-based classification is an attractive approach, it is not known at present whether this provides a better method for classifying neuropathic pain. However, it will be of interest to determine the possible additional clarification provided by a hierarchical structured system that classifies pain on the basis of: (1) symptoms, (2) symptoms plus signs, (3) symptoms plus signs plus mechanisms, and (4) symptoms plus signs plus mechanisms plus pharmacological analysis. Such studies are currently under way.

ONGOING AND EVOKED PAIN

From a clinical point of view, it is often helpful to distinguish between stimulus-independent and stimulus-dependent types of pains (Table 8.2).

Stimulus-independent pain

These pains are spontaneous and may be continuous or paroxysmal. Their character differs, but can be shooting, shock-like, aching, cramping, crushing, smarting, burning, etc. Episodic, paroxysmal types of pain are brief and shooting, electric, shock-like, or stabbing in their character. In its most typical form paroxysmal pain is seen in tic douloureux, in entrapment neuropathies, in amputees, and in luetic diseases. For example, in tabes dorsalis, shooting pains are described often in the form of transverse lightning pains in the legs and are provoked by emotional stress. Shooting pains can also occur in cases with a nerve compression (e.g. slipped disk, vertebral compression, neoplastic nerve compression, and entrapment syndromes).[4,22]

The mechanism underlying these pains is assumed to reflect an increased discharge in sensitized C-nociceptors, but occasionally the pains may reflect increased activity in sensitized receptors associated with large myelinated A-fibers, giving a sensation of burning or dysesthesia.[23]

Table 8.1 *Classification of neuropathic pain according to location and cause*

Peripheral	Spinal	Brain
Neuropathies	Multiple sclerosis	Stroke
Herpes zoster	Spinal cord injury	Multiple sclerosis
Nerve injuries	Arachnoiditis	Neoplasms
Amputations	Neoplasms	Syringomyelia
Plexopathies	Syringomyelia	Parkinson's disease?
Radiculopathies	Spinal stroke	Epilepsy?
Avulsions		
Neoplasms		
Trigeminal neuralgia		

Table 8.2 *Recording of various parameters in neuropathic pain*

Stimulus independent	Stimulus dependent
Pain character	Stimulus type(s)
Pain duration	Pain character
Pain intensity of different pain types	Pain intensity evoked by different stimuli
Pain unpleasantness	Pain radiation
Pain radiation	Pain aftersensation
Pain distribution	Pain summation
Pain area	Pain area

Stimulus-dependent pains

Stimulus-evoked pains are classified according to the stimulus type that provokes them: mechanical, thermal, or chemical.[1,10,14,17–19,24,25]

In some patients several of these phenomena may be present, whereas in others only one type of hyperalgesia is present. For example, patients with nerve injury pain or amputation may have trigger points to mechanical stimuli, but with entirely normal thermal sensation. In some patients with neuropathy, cold allodynia may be the only abnormality present. Therefore, a series of stimuli have to be used to document or exclude abnormality. The evoked pains are usually brief, lasting only for the period of stimulation, but sometimes they can persist even after cessation of stimulation, causing aftersensations (see below), which can last for hours. In such cases distinction between evoked and spontaneous types of pain can be difficult.

FINDINGS IN NEUROPATHIC PAIN

Sensory deficit and pain

An essential part of neuropathic pain is a loss (partial or complete) of afferent sensory function and the paradoxical presence of certain hyperphenomena (see below) in the painful area. In some patients the sensory deficit may be gross, whereas in others it may be subtle and difficult to detect with bedside methods, but quantitative measures can usually reveal minor changes.[19,26,27] The sensory loss may involve all sensory abnormalities, but a loss of spinothalamic functions (cold, warmth, pinprick) appears to be crucial and the possibility that such spinothalamic loss is a requirement has been raised.[28] For example, in poststroke pain, large-scale studies have suggested that sensory deficit is a necessary, albeit insufficient, condition for the occurrence of pain.[29,30] In central pain due to spinal cord injury, recent studies indicate that sensory loss and areas with hypersensitivity are also characteristic features. It remains to be seen whether similar patterns also occur in other neuropathic pain states.

Allodynia and hyperalgesia

Hyperalgesia (the lowering of the pain threshold and an increased response to noxious stimuli) and allodynia (the evocation of pain by non-noxious stimuli) are typical elements of neuropathic pain. Three types of mechanical hyperalgesia can be distinguished:

- Static hyperalgesia: gentle pressure on skin evokes pain.
- Punctate hyperalgesia: punctate stimuli such as pinprick-evoked pain.

- Dynamic hyperalgesia: light brush evokes a sensation of pain.

For thermal stimuli, both cold and heat can evoke abnormal pain:

- Cold hyperalgesia: cold stimuli evoke a sensation of pain (the underlying mechanism is unclear, but cortical reorganization due to a loss of cold Aδ-fibers is one possibility).
- Heat hyperalgesia: warm and heat stimuli evoke pain (sensitization of C-nociceptors and a corresponding sensitization of second-order neurons).

The dynamic mechanical-type allodynia is mediated by Aβ-fibers, whereas the static high-threshold type of hyperalgesia, which is evoked by blunt pressure, appears to be mediated by sensitized C-nociceptors.[31,32] The static type of hyperalgesia would also be expected to be associated with thermal hyperalgesia, however this is not always the case.[26] Punctate hyperalgesia evoked by pinprick, usually a stiff von Frey hair, is mediated by sensitized Aδ-nociceptors. While certain types of hyperalgesia reflect sensitization of receptors, allodynia is always a central phenomenon mediated by large myelinated fibers.[18]

Allodynia is considered to be exclusively a cutaneous disorder, but recent findings suggest that it can be a manifestation of deep tissue pathology. For example, in poststroke pain, which is a central neuropathic disorder, deep pain may be associated with a lowering of pain threshold to mechanical pressure and with an exaggerated response to a challenge of i.m. 0.5-ml 9% hypertonic saline into the painful deep tissue (unpublished observations). In patients with sciatica or Guillain–Barré syndrome, proximal limb pain is often accompanied by soreness on palpation. Allodynia can usually be separated from the tenderness seen in musculoskeletal pain conditions. In patients with allodynia, a firm pressure in the allodynic area can sometimes relieve their pain. These findings indicate that at the receptor level separate mechanisms are involved, e.g. touch allodynia is elicited by rapidly adapting mechanoreceptors, while the pressure-induced pain relief may be related to the recruitment of slowly adapting mechanoreceptors in addition to other deeply located receptors.

When present, allodynia or hyperalgesia can be quantified by measuring intensity, threshold for elicitation, duration, and area of allodynia.[33] The evocation of pain by a stimulus implies that a complete abolition of afferent information does not give rise to allodynia. Nevertheless, on occasions, in spite of a complete injury, abnormal sensations may develop subsequently and present as anesthesia dolorosa in the deafferented body part. This phenomenon can probably be ascribed to spontaneous firing in nerve sprouts, to alteration in peripheral innervation territory, to an expansion of receptive fields of sensitized central neurons that have lost their normal innervation, or to a combination of such mechanisms. Hyperalgesia can be provoked in normal subjects following blockade of large-diameter afferent fibers. Pinprick or cold is now perceived as burning or squeezing pain, suggesting that afferent fibers under normal conditions exert an inhibitory input on dorsal horn neuronal activity. In neuropathic pain, this inhibition may be disrupted. The chemical mediators of this inhibition are unknown, but γ-aminobutyric acid (GABA) and glycine are likely candidates.

Hyperpathia

Hyperpathia is a variant of hyperalgesia and allodynia and is the archetypal disorder in neuropathic pain whenever there is axonal loss. In these cases, an explosive pain response is suddenly evoked from cutaneous areas with an increased sensory detection threshold when the stimulus intensity exceeds that sensory threshold.[3,18,27] Hyperpathia is a reflection of peripheral or central deafferentation leading to an elevation of threshold on one hand and a central hyperexcitability on the other as a result of lost or abnormal input from afferents.

Paroxysms

Distinct from the above types of evoked pain, some patients complain of shooting, electric, shock-like, or stabbing pain that occurs spontaneously or, more often, following stimulation. These types of pain are termed paroxysms and can be elicited by an innocuous tactile stimulus or by blunt pressure. In their most typical form, paroxysms are seen in tic douloureux, where they dominate the clinical picture; it is characteristic that non-noxious tactile inputs elicit these paroxysms, while noxious stimuli fail to do so.

Paresthesiae

Paresthesiae are abnormal but nonpainful sensations which can be spontaneous or evoked. They are often described as "pins and needles" and are assumed to reflect spontaneous bursts of activity in Aβ-fibers.

Dysesthesiae

Dysesthesiae are abnormal, unpleasant, but not necessarily painful sensations, which can be spontaneous or provoked by external stimuli. These are probably due to sensitization of the C-nociceptors and it is unlikely that there is any qualitative difference between evoked dysesthesiae and evoked hyperalgesia.

Referred pain and abnormal pain radiation

In neuropathic pain, an abnormal spread of pain can be seen following both peripheral and central lesions. In painful myelopathic disorders patients may experience a circular spreading sensation following single punctate stimulation, with a relationship between the spread of the pain and the intensity of the perceived pain. Similarly, there is a relationship between the magnitude of deep muscle pain and the area of referred cutaneous pain from such deep structures.[34-37] While referral generally is described from deep to cutaneous structures, the reverse is far less common. Referral can be seen following skin sensitization, e.g. in capsaicin-induced hyperalgesia.[38] There is a link between pain intensity, pain radiation, and pain referral. The magnitude of pain from, for example, deep tissue is proportional to the extent of referral in cutaneous tissue both experimentally and clinically.[34,37] Similarly, in experimental pain induced by intradermal capsaicin the spread increases with increasing pain intensity.[39]

Experimental studies in humans and animals[40] have shown that such abnormal radiation may be related to changes in spinal wide dynamic range (WDR) neurons encoding noxious information. WDR cells are in part characterized by small receptive zones that can be excited by non-noxious stimuli (touch, gentle pressure) surrounded by a much larger zone from which noxious stimuli (pinch, firm pressure, temperature > 45°C) can evoke neuronal discharges. These large receptive field zones are overlapping, extend over several dermatomes, and their receptive fields are a reflection of synaptic propriospinal interconnections in the spinal dorsal horn that extend over several segments. Therefore, a noxious stimulus will in contrast to a non-noxious stimulus activate several WDR neurons, and increasing the stimulus intensity will result in activation of further WDR neurons in a rostrocaudal distribution manner. Since increasing stimulus intensity has the effect of recruiting more dorsal horn neurons, the degree of radiation and referral is likely to be a reflection of a progressive recruitment of WDR neurons spreading along the spinal cord. A similar mechanism may be involved in the sensory abnormalities seen in patients with nerve injury and in the extensive spread of sensory dysfunction to the contralateral side as well as proximally and distally to the lesion.

Windup-like pain and aftersensations

Windup-like pain, or abnormal temporal summation, is the clinical equivalent to increasing neuronal activity following repetitive C-fiber stimulation of more than 0.3 Hz.[41,42] In humans, such pains may be evoked by either repetitive noxious or non-noxious stimulation from normal or hyperalgesic cutaneous areas respectively. When repetitive low-threshold stimuli, which exclusively activate Aβ-fibers, are applied at intervals of less than 3 s, they give rise to pain, which means that these stimuli have gained access to central windup mechanisms that are normally reserved for nociceptors and C-fiber input. The windup-like pain can be produced by a variety of stimuli, including mechanical, thermal, and electrical types, and can be elicited not only from skin but also from other tissues, e.g. muscle.[42] It is now clear that abnormal temporal summation with windup-like phenomena is a characteristic feature of many chronic pain conditions, including neuropathic pain,[14,22,30,43–45] and that this can blocked or attenuated by compounds that affect windup.[46–51] Aftersensations – the persistence of pain long after termination of a painful stimulus – are another characteristic feature of neuropathic pain[27] and correlate with existing evoked pain; aftersensations are, therefore, possibly mediated by the same mechanisms (unpublished observations). Because of the relationship between windup-like pain and aftersensations, it is thought that both of these phenomena may reflect neuronal discharges in WDR neurons.

ASSESSMENT OF NEUROPATHIC PAIN

History

The examination of a patient with suspected neuropathic pain begins with taking the history. Patients may describe their pains in a variety of ways: they may complain of unpleasant pricking or sticking sensations in parts of the body. They may have a burning, scalding, aching, or deep sore pain. A characteristic in many neuropathic pain conditions is the presence of allodynia following exposure to nonpainful cold. In such cases, patients may describe their pain in a paradoxical manner as burning hot or ice-burning or as if holding a snowball in the hand. Some patients with central pain complain of pain evoked by movement in which the movement itself elicits a tightening, squeezing, or burning sensation in the skin. At other times the pain is one of paroxysms with stabbing, shooting, lancinating types of pain. Paroxysms last seconds, but can be repeated with ultrashort intervals, giving a false impression of continuous types of pains.

An important point concerns the possible classification of pain just on the basis of symptoms. While there are no data supporting this view, Galer and Jensen[52] have presented a neuropathic pain scale in which presumed common symptoms encountered in neuropathic pain are recorded and scored as: intense, sharp, hot, dull, cold, or itchy skin sensitivity. While this test has shown validity in normal volunteers and in response to treatment it remains to be seen whether it can distinguish neuropathic pain patients from other chronic pain patients.

Distribution of sensory abnormalities on a map

Plotting the distribution of various types of pain on a template body map is an important initial step in pain assessment. The area in which pain is felt can be quantified and any temporal variation in the size of that area over time as a result of, for example, therapy or the natural history of the disease can be measured. Such procedures are useful, e.g. when recording the effects of drugs. Automatic drawing systems have been proposed, which may be of value for more accurate measurements.

Clinical examination

All patients should be subjected to a general physical and neurological examination. Sensory abnormalities can be specifically assessed and quantified using simple bedside equipment (Fig. 8.1). The sensory modalities tested most commonly at the bedside include pinprick, touch, cold, heat, and vibration sensation. Pinprick sensation is assessed by the response to pinprick stimuli. Touch is examined by gently touching the involved skin area with a cotton swab – it is important to distinguish between dynamic stimuli in which the area is stroked and a static stimulus in which the skin is exposed to a static, i.e. a nondynamic, stimulus. Cold and warm sensations are recorded by measuring the response to a specific cold or warm thermal stimulus, e.g. thermorollers maintained at 20°C and 40°C respectively. Cold sensation can also be assessed by the response to a drop of acetone on the skin. Vibration is assessed by a tuning fork placed at strategic points (malleol, interphalangeal joints, etc.). At present there is no consensus about the site where such activity should be measured, but it is generally agreed that this is best performed in the area with maximal abnormality using the contralateral area as control. However, this needs to be qualified by understanding that some studies have described contralateral segmental sensory abnormalities following a unilateral nerve or root lesion. An examination of the mirror image area of a nerve injury may therefore not represent a true control, but without a body of validated "normal values" for the various psychophysical modalities this appears to be the best option at present. For all types of stimuli, the response can be graded simply as:[53]

- normal;
- decreased;
- increased.

If the response is hyperesthetic, it is classified as dysesthetic, hyperalgesic, or allodynic. A correlation between spontaneous pain and sensory response in the painful area suggests that the two phenomena are reflections of the same cause: a central sensitization of dorsal horn neurons.[23,31]

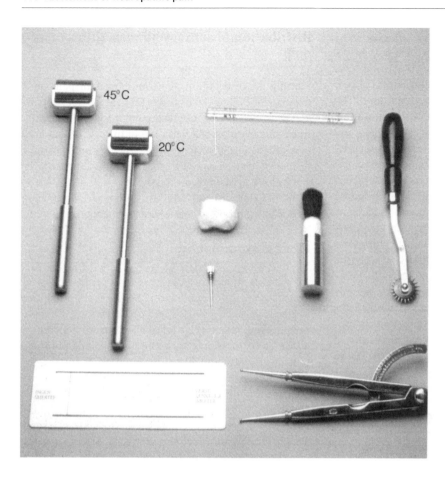

Figure 8.1 *Bedside equipment for analyzing sensory function in humans: metal thermorollers (kept at specific temperatures), von Frey hair, cotton wool, brush, pinprick roller, two-point discriminator, and a visual analog scale (VAS) meter.*

An essential point concerns the detailed description of what the sensory abnormalities reflect: does the distribution correspond to the innervation territory of a sensory nerve, to fascicles, to roots, to cord segment, or to a cerebral structure? This is not always an easy task and may require detailed neurological knowledge. However, this is important because a distinction has to be made between the sensory abnormalities seen in, for example, somatization disorders and those seen in diseases of the nerves or central nervous system (CNS).

LABORATORY AND EXPERIMENTAL EXAMINATION

More detailed and accurate testing can be carried out using various methods. These include mechanical, thermal, and chemical tools, and the practical aspects of these methods of quantitative sensory testing are discussed by Jorum and Arendt-Nielsen in Chapter P3.

Mechanical stimuli

The standard tools for mechanical testing in the experimental laboratory are von Frey hairs and blunt pres-

sure. von Frey hairs bend at different forces, permitting both a stimulus-dependent (threshold to detection and threshold to pain perception) and a response-dependent (evoked sensation to a particular stimulus) pain assessment. This can be performed for single and for repetitive pinprick stimuli. For a dynamic brush, camel hair paintbrushes can be used.

Determination of the area of abnormality may also be a useful outcome measure because such an area of cutaneous abnormality probably reflects the expansion of receptive fields of sensitized dorsal horn neurons.[1,22]

Thermal stimuli

Thermal testing is often carried out using probes or thermodes and several instruments are commercially available. Lasers, with argon or CO_2 stimuli, have also been used. The size and duration of the thermal stimulus seem to be important because temporal and spatial summation is pronounced for C-fibers, but is only weak for Aδ-fibers. While short-lasting heat stimuli on small areas normally evoke a pinprick sensation (indicating Aδ-fiber activation), heat stimuli of long duration on larger areas give rise to a burning sensation (indicating C-fiber activation). To what extent this observation is also present in neuropathic skin is unclear.

Chemical stimuli

Chemical stimuli can be used to determine the threshold of the evoked response. Capsaicin, applied either topically or intradermally, has been widely used in normal volunteers to show that an area of primary and secondary hyperalgesia develops as a result of an explosive discharge from activated C-nociceptors.[24,39,54–56] A similar approach has been used in patients with postherpetic neuralgia to test C-fiber activity and to assess the degree of surviving sensitized C-nociceptors compared with the degree of deafferentation.[57] It remains to be seen whether this technique can differentiate between peripheral and central sensitization.

A characteristic and central feature in many patients with neuropathic pain is a paradoxical sensibility, with an increased detection threshold to cold/heat and a reduced pain threshold to the same stimuli. Such a response pattern reflects both a loss of afferent fibers/disturbance of central pathways and a sensitization of peripheral receptors/central neurons along the somatosensory pathway.[1,3,4,17–19,26,58–63]

Alterations in the spatial and temporal characteristics of these stimuli may add another dimension to the pain experience, e.g. the presence of spatial and temporal summation. In addition to the above measures, various physiological correlates can be used in the analysis of neuropathic pain. These include microneurographic recordings, electromyogram (EMG) activity, brain imaging techniques, evoked potentials, and measurement of "pain substances" in body fluids. There is at present insufficient information to determine the most useful pain correlate, but in time it is possible that some of these experimental techniques may be added to the portfolio of measures used in the routine clinical assessment of neuropathic pain and may even permit a further elucidation of the underlying mechanisms in neuropathic pain.

For sensory modality (mechanical, thermal, chemical, electrical), it is possible to determine threshold, summation threshold, response function, and area of abnormality (Table 8.3).

Assessment of sympathetic activity

Sympathetic hyperactivity may be present in some peripheral neuropathic pain states as part of complex regional pain syndrome (CRPS; formerly known as causalgia or reflex sympathetic dystrophy) type I or type II. The clinical aspects of sympathetic hyperactivity include a perception of burning-type pain immediately (hours or days) after injury together with the demonstration of swelling, smooth glossy skin, and vasomotor instability. Later, a characteristic localized osteoporosis can be observed in the hands and fingers (Sudeck's atrophy). These features may exist alone or in combination. Sweating may be affected, producing either wet or dry skin. Similarly, the skin may be cooler or warmer, depending on the degree of cutaneous vasoconstriction. In patients suspected of sympathetic dysfunction, tests can be useful to document the degree of sympathetic involvement. These include sweat testing, galvanic skin resistance, plethysmography, skin blood flow measurement (laser Doppler test, thermography), and cutaneous histamine response. Diagnostic sympathetic blocks may also be used to determine the possible involvement of the sympathetic nervous system in a particular pain condition.[63] There is at present no single test that can be used to exclude sympathetically maintained pain and there are no known symptoms that predict it.[60]

OUTCOME MEASURES

In the evaluation of a pharmacological or nonpharmacological intervention, therapeutic success is often equated with pain reduction. As a result, many clinicians limit themselves to the measurement of pain and pain relief, thereby overlooking other important aspects of the therapeutic outcome, such as functional improvement or improvement in quality of life. In order to assess mechanisms it is important that the measures used in experimental research reflect the pain measures used in humans.[64,65] These are discussed in more detail in other chapters, and only the elements immediately relevant to

Table 8.3 *Stimulus and response measures in neuropathic pain patients*

Stimulus modality	Threshold	Summation	Stimulus response	Area of abnormality
Touch	Detection	Touch-evoked allodynia	+	+
von Frey hair	Detection Pain	Repetitive stimulation > 2 Hz	+	+
Thermal	Detection Pain	Repetitive stimulation	+	+
Mechanical pressure	Pain	Repetitive stimulation	+	+
Capsaicin	Pain	Repetitive stimulation	+	+
Electrical stimuli	Detection Pain	Repetitive stimulation	+	+ (Referred pain)

the patient suffering from neuropathic pain will be discussed here.

Clinical pain measures

These can be divided into the recording of spontaneous ongoing pain and that of evoked pain. For this purpose, visual analog scaling as well as multidimensional descriptor (e.g. the McGill Pain Questionnaire) and cross-modality matching scales have been used. In certain pain conditions, for example neuropathic pain, it may also be important to assess specific measures, e.g. aftersensations, windup-like pain, radiation, and area of allodynia to specific stimuli. Recording of pain intensity is still the most frequently assessed dimension of therapeutic outcome The visual analog scale (VAS), verbal category scales, and numerical rating scales are the most commonly used scales. An example of a numerical rating scale is the 11-point Lickert rating scale, whereby the subject is asked to rate his pain by giving a number between "0" (no pain) and "10" (most intense pain). A widely used category scale is the four-point intensity scale (none, mild, moderate, and severe pain). However, this scale usually does not have enough levels to describe accurately the effects of treatment. Improved category scales with more descriptors are available. In many clinical pain conditions, pain intensity fluctuates over time. In these cases it may be necessary to rate the percentage of time that the patient's pain falls within certain intensity categories. A slightly different approach has been taken in the Brief Pain Inventory of Wisconsin (BPI), which involves measurement of the pain intensity when it is at its worst, when it is at its least, and the average pain intensity.

A unidimensional recording of pain intensity or pain relief may overlook other important aspects of a therapeutic outcome, such as functional improvement or improvement in quality of life. It is also possible that certain therapies can reduce pain intensity, while their associated side-effects result in a diminished quality of life. If pain intensity or relief measures are used in isolation in this situation, then a falsely optimistic view of the effect of that therapy may be formed by the clinician.

In neuropathic pain it is not sufficient to record one single pain condition; the various other neuropathic phenomena such as paroxysms, spontaneous ongoing pain, touch-evoked pain, and cold allodynia are equally important. Each pain component in a particular neuropathic pain condition may have its own magnitude and each may be influenced separately by a particular drug.

Whereas pain intensity scales focus on the present pain experience, pain relief scores rely on the patient's memory of pain. Since patients tend to overestimate their past pain, the use of pain relief scores may lead to an overestimation of the effects of the treatment, certainly in cases of prolonged follow-up. On the other hand, it has been suggested that pain relief category scales are more sensitive to small reductions in pain. A neuropathic pain scale has recently been introduced and validated.[52] It remains to be seen whether this scale offers any additional value in neuropathic pain assessment and in measuring outcome.

Assessment of quality of life and health status

An increasing number of clinical trials include measures of quality of life in the evaluation of the treatment of chronic pain. These measures have become an important indicator of treatment "success." Among the measures of quality of life, the Sickness Impact Profile (SIP), the SIP Roland, the West Haven–Yale Multidimensional Pain Inventory, the Nottingham Health Profile, and the SF-36 have been validated (for further details of pain measures, see Chapter P1).

Treatment as a tool to assess neuropathic pain

Specific treatments have been designed and tried for different pain conditions, including neuropathic pain. They will be described in detail in other chapters. These treatments, which currently include tricyclic antidepressants, sodium channel blockers (such as carbamazepine and lamotrigine), gabapentin, opioids, and N-methyl-D-aspartate (NMDA) channel blockers among others, all have specific targets for their mode of action. It has been suggested that this may help to unravel the mechanisms of neuropathic pain based on the specific action of these drugs. Previous studies have shown that such drugs may have an action not only on pain intensity but also on specific aspects of pain, such as evoked pain. Studies have shown that in patients with neuropathic pain due to nerve injury and amputation NMDA receptor antagonists can block both pain and evoked pain produced by touch stimuli, indicating that these phenomena are probably produced by the same mechanism, i.e. a central sensitization mediated by excess activity at NMDA receptor channels. An additional example would be the joint blockade of pain by sodium channel-blocking agents and NMDA receptor-blocking drugs, suggesting that at least two different mechanisms may operate in concert.

The introduction of the concept of "number needed to treat" (NNT) from systematic reviews has made it possible to compare the efficacy (NNT) and side-effect profile (NNH; number needed to harm) for a particular therapy in different pain conditions,[66] and thus to determine whether a drug with a known mechanism of action is effective in specific neuropathic pain conditions. In theory, this could enable the determination of the pain mechanisms involved for certain types of neuropathic pains. The same principle could also be applied using separate drugs for the same pathological condition to determine whether distinct or identical mechanisms may be in operation.[6,7] However, at present, this principle has not yet been applied, partly because of the crude measures that are used for quantifying efficacy in chronic pain, i.e. global pain intensity or global pain relief.

Chronic low back pain

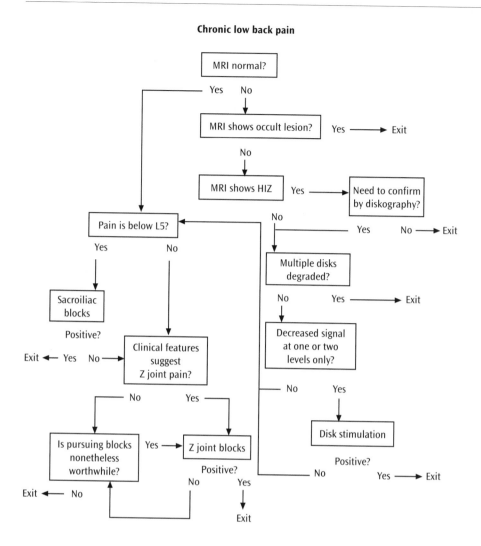

Figure 9.3 *An algorithm for the investigation of back pain, using diagnostic blocks. Z joint, zygapophysial joint; MRI, magnetic resonance imaging; HIZ, high-intensity zone.*

are more appropriate if the subsequent treatment is to be radiofrequency neurotomy. In that event, medial branch blocks are not only diagnostic but also prognostic.

Blocks should be initiated at the L5–S1 level, as this is the level most commonly symptomatic. If the response is negative, the L4–5 level should next be tested. Pain from L3–4 is uncommon, and the investigator should consider carefully before wantonly continuing investigations to this and higher levels.

A single positive response is not diagnostic of lumbar zygapophysial joint pain. The false-positive rate of single blocks[87] and the placebo-response rate[122] are high. Consequently, any positive response should be tested with a control block.

If the MRI shows an unexpected, occult lesion, investigation by diagnostic blocks is not warranted. Management can be implemented on the basis of the nature of the lesion identified.

The MRI may show a high-intensity zone (HIZ) in an annulus fibrosus. This sign should not be confused with fissure or unremarkable spots in the annulus. It consists of a bright signal, seen on carefully acquired T2-weighted images, with a brightness greater than that of the nucleus and at least equivalent to that of the cerebrospinal fluid.[126–129] When present in patients with back pain, it implicates the affected disk as the source of the patient's pain, with a positive likelihood ratio of 6.[126,130] The sign is not common, being found in fewer than 30% of patients.[126–129] However, when present, its high likelihood ratio renders it a diagnostic sign. For the diagnosis of internal disk disruption, a likelihood ratio of 6 converts the pretest likelihood of 40% to a diagnostic confidence of 80%. In that event, internal disk disruption can be diagnosed on the basis of MRI alone, and further investigation may not be necessary if all that is required is a diagnosis. Confirmation of diskogenic pain by diskography would be required only if destructive treatment is being entertained.

If the MRI does not show an HIZ, a critical consideration is whether multiple disks are degraded. If that is the case, pursuit of diskogenic pain is questionable, for if multiple disks are likely to be symptomatic there is no available, efficient treatment for multilevel disk disease.

If, however, only one, or perhaps two, disks are abnormal, it is potentially profitable to establish a diagnosis of diskogenic pain. This can be achieved by disk stimulation complemented by postdiskography CT scanning.[121]

Disk stimulation establishes whether or not the disk is symptomatic. For the diagnosis to be valid, the criteria prescribed by the IASP should be satisfied. They are that stimulation of the target disk reproduces the patient's pain, but stimulation of adjacent disks does not, and that CT scanning has established the internal morphology of the disk and whether or not a fissure characteristic of internal disk disruption is present.

If disk stimulation is negative or not indicated, the utility of reverting to sacroiliac and zygapophysial joint blocks should be considered. These may or may not be the source of pain despite the appearance of the disks on MRI. However, the positive yield of the foregoing steps in the algorithm should reduce the need for this consideration to only a minority of patients.

The utility of undertaking diagnostic blocks and disk stimulation is that target-specific treatment can be implemented if a positive diagnosis is found. There is no established treatment for sacroiliac joint pain, but the utility of establishing a diagnosis of sacroiliac joint pain is that it eliminates the need for futile pursuit of the pain with zygapophysial joint blocks or diskography. For zygapophysial joint pain and diskogenic pain there are treatments.

Lumbar zygapophysial joint pain can be treated effectively by percutaneous radiofrequency neurotomy.[89**] By careful attention to operative technique, complete relief of pain can be provided in the majority of patients for periods in excess of 12 months.[89**] The cardinal preoperative requirement is complete relief of pain following controlled diagnostic blocks.

Although fusion has been the mainstay for treatment of lumbar diskogenic pain, its results have been contentious.[131] A less destructive alternative is now available. In rigorously diagnosed patients with internal disk disruption, dramatic pain relief and decrease in disability can be achieved by intradiskal electrothermal annuloplasty (IDET).[132*] Although in its infancy, this procedure holds promise as a palatable alternative to major surgery in the treatment of diskogenic pain.

REFERENCES

1. Last JM ed. *A Dictionary of Epidemiology*, 3rd edn. New York, NY: Oxford University Press, 1995: 171.
2. Sackett DL, Haynes RB, Guyatt GH, Tugwell P. *Clinical Epidemiology: A Basic Science for Clinical Medicine*, 2nd edn. Boston, MA: Little, Brown & Co., 1991: 119–39.
3. Gore DR, Sepic SB, Gardner GM. Roentgenographic findings of the cervical spine in asymptomatic people. *Spine* 1986;1: 521–4.
4. Elias F. Roentgen findings in the asymptomatic cervical spine. *NY State J Med* 1958; **58**: 3300–3.
◆ 5. Heller CA, Stanley P, Lewis-Jones B, Heller RF. Value of x ray examinations of the cervical spine. *Br Med J* 1983; **287**: 1276–8.
◆ 6. Fridenberg ZB, Miller WT. Degenerative disc disease of the cervical spine: a comparative study of asymptomatic and symptomatic patients. *J Bone Joint Surg* 1963; 45A: 1171–8.
7. Torgerson WR, Dotter WE. Comparative roentgenographic study of the asymptomatic and symptomatic lumbar spine. *J Bone Joint Surg* 1976; 58A: 850–3.
◆ 8. Magora A, Schwartz A. Relation between the low back pain syndrome and x-ray findings. *Scand J Rehabil Med* 1976; **8**: 115–26.
9. Fullenlove TM, Williams AJ. Comparative roentgen findings in symptomatic and asymptomatic backs. *Radiology* 1957; **68**: 572–4.
10. Splithoff CA. Lumbosacral junction: roentgenographic comparison of patients with and without backaches. *JAMA* 1953; **152**: 1610–13.
11. Witt I, Vestergaard A, Rosenklint A. A comparative analysis of x-ray findings of the lumbar spine in patients with and without lumbar pain. *Spine* 1984; **9**: 298–300.
◆ 12. Lawrence JS, Bremner JM, Bier F. Osteo-arthrosis: prevalence in the population and relationship between symptoms and x-ray changes. *Ann Rheum Dis* 1966; **25**: 1–24.
13. McAlindon TE. The knee. *Bailliere's Clin Rheumatol* 1999; **13**: 329–44.
14. Croft P. Diagnosing regional pain: the view from primary care. *Bailliere's Clin Rheumatol* 1999; **13**: 231–42.
15. Lane NE, Thompson JM. Management of osteoarthritis in the primary care setting: an evidence-based approach to treatment. *Am J Med* 1997; **103**: 25S–30S.
16. Hadler NM. Knee pain is the malady – not osteoarthritis. *Ann Int Med* 1992; **116**: 598–9.
17. Wiesel SW. A study of computer-assisted tomography. 1. The incidence of positive CAT scans in an asymptomatic group of patients. *Spine* 1986; **9**: 549–51.
18. Mont M, Hungerford DS. Non-traumatic avascular necrosis of the femoral head. *J Bone Joint Surg* 1995; 77A: 459–74.
◆ 19. Boden SD, Davis DO, Dina TS, *et al.* Abnormal magnetic-resonance scans of the lumbar spine in asymptomatic subjects. *J Bone Joint Surg* 1990; 72A: 403–8.
◆ 20. Jensen MC, Bran-Zawadzki MN, Obucjowski N, *et al.* Magnetic resonance imaging of the lumbar spine in people without back pain. *N Engl J Med* 1994; **331**: 69–73.
◆ 21. Boden SD, McCowin PR, Davis DG, *et al.* Abnormal magnetic-resonance scans of the cervical spine in asymptomatic subjects: a prospective investigation. *J Bone Joint Surg* 1990; 72A: 1178–84.
◆ 22. Teresi LM, Lufkin RB, Reicher MA, *et al.* Asymptomatic degenerative disk disease and spondylosis of the cervical spine: MR imaging. *Radiology* 1987; **164**: 83–8.
23. Modic MT, Masaryk TJ, Mulopulos GP, *et al.* Cervical radiculopathy: prospective evaluation with surface coil

MR imaging, CT with metrizamide, and metrizamide myelography. *Radiology* 1986; **161:** 753–9.

24. Yousem DM, Atlas SW, Goldberg HI, Grossman RI. Degenerative narrowing of the cervical spine neural foraminal evaluation with high-resolution 3-DFT gradient echo MR imaging. *Am J Roentgenol* 1991; **156:** 1229–36.

25. Kaiser JA, Holland BA. Imaging of the cervical spine. *Spine* 1998; **23:** 2701–12.

26. Brown BM, Schwartz RH, Frank E, Blank NK. Preoperative evaluation of cervical radiculopathy and myelopathy by surface-coil MR imaging. *Am J Roentgenol* 1988; **151:** 1205–12.

27. Hedberg MC, Drayer BP, Flom RA, *et al.* Gradient echo (GRASS) MR imaging in cervical radiculopathy. *Am J Roentgenol* 1988; **150:** 683–9.

28. Tyson LL. Imaging of the painful shoulder. *Curr Probl Diagn Radiol* 1995; **24:** 110–40.

29. Norris TR, Green A. Imaging modalities in the evaluation of shoulder disorders. In: Matsen FA, Fu FH, Hawkins RJ eds. *The Shoulder: A Balance of Mobility and Stability*. Rosement, IL: American Academy of Orthopedic Surgeons, 1993: 353–67.

30. Stiles RG, Otte MT. Imaging of the shoulder. *Radiology* 1993; **188:** 603–13.

◆ 31. Sher JS, Uribe JW, Posada A, *et al.* Abnormal findings on magnetic resonance images of asymptomatic shoulders. *J Bone Joint Surg* 1995; **77A:** 10–15.

32. Milgrom C, Schaffler M, Gilbert S, van Holsbeeck M. Rotator-cuff changes in asymptomatic adults. *J Bone Joint Surg* 1995; **77B:** 296–8.

33. Chandnani V, Ho C, Gerharter J, *et al.* MR findings in asymptomatic shoulders: a blind analysis using symptomatic shoulders as controls. *Clinical Imaging* 1992; **16:** 25–30.

34. Lowe J, Schachner E, Hirschberg E, *et al.* Significance of bone scintigraphy in symptomatic spondylolysis. *Spine* 1984; **9:** 654–5.

35. Elliot S, Huitson A, Wastie ML. Bone scintigraphy in the assessment of spondylolysis in patients attending a sports injury clinic. *Clin Radiol* 1988; **39:** 269–72.

36. Jackson DW, Wiltse LL, Dingeman RD, Hayes M. Stress reactions involving the pars interarticularis in young athletes. *Am J Sports Med* 1981; **9:** 304–12.

37. Van den Oever M, Merrick MV, Scott JHS. Bone scintigraphy in symptomatic spondylolysis. *J Bone Joint Surg* 1987; **69B:** 453–6.

38. Harden RN, Bruehl S, Galer BS, *et al.* Complex regional pain syndrome: are the IASP diagnostic criteria valid and sufficiently comprehensive? *Pain* 1999; **83:** 211–19.

39. Littenberg B, Siegel A, Tosteson ANA, Mead T. Clinical efficacy of SPECT bone imaging for low back pain. *J Nucl Med* 1995; **36:** 1707–13.

40. von Rossum J, Brauma OJ, Kamphuisen HA, Onvlee GJ. Tennis elbow: a radial tunnel syndrome? *J Bone Joint Surg* 1978; **60B:** 197–8.

41. Rozmaryn LM. Carpal tunnel syndrome: a comprehensive review. *Curr Opin Orthop* 1997; **8:** 33–43.

42. Buch-Jaeger N, Foucher G. Correlation of clinical signs with nerve conduction tests in the diagnosis of carpal tunnel syndrome. *J Hand Surg* 1994; **19B:** 720–4.

43. Nathan PA, Keniston RC, Myers LD, Meadows KD. Longitudinal study of median nerve sensory conduction in industry: relationship to age, gender, hand dominance, occupational hand use, and clinical diagnosis. *J Hand Surg* 1992; **17A:** 850–7.

44. Katz JN, Larson MG, Fossel AH, Liang MH. Validation of surveillance case definition of carpal tunnel syndrome. *Am J Public Health* 1991; **81:** 189–93.

◆ 45. Hadler NM. Carpal tunnel syndrome, diagnostic conundrum. *J Rheumatol* 1997; **24:** 417–19.

◆ 46. Knutsson B. Comparative value of electromyographic myelographic and clinical–neurological examinations in diagnosis of lumbar root compression syndrome. *Acta Orthop Scand* 1961; **49:** 1–135.

47. Tullberg T, Svanborg E, Isacsson J, Grane P. A preoperative and postoperative study of the accuracy and value of electrodiagnosis in patients with lumbosacral disc herniation. *Spine* 1993; **18:** 837–42.

48. La Joie WJ. Nerve root compression: correlation of electromyographic, myelographic and surgical findings. *Arch Phys Med Rehab* 1972; **53:** 390–2.

● 49. Dvorak J. Neurophysiologic tests in diagnosis of nerve root compression caused by disc herniation. *Spine* 1996; 21 (Suppl. 24S): 39S–44S.

● 50. Andersson GBJ, Brown MD, Dvorak J, *et al.* Consensus summary on the diagnosis and treatment of lumbar disc herniation. *Spine* 1996; 21 (Suppl. 24S): 75S–78S.

● 51. Dvorak J. Epidemiology, physical examination and neurodiagnostics. *Spine* 1998; **23:** 2663–73.

52. Dumitru D, Dreyfuss P. Dermatomal/segmental somatosensory evoked potential evaluation of L5/S1 unilateral/unilevel radiculopathies. *Muscle Nerve* 1996; **19:** 442–9.

53. Thomas D, McCullum D, Siahamis G, Langlois S. Infrared thermographic imaging, magnetic resonance imaging, CT scan and myelography in low back pain. *Br J Rheumatol* 1990; **29:** 268–73.

54. Uematsu S, Hendler N, Hungerford D, *et al.* Thermography and electrode-myography in the differential diagnosis of chronic pain syndromes and reflex sympathetic dystrophy. *Electromyog Clin Neurophysiol* 1981; **21:** 165–82.

55. Lofstrom JB, Cousins MJ. Sympathetic neural blockade of upper and lower extremity. In: Cousins MJ, Bridenbaugh PO eds. *Neural Blockade in Clinical Anesthesia and Management of Pain*, 2nd edn. Philadelphia, PA: Lippincott, 1988: 461–500.

56. Verril P. Sympathetic ganglion lesions. In: Wall PD, Melzack R eds. *Textbook of Pain*, 2nd end. Edinburgh: Churchill Livingstone, 1989: 773–83.

57. Bonica JJ. Causalgia and other reflex sympathetic dystrophies. In: Bonica JJ ed. *The Management of Pain*, 2nd

edn, vol. 1. Philadelphia, PA: Lea and Febiger, 1990: 220–43.

58. Haddox JD. A call for clarity. In: Campbell JN ed. *Pain 1996. An Updated Review. Refresher Course Syllabus.* Seattle, WA: IASP Press, 1996: 97–9.

♦ 59. Price DD, Long S, Wilsey B, Rafii A. Analysis of peak magnitude and duration of analgesia produced by local anesthetics injected into sympathetic ganglia of complex regional pain syndrome patients. *Clin J Pain* 1998; **14:** 216–26.

60. Rocco AG, Kaul AF, Reisman RM, *et al.* A comparison of regional intravenous guanethidine and reserpine in reflex sympathetic dystrophy: a controlled, randomized, double-blind cross-over study. *Clin J Pain* 1989; **51:** 205–9.

61. Blanchard J, Ramamurthy S, Walsh N, *et al.* Intravenous regional sympatholysis: a double-blind comparison of guanethidine, reserpine, and normal saline. *J Pain Symptom Manage* 1990; **5:** 357–61.

62. Ramamurthy S, Hoffman J, Group GS. Intravenous regional guanethidine in the treatment of reflex sympathetic dystrophy/causalgia: a randomized, double-blind study. *Anesth Analg* 1995; **81:** 718–23.

♦ 63. Jadad AR, Caroll D, Glynn CJ, McQuay HJ. Intravenous regional sympathetic blockade for pain relief in reflex sympathetic dystrophy: a systematic review and a randomized double-blind crossover study *J Pain Sympt Manage* 1995; **10:** 13–20.

♦ 64. Fine PG, Roberts WJ, Gillete RG, Child TR. Slowly developing placebo responses confound tests of intravenous phentolamine to determine mechanisms underlying idiopathic chronic low back pain. *Pain* 1994; **56:** 235–42.

65. Verdugo RJ, Ochoa JL. "Sympathetically maintained pain." I. Phentolamine block questions the concept. *Neurology* 1994; **44:** 1003–10.

66. Verdugo RJ, Campero M, Ochoa JL. Phentolamine sympathetic block in painful polyneuropathies. II. Further questioning of the concept of "sympathetically maintained pain." *Neurology* 1994; **44:** 1010–14.

67. Hogan QH, Abram SE. Diagnostic and prognostic neural blockade. In: Cousins MJ, Bridenbaugh PO eds. *Neural blockade in Clinical Anesthesia and Management of Pain.* Philadelphia, PA: Lippincott-Raven, 1998: 837–977.

● 68. Bogduk N, Aprill C, Derby R. Diagnostic blocks of synovial joints. In: White AH ed. *Spine Care.* Vol. 1. *Diagnosis and Conservative Treatment.* St Louis, MO: Mosby, 1995: 298–321.

69. Dreyfuss P, Michaelsen M, Fletcher D. Atlanto-occipital and lateral atlanto-axial joint pain patterns. *Spine* 1994; **19:** 1125–31.

70. Busch E, Wilson PR. Atlanto-occipital and atlanto-axial injections in the treatment of headache and neck pain. *Reg Anesth* 1989; 14 (Suppl. 2): 45.

71. McCormick CC. Arthrography of the atlanto-axial

(C1–C2) joints: technique and results. *J Intervent Radiol* 1987; **2:** 9–13.

72. Dreyfuss P, Rogers J, Dreyer S, Fletcher D. Atlanto-occipital joint pain: a report of three cases and description of an intra-articular joint block technique. *Reg Anesthesia* 1994; **19:** 344–53.

♦ 73. Bogduk N, Lord SM. Cervical zygapophysial joint pain. *Neurosurg Q* 1998; **8:** 107–17.

74. Barnsley L, Bogduk N. Medial branch blocks are specific for the diagnosis of cervical zygapophysial joint pain. *Reg Anesth* 1993; **18:** 343–50.

75. Barnsley L, Lord S, Wallis B, Bogduk N. False-positive rates of cervical zygapophysial joint blocks. *Clin J Pain* 1993; **9:** 124–30.

76. Barnsley L, Lord S, Bogduk N. Comparative local anaesthetic blocks in the diagnosis of cervical zygapophysial joints pain. *Pain* 1993; **55:** 99–106.

♦ 77. Lord SM, Barnsley L, Bogduk N. The utility of comparative local anaesthetic blocks versus placebo-controlled blocks for the diagnosis of cervical zygapophysial joint pain. *Clin J Pain* 1995; **11:** 208–13.

♦ 78. Lord SM, McDonald GJ, Bogduk N. Percutaneous radiofrequency neurotomy of the cervical medial branches: a validated treatment for cervical zygapophysial joint pain. *Neurosurg Q* 1998; **8:** 288–308.

79. Lord SM, Barnsley L, Wallis BJ, *et al.* Percutaneous radio-frequency neurotomy for chronic cervical zygapophysial-joint pain. *N Engl J Med* 1996; **335:** 1721–6.

80. McDonald G, Lord SM, Bogduk N. Long-term follow-up of cervical radiofrequency neurotomy for chronic neck pain. *Neurosurgery* 1999; **45:** 61–8.

81. Schwarzer AC, Aprill CN, Bogduk N. The sacroiliac joint in chronic low back pain. *Spine* 1995; **20:** 31–7.

♦ 82. Maigne JY, Aivaliklis A, Pfefer F. Results of sacroiliac joint double block and value of sacroiliac pain provocation tests in 54 patients with low-back pain. *Spine* 1996; **21:** 1889–92.

83. Dreyfuss P, Michaelsen M, Pauza K, *et al.* The value of history and physical examination in diagnosing sacroiliac joint pain. *Spine* 1996; **21:** 2594–602.

♦ 84. Schwarzer AC, Aprill CN, Derby R, *et al.* Clinical features of patients with pain stemming from the lumbar zygapophysial joints: is the lumbar facet syndrome a clinical entity? *Spine* 1994; **19:** 1132–7.

85. Dreyfuss P, Schwarzer AC, Lau P, Bogduk N. Specificity of lumbar medial branch and L5 dorsal ramus blocks: a computed tomographic study. *Spine* 1997; **22:** 895–902.

86. Kaplan M, Dreyfuss P, Halbrook B, Bogduk N. The ability of lumbar medial branch blocks to anesthetize the zygapophysial joint. *Spine* 1998; **23:** 1847–52.

87. Schwarzer AC, Aprill CN, Derby R, *et al.* The false-positive rate of uncontrolled diagnostic blocks of the lumbar zygapophysial joints. *Pain* 1994; **58:** 195–200.

88. van Kleef M, Barendse GAM, Kessels A, *et al.* Random-

ized trial of radiofrequency lumbar facet denervation for chronic low back pain. *Spine* 1999; **24:** 1937–42.

◆ 89. Dreyfuss P, Halbrook B, Pauza K, *et al*. Efficacy and validity of radiofrequency neurotomy for chronic lumbar zygapophysial joint pain. *Spine* 2000; **25:** 1270–7.

● 90. Merskey H, Bogduk N eds. *Classification of Chronic Pain. Descriptions of Chronic pain Syndromes and Definitions of Pain Terms*, 2nd edn. Seattle, WA: IASP Press, 1994.

● 91. Bogduk N, Aprill C, Derby R. Discography. In: White AH ed. *Spine Care.* Vol. 1. *Diagnosis and Conservative Treatment.* St Louis, MO: Mosby 1995: 219–38.

92. Walsh TR, Weinstein JN, Spratt KF, *et al*. Lumbar discography in normal subjects. *J Bone Joint Surg* 1990; 72A: 1081–8.

93. Schellhas KP, Smith MD, Gundry CR, Pollei SR. Cervical discogenic pain: prospective correlation of magnetic resonance imaging and discography in asymptomatic subjects and pain sufferers. *Spine* 1996; **21:** 300–12.

94. Mercer S, Bogduk N. The ligaments and anulus fibrosus of human adult cervical intervertebral discs. *Spine* 1999; **24:** 619–26.

95. Lord SM. Commentary on cervical diskogenic pain. *Pain Med J Club J* 1996; **2:** 213–15.

96. Cherry DA, Gourlay GK, McLachlan M, Cousins MJ. Diagnostic epidural opioid blockade and chronic pain: preliminary report. *Pain* 1985; **21:** 143–52.

97. Yousem DM, Atlas SW, Grossman RI, *et al*. MR imaging of Tolosa–Hunt syndrome. *AJNR* 1989; **10:** 1181–4.

98. Goto Y, Hosokawa S, Goto I, *et al*. Abnormality in the cavernous sinus in three patients with Tolosa–Hunt syndrome: MRI and CT findings. *J Neurol Neurosurg Psychiatry* 1990; **55:** 231–4.

99. Rowed DW, Kassel EE, Lewis AJ. Transorbital intracavernous needle biopsy in painful ophthalmoplegia. *J Neurosurg* 1985; **62:** 776–80.

◆100. Deyo RA, Diehl AK. Cancer as a cause of back pain: frequency, clinical presentation and diagnostic strategies. *J Gen Intern Med* 1988; **3:** 230–8.

101. Bachulis BL, Long WB, Hynes GD, Johnson MC. Clinical indications for cervical spine radiographs in the traumatized patient. *Am J Surg* 1987; **153:** 473–7.

102. Kreipke DL, Gillespie KR, McCarthy MC, *et al*. Reliability of indications for cervical spine films in trauma patients. *J Trauma* 1989; **29:** 1438–9.

103. Hoffman JR, Schriger DL, Mower W, *et al*. Low-risk criteria for cervical-spine radiography in blunt trauma: a prospective study. *Ann Emerg Med* 1992; **21:** 1454–60.

104. Gerrelts BD, Petersen EU, Mabry J, Petersen SR. Delayed diagnosis of cervical spine injuries. *J Trauma* 1991; **31:** 1622–6.

105. Johnson MJ, Lucas GL. Value of cervical spine radiographs as a screening tool. *Clin Orthop* 1997; **340:** 102–8.

106. Deyo RA, Diehl AK. Lumbar spine films in primary care: current use and effects of selective ordering criteria. *J Gen Intern Med* 1986;1: 20–5.

107. Nice DA, Riddle DL, Lamb RL, *et al*. Intertester reliability of judgements of the presence of trigger points in patients with low back pain. *Arch Phys Med Rehabil* 1992; **73:** 893–8.

108. Njoo KH, Van der Does E. The occurrence and interrater reliability of myofascial trigger points in the quadratus lumborum and gluteus medius: a prospective study in non-specific low back pain patients and controls in general practice. *Pain* 1994; **58:** 317–23.

109. Bogduk N. *Clinical Anatomy of the Lumbar Spine and Sacrum*, 3rd edn. Edinburgh: Churchill Livingston, 1997: 215–25.

110. Silbert PL, Makri B, Schievink WI. Headache and neck pain in spontaneous internal carotid and vertebral artery dissections. *Neurology* 1995; **45:** 1517–22.

111. Dvorak J, Hayek J, Zehnder R. CT-functional diagnostics of the rotatory instability of the upper cervical spine. Part 2. An evaluation on healthy adults and patients with suspected instability. *Spine* 1987; **12:** 725–31.

◆112. Bogduk N. International Spinal Injection Society guidelines for the performance of spinal injection procedures. Part 1. Zygapophysial joint blocks. *Clin J Pain* 1997; **13:** 285–302.

113. Barnsley L, Lord SM, Wallis BJ, Bogduk N. The prevalence of chronic cervical zygapophysial joint pain after whiplash. *Spine* 1995; **20:** 20–6.

◆114. Lord S, Barnsley L, Wallis BJ, Bogduk N. Chronic cervical zygapophysial joint pain after whiplash: a placebo-controlled prevalence study. *Spine* 1996; **21:** 1737–45.

115. Lord SM, Bogduk N. The cervical synovial joints as sources of post-traumatic headache. *J Musculoskeletal Pain* 1996; **4:** 81–94.

◆116. Lord S, Barnsley L, Wallis B, Bogduk N. Third occipital headache: a prevalence study. *J Neurol Neurosurg Psychiatry* 1994; **57:** 1187–90.

117. Dwyer A, Aprill C, Bogduk N. Cervical zygapophysial joint pain patterns. I. A study in normal volunteers. *Spine* 1990; **15:** 453–7.

118. Joseph B, Kumar B. Gallie's fusion for atlantoaxial arthrosis with occipital neuralgia. *Spine* 1994; **19:** 454–5.

119. Ghanayem AJ, Leventhal M, Bohlman HH. Osteoarthrosis of the atlanto-axial joints – long-term follow-up after treatment with arthrodesis. *J Bone Joint Surg* 1996; 78A: 1300–7.

120. Grubb SA, Kelly CK. Cervical discography: clinical implications from twelve years experience. *Spine* 2000; **25:** 1382–9.

◆121. Schwarzer AC, Aprill CN, Derby R, *et al*. The prevalence and clinical features of internal disc disruption in patients with chronic low back pain. *Spine* 1995; **20:** 1878–83.

122. Schwarzer AC, Wang S, Bogduk N, *et al*. Prevalence and clinical features of lumbar zygapophysial joint pain: a study in an Australian population with chronic low back pain. *Ann Rheum Dis* 1995; **54:** 100–6.

123. Schwarzer AC, Derby R, Aprill CN, *et al*. Pain from the

lumbar zygapophysial joints: a test of two models. *J Spinal Disord* 1994; **7:** 331–6.

124. Revel M, Poiraudeau S, Auleley GR, *et al*. Capacity of the clinical picture to characterize low back pain relieved by facet joint anesthesia: proposed criteria to identify patients with painful facet joints. *Spine* 1998; **23:** 1972–7.

125. Bogduk N. Commentary on the capacity of the clinical picture to characterize low back pain relieved by facet joint anesthesia. *Pain Med J Club J* 1998; **4:** 221–2.

◆126. Aprill C, Bogduk N. High intensity zone: a diagnostic sign of painful lumbar disc on magnetic resonance imaging. *Br J Radiol* 1992; **65:** 361–9.

127. Schellhas KP, Pollei SR, Gundry CR, Heithoff KB. Lumbar disc high-intensity zone: correlation of mag-netic resonance imaging and discography. *Spine* 1996; **21:** 79–86.

◆128. Ito M, Incorvaia KM, Yu SF, *et al*. Predictive signs of dis-cogenic lumbar pain on magnetic resonance imaging with discography correlation. *Spine* 1998; **23:** 1252–8.

129. Saifuddin A, Braithwaite I, White J, *et al*. The value of lumbar spine magnetic resonance imaging in the dem-onstration of anular tears. *Spine* 1998; **23:** 453–7.

130. Bogduk N. Point of view. *Spine* 1998; **23:** 1259–60.

●131. Turner JA, Ersek M, Herron L, *et al*. Patient outcomes after lumbar spinal fusions. *JAMA* 1992; **268:** 907–11.

132. Karasek M, Bogduk N. Twelve-month follow up of a controlled trial of intradiscal thermal anuloplasty for back pain due to internal disc disruption. *Spine* 2000; **25:** 2601–7.

10

Outcome measurement in chronic pain

CHRISTOPHER D SLETTEN

The task of measuring outcomes is critical for all health care endeavors. Some outcome measures are rather self-evident, such as mortality rates of specific interventions. Chemotherapies for cancer can be specifically evaluated for their effectiveness in ameliorating the disease. Surgeries for joint replacement, glaucoma, hernias, etc. can be evaluated for their effectiveness in health recovery. The treatment of chronic pain, however, is not afforded the clarity of survival or disease recovery as a gold standard for outcome. This field has many variables that seem important and many variables that are hard to quantify.

The issue of outcome measurement in chronic pain is complicated by several additional factors. These include goals for treatment, the targeted symptoms, and the nature of the treatment. In most cases of chronic pain, the patient's preeminent goal is pain relief. Secondarily, patients also seek relief from emotional distress and return to better levels of functioning. Health care providers may have a number of goals: improvement in overall health, increased functional capacity, as well as pain relief. Finally, other involved parties – employers, insurance providers, government agencies – have goals directed at the economic aspects of the pain problem.

The target of the specific intervention affects the focus on which outcomes are important. The surgeon seeks a goal of structural restoration to relieve pain. Therefore, he or she may view a successful outcome as improved physiologic functioning as measured by tests such as magnetic resonance imaging (MRI), computed tomography (CT), and electromyogram (EMG). The pain physician's focus is on identifying and treating the physiologic mechanisms of pain. Successful treatment from this perspective would include reduction or elimination of pain and restoration of function. Pain rehabilitation specialists (phy-

sicians, psychologists) have a treatment focus that gives greatest attention to improved physical and emotional functioning and a restoration of a more normal lifestyle. This last approach gives least emphasis to reduction in pain levels.

In each of the treatments mentioned, the treatment itself can have a direct effect on outcomes. Presumably, after a period of postoperative recovery, surgical interventions can be judged based on the level of structural and physiologic improvement. Various pain interventions such as injections, nerve blocks, and medications may have their effects immediately or over time. Therefore, the timing of outcome measurement is a necessary consideration to accurately measure the success of a given treatment. Finally, in a rehabilitation setting, the initial gains of treatment may only be the beginning of improvement and longer follow-up intervals may be needed to demonstrate treatment effectiveness and durability.

Given these factors, this chapter has as its goal to present several of the most appropriate and useful outcome measures for chronic pain treatment. Other chapters in this text focus on assessment of distress, impairment, and other psychological factors seen in chronic pain populations. This chapter will focus on the use of various measures to assess the outcome of treatment.

For the sake of clarity, this discussion will be broken down according to the purpose of the measurement, and will generally cover the areas of physical capacity, psychological functioning, and socioeconomic impact. There are many components to each of these areas, and an in-depth review of measurement properties and specific measures is beyond the scope of this chapter. However, it will provide an overview of these areas and their use in evaluating chronic pain treatments.

PHYSICAL CAPACITY

Chronic painful conditions differ in their impact on physical capacity and functioning. For example, disorders that lead to chronic low back pain may be more strongly associated with physical incapacity than other chronic painful conditions (e.g. headache, abdominal pain, fibromyalgia). Because of this, outcome measurement of physical capacity has been most widely studied in populations with musculoskeletal pain problems such as low back pain.[1**,2*,3**] The most common physical outcome measures are range of motion, strength, lifting capacity, and general functional capacity.[1**,4***]

Range of motion

Range of motion has long been a widely accepted measure of physical functioning for patients with musculoskeletal pain.[4***] Several methods have been used to determine spine range of motion. The Schober Technique involves placing several marks along the back with the patient in the neutral position, these marks are then measured with the back in full flexion.[1**] This has been shown to be only marginally reliable because of the variability of landmarks. A simpler method of determining range of motion is to have the patient bend over toward the ground and measure the distance from their fingertips to the ground.[1**,4***] This method is easily applied; however, variability in patient effort and measurement error lead to significant reliability problems.[5] Other methods include photographic or computerized video to analyze spine range of motion, and the use of three-dimensional radiography.[1**] The most widely accepted method for spine range of motion is inclinometry. This method uses a hand-held device – the inclinometer – placed at the first lumbar and sacral levels to measure sagittal and axial motion of the spine.[4***,6*] This method has been accepted by the American Medical Association, and is included in its *Guides to the Evaluation of Permanent Impairment*.[7]

Strength

The second type of physical assessment that can be used for treatment outcome measurement is strength. Many patients with chronic pain are observed to have diminished strength. Like range of motion, most of the research in this area has focused on spine pain.[4***] There are a number of commercially available machines that incorporate computer technology to measure isometric, isokinetic, and isodynamic parameters of strength.[1**] The area of focus of these machines is typically the trunk – specifically, the trunk extensor and abdominal flexor muscles.

Lifting capacity

Lifting capacity assesses the individual's physical functioning at a more complex level. In general, lifting tasks incorporate aspects of both range of motion and strength. They have been used to simulate work demands and to give a general marker of physical rehabilitation in the treatment setting.[3**] As with strength measures, there has been a variety of machines and computer applications designed to assess lifting capacity.[1**] Like other measures of physical capacity, even the most sophisticated machine is unable to neutralize factors of motivation and perception on the part of the subject. One lifting performance task has been designed to account for both isoinertial performance and psychophysical components of lifting. The Progressive Isoinertial Lifting Evaluation (PILE) is a relatively simple test that measures lifting capacity.[8**] The basic format of the PILE is to have the subject lift weights in a covered plastic box that hides the amount of weight lifted. The weight is lifted from the floor to waist height, from waist height to shoulder height and placed on a shelf, then from the shelf to the floor. This repeated 10 times in a minute before additional weight is added. The PILE is stopped when the individual reports fatigue or pain.[8**,9]

Functional capacity

General functional capacity can be defined and measured in a number of ways. The most commonly used system is the Functional Capacity Evaluation (FCE). The FCE can range from a global assessment of functioning to quite specific, job-related assessments. The standard format for FCE is a series of lifting and endurance tasks conducted in a controlled, standardized setting. The person receives a rating of overall capacity that can be compared with standard levels of job demands.[10***] Broad application of FCE for outcome measurement is difficult owing to the labor-intensive nature of the testing, cost of equipment, and difficulties with reliability. Harding *et al.* have developed a system of measuring general capacity that is less labor intensive yet broad in scope.[11] This system uses a series of tasks to measure overall fitness and strength. The tasks include a 10-min walk, a 20-m speed walk, a 2-min stair climbing, a stand-up test, a sit-up tolerance, and arm endurance, grip, and peak respiratory flow tests. These measures have been shown to be reliable and well correlated with other measures of functioning.[12**]

In evaluating the efficacy and utility of outcome measures it is tempting to place great faith in measures of physical functioning. These measures seem to be quite objective, after all they are measuring a "physical phenomenon." However, several cautions are important. As mentioned above, the perspective and/or intended use of physical capacity data must be considered. From the patient's perspective, there may be motivation to exert excessive or minimal effort during physical testing. Exces-

measures. Since most of the outcome measures rely on self-report, there is the clear possibility of patient bias and influence on the measures. Health care providers may also introduce bias based on their theoretical approach to pain. Finally, third-party consumers (employers, insurance carriers) may care less about patient health and satisfaction and more about the financial bottom line. All of these influences should be accounted for when considering treatment outcomes. It is highly unlikely that all of these goals will be attained. The patient may not get complete pain relief but may have improved emotional and occupational functioning. In some cases, unrestricted return to work may not be feasible. Despite this, a comprehensive view of treatment outcome can provide the best estimate of a specific treatment's effectiveness and utility.

The clinical significance of a treatment is a growing area of focus for many outcome studies.[4***] Many studies report statistically significant changes in outcome measures that may not represent any meaningful change clinically. To begin to address this need, pretreatment and outcome data should not only be looked at in terms of statistical change but comparisons should be made with "normal" or nonpatient levels of functioning.[56***] With respect to economic and occupational outcomes, this may mean more specifically defined behavioral markers of functioning.[4***] The difficulty of these changes is that they bring increased complexity and cost to studying outcomes. The more data that are required, the more chance there is for erroneous or missing data and decreased levels of compliance.

The generalizability of outcome studies is of obvious importance. If a study is so unique and specific in the type of patient treated or the study design, it is probably of little use for broader clinical application. Factors that can aid in the applicability of an outcome study are careful definition of patient selection criteria and patient characteristics, using well-disseminated measures, adequate sample size, careful methodology, and adequate follow-up measurement.

Outcome studies in the chronic pain literature have significantly added to our understanding of the treatment process and effectiveness. The vast majority of these studies have been conducted in multidisciplinary treatment settings, often with a rehabilitation focus. Rehabilitation settings have fostered the use of a broad range of measures, both physical and psychological. These studies have been limited, however, because of the difficulty of achieving true randomization, limitations on use of control groups, and subject attrition at follow-up. The goal for future studies should be a broader application of outcome measures across treatment settings, surgeon's office, pain clinic, medical clinic, and continued attention to increasing compliance with follow-up assessments. Once we have achieved a more universal set of standards, we will be better able to serve our patients and colleagues with timely and effective care.

REFERENCES

1. Flores L, Gatchel RJ, Polatin PB. Objectification of functional improvement after nonoperative care. *Spine* 1997; **22:** 1622–33.

2. Beurskens AJHM, de Vet HCW, Koke AJA. Responsiveness of functional status in low back pain: a comparison of different instruments. *Pain* 1996; **65:** 71–6.

3. Mayer TG, Gatchel RJ, Mayer H, *et al*. A prospective two-year study of functional restoration in industrial low back injury: an objective assessment procedure. *JAMA* 1987; **13:** 1763–7.

4. Tait RC. Evaluation of treatment effectiveness in patients with intractable pain: measures and methods. In: Gatchel RJ, Turk DC eds. *Psychosocial Factors in Pain: Critical Perspectives*. New York, NY: The Guilford Press, 1999: 457–80.

5. Robinson ME, Greene AF, O'Connor P, *et al*. Reliability of lumbar isometric torque in patients with chronic low back pain. *Phys Ther* 1992; **72:** 186–90.

6. Hildebrandt J, Pfingsten M, Saur P, Jansen J. Prediction of success from a multidisciplinary treatment program for chronic low back pain. *Spine* 1997; **22:** 990–1001.

7. American Medical Association. *Guides to the Evaluation of Permanent Impairment*, 5th edn. Chicago, IL: AMA, 2000.

8. Mayer TG, Barnes D, Kishino N, *et al*. Progressive isoinertial lifting evaluation. I. A standardized protocol and normative database. *Spine* 1988; **13:** 993–7.

9. Burns JW, Johnson BJ, Devine J, *et al*. Anger management style and the prediction of treatment outcome among male and female chronic pain patients. *Behav Res Ther* 1998; **36:** 1051–62.

10. Isernhagen S. Contemporary issues in functional capacity evaluation. In: Isernhagen S ed. *The Comprehensive Guide to Work Injury Management*. Gaithersburg, MD: Aspen, 1994: 410–29.

11. Harding VR, Williams ACC, Richardson PH, *et al*. The development of a battery of measures for assessing physical functioning of chronic pain patients. *Pain* 1994; **58:** 367–75.

12. Williams AC, Richardson PH, Nicholas MK, *et al*. Inpatient vs. outpatient pain management: results of a randomised controlled trial. *Pain* 1996; **66:** 13–22.

13. Kerns RD. Psychosocial factors: primary or secondary outcomes? In: Cohen MJM, Campbell JN eds. *Pain Treatment at a Crossroads: A practical and Conceptual Reappraisal*. Seattle, WA: IASP Press, 1996: 183–92.

14. Turk DC, Flor H. Chronic pain: a biobehavioral perspective. In: Gatchel RJ, Turk DC eds. *Psychosocial Factors in Pain*. New York, NY: Guilford Press, 1999: 18–34.

15. Carlsson AM. Assessment of chronic pain. I. Aspects of reliability and validity of the visual analogue scale. *Pain* 1983; **16:** 87–101.

16. Jensen MP, Karoly P, Braver S. The measurement of clinical pain intensity: a comparison of six methods. *Pain* 1986; **27:** 117–26.

17. Jensen MP, Turner JA, Romano JM, Fisher LD. Comparative reliability and validity of chronic pain intensity measures. *Pain* 1999; **83:** 157–62.

18. Rybstein-Blinchik E. Effects of different cognitive strategies on chronic pain experience. *J Behav Med* 1979; **2:** 93–101.

◆ 19. Melzack R. The McGill Pain Questionnaire: major properties and scoring methods. *Pain* 1975; **1:** 277–99.

20. Burchiel KJ, Anderson VC, Wilson BJ, *et al*. Prognostic factors of spinal cord stimulation for chronic back and leg pain. *Neurosurgery* 1995; **36:** 1101–10.

21. Salovey P, Smith AF, Turk DC, *et al*. The accuracy of memory for pain: not so bad most of the time. *Am Pain Soc J* 1993; **2:** 184–91.

22. Jensen MP, Turner JA, Romano JM, Lawler BK. Relationship of pain-specific beliefs to chronic pain adjustment. *Pain* 1994; **57:** 301–9.

23. Jensen MP, Karoly P. Pain-specific beliefs, perceived symptom severity, and adjustment to chronic pain. *Clin J Pain* 1992; **8:** 123–30.

24. Jensen MP, Karoly P. Control beliefs, coping efforts, and adjustment to chronic pain. *J Consult Clin Psychol* 1991; **59:** 431–8.

25. DeGood DE, Shutty Jr MS. Assessment of pain beliefs, coping, and self-efficacy. In: Turk DC, Melzack R eds. *Handbook of Pain Assessment*. New York, NY: Guilford Press, 1992: 214–34.

26. Bandura A. Self-efficacy: toward a unifying theory of behavioral change. *Psychol Rev* 1977; **84:** 191–215.

27. Lorig K, Chastain RL, Ung E, *et al*. Development and evaluation of a scale to measure perceived self-efficacy in people with arthritis. *Arthritis Rheumatol* 1987; **32:** 37–44.

28. Anderson KO, Dowds BN, Pelletz RE, *et al*. Development and initial validation of a scale to measure self-efficacy beliefs in patients with chronic pain. *Pain* 1995; **69:** 231–6.

◆ 29. Rosenstiel AK, Keefe FJ. The use of coping strategies in chronic low back pain patients: relationship to patient characteristics and current adjustment. *Pain* 1983; **17:** 33–44.

30. Dozois DJA, Dobson KS, Wong M, *et al*. Predictive utility of the CSQ in low back pain: individual vs. composite measures. *Pain* 1996; **66:** 171–80.

31. Pfingsten M, Hildebrandt J, Leibing E, *et al*. Effectiveness of a multimodal treatment program for chronic low-back pain. *Pain* 1997; **73:** 77–85.

32. Fairbank JC, Cooper J, Daview JB, O'Brien JP. The Oswestry Low Back Pain Disability Questionnaire. *Physiotherapy* 1980; **66:** 271–3.

33. Roland M, Morris R. A study of the natural history of back pain. I. Development of a reliable and sensitive measure of disability in low-back pain. *Spine* 1983; **8:** 141–4.

34. Pollard CA. Preliminary validity study of the Pain Disability Index. *Percept Motor Skills* 1984; **59:** 974.

35. Chibnall JT, Tait RC. The Pain Disability Index: factor structure and normative data. *Arch Phys Med Rehabil* 1994; **75:** 1082–6.

◆ 36. Kerns RD, Turk DC, Rudy TE. The West Haven–Yale Multidimensional Pain Inventory (WHYMPI). *Pain* 1985; **21:** 345–56.

37. Rudy TE, Turk DC, Kubinski JA, Zaki HS. Differential treatment responses of TMD patients as a function of psychological characteristics. *Pain* 1995; **61:** 103–12.

38. Butcher JN, Dahlstrom WG, Graham JR, *et al*. *MMPI-2: Manual for Administration and Scoring*. Minneapolis, MN: University of Minnesota Press, 1989.

39. Dvorak J, Valach L, Fuhrimann P, Heim E. The outcome of surgery for lumbar disc herniation. II. A 4–17 year's follow-up with emphasis on psychosocial aspects. *Spine* 1988; **13:** 1423–7.

40. Barnes D, Gatchel RJ, Mayer TG, Barnett J. Changes in MMPI profiles of chronic low back pain patients following successful treatment. *J Spinal Disord* 1990; **3:** 353–5.

41. Buckelew SP, DeGood DE, Schwartz DP, Kerler RM. Cognitive and somatic item response patterns of pain patients, psychiatric patients, and hospital employees. *J Consult Clin Psychol* 1986; **42:** 852–60.

42. Wallis BJ, Lord SM, Bogduk N. Resolution of psychological distress of whiplash patients following treatment by radiofrequency neurotomy: a randomised, double-blind, placebo-controlled trial. *Pain* 1997; **73:** 15–22.

◆ 43. Dworkin RH, Gitlin MJ. Clinical aspects of depression in chronic pain patients. *Clin J Pain* 1991; **7:** 79–94.

44. McCracken LM, Gross RT, Sorg PJ, Edmands TA. Prediction of pain in patients with chronic low back pain: effects of inaccurate prediction and pain-related anxiety. *Behav Res Ther* 1993; **31:** 647–52.

● 45. Turk DC, Okifuji A. Detecting depression in chronic pain patients: adequacy of self-reports. *Behav Res Ther* 1994; **32:** 9–16.

46. Geisser ME, Roth RS, Robinson ME. Assessing depression among persons with chronic pain using the Center for Epidemiological Studies – Depression scale and the Beck Depression Inventory: a comparative analysis. *Clin J Pain* 1997; **13:** 163–70.

47. Radloff L. The CES-D scale: a self-report depression scale for research in the general population. *J Appl Psychol Meas* 1977; **1:** 385–401.

48. Bergner M, Bobbitt RA, Pollard WE, *et al*. The Sickness Impact Profile: validation of a health status measure. *Med Care* 1976; **14:** 56–67.

49. Radosevich DM, Wetzler H, Wilson SM. *Health Status Questionnaire (HSQ) 2.0: Scoring Comparisons and Reference Data*. Bloomington, MN: Health Outcomes Institute, 1994.

50. Becker N, Hojsted J, Sjogren P, Eriksen J. Sociodemographic predictors of treatment outcome in chronic nonmalignant pain patients: do patients receiving or applying for disability pension benefit from multidisciplinary pain treatment? *Pain* 1998; **77:** 279–87.

● 51. Okifuji A, Turk DC, Kalauokalani D. Clinical outcome

Resources[1,2]

- Ideally, there should be dedicated accommodation, with all staff and facilities within a single area. This should include interview, examination, and minor treatment rooms. Secretarial and administrative staff should be within the unit accommodation. As most UK hospitals predate properly developed pain management units, this is not always possible. Pragmatic solutions may be needed in sharing accommodation used by other units.
- Access to outpatient and inpatient beds for treatment purposes is important.
- There should be dedicated access to shared facilities such as operating room and radiology services for major invasive procedures.
- Pain management programs will require more extensive space and facilities.[3]
- Appropriate equipment for treatment should be available.

Table 11.1 shows the size and costs for a teaching hospital clinic, a pain management program (PMP), and a district hospital. The figures relate to 1994 and are the most recent available. A multiplier of 19% will give current costs based on cost of living increases in the UK to December 2001. The numbers of staff are shown as whole-time equivalents (WTEs) and costs shown on a *pro rata* basis. In virtually every clinic, staff numbers will have increased from those shown (P. J. D. Evans, J. Watt, and J. E. Charlton, personal communication).

Expenditure

The major cost to any pain management unit is staff salaries. The extent of these will depend upon the size of

the unit and the scope of the services offered. One of the many debates that surround the provision of health care under a system such as the NHS is the cost of new treatments that are, as yet, unproven in terms of cost benefit. Examples might be the use of implanted drug delivery systems or spinal cord stimulators. There are strong arguments that treatments like these may benefit individuals with particularly intractable and malefic problems. However, evidence for cost benefit is lacking and the paymasters of the NHS are unwilling to unloose the purse strings for expensive therapy of this nature without such evidence.

Apart from salaries other costs include:

- Accommodation.
- Purchase and capital cost for major equipments such as radiofrequency lesion generators.
- Purchase and capital cost of minor equipment such as transcutaneous electrical nerve stimulators (TENS), computers, and facsimile and answering machines.
- Supply, maintenance, and replacement costs of all equipment.
- A regular maintenance program and a rolling replacement program for all equipment. The timing will vary with the equipment concerned.
- Medication costs.
- Stationery, printing, photocopying, postage, telephone, and facsimile costs.
- Charges for other hospital services such as radiology and laboratory costs.
- Internal hospital charges for consultation with other services.
- Teaching and educational materials and expenses.

Table 11.2 shows the costs associated with a teaching hospital pain clinic, a pain management program, and a district hospital. These are by no means comprehensive and do not include any shared costs that might be

Table 11.1 *Salary costs of a teaching hospital (Hospital 1), a similar hospital with a pain management unit (Hospital 2), and a district hospital (Hospital 3)*

Staff	Hospital 1			Hospital 2 PMP			Hospital 3 district		
	Number	WTEs	Cost £	Number	WTEs	Cost £	Number	WTEs	Cost £
Consultants	2	0.7	52,120	2	0.7	39,200	2	1	58,000
Trainee doctors	2		25,100				1	0.2	5,000
Other MDs	1	2	9,300	2	2	60,000	2	0.4	10,000
Chief nurse	1	2	14,000	2	2	44,900	1	1	24,000
Nurses	3		25,500				1	0.4	6,000
Ancillary staff	1		8,100						
Acupuncturist	1		10,400			15,000	1	0.1	3,000
Psychologist		3		3	3	76,000			
Physiotherapist	1	2.5	7,100	2.5	2.5	52,000			
Occupational therapist		1		1	1	22,400			
Clerk/ancillary	1	1.5	9,500	2	1.5	20,000	1	0.8	8,000
Secretarial	1	2	14,100	2	2	26,000	1	0.4	4,000
Computing assistant	1		11,500						

WTEs, whole-time equivalents; PMP, pain management program.

Table 11.2 *Costs of facilities, consumables, and other central charges for a teaching hospital (Hospital 1), a similar hospital with a pain management program (Hospital 2), and a district hospital (Hospital 3)*

	Hospital 1 teaching			Hospital 2 PMP			Hospital 3 district		
	Number	Area m²	Cost £	Number	Area m²	Cost £	Number	Area m²	Cost £
Facilities									
Office	2	14	1,400	10	9	4,500	1	16	N/A
Consulting	1	12	600	1	14	700	3	12	N/A
Treatment	0.5	25	625	2	10	1,000	1	20	N/A
Radiograph room	0.2	30	300						
Bed space (per person)	12	72	43,200	30	15	22,500	6	N/A	N/A
Waiting room	1	20	1,000	1	25	1,250	1	20	N/A
Reception	0.5	30	750	2	30	3,000			
Other				1	24	1,200			
Consumables									
Small items			10,000			15,000			2,000
Leasing			22,000			30,000			
Capital acquisitions									
Intensifier			65,000						
Other			12,500						
TENS	60		3,600						
Acupuncture needles	40,000		5,600						
Central charges									
Outpatients			N/A			8,400			72,000
Inpatient facilities			12,000			58,000			5,000
Management			8,000			8,000			5,000
Pharmacy/radiology/ operating room costs									78,000
Computing/records			13,000						N/A

N/A, not available; PMP, pain management program.

associated with a pain management subdirectorate that is providing acute pain management services as part of a comprehensive service. A multiplier of 19% will give current costs based on cost of living increases in the UK to December 2001 (P. J. D. Evans, J. Watt, and J. E. Charlton, personal communication).

CLINICAL ACTIVITY FOR THE AVERAGE YEAR

It is difficult to make comparisons between clinics in terms of clinical activity as local working practices are influenced by many factors. The pattern of work shown in Table 11.3 are averages obtained in a survey of teaching and district hospital pain clinics in the early 1990s. These have been averaged to a consultant equivalent which is the number of cases and procedures undertaken by a consultant with four half-days dedicated to chronic pain work (P. J. D. Evans, J. Watt, and J. E. Charlton, personal communication).

The marked differences in these figures probably reflect variation in the philosophy of clinical practice as well as the type of patient referred to the clinics. The higher number seen in the district hospital may reflect simpler cases referred because there are specific procedures that the pain clinic can carry out (e.g. nerve blocks, TENS trials). This leads to a higher clinic census and a greater number of procedures. The activity in the teaching hospital may conceivably reflect the leisurely pace of life in the marbled halls of academe, but it is more likely to be a reflection of the complexity of the cases referred and recognition that many chronic pain patients have already had too many invasive procedures. The difference between the new patient numbers and the inpatient numbers on the pain management program numbers represents the number of patients screened initially for their suitability to participate and those admitted to the inpatient part of the program.

The Clinical Standards Advisory Group (CSAG) report noted large variations in the numbers of new patients seen each month.[7] These varied between 15 and 80, and follow-up visits varied between 5 and 160. The ratio of follow-up visits to new patients varied between 0.33 and 7.1.

Treatments used in chronic pain services also varied widely, and Table 11.4 shows the proportion of clinics where the listed treatments were available. This was based on a sample of 122 clinics throughout the UK (data from Pain Society files).

Activity for the year	Hospital 1	Hospital 2 PMP	Hospital 3 district
New patients	270	240	455
Follow ups	550	32	1,075
Outpatient procedures	210	0	550
Day-case procedures	160	0	40
Inpatients	4	110	30

Table 11.3 *Clinical activity in a teaching hospital (Hospital 1), a similar hospital with a pain management program (Hospital 2), and a district hospital (Hospital 3)*

PMP, pain management program.

Table 11.4 *Treatments used in chronic pain services*

Treatments available	Proportion of clinics (%)
Nerve blockade	99
TENS	98
Radiograph-assisted treatments	96
One-shot epidural	96
Acupuncture	86
Physiotherapy	82
Opioids for noncancer pain	75
Continuous epidural	73
Subcutaneous drug delivery systems	71
Psychology	66
Intravenous drug delivery systems	60
Radiofrequency lesioning	51
Pain management program	40
Spinal cord stimulation	26
Hypnotherapy	20

TENS, transcutaneous electrical nerve stimulation.

DISTRICT HOSPITAL PAIN CLINIC

A typical district hospital pain clinic would have the following staff:

- Two consultant anesthesiologists with a minimum of three half-day sessions for acute and chronic pain work. This will provide for continuity of cover.
- Another physician at an intermediate grade carrying out screening or follow-up clinics for two half-days per week.
- An anesthesiologist in training (attending on an intermittent basis).
- The equivalent of a full-time senior nurse specializing in acute pain relief.
- Two part-time nurses or ancillary care workers to help with outpatient clinics and procedure sessions.
- Two specialist cancer care nurses.
- Access to clinical psychology services
- Two part-time secretaries and/or filing clerks.

The consultant anesthesiologists will act as supervisors and back-up for the nurse-led acute pain team. This part of their duties may account for about one half-day per week, the majority of the ward work being undertaken by the nurses. For the chronic pain part of the workload, they will each contribute one or two outpa-

tient clinics per week and undertake one treatment session per week. Each session will be the equivalent of half a day. By and large, administration and the management of the day-to-day running of the clinic (note reviews, checking laboratory and radiological investigations) is done out of hours. The same applies to additional duties, such as seeing inpatients with pain problems in the care of other services in the hospital and the assessment and treatment of patients with pain arising from cancer that is not responding to conventional treatment. These patients may be in the hospital, at home, or in a local hospice.

There is a network of nurses specializing in domiciliary and hospital-based care of patients with advanced cancer throughout the UK. These nurses are not specially trained in pain relief but have wide experience and provide a skilled resource for patient management. Many consultants specializing in pain management have links with these cancer care nurses and local hospices and provide a *pro bono* service of advanced pain relief techniques and invasive treatment. At the district hospital level, until recently, it has been rare for any contractual recognition of the additional burden and expense that can result from this sort of work. Prior to this, work carried out in the palliative care setting has been a donation of time and expertise on the part of the specialist and has been subsidized by other parts of the pain clinic funding.

The overall incidence of pain on admission to a local hospice is 40%; however, only 11% of admissions require further advice about pain treatment and fewer than 4% require invasive treatment by the pain management service (J. E. Charlton, personal communication). The percentage of patients requiring invasive treatment will vary with local practice, but rarely reaches more than 6%.

TEACHING HOSPITAL PAIN CLINIC

The larger teaching hospitals will have greater numbers of personnel and better facilities:

- Four consultant anesthesiologists with a minimum of three half-day sessions for acute and chronic pain work.
- A consultant in another discipline with a regular input into the clinic (e.g. rehabilitation, psychiatry).
- Two physicians at an intermediate grade doing screening or follow-up clinics for two half-days a week.

- A medical academic and/or a Fellow.
- Trainees from various disciplines present all the time (chiefly drawn from anesthesiologists in training).
- One senior nurse specialist in chronic pain relief running some independent clinics.
- The equivalent of two full-time senior nurses specializing in acute pain relief.
- The equivalent of three full-time nurses or ancillary care workers to help with outpatient clinics and procedure sessions.
- Two specialist cancer care nurses based in the hospital.
- Regular links with community-based palliative care nurses and hospice staff.
- One or two full-time clinical psychologists.
- A part-time physiotherapist.
- Two or three whole-time equivalent secretaries and/or filing clerks.
- Managerial and accountancy staff with part-time responsibility to pain clinic.

Clinical activity for a teaching hospital unit is broadly the same as that for a district hospital. The case mix, however, may be very different. Where a pain clinic has been established a long time, the level of expertise in community-based medicine is likely to be high as a consequence of the teaching activity and previous experience of patients treated by the unit. The "easy cases" are no longer referred to the pain clinic as the primary care physicians can treat them effectively. Cases are more difficult to assess and therapy may need to be more prolonged and more complex, and this is reflected in the smaller numbers of patients seen and differences in the number of procedures carried out.

There are, however, many similarities in the clinical work. The teaching hospital pain clinic will take a far greater role in terms of teaching, research, audit, and appraisal. In addition to their greater resources, they will be able to utilize the skills of colleagues in other disciplines such as neurosurgery, rehabilitation, and behavioral medicine. In addition, "rationalization" of some hospital-based services may mean that pediatric and oncology services in the UK are largely found in teaching hospitals and this may generate specialist referrals.

The core activities for all hospital-based pain management units are as follows:

- Medication: control and rationalization of drug therapy is frequently desirable.
- Diagnostic and therapeutic nerve blocks: these may include neurolytic procedures and radiofrequency lesioning.
- Stimulation-produced analgesia such as acupuncture and TENS: physical therapy.
- Psychological approaches.

More advanced treatment methods found in larger units (but not necessarily exclusively) are:

- Sophisticated methods of drug delivery such as implanted drug delivery systems: drug control and detoxification regimes.
- More complicated nerve blocks using modern imaging methods: expertise in these techniques may be found in only a few centers as they decrease in popularity.
- Invasive and expensive techniques such as spinal cord stimulation: techniques of central stimulation and neurosurgery.
- Early triage schemes for injury such as "back schools" and rehabilitation programs.
- Pain management programs and advanced psychological techniques.
- Educational and self-help schemes.

INCOME

As has been suggested earlier, a major issue for pain treatment in the UK is the amount of work that is done without income generation. The majority of pain clinic work is covered by contracts between the hospital (NHS Trust) and the Health Authority. However, these are usually "broad brush" in their approach and have been concluded between administrators. As a consequence, much detail of clinical activity goes unrecognized and it is important to try and get quality issues as part of any contract for pain management. Areas that require special attention include:

- Tracking and recovering income from outpatient consultations, treatment sessions, and follow-up visits.
- Tracking and recovering income from external contracts (referrals from outside the local Health Authority).
- Tracking and recovering income from work carried out within the hospital (inpatient consultations).
- Charging for consultations and interventions carried out at the request of local palliative care teams and hospices.
- Tracking and recovering income from "nonphysician members" of the pain team such as nurses, psychologists, and physiotherapists.
- Recovering the cost of equipment used in invasive therapies, such as implantable devices.
- Charging for educational material and activity and the associated bureau costs.

The best way of ensuring that pain clinic income is maintained is to insist that clinicians are involved in the process of negotiating contracts. This has become of far greater importance because the most recent of a series of reorganizations of the NHS has devolved funding for 75% of the hospital work to primary care. The practical effects of this latest change have yet to be assessed, but it is likely that the purchase of pain management services will

approach. *Best Pract Res Clin Rheumatol* 1999; **13:** 493–506.

● 12. Morley S, Ecclestone C, Williams A. Systematic review and meta-analysis of randomized controlled trials of cognitive behaviour therapy and behaviour therapy for chronic pain in adults, excluding headache. *Pain* 1999; **80:** 1–13.

● 13. Fishbain DA, Cutler RB, Rosomoff HL, *et al*. What is the quality of the implemented meta-analytic procedures in chronic pain treatment meta-analyses? *Clin J Pain* 2000; **16:** 73–85.

● 14. Wittink H. Physical fitness, function and physical therapy in patients with pain: clinical measures of aerobic fitness and performance in patients with chronic low back pain. In: IASP eds. *IASP Refresher Course on Pain Management*. Seattle, WA: IASP Press, 1999: 137–44.

15. Okifuji A, Turk DC, Curran SL. Anger in chronic pain: investigations of anger targets and intensity. *J Psychosomatic Res* 1999; **47:** 1–12.

16. Finestone HM, Stenn P, Davies F, *et al*. Chronic pain and health care utilization in women with a history of childhood sexual abuse. *Child Abuse Neglect* 2000; **24:** 547–56.

17. Liebschutz JM, Feinman G, Sullivan L, *et al*. Physical and sexual abuse in women infected with the human immunodeficiency virus: increased illness and health care utilization. *Arch Intern Med* 2000; **160:** 1659–64.

18. Coker AL, Smith PH, Bethea L, *et al*. Physical health consequences of physical and psychological intimate partner violence. *Arch Fam Med* 2000; **9:** 451–7.

19. Maruta T, Osborne D, Swanson DW, Halling JM. Chronic pain patients and spouses: marital and sexual adjustment. *Mayo Clin Proc* 1981; **56:** 307–10.

◆ 20. Pilowsky I. Abnormal illness behaviour: a 25th anniversary review. *Aust NZ J Psychiatry* 1994; **28:** 566–73.

21. Jensen MP, Nielson WR, Romano JM, *et al*. Further evaluation of the pain stages of change questionnaire: is the transtheoretical model of change useful for patients with chronic pain? *Pain* 2000; **86:** 255–64.

● 22. Turner JA, Keefe FJ. Cognitive–behavioral therapy for chronic pain. In: IASP eds. *IASP Refresher Course on Pain Management*. Seattle, WA: IASP Press, 1999: 523–33.

23. Turner JA, Jensen MP, Romano JM. Do beliefs, coping, and catastrophizing independently predict functioning in patients with chronic pain? *Pain* 2000; **85:** 115–25.

24. Currie SR, Wilson KG, Pontefract AJ, deLaplante L. Cognitive–behavioral treatment of insomnia secondary to chronic pain. *J Consult Clin Psychol* 2000; **68:** 407–16.

25. McQuay H. Opioids in pain management. *Lancet* 1999; **353:** 2229–32.

● 26. Savage SR. Chronic pain and the disease of addiction: the interfacing roles of pain medicine and addiction medicine. In: IASP eds. *IASP Refresher Course on Pain Management*. Seattle, WA: IASP Press, 1999: 115–23.

◆ 27. American Academy of Pain Medicine, American Pain Society. *Joint Consensus Statement Regarding the Use of Opioids for the Treatment of Pain*. Glenview, IL: AAPM, 1996.

28. American Society for Addiction Medicine. Public policy statement: rights and responsibilities of physicians who use opioids for the treatment of pain. *J Addict Dis* 1998; **17:** 131–2.

29. Portenoy RK. Chronic opioid therapy in nonmalignant pain. *J Pain Symptom Ther* 1990; **5:** 1–12.

◆ 30. Fishman SM, Bandman TB, Edwards A, *et al*. The opioid contract in the management of chronic pain. *J Pain Symptom Manage* 1999; **18:** 27–37.

◆ 31. United States Federation of State Medical Boards. Model guidelines for the use of controlled substances in the treatment of pain. *USFSMB Fed Bull* 1998; **85** (2): 84–7.

32. Fishbain DA, Cutler RB, Rosomoff HL, *et al*. Validity of self-reported drug use in chronic pain patients. *Clin J Pain* 1999; **15:** 184–91.

● 33. Wesson D, Ling W, Smith D. Prescription of opioids for treatment of pain in patients with addictive disease. *J Pain Symptom Manage* 1993; **8:** 289–96.

34. Jamison RN, Kauffman J, Katz NP. Characteristics of methadone maintenance patients with chronic pain. *J Pain Symptom Manage* 2000; **19:** 53–62.

◆ 35. Portenoy RK. Current pharmacotherapy of chronic pain. *J Pain Symptom Manage* 2000; **19** (Suppl. 1): S16–S20.

36. Maruta T, Swanson DW, McHardy MJ. Three year follow-up of patients with chronic pain who were treated in a multidisciplinary pain management center. *Pain* 1990; **41:** 47–53.

37. Maruta T, Malinchoc M, Offord KP, Colligan RC. Status of patients with chronic pain 13 years after treatment in a pain management center. *Pain* 1998; **74:** 199–204.

38. Fishbain DA, Cutler RB, Rosomoff HL, *et al*. Prediction of "intent," "discrepancy with intent" and "discrepancy with non-intent" for the patient with chronic pain to return to work after treatment at a pain facility. *Clin J Pain* 1999; **15:** 141–50.

39. Turk DC. Here we go again: outcomes, outcomes, outcomes. *Clin J Pain* 1999; **15:** 241–3.

● 40. Turk DC, Okifuji A. Treatment of chronic pain patients: clinical outcomes, cost-effectiveness, and cost-benefits of multidisciplinary pain centers. *Crit Rev Phys Med Rehabil* 1998; **10:** 181–208.

41. Donovan MI, Evers K, Jacobs P, *et al*. When there is no benchmark: designing a primary care-based chronic pain management program from the scientific basis up. *J Pain Symptom Manage* 1999; **18:** 38–48.

13

Medicolegal aspects of chronic pain

GEORGE MENDELSON, DANUTA MENDELSON, AND NORTIN M HADLER

Chronic pain will test the coping abilities of any sufferer and the artfulness of any physician recruited to pursuit of palliation. Whenever the experience of chronic pain is confounded by medicolegal issues, the challenges are compounded. Such is increasingly the case. In this chapter, we shall provide overviews of three such arenas: (1) the international controls over the distribution and the current legal requirements concerning the prescription of opioid analgesics in a number of jurisdictions; (2) the issue of consent and malpractice in relation to the potential risks of certain types of treatment and procedures undertaken for pain relief; and (3) some aspects of personal injury claims in which pain is a significant complaint.

LEGAL CONTROLS AND USE OF OPIOID ANALGESICS

In this chapter the terms "opioid" or "narcotic" will be used to refer to the therapeutically used drugs prescribed for the relief of severe pain, of which morphine is a typical representative (for an extensive discussion of the pharmacology of this class of agents, see Chapters A3 and P6). All opioids utilized in the management of patients with severe pain are classified as drugs of addiction (termed "drugs of dependence," "dangerous drugs," or "controlled substances" in some legislation). In nearly all jurisdictions in the industrialized world, the prescription of these medications is controlled by legislation. Furthermore, compliance with the relevant legal provisions by the prescribing medical practitioner is monitored. Therefore, practitioners must be familiar with relevant legal requirements so as to comply at all times.

History of legislative controls

The legal control of opioids has been traced by Manderson[1] to "the anti-Chinese hysteria" which, in his view, motivated the enactment of the first "opium laws" in Canada, Australia, and the USA. International cooperation in the control of the manufacture and distribution of opioids – particularly opium itself – was initiated at the time of the Shanghai Opium Commission, which convened in February 1909 with 13 nations represented. In December 1911, the International Conference on Opium, held at The Hague with only 12 nations represented, called for "control of all phases of the preparation and distribution of medicinal opium, morphine, heroin, cocaine, and any new derivative that could be scientifically shown to offer similar dangers."[2] By the Third Conference, in June 1914, Serbia and Turkey were the only governments of the 46 represented to refuse to sign.[2] Later that year, the Harrison Act to control traffic in opioids and cocaine was passed into law by both houses of the US Congress. Following the First World War, the League of Nations constituted an Opium Advisory Committee that was superseded in 1925 by a Permanent Central Board "to oversee the traffic and treaties with regard to narcotics."[2]

It was not until 1961 that further coordinated international action was taken with respect to the control of opioid drugs. At an international conference held in New York that year, 73 countries adopted the Single Convention on Narcotic Drugs. This convention established the International Narcotics Control Board (INCB) to "receive reports from governments about the movement of opioids and would work with national authorities to spot and halt diversion of these substances into illicit channels."[3] (The Single Convention included "cocaine" with the narcotic drugs, although its structure and pharmacology are unrelated to the opioids.)

The second principal aim of the Single Convention was "to codify the treaties that had placed controls over the production, distribution and consumption" of narcotic drugs.[3] The INCB was also to "ensure that supply and demand for licit opioid drugs were in balance, thus preventing undersupply of these medications for legitimate purposes." The INCB, located in Vienna, provides annual reports as well as special reports, such as that on "Availability of opiates for medical needs" published in 1996. It is of concern to read in the report that "most governments in the world did not respond to its questionnaire; thus, the Board did not have sufficient information concerning approximately one half of the world's population."[4] The report noted that there were continuing "unmet medical needs for narcotic drugs particularly but not only in less developed countries."

Current legislative controls

A comprehensive transnational discussion of the statutory controls over the possession, storage, prescription, and administration of drugs of addiction in general, and the opioids in particular, would serve little purpose other than to illustrate the sociopolitical debate the topic generates. It is important for medical practitioners treating patients with chronic pain to be familiar with the provisions of the relevant legislation and the regulations made under the terms of these statutes. We will focus on some of the issues that generalize.

The statutes that govern the prescription and administration of "controlled" substances generally categorize medications as well as other drugs and poisons as "schedules." Opioid analgesics, which are considered capable of producing physical dependence or addiction, are usually singled out. Other drugs of addiction such as cocaine, dexamphetamine, and methylphenidate are often separately scheduled, as are agents such as the benzodiazepines and chloral hydrate which can produce dependence. Although psychostimulants have been used in controlled studies for pain relief, legal restrictions on their prescription preclude their use for this indication in Australia but not necessarily in other countries.[5,6]

The legislation in the various jurisdictions generally provides that medical practitioners and dentists (as well as veterinary surgeons who, however, may only prescribe such a drug for the treatment of an animal) are the only persons entitled to prescribe narcotics. Generally, these substances have to be stored locked separately from other drugs. Often, as in the various Australian states and territories, a register must be kept to record the administration of controlled substances. In some jurisdictions, it is a legal requirement that administration of opioids be witnessed as a safeguard against self-administration of narcotics by nursing or medical staff.

Specific provisions, which vary dramatically transnationally, apply if the patient is considered to be addicted to an opioid. In Australia, the medical practitioner must obtain a permit before prescribing for a person believed to be drug dependent. Methadone is the only opioid sanctioned, and is only permitted if the patient is being treated at a methadone program treatment center. In South Australia, such drugs can only be prescribed for maintaining or treating addiction with authorization by the Health Commission.

In the USA, the prescription of opioids is regulated by the federal Controlled Substances Act (CSA) and the Federal Food, Drug, and Cosmetic Act (FFDCA).[7] The legislation requires registration, record-keeping, and reporting of the use of opioids. According to Joranson,[7] there are six aspects to the CSA control of the use of opioids: (1) opioids are necessary to public health; (2) opioid availability is guaranteed; (3) the federal definition of addict does not include chronic pain patients; (4) federal regulations specifically recognize opioid treatment of intractable pain; (5) the amount of opioid provided is not restricted; and (6) medical and scientific matters are considered in making drug control decisions.

In the USA, most state laws regulating opioid prescription are modeled on the Uniform Controlled Substances Act developed by the National Conference on Uniform State Laws.[7] In some states, physicians are required to report "addicts" and those who require extended treatment with controlled substances. Although federal law in the USA does not restrict the amount of opioid which may be prescribed, several states do, including New York, New Jersey, Utah, and Wisconsin.[7] Ten states require that a copy of each prescription for a controlled substance be sent to the state agency which monitors the prescribing of such substances.[8,9] Because of concern that such programs may discourage the physician from prescribing opioids for patients who have a legitimate medical need for the medication, the Rhode Island medical association advised its members that the multiple copy prescription system "is not to be used as the excuse for not prescribing and that the doctor will be liable under malpractice statutes" for failure to provide necessary medication, and the state legislature was reported in 1995 to have drafted a bill to eliminate the duplicate copy prescription program.[10]

In Texas, the Intractable Pain Treatment Act 1989 has defined intractable pain as "a pain state in which the cause of the pain cannot be removed or otherwise treated and for which in the generally accepted course of medical practice no relief or cure of the cause of the pain is possible or none has been found after reasonable effort." The Act provides that, subject to certain safeguards and provisions concerning nontherapeutic prescription, "physicians in Texas may treat intractable pain with opioids as they may under federal law, that hospitals or other facilities may not interfere with a physician's treatment of intractable pain, and that a physician is not subject to disciplinary action solely for treating intractable pain."[7] Similar legislation has been adopted by California, Missouri, Nevada, North Dakota, Oregon, Virginia, and Washington. The Oregon statute requires the patient's written consent to pain medication. The need for such legislation protecting physicians who utilize opioids for treatment of chronic noncancer pain has been demonstrated by a series of cases in a number of states of the USA, where doctors had been charged by state authorities for "inappropriately and excessively" prescribing Schedule II controlled substances.[11,12]

A model Pain Relief Act has been developed under the sponsorship of the American Society of Law, Medicine and Ethics,[13] and with continued efforts from the various Cancer Pain Initiatives in the United States it could be that this will become the basis for legislation in some states. The purpose of such proposed legislative changes is to ensure that "with new standards of care, prescriptions for opioids written in good faith for the treatment of pain should survive legal scrutiny."[14]

In 1996, the Canadian Parliament enacted the Controlled Drugs and Substances Act which came into force on 14 May 1997. Under this statute, a patient seeking to obtain an opioid analgesic from a medical practitioner must disclose to the practitioner particulars relating to the acquisition by him or her of every substance listed in the schedules to the Act, and of every authorization to obtain such substances from other practitioners, within the preceding 30 days.

The Canadian Centre on Substance Abuse Act 1988 appears to be a unique legislation that established a center for the promotion of increased awareness of alcohol and drug abuse, education, and the development of harm minimization policies.

In the UK, the Misuse of Drugs Act 1971 and the Criminal Justice (International Co-operation) Act 1990 provide, respectively, for the control and regulation of narcotics in accordance with the Single Convention and for cooperation in implementation of the Vienna Convention against Illicit Traffic in Narcotic Drugs and Psychotropic Substances.

The use of opioids in pain management

Discussion of the clinical indications for the prescription of narcotic analgesics for patients with chronic pain can be found in many of the chapters in this text. In the management of patients with cancer pain, the use of analgesics should follow the principles recommended by the World Health Organization.[15] This allows for the gradual introduction of narcotic analgesics if inadequate pain relief is obtained from mild analgesics and other treatments, according to well-established clinical practice of dose titration.[16]

Although the role of narcotic analgesics in the management of cancer pain is well recognized, the use of these agents in the treatment of patients with chronic noncancer pain remains controversial. It has been claimed that "fear of addiction limits opioid use by both physicians and patients,"[17] and the term "opiophobia" has been used to describe this phenomenon.[18] Zenz and Willweber-Strumpf have commented specifically on opiophobia and the widespread phenomenon of undertreatment of cancer pain in a number of European countries.[19] On the other hand, systematic attempts to demonstrate important benefit from opioids in chronic noncancer back pain provide little compelling rationale for opioid prescription.[20] Such data fuel the controversy.

The influence of the laws that regulate the prescription of opioids on the treatment of cancer pain has been commented on by several authors. According to Weissman, there are four "potential ways" in which such laws and regulations can affect medical care. These are (1) by placing restrictions on physician practice; (2) by affecting patient access to opioid analgesics; (3) by stigmatizing patients; and (4) indirectly through physicians' perceptions of regulations, resulting in modified medical practices.[21]

Weissman cited data which indicated that, in the USA, in states with a multiple copy prescription program only 21–35% of registered physicians had ordered the necessary prescription blanks, in effect "restricting patient access" to effective opioid analgesics. The requirement in some states that patients receiving opioids long-term, even for cancer pain, must be registered as drug addicts is stigmatizing, and responsible for reluctance by patients who might be benefited. In response, some medical boards have published clinical guidelines to try to overcome any unfounded concerns and fears.[22,23]

The introduction of a multiple copy prescription program in Texas in 1982 led to a 63.6% reduction in prescriptions for opioids, suggesting that less potent medications had been substituted. Other data cited by Weissman indicated that a survey of physicians in Minnesota found that they were reluctant to prescribe opioids for both acute and chronic pain owing to the then "current Minnesota regulatory climate" and also "indicated a reduced willingness to accept new patients who may require controlled substances."[21] Similarly, a survey of French oncologists and primary care physicians showed that "the constraints of prescription forms" as well as "perceptions that morphine has a poor image in public opinion" were among factors that inhibited the prescription of morphine for cancer pain.[24]

The influence of governmental regulations was also highlighted by Hill to be among factors that lead to undertreatment of pain, among other societal barriers to adequate pain management.[25,26] Such barriers affect the treatment of pain due to cancer as well as chronic noncancer pain.[27]

LEGAL LIABILITY AND PAIN MANAGEMENT

Shapiro[28] has discussed liability issues that may arise in the management of pain under the following five headings:

1 liability to patients and/or exposure to professional discipline for inappropriate pain management;
2 liability to third parties for injury caused by patients treated for pain;
3 the legal distinction between pain management and euthanasia or physician-assisted suicide;
4 health care payors' liability to patients for cost-containment decisions that impact on pain management;
5 manufacturers' and health care providers' liability for the risks and side-effects of prescription drugs and pain-management devices.

Other legal issues in pain management relate to the use of placebo medications,[29] generally in a misguided attempt to demonstrate that the pain "is not real."

The impact of cost-containment decisions, responsibility to third parties, and product liability issues will not be discussed in this chapter. Euthanasia and physician-assisted suicide have been the topic of numerous articles and symposia over the past few years, and the interested reader is referred to articles which discuss the legislation in the Northern Territory of Australia,[30–32] [now overridden by the federal Euthanasia Laws Act 1997 (Cth)], and the medical,[33] psychiatric,[34] coronial,[35] and moral[36,37] issues which it raised. Other recent reviews have considered the current position in the USA,[38] including constitutional,[39] legal,[40] regulatory,[41,42] and nursing[43] concerns.

This section will discuss issues involving direct liability to patients, such as obtaining valid consent to treatment, and malpractice claims related to pain management. We shall not discuss issues relevant to the misdiagnosis of acute pain in emergency settings (such as myocardial infarction or acute appendicitis[44]), as these generally are pertinent to acute care and emergency physicians[45] rather than those working in specialized pain clinics.

Valid consent to treatment and medical duty of adequate disclosure

In the UK, Australia, and Canada, the law considers consent to medical treatment as "real" or "valid" for the purposes of a defense against the allegation of battery if it is given by a competent person who has made the decision voluntarily upon being informed in broad terms of the nature and effects of the "general surgical procedure or treatment."[46] It is in this sense of validity of the patient's consent that the Australian law requires consent to be "informed." Consequently, in the case of Rogers v. Whitaker[46] the High Court of Australia rejected the American doctrine of informed consent[47] in the context of the law of negligence, noting that the expression "the patient's right to self-determination" is "perhaps suitable to cases where the issue is whether a person has agreed to the general surgical procedure or treatment." In rejecting the American doctrine of informed consent in negligence, the High Court of Australia followed the majority of the House of Lords in Sidaway's case (see below), and the decision in the Canadian case of Reibl v. Hughes.[48]

In the UK case of In re W,[49] Lord Donaldson MR provided a most insightful explanation of the importance and purpose of consent to medical treatment when he wrote that:

[consent] has two purposes, the one clinical and the other legal. The clinical purpose stems from the fact that in many instances the cooperation of the patient and the patient's faith or at least confidence in the efficiency of the treatment is a major fact contributing to the treatment's success. Failure to obtain such consent will not only deprive the patient and the medical staff of this advantage, but will usually make it more difficult to administer the treatment … The legal purpose is quite different. It is to provide those concerned in the treatment with a defence to a criminal charge of assault or battery or a civil claim for damages for trespass to the person. It does not, however, provide them with any defence to a claim that they negligently advised a particular treatment or negligently carried it out.

Prosecution for criminal battery, or a civil action for trespass to the person, in relation to nonconsensual treatment for the purpose of pain relief would probably only occur in exceptional circumstances. Laskin CJ, of the Canadian Supreme Court, in the case of Reibl v. Hughes,[48] noted that he could "appreciate the temptation to say that the genuineness of consent to medical treatment depends on proper disclosure of the risks which it entails, but … unless there has been misrepresentation or fraud to secure consent to the treatment, a failure to disclose the attendant risks, however serious, should go to negligence rather than to battery."

It is worth noting that some statutes which enshrine a patient's right to refuse medical treatment exclude pain relief and palliative care from the definition of medical treatment that can be refused. This means that, under such a statute, neither the patient nor the patient's agent can refuse palliative care which includes "the provision of reasonable medical procedures for relief of pain, suffering and discomfort."[50]

As Lord Donaldson pointed out, however, the patient's consent of itself will not provide the physician with a defense to a claim that he or she "negligently advised a particular treatment or negligently carried it out." Under the law of negligence, where there exists a legal duty of care toward another person, one must guard against creating risks that may result in an injury to that person. If a particular risk cannot be eliminated or minimized, then the risk ought to be disclosed to those who may be harmed by it. However, the patient can only sue in negligence for nondisclosure of the particular risk if the risk actually eventuates causing an injury. The duty of medical practitioners toward their patients involves the exercise of reasonable care and skill in the provision of diagnosis, advice, and treatment to the patient. The breach of duty may involve a failure to disclose a reasonably foreseeable material risk inherent in the proposed treatment.

The medical duty of adequate disclosure is based upon acknowledgment that, while provision of information in broad terms about the nature of the intended procedure is sufficient to satisfy the legal standard of valid consent as a defense to a possible claim of battery, it falls short of satisfying the concept of consent as an expression of the patient's considered choice.

The issue of consent in negligence is thus relevant in so far as it helps to establish the standard of care expected of a medical practitioner in relation to advice and provision of information – did the medical practitioner, for example, provide sufficient information to enable the patient to choose between undergoing or not undergoing the risky treatment in question? The patient's "choice is, in reality, meaningless unless it is made on the basis of relevant information and advice."[46] The principles relating to the medical duty to provide adequate advice are the same irrespective of the nature of the proposed operation; the two cases described below were chosen because they deal with surgery undertaken for relief of chronic pain.

In the Sidaway case, the plaintiff, aged 64 years, had a laminectomy at the C4–5 level for the relief of pain in the right shoulder and arm. Following the operation, Mrs Sidaway developed "a severe impairment of movement on her right side and some ill effects on the left" which were attributed to damage to the spinal cord at the time of the operation.[51]

The subsequent legal proceedings were appealed to the House of Lords. In a majority decision, the Law Lords accepted that the decision as to what degree of disclosure of risks is best calculated to assist a particular patient to make a rational choice whether or not to undergo a specific treatment is a matter of clinical judgment. Their Lordships applied the test of liability first adopted by McNair J in the case of Bolam v. Friern Hospital Management Committee,[52] according to which doctors would not be found in breach of the duty in the matters of diagnosis and treatment if they had acted in accordance with a practice accepted at the time as proper by a reasonable body of medical opinion even though other physicians may have adopted a different practice.

In Sidaway's case, the court considered that the risk of serious complications following an operation of the type which the plaintiff had was in the range of 1–2%, and that the surgeon was therefore not under a legal duty to disclose such low-level risk. It was noted, however, that "the court must decide whether the information afforded to the patient was sufficient to alert the patient to the possibility of serious harm of the kind in fact suffered." In a dissenting judgment, Lord Scarman stated:[53]

> English law must recognize a duty of the doctor to warn his patient of the risk inherent in the treatment which he is proposing; and especially so if the treatment is going to be surgery. The critical limitation is that the duty is confined to material risk. The test of materiality is whether in the circumstances of the particular case the court is satisfied that a reasonable person in the patient's position would be likely to attach significance to the risk.

In the Australian case of Ellis v. Wallsend District Hospital,[54] the plaintiff, Mrs Ellis, had for many years suffered from apparently intractable neck pain. She became addicted to a prescription drug. Problems resulting from her drug dependence led to hospital admissions on at least three occasions. In 1974, she took what was described as "a serious drug overdose." In 1975, Mrs Ellis underwent a cervical posterior rhizotomy (involving the C2–C6 nerve roots) at Wallsend District Hospital, for the relief of her chronic neck pain. Six days after the operation, she became quadriplegic. The surgeon died in 1986. In 1988, Mrs Ellis brought proceedings in assault, negligence, and breach of contract against the surgeon's estate and Wallsend District Hospital. She alleged that the surgeon was negligent in: (1) advising her to undergo the operation; (2) failing to warn her of the risks attendant on the type of surgery performed; (3) failing to obtain her consent to the operation; and (4) performing the operation.

These allegations against the surgeon and the hospital were originally heard by Cole J, who held that the late surgeon and the hospital were not liable. With respect to the allegation of negligence, His Honour found that the surgeon breached the duty of care when he failed to warn Mrs Ellis of the risk of paralysis due to the close proximity of the site of the operation to the spinal cord, and of the risk that there was only a 30% chance of success in achieving long-term pain relief.

Rogers v. Whitaker[55] remains the major Australian case dealing with the medical duty of disclosure of material risks. The defendant ophthalmic surgeon, Dr Rogers, performed surgery upon the plaintiff, Mrs Whitaker, who had lost vision in her right eye at the age of 9 years. She had retained normal vision in her left eye. In 1984, at the age of 47 years, she went to Dr Rogers to surgically improve the appearance of the right eye by removing scar tissue. It was also hoped that the operation would restore significant sight to that eye and also assist in managing the plaintiff's early glaucoma. Mrs Whitaker was apparently very nervous and "keenly interested" to know of possible complications which might attend the operation. Dr Rogers told her about some risks, but failed to mention the possibility of the admittedly remote risk (1: 14,000) of sympathetic ophthalmia occurring in her left eye. Mrs Whitaker agreed to the operation, which was carried out without negligence. Nevertheless, the plaintiff did develop sympathetic ophthalmia in her left eye and as a result became virtually blind in 1986. She sued Dr Rogers for a negligent failure to respond to her questions about possible complications by warning her of the risk, albeit remote, of sympathetic ophthalmia. The court held that he was liable.

The majority in the High Court adopted the approach of Lord Scarman in the Sidaway case and of Laskin CJ in the Canadian case, Reibl v. Hughes.[56] Their Honours explained that although the duty of a medical practitioner to exercise reasonable care and skill in the provision of professional advice and treatment is a single and comprehensive duty, there are distinctions among diagnosis, treatment, and advice. The first two elements of the doctor–patient relationship are regarded as the essence of clinical function, with the patient's contribution limited to the narration of symptoms and relevant history enabling the medical practitioner to provide diagnosis and treatment according to his or her level of skill. However, in the area of provision of advice to the patient, the court can make its own assessment of whether the extent of the disclosure is sufficient, because, "except in cases of emergency or necessity, all medical treatment is preceded by the patient's choice to undergo it."[55] Such choice will be meaningless unless it is made on the basis of disclosure of the material risks inherent in the proposed treatment. The High Court held that the risk is material if:[55]

> in the circumstances of the case, a reasonable person in the patient's position, if warned of the risk, would be likely to attach significance to it or if the medical practitioner is or should reasonably be aware that the particular patient, if warned of the risk, would be likely to attach significance to it. This duty is subject to therapeutic privilege.

It is incumbent on the physician to make sure that the patient understands the information, particularly where it appears that the patient may have some difficulty with the language spoken by the doctor.[57] The concept of therapeutic privilege allows the physician discretion in respect of whether or not and, if so, when to disclose disturbing information directly to the patient. Therapeutic privilege operates in those cases where there is a particular danger that the provision of all relevant information will harm an unusually nervous, disturbed, or volatile patient.

Guidelines formulated by the National Health and Medical Research Council of Australia suggest that known risks should be disclosed when an adverse outcome is common even though the detriment is slight; known risks should be disclosed where the potential injury or damage is severe even though the occurrence of such an adverse outcome is rare.[58]

Similar considerations concerning disclosure of potential material risks apply to other treatment procedures undertaken for pain management, e.g. nerve blocks. Swerdlow[59] has reviewed a variety of problems following such procedures which have led to legal action, and found that lack of consent was one of the five grounds on which such litigation had arisen. Others were medical complications due to the procedure, incompetence in carrying out the specific procedure, the wrong procedure being performed, and inadequate treatment of the complication.

The law in relation to consent and the duty of disclosure was again considered by the High Court of Australia in the case of Chappel v. Hart.[60] Mrs Hart had a wide-necked pharyngeal diverticulum (pharyngeal pouch). Because of this condition, small scraps of food which she swallowed collected in the pouch, causing infection and inflammation. It was acknowledged that Mrs Hart's condition was painful and very distressing, with surgery providing the only prospect of a cure. She was referred to the defendant surgeon, who advised that she should undergo a procedure for removal of the pharyngeal pouch. The court accepted that the perforation of the esophagus, a well-recognized complication of this procedure, can and does occur without any negligence on the part of the surgeon.

In the great majority of cases, the perforation will have no lasting adverse effects. However, on rare occasions bacteria may be present in the esophagus. Such presence occurs at random. If this happens, there is a risk that the bacteria may escape through the perforation into the mediastinum and cause inflammation of the tissues of the mediastinum (mediastinitis). Mediastinitis may in turn lead to a number of further complications, including inflammation of laryngeal nerves, which may, on a rare occasion, cause the loss of function of a vocal cord. Her surgeon, Mr Chappel, warned Mrs Hart of the inherent risk of esophageal perforation, but did not warn her about the risk of mediastinitis and laryngeal nerve damage. This risk eventuated following a procedure undertaken on 10 June 1983, when part of the pouch was excised. While her condition was not thereby aggravated, the distressing problem associated with swallowing food persisted. In February 1985, a grape stuck in Mrs Hart's throat and had to be surgically removed. Subsequently, another surgeon successfully carried out the second stage of surgery to remove the pouch.

However, owing to the laryngeal nerve damage, Mrs Hart was unable to shout, and so she resigned from her work as a school librarian. She sued Mr Chappel in negligence and in contract, claiming that he was negligent, *inter alia*, in his failure to warn her that the procedure involved an inherent risk of mediastinitis and the risk of possible injury to the laryngeal nerve. This information, Mrs Hart submitted, related to material risks of which the defendant ought to have warned her. The majority determined that Dr Chappel's failure to warn the plaintiff about these risks constituted a breach of duty of care.

In Australia, there has been adverse publicity in the media concerning the epidural injection of steroids, although the accepted view in the medical literature has been that such injections are both safe and effective in the management of specific conditions.[61,62] Claims to the contrary have been made by Nelson,[63] whose article has been criticized and attention has been drawn to his misquotation of the relevant literature.[64,65] The Health Department of Western Australia[66] has issued guidelines for the use of epidural steroids, which set out the indications for this treatment and the appropriate procedure for obtaining valid consent, including relevant information which

although drawing attention to the hazards of the loose and imprecise usage of medical terminology in the medicolegal field, itself has been criticized for vague and in some instances even incorrect (e.g. its description of sciatica) discussion of certain terms. In a discussion of the possible relationships between chronic pain and litigation, Weintraub[110] drew attention to what he termed "the surge in fraudulent claims" in the USA. There are, however, no objective tests to determine whether or not an individual does or does not subjectively experience pain, and each patient with a complaint of pain, whether or not involved in litigation or in receipt of compensation benefits, requires a comprehensive evaluation. It is ultimately for the court to determine whether or not a claim is fraudulent. As we have argued elsewhere, there is no such diagnosis as "malingering,"[111] and any such putative "diagnosis" offered by a clinician usurps the function of the trier of fact.

Of relevance in this context is the trend identified by Merskey and Teasell that they have described as "the disparagement of pain."[112] According to these authors, there are three factors that encourage physicians to underestimate patients' pain. These are: the requirement for doctors to control the issue of narcotics; circumstances in which patients may benefit from compensation by exaggeration of pain severity; and the development of attitudes that understate the importance of the relief of pain and overstate the importance of activity, exercise, and not complaining.

Despite anecdotal and single-case reports, whether or not fibromyalgia can be caused by traumatic injury remains unresolved, and similarly it is unclear whether it can be considered to be a cause of work disability.[113,114] The apparent increasing prevalence may be attributable to the new-found respectability and validation, both medical and social, of the diagnostic term.

The effect of compensation on pain treatment outcome

Having no recourse that seems more ready or more appealing than to be a claimant seeking redress under workers' compensation for a regional musculoskeletal disorder, as we discussed above, is a reproach to the psychosocial milieu of the workplace. True, the vast majority of such claimants return to work as rapidly as if they had sought care in the context of health insurance but they do not feel as well when they return.[115] And once a claimant, they are more likely to seek similar recourse with the next regional musculoskeletal disorder and to recover even less rapidly. Emerging from this population are those who do not return to work at all. These are the chronic pain patients for whom Workers' Compensation bureaucracies spend so much in the quest for maximal medical improvement and more, yet, in disability determination. The care of these claimants underwrites

a goodly percentage of the establishment devoted to the management of chronic noncancer pain. Many of these claimants feel better for the effort. Few feel well enough to return to their prior level of performance so that there is no compromise in their income. For example, Fowler and Mayfield,[116] in a study comparing 327 patients receiving disability compensation with 613 patients not in receipt of compensation, commented that compensation beneficiaries – although manifesting fewer symptoms – had a significantly poorer occupational adjustment than the no-compensation group.

In a similar study of the duration of time off work due to low back pain, Leavitt[117] found that among a group of 1,373 patients with pain following a work injury 23.7% were disabled for longer than 12 months, whereas among 417 patients with similar pain not receiving compensation benefits 13.2% were off work for longer than 12 months.

The surgical literature is replete with the observation that elective orthopedic procedures are met with less success when the patient is a workers' compensation claimant. That has been shown repeatedly in lumbar spine and carpal tunnel surgery.[118]

Although the studies reviewed above have indicated that the receipt of compensation has a negative effect on treatment outcome and tends to prolong work disability, it has been demonstrated that specific treatment programs can reduce the likelihood of progression to pain chronicity following work injuries.[119,120] Similarly, Fordyce et al.[121] have shown that a treatment program for low back pain, which incorporates behavioral methods, is more effective than traditional management. Thus, the adverse effect of compensation on the outcome of treatment for acute pain following work injuries can be modified by specific programs which stress early mobilization and return to the work-place, appropriate activity and exercises, and avoidance of other factors which may promote "learned pain behavior."

The rating of pain-related impairment

Sensible or not, in the context of the medicolegal evaluation of a compensation recipient or litigant with chronic pain, it is important to distinguish between the concepts of impairment and disability, as defined by the World Health Organization.[122] Impairment is defined as the "loss or abnormality of psychological, physiological, or anatomical structure or function," whereas disability is defined as the "restriction or lack (resulting from an impairment) of ability to perform an activity in the manner or within the range considered normal for a human being."

It is generally accepted that the evaluation and rating of impairment is the task of the clinician, whereas the determination of disability is an administrative and legal issue that depends upon the specific circumstances of the claimant and the relevant statutory provisions.

These considerations have been summed up in the following terms by Curran et al.:[123]

[I]t is desirable that "impairment" and "disability" not be used interchangeably. The evaluation of impairment is alone a medical responsibility, while the evaluation of disability is essentially an administrative responsibility. While the uniquely medical character of the former is self-evident, the determination of disability involves review, not only of medical factors but of legal, psychological, social, and vocational considerations as well.

Guidelines for the evaluation and rating of permanent impairment due to pain had been included in the fourth edition of the Guides published by the American Medical Association.[124] The Guides stated that "chronic pain and pain-related behavior are not, per se, impairments, but they should trigger assessments with regard to ability to function and carry out daily activities." This statement suggests that pain may be a cause of disability, although it is not "per se" an impairment.

The Guides also noted that in the USA the Social Security Administration "gives credence to pain only insofar as it relates to an underlying physical or mental impairment," and that similarly the US Department of Veterans' Affairs "generally does not consider pain, except as a manifestation of a physical or mental impairment."

Despite these caveats, the Guides repeatedly referred to "pain impairment," yet offered little practical assistance beyond stating that "chronic pain in the absence of objectively validated diseases or impairments, such as those that are described in the Guides, should be evaluated on a multidisciplinary basis." The "pain intensity–frequency grid" provided no indication as to how impairment could be evaluated on the basis of that grid. The three examples provided in this chapter were similarly unhelpful, and in each instance the reader was referred to the appropriate section for an impairment assessment based on the underlying physical disorder.

This edition of the Guides, like its predecessors, lacked specific criteria for the rating of impairment due to chronic pain in the absence of a demonstrable organic abnormality.

In the fifth edition of the AMA Guides, published in 2000, the chapter dealing with pain-related impairment was entirely rewritten by Turk, Loeser, and Robinson, all from the University of Washington's multidisciplinary pain clinic.

In previous writings, Turk et al.[125] had suggested a set of multiaxial criteria for the determination of "impairment due primarily to pain." The criteria they had proposed combined both physical findings or behavioral manifestations and functional loss. Thus, whether or not abnormal physical findings were present, there would need also to be significant functional loss in the areas of "daily living, social functioning, time efficiency in completing routine tasks of living, and the performance of basic work behaviors."

These authors also discussed the various procedures used in the evaluation of pain patients, and recommended that additional measures such as observation of pain behaviors, assessment of coping skills, cognitive style, and vocational factors be utilized in the determination of impairment due primarily to chronic pain.

In a subsequent article, Turk and Rudy further discussed the problems in assessment due to the "minimal association between the extent of impairment and degree of disability, and between the magnitude of physical pathology and severity of the pain report."[126]

They commented that "the most prominent behavioral component of persistent pain and disability is associated with the principles of operant conditioning." In relation to pain complaints that are attributed to work injuries, Turk and Rudy observed that:[126]

[A]nother operant conditioning principle that is relevant to persistent pain is that of response costs that can operate to decrease "well behaviors,'" for example, when injured workers are told by attorneys, employers, or union representatives that they will lose their pending litigation cases or compensation benefits if they are observed engaging in normal activities. Because of established reinforcement contingencies, pain behaviors persist long after the initial tissue pathology is resolved or greatly reduced. These behaviors then become an important set of factors in understanding reports of pain and disability and thus are among the targets of assessment and elimination.

Turk and Rudy[126] suggested that the focus of impairment and disability evaluation be on the injured worker rather than on biomedical diagnosis, and that psychological, behavioral, and job-related factors also need to be considered.

The benefits of such an approach in the vocational rehabilitation of injured workers have been demonstrated by the success of functional restoration[127,128] and work-hardening programs.[129] In relation to such programs, it is relevant to note that "disability exaggeration" is a poor predictor of the success of functional restoration program for patients with chronic low back pain.[130] These authors have commented that, in fact, when disability exaggeration did correlate significantly with a positive treatment outcome, the correlation was negative.

It is clear that any proposed system of rating of impairment due to chronic pain needs to take into consideration relevant occupational factors in translating impairment into disability. McBride,[131] in an important yet relatively neglected work on the evaluation of disability, provided an extensive listing of various occupations, indicating those parts of the body which may be functionally impaired and the individual "still work at the designated job." Nachemson[132] emphasized that, with respect to chronic low back pain, return to work is possible and indeed "well justified from a medical, psychological, and economic point of view" for the approximately 80% of patients who do not have an objectively demonstrable organic cause for the pain complaint or significant physical impairment.

There is an urgent need for the type of classification of suitable occupations initially devised by McBride to be updated. Robinson[133] has presented a list of 89 occupations that he termed "potentially appropriate" for individuals who are unable to return to their usual work because of low back pain. The approach that he used to identify these occupations, based on the Worker Rehabilitation Questionnaire, is a promising one, and deserves further evaluation.

In discussing the concepts of impairment and disability due to chronic pain, it must also be noted that the Committee on Pain, Disability, and Chronic Illness Behavior of the Institute of Medicine, in an important report, recommended that "'chronic pain' alone should not be added to the SSA [Social Security Administration, USA] regulatory listing of impairments that allow a presumption of disability, nor should 'chronic pain syndrome' be added to the listings. Likewise, 'illness behavior' should be neither a diagnosis nor a listing."[133] Thus, the Committee recommended that the complaint of chronic pain "*per se*," in the absence of a specific diagnosable physical disease or mental disorder, should not be accepted as a cause of work incapacity leading to entitlement to disability benefits.

If it is considered that the pain complained of by the patient cannot be attributed to a specific demonstrable physical cause, the problem of determining the extent of any pain-related impairment thus becomes a difficult one, and the method initially suggested by Turk *et al.*,[125,126] and now incorporated with minimal modifications in the fifth edition of the AMA Guides,[103] appears the most appropriate. As set out in Chapter 18 of the fifth edition of the AMA Guides, the evaluation of pain-related impairment involves six steps. Three of these utilize questionnaires, and thus rely on the individual's self-report. These questionnaires rate pain severity, activity limitation, and effect of pain on mood. The examiner rates the individual on the presence of pain behaviors, and is also required to make "a global assessment of the person's credibility." The final step involves the calculation of the "total pain-related impairment score" and the determination of the "impairment class" on the basis of that score.

It will be apparent that the method of assessment of pain-related impairment in the fifth edition of the AMA Guides is quite different from those in relation to other conditions. One of the principles of impairment assessment is that it should have an objective basis. Although Chapter 18 is an improvement on its predecessors in earlier editions of the AMA Guides, it is crucially dependent not only on the subjective responses of the person being evaluated but also on the subjective responses of the examiner, both in relation to observations of pain behavior and in deciding that person's credibility.

There are indications that in many jurisdictions the

courts and tribunals are becoming increasingly familiar with the recent advances in the understanding of pain mechanisms, and are beginning to utilize this knowledge in the decision-making process.[135] It is therefore equally important that clinicians who treat patients with chronic pain and who are likely therefore to become involved as expert witnesses in the legal process keep abreast of new developments in the understanding and management of chronic pain problems.

REFERENCES

1. Manderson D. An archaeology of drug laws. *Int J Drug Policy* 1994; **5:** 235–45.
2. Musto DF. *The American Disease: Origins of Narcotic Control* (expanded edition). New York, NY: Oxford University Press, 1987.
3. Angarola RT. National and international regulation of opioid drugs: purpose, structures, benefits and risks. *J Pain Symptom Manage* 1990; **5:** S6–S11.
4. International Narcotics Control Board. *Availability of Opiates for Medical Needs*. Vienna: INCB, 1996.
5. Bruera E, Watanabe S. Psychostimulants as adjuvant analgesics. *J Pain Symptom Manage* 1994; **9:** 412–15.
6. Yee JD, Berde CB. Dextroamphetamine or methylphenidate as adjuvants to opioid analgesia for adolescents with cancer. *J Pain Symptom Manage* 1994; **9:** 122–5.
7. Joranson DE. Federal and state regulation of opioids. *J Pain Symptom Manage* 1990; **5:** S12–S23.
8. Wastila LJ, Bishop C. The influence of multiple copy prescription programs on analgesic utilization. *J Pharm Care Pain Symptom Control* 1996; **4** (3): 3–19.
9. Angarola RT, Bormel FG. The potential negative impact of multiple copy prescription programs on patient care. *J Pharm Care Pain Symptom Control* 1996; **4** (3): 53–6.
10. Angarola RT. DEA proposes controlled substances monitoring act. *APS Bull* 1995; **5** (3): 3–5, 22.
11. Hoover v. The Agency for Health Care Administration, 676 So.2d 1380 (Fla. 3rd DCA 1996).
12. Reese v. Department of Professional Registration, Board of Medical Examiners, 471 So.2d 601 (Fla. 1st DCA 1985).
13. Dubler N, Levine R, Johnson SH. Project on legal constraints on access to effective pain relief. In: *Syllabus of National Meeting on Legal, Ethical and Institutional Issues in Pain Relief*. Cambridge, MA, 1996.
14. Clark HW, Sees KL. Opioids, chronic pain and the law. *J Pain Symptom Manage* 1993; **8:** 297–305.
15. Swerdlow M, Stjernsward J. Cancer pain relief – an urgent problem. *World Health Forum* 1982; **3:** 325–30.
16. Foley KM. The treatment of cancer pain. *N Engl J Med* 1985; **313:** 84–95.
17. Foley KM. The "decriminalization" of cancer pain. In: Hill CS, Fields WS eds. *Drug Treatment of Cancer Pain in a Drug-oriented Society*. New York, NY: Raven Press, 1989: 5–18.

◆ 18. Morgan JP. American opiophobia: customary under-utilization of opioid analgesics. In: Hill CS, Fields WS eds. *Drug Treatment of Cancer Pain in a Drug-oriented Society*. New York, NY: Raven Press, 1989: 175–89.

19. Zenz M, Willweber-Strumpf A. Opiophobia and cancer pain in Europe. *Lancet* 1993; **342**: 1075–6.

● 20. Jamison RN, Raymond SA, Slawsby EA, *et al*. Opioid therapy for chronic noncancer back pain. *Spine* 1998; **23**: 2591–600.

21. Weissman DE. Doctors, opioids and the law: the effect of controlled substances regulations on cancer pain management. *Semin Oncol* 1993; **20** (2 Suppl. 1): 53–8.

22. California Medical Board. Guideline for prescribing controlled substances. *J Pharm Care Pain Symptom Control* 1995; **3** (2): 117–21.

23. Robinson DE. Prescribing controlled substances for cancer pain: position paper of the Utah Division of Occupational and Professional Licensing. *J Pharm Care Pain Symptom Control* 1993; **1**: 109–112.

24. Larue F, Colleau SM, Fontaine A, Brasseur L. Oncologists and primary care physicians' attitudes toward pain control and morphine prescribing in France. *Cancer* 1995; **76**: 2375–82.

◆ 25. Hill CS. The negative influence of licensing and disciplinary boards and drug enforcement agencies on pain treatment with opioid analgesics. *J Pharm Care Pain Symptom Manage* 1993; **1**: 43–62.

26. Hill CS. The barriers to adequate pain management with opioid analgesics. *Semin Oncol* 1993; **20** (Suppl. 1): 1–5.

27. Hill CS. Government regulatory influences on opioid prescribing and their impact on the treatment of pain of nonmalignant origin. *J Pain Symptom Manage* 1996; **11**: 287–98.

28. Shapiro RS. Liability issues in the management of pain. *J Pain Symptom Manage* 1994; **9**: 146–52.

29. Rushton CH. Placebo pain medication: ethical and legal issues. *Pediatr Nurs* 1995; **21**: 166–8.

30. Mendelson D. The Northern Territory's euthanasia legislation in historical perspective. *J Law Med* 1995; **3**: 136–44.

31. Mendelson D. Euthanasia. In: Smith R ed. *Health Care Crime and Regulatory Control*. Sydney: The Australian Institute of Criminology, Hawkins Press, 1998: 149–66.

32. Gillett G. Ethical aspects of the Northern Territory euthanasia legislation. *J Law Med* 1995; **3**: 145–51.

33. Ashby M. Hard cases, causation and care of the dying. *J Law Med* 1995; **3**: 152–60.

34. Buchanan J. Euthanasia: the medical and psychological issues. *J Law Med* 1995; **3**: 161–8.

35. Ranson D. The coroner and the Rights of the Terminally Ill Act 1995 (NT). *J Law Med* 1995; **3**: 169–76.

36. Mullen PE. Euthanasia: an impoverished construction of life and death. *J Law Med* 1995; **3**: 121–8.

◆ 37. Kuhse H, Singer P. Active voluntary euthanasia, morality and the law. *J Law Med* 1995; **3**: 129–35.

◆ 38. Thomasma DC. When physicians choose to participate

in the death of their patients: ethics and physician-assisted suicide. *J Law Med Ethics* 1996; **24**: 183–97.

39. Linville JE. Physician-assisted suicide as a constitutional right. *J Law Med Ethics* 1996; **24**: 198–206.

40. Schwartz J. Writing the rules of death: state regulation of physician-assisted suicide. *J Law Med Ethics* 1996; **24**: 207–16.

41. Miller FG, Brody H, Quill TE. Can physician-assisted suicide be regulated effectively? *J Law Med Ethics* 1996; **24**: 225–32.

42. Coleman CH, Fleischman AR. Guidelines for physician-assisted suicide: can the challenge be met? *J Law Med Ethics* 1996; **24**: 217–24.

43. Kjervik DK. Assisted suicide: the challenge to the nursing profession. *J Law Med Ethics* 1996; **24**: 237–42.

44. Rusnak RA, Borer JM, Fastow JS. Misdiagnosis of acute appendicitis: common features discovered in cases after litigation. *Am J Emerg Med* 1994; **12**: 397–402.

45. Karcz A, Korn R, Burke MC, *et al*. Malpractice claims against emergency physicians in Massachusetts: 1975–1993. *Am J Emerg Med* 1996; **14**: 341–5.

◆ 46. Rogers v. Whitaker [1992] 175 CLR 479 at 490. See also: Chatterton v. Gerson [1981] 1 QB 432; Sidaway v. The Board of Governors of the Bethlem Royal Hospital and the Maudsley Hospital [1985] 1 AC 871 (Lord Scarman dissenting); Secretary, Department of Health & Community Services (NT) v. JWB and SMB [1992] 175 CLR 218; Malette v. Shulman [1990] 67 DLR (4th) 321.

◆ 47. Faden RR, Beauchamp TL. *A History and Theory of Informed Consent*. New York, NY: Oxford University Press, 1986.

48. Reibl v. Hughes [1980] 2 Supreme Court Reports (Canada) 880.

49. In re W (a Minor) [1992] 3 WLR 758 at 765.

50. Medical Treatment Act 1988 (Vic). See also: Medical Treatment (Enduring Power of Attorney) Act 1990 (Vic), ss 5(1); 7(3); Schedule 1 Note; Consent to Medical Treatment and Palliative Care Act 1995 (SA) s 8(7).

51. Sidaway v. The Board of Governors of the Bethlem Royal Hospital and the Maudsley Hospital [1985] 1 AC 871.

52. Bolam v. Friern Hospital Management Committee [1957] WLR 582 at 587.

53. Sidaway v. The Board of Governors of the Bethlem Royal Hospital and the Maudsley Hospital [1985] 1 AC 871, at 890–1, per Lord Scarman.

54. Ellis v. Wallsend District Hospital [1989] Australian Torts Reports pp. 80–289.

55. Rogers v. Whitaker [1992] 175 CLR 479 pp. 483, 490.

56. Reibl v. Hughes [1980] 2 Supreme Court Reports (Canada) 880.

57. Reibl v. Hughes [1980] 2 Supreme Court Reports (Canada) 880, per Laskin CJ.

58. National Health and Medical Research Council. *General Guidelines for Medical Practitioners on Providing Information to Patients*. Canberra: Australian Government Publishing Service, 1993.

59. Swerdlow M. Medico-legal aspects of complications following pain relieving blocks. *Pain* 1982; **13:** 321–31.

60. Chappel v. Hart [1998] 55 HCA at 93(viii); (1998) 72 ALJR 1344.

61. Pawl RP, Anderson W, Shulman M. Effect of epidural steroids in the cervical and lumbar region on surgical intervention for discogenic spondylosis. *Adv Pain Res Ther* 1985; **9:** 791–8.

62. Benzon HT. Epidural steroid injections for low back pain and lumbosacral radiculopathy. *Pain* 1986; **24:** 277–95.

63. Nelson DA. Dangers from methylprednisolone acetate therapy by intraspinal injection. *Arch Neurol* 1988; **45:** 804–6.

64. Wilkinson H. Dangers from methylprednisolone acetate therapy by intraspinal injection [letter]. *Arch Neurol* 1989; **46:** 721.

65. Abram SE. Perceived dangers from intraspinal steroid injections [letter]. *Arch Neurol* 1989; **46:** 719–20.

66. Health Department of Western Australia. *Guidelines for Medical Practitioners for the Epidural Administration of Depo-Medrol*. Perth, Australia: Health Department of Western Australia, 1990.

● 67. Tennant FS, Uelmen GF. Narcotic maintenance for chronic pain: medical and legal guidelines. *Postgrad Med* 1983; **73:** 81–94.

68. Savage SR. Long-term opioid therapy: assessment of consequences and risks. *J Pain Symptom Manage* 1996; **11:** 274–86.

● 69. Portenoy RK, Foley KM. Chronic use of opioid analgesics in non-malignant pain: report of 38 cases. *Pain* 1986; **25:** 171–86.

70. Porter J, Jick H. Addiction rare in patients treated with narcotics [letter]. *N Engl J Med* 1980; **302:** 123.

● 71. Medina JL, Diamond S. Drug dependency in patients with chronic headache. *Headache* 1977; **17:** 12–14.

72. Wesson DR, Ling W, Smith DE. Prescription of opioids for treatment of pain in patients with addictive disease. *J Pain Symptom Manage* 1993; **8:** 289–96.

73. Musto DF. Iatrogenic addiction: the problem, its definition and history. *Bull NY Acad Med* 1985; **61:** 694–705.

74. Steven ID. Opioid dependence in 15 patients after a work injury. *Med J Aust* 1995; **163:** 193–6.

75. McCarroll v. Reed 679 P.2d 851 (Okl. App. 1983).

76. Ballenger v. Crowell 247 S.E.2d 287 (1978).

77. AB and Others v. John Wyeth and Brothers Ltd; AB and Others v. Roche Products Ltd (unreported, Court of Appeal (Civil Division) 13 December 1996; Stuart-Smith, Aldous, Brooke LJJ.

78. Fisher v. Bristol-Myers Squibb Co., 181 FRD 365 (ND Ill. May 28, 1998) and Dhamer v. Bristol-Myers Squibb Co. and Cephallon Laboratories 183 FRD 520 (ED Ill. November 18, 1998).

79. Smith v. Healthscope Pty Ltd and Ors (unreported, Supreme Court of Victoria, 30 June 1994; Eames J).

80. Los Alamos Medical Center, Inc. v. Coe 275 P.2d 175 (1954).

81. Rigelhaupt JL. Physician's liability for causing patient to become addicted to drugs. 16 ALR 4th 999 (1982).

82. R. v. Adams [1957] Crim LR 365.

83. Devlin P. *Easing the Passing: The Trial of Dr John Bodkin Adams*. London: Faber and Faber, 1986: 71.

84. Cherny NI, Catane R. Professional negligence in the management of cancer pain. *Cancer* 1995; **76:** 2181–5.

85. Angarola RT, Donato BJ. Inappropriate pain management results in high jury award [letter]. *J Pain Symptom Manage* 1991; **6:** 407.

◆ 86. Rich BA. Pain management: legal risks and ethical responsibilities. *J Pharm Care Pain Symptom Control* 1997; **5:** 5–20.

87. Doctor liable for not giving enough pain medicine. http://www.cnn.com/2001/LAW/06/13/elderabuse.lawsuit/index.html. Accessed 17 June 2001. Copy on file with authors.

88. Hermes ER, Hare BD. Meperidine neurotoxicity: three case reports and a review of the literature. *J Pharm Care Pain Symptom Control* 1993; **1** (3): 5–20.

89. Dula DJ, Anderson R, Wood GC. A prospective study comparing I.M. ketorolac with I.M. meperidine in the treatment of acute biliary colic. *J Emerg Med* 2001; **20:** 121–4.

90. Sandhu DP, Iacovou JW, Fletcher MS, *et al.* A comparison of intramuscular ketorolac and pethidine in the alleviation of renal colic. *Br J Urol* 1994; **74:** 690–3.

91. Koenig KL, Hodgson L, Kozak R, *et al.* Ketorolac vs meperidine for the management of pain in the emergency department. *Acad Emerg Med* 1994; **1:** 544–9.

92. Thompson DR. Narcotic analgesic affects on the sphincter of Oddi: a review of the data and therapeutic implications in treating pancreatitis. *Am J Gastroenterol* 2001; **96:** 1266–72.

93. Dwyer v. Roderick and Others [1983] 127 Sol Jo 805; [1983] 80 Law Soc Gaz 3003.

94. Hadler NM. *Occupational Musculoskeletal Disorders*, 2nd edn. Philadelphia, PA: Lippincott Williams & Wilkins, 1999.

95. Hadler NM. Regional back pain: predicament at home, nemesis at work. *J Occup Environ Med* 1996; **38:** 973–8.

96. Hadler NM. Back pain in the workplace: what you lift and how you lift matters far less than whether you lift or when. *Spine* 1997; **22:** 935–40.

97. Hadler NM. Repetitive upper extremity motions in the workplace are not hazardous. *J Hand Surg* 1997; **22A:** 19–29.

98. Hadler NM. Workers with disabling back pain. *N Engl J Med* 1997; **337:** 341–43.

99. Mendelson G. Chronic pain. In: *Psychiatric Aspects of Personal Injury Claims*. Springfield, IL: Charles C. Thomas, 1988: 91–111.

100. Mendelson G. Chronic pain and compensation: a review. *J Pain Symptom Manage* 1986; **1:** 135–44.

101. Hadler NM. If you have to prove you're ill, you can't get

well. The object lesson of fibromyalgia. *Spine* 1996; **21:** 2396–400.

102. Hendler N, Bergson C, Morrison C. Overlooked physical diagnoses in chronic pain patients involved in litigation. Part 2. The addition of MRI, nerve blocks, 3-D CT, and qualitative flow meter. *Psychosomatics* 1996; **37:** 509–17.

103. American Medical Association. *Guides to the Evaluation of Permanent Impairment*, 5th edn. Chicago, IL: American Medical Association, 2000.

104. Babitsky S, Sewall HD. *Understanding the AMA Guides in Workers' Compensation*. New York, NY: John Wiley & Sons, 1992.

105. Babitsky S, Mangraviti J. *Understanding the AMA Guides: a Comparison of the Fourth Edition to the Third Edition Revised*. New York, NY: John Wiley & Sons, 1994.

106. Tyrer SP. Learned pain behaviour. *Br Med J* 1986; **292:** 1–2.

107. World Health Organization. *The ICD-10 Classification of Mental and Behavioural Disorders: Clinical Descriptions and Diagnostic Guidelines*. Geneva: WHO, 1992.

108. American Psychiatric Association. *Diagnostic and Statistical Manual of Mental Disorders*, 4th edn, text revision. Washington, DC: American Psychiatric Association, 2000.

109. Reilly PA, Littlejohn GO. A glossary of pain terms for medicolegal work. *Med J Aust* 1991; **155:** 264–6.

110. Weintraub MI. Chronic pain in litigation. What is the relationship? *Neurol Clin* 1995; **13:** 341–9.

●111. Mendelson G, Mendelson D. Legal and psychiatric aspects of malingering. *J Law Med* 1993; **1:** 28–34.

●112. Merskey H, Teasell RW. The disparagement of pain: social influences on medical thinking. *Pain Res Manage* 2000; **5:** 259–70.

113. Wolfe F, Aarflot T, Bruusgaard D, *et al.* Fibromyalgia and disability. Report of the Moss International Working Group on medico-legal aspects of chronic widespread musculoskeletal pain complaints and fibromyalgia. *Scand J Rheumatol* 1995; **24:** 112–18.

114. Hadler NM. Fibromyalgia: La maladie est morte. Vive le Malade! *J Rheumatol* 1997; **24:** 1250–1.

115. Hadler NM, Carey TS, Garrett J. The influence of indemnification by compensation insurance on recovery from acute backache. *Spine* 1995; **20:** 2710–15.

116. Fowler DR, Mayfield DG. Effect of disability compensation: disability symptoms and motivation for treatment. *Arch Environ Health* 1969; **19:** 719–25.

117. Leavitt F. The role of psychological disturbance in extending disability time among compensable back injured industrial workers. *J Psychosom Res* 1990; **34:** 447–53.

118. Higgs PE, Edwards D, Martin DS, Weeks PM. Carpal tunnel surgery outcomes in workers: effect of workers' compensation status. *J Hand Surg (Am)* 1995; **20:** 354–60.

119. Wiesel SW, Feffer HL, Rothman RH. Industrial low back pain: a prospective evaluation of a standardized diagnostic and treatment protocol. *Spine* 1984; **9:** 199–203.

120. Ryan WE, Krishna MK, Swanson CE. A prospective study evaluating early rehabilitation in preventing back pain chronicity in mine workers. *Spine* 1995; **20:** 489–91.

121. Fordyce WE, Brockway JA, Bergman JA, Spengler D. Acute back pain: a control group comparison of behavioral vs. traditional management methods. *J Behav Med* 1986; **9:** 127–40.

122. World Health Organization. *International Classification of Impairments, Disabilities, and Handicaps*. Geneva: WHO, 1980.

123. Curran WJ, Hall MA, Kaye DH. *Health Care Law, Forensic Science, and Public Policy*, 4th edn. Boston, MA: Little, Brown, 1990.

124. *American medical Association Guides to the Evaluation of Permanent Impairment*, 4th edn. Chicago, IL: American Medical Association, 1993.

125. Turk DC, Rudy TE, Stieg RL. The disability determination dilemma: toward a multiaxial solution. *Pain* 1988; **34:** 217–29.

◆126. Turk DC, Rudy TE. Pain and the injured worker: integrating biomedical, psychosocial and behavioral factors in assessment. *J Occup Rehabil* 1991; **1:** 159–79.

127. Mayer T, Gatchel R, Mayer H, *et al.* A prospective two year study of functional restoration in industrial low back injury: an objective assessment procedure. *JAMA* 1987; **258:** 1763–7.

128. Moreno R, Cunningham AC, Gatchel RJ, Mayer TG. Functional restoration for chronic low back pain: changes in depression, cognitive distortion, and disability. *J Occup Rehabil* 1991; **1:** 207–16.

129. Matheson LN, Ogden LD, Violette K, Schultz K. Work hardening: occupational therapy in vocational rehabilitation. *Am J Occup Ther* 1985; **39:** 314–21.

130. Hazard RG, Bendix A, Fenwick JW. Disability exaggeration as a predictor of functional restoration outcomes for patients with chronic low-back pain. *Spine* 1991; **16:** 1062–7.

131. McBride ED. *Disability Evaluation and Principles of Treatment of Compensable Injuries*, 6th edn. Philadelphia, PA: J. B. Lippincott, 1963.

132. Nachemson A. Work for all – for those with low back pain as well. *Clin Orthop* 1983; **179:** 77–85.

133. Robinson DD. Occupations potentially appropriate for persons with low back pain [abstract]. *Pain* **5** (Suppl.): S394.

134. Osterweis M, Kleinman A, Mechanic D eds. *Pain and Disability: Clinical, Behavioral, and Public Policy Perspectives*. Washington, DC: National Academy Press, 1987.

135. Ontario Workers' Compensation Appeals Tribunal. *Decision no. 915*. Toronto: Research Publications Department, WCAT, 1987.

14

Applied physiology of neuropathic pain: experimental models and their application in the study of mechanisms and treatments

XIAO-JUN XU AND ZSUZSANNA WIESENFELD-HALLIN

Chronic pain has been gaining recognition in recent decades as a major medical and social problem. This can be attributed – but not limited – to several factors, such as improved medical treatment of acute diseases, increased life expectancy of chronically ill patients, a general increase in the age of the population, and changes in the attitude of patients and physicians toward pain. Although only present in a minority of chronic pain patients, neuropathic pain after injury, i.e. diseases of dysfunction of the nervous system, represents a significant clinical problem because of its complexity, chronicity, and resistance to conventional treatments.[1] Moreover, our understanding of the pathophysiological mechanisms of neuropathic pain is still limited. In the last two decades, increasing efforts have been made by scientists working in the field of basic pain research to develop relevant animal models of neuropathic pain.[2–4] Studies with these models have greatly advanced our knowledge of the plasticity of the nervous system after injury, of the possible relationship between these plastic changes and the development of neuropathic pain, and of the pharmacological modulations of these conditions.[3,5] The aim of this chapter is to provide an account of some of these animal models of neuropathic pain. We will also briefly discuss what the animal models have taught us about the mechanisms and treatments of neuropathic pain.

ON THE RATIONALE AND ETHICAL CONSIDERATIONS IN DEVELOPING ANIMAL MODELS OF NEUROPATHIC PAIN

Clinical research on neuropathic pain states is difficult as these are not common disorders. Furthermore, assembling homogeneous patient populations for the systematic study of important variables underlying the pain states is difficult.[1,3] Moreover, in order to produce neuropathic pain in an experimental setting, identical injuries need to be introduced to nervous tissues, a procedure that cannot be carried out in humans. In addition, invasive methods are usually used to study underlying mechanisms and to test novel, unproven treatments, which are also procedures that cannot be carried out in patient populations. All of these factors point to a requirement for analogs of human neuropathic pain conditions in laboratory animals. However, it has to be acknowledged that inflicting pain and suffering in animals poses ethical concerns that need to be carefully considered by scientists involved in research in this field. The ethical guidelines concerning animal research in institutions, at local and national levels, which have been set up specifically for experimental pain research by the International Association for the Study of Pain (IASP), should always be observed.[6]

More practical guidelines concerning neuropathic pain research are also available.[4] Another important question in the evaluation of animal models for neuropathic pain is: "If such models are available, how relevant are they to our understanding of human conditions?" Several considerations clearly suggest that they are relevant:

- Nerve injury of various types can consistently be produced in animals. Several of the established animal models have direct relevance to different human conditions of nerve injury or neuropathy in terms of etiology and characterization.[3,4]
- Animals exhibit pain-like behaviors after experimentally inflicted nerve injury, many of which are similar to the responses of patients with neuropathic pain.[3,4]
- The behavioral responses to innocuous stimuli and analgesics by some of these animal models of neuropathic pain are similar to the responses shown by patients.
- Existing animal models of neuropathic pain show marked diversity which likely reflects the complex nature of human pathophysiology.

ANIMAL MODELS OF PERIPHERAL NEUROPATHIC PAIN

Neuropathic pain after complete peripheral nerve injury

From a historical perspective, one of the earliest experimentally induced nerve injuries was probably produced by Head when he allowed his own superficial branch of the radial nerve to be cut for the purposes of studying nerve regeneration and cutaneous sensibility.[7] The matter of neuropathic pain was not, however, under investigation at that time. Similarly, although in many animal experiments a variety of injuries to the peripheral and central nervous system (CNS) were produced, they were neither intended to be nor studied as models of chronic neuropathic pain. This changed in the late 1970s when several groups started to tackle this issue. The most influential study was probably that of Wall and Devor, in which they proposed that self-mutilation behaviors in mice and rats reflect reactions by animals to abnormal sensations resulting from chronic lesions of peripheral nerves and thus may be regarded as animal models of anesthesia dolorosa.[2,8] This finding followed their description of the electrophysiological properties of neuromas, which to some extent also provided physiological mechanisms for autotomic behavior.[9,10] Autotomy can also be observed after other injuries that lead to substantial deafferentation, such as multiple dorsal root rhizotomy or spinal cord injury.[11–13]

The autotomy model has been one of the most debated in the field of pain research.[13–16] This may largely be the result of the nature of the behavior, although the assertion that humans do not perform autotomy except in rare conditions, such as hereditary sensory neuropathy, do not appear to be completely true. It has been shown that humans with normal intelligence may exhibit compulsive, targeted, self-injurious behavior when experiencing neuropathic pain.[13,17] This realization along with many reports in animal literature clearly support the notion that autotomy after experimentally induced nerve injury represents an animal model of neuropathic pain in which pain is referred to deafferented body regions following the injury.[13,14,18]

The method of complete transection of a major peripheral nerve, such as the sciatic nerve, has been widely used in studies of neural plasticity[4,5] for historical reasons, since the axotomy model has been used for some time. Also, axotomy has practical advantages over recently developed partial nerve-injured models (see below) as the injury is relatively easy to produce and the result of the injury, as long as regeneration is prevented, is usually consistent.[4] Many data concerning morphological, biochemical, and physiological plasticity occurring after peripheral nerve injury have been accumulated using the axotomy model, which may be critical to our understanding of the mechanisms of neuropathic pain.[5]

Animal models of neuropathic pain after partial peripheral nerve injury

In the clinical situation, the complete section of a major peripheral nerve is uncommon and the majority of neuropathic pain cases involve partial or minor nerve injury.[1] Furthermore, the features of neuropathic pain include allodynia and hyperalgesia, which are difficult to study with the axotomy model since, with this model, the peripheral area affected by the nerve injury is totally deafferentated.[1] For this reason, the initial development of a partial nerve injury model by Bennett and Xie[19] was a significant step forward in this field. This model is produced by a moderate constriction of the sciatic nerve in rats, leading to partial degeneration and demyelination of the nerve by mechanical, ischemic, and/or chemical lesions.[19–22] Along with the injury, there is a period (weeks to months) of behavioral abnormalities that is characterized by mechanical and cold allodynia as well as by heat hyperalgesia.[19,23] Behaviors suggesting the presence of spontaneous pain are also present,[19,23] although definite proof of such an assertion, as in the case of autotomy, is perhaps unattainable.

Two other rat models of partial nerve injury have also gained considerable popularity. These are the Seltzer model, which involves a partial ligation of the sciatic nerve in the upper thigh,[24] and the Chung model, which involves ligation and section of one or two spinal nerves innervating the lumbar spinal cord.[25] These two models eliminate sensory innervation evenly across the paw, as the sciatic nerve in the upper thigh and spinal nerves are nonfasciculated. Thus, it is ensured that no areas of hypoalgesic or anesthetic skin are present. Again, various sensory abnormalities can be detected with these two models that usually persist for weeks or months.[24-26] One of the features of the Seltzer model is the presence of pain-like symptoms on the unoperated contralateral side, which may be similar to the so-called "mirror image" pain observed in some patients with sympathetically maintained pain.[27]

Other animal models of neuropathic pain after peripheral nerve injury or disease

Peripheral neuropathic pain has an extremely widespread spectrum of etiology.[1] Peripheral neuropathies of various origins constitute a major cause of pain, e.g. following herpes zoster infection or diabetic neuropathy.[28,29] Efforts have been made in recent years to develop specific animal models for many of these conditions, with varying degrees of success. Animal models of diabetes have been available for many years for the purpose of studying the disease itself. It has been well established that hyperalgesia to thermal, mechanical, and noxious chemical stimulation can be observed in diabetic rats,[30-32] as can tactile allodynia, which was demonstrated in a study by Calcutt et al.[33] The problem with these models, especially the widely used selective β-cell toxin streptozotocin (STZ) model, which induces rapid insulin-deficiency diabetes, is that they do not produce the major structural changes found in human diabetic neuropathy.[34] Hence, the relevance of the behavioral abnormalities observed in STZ-treated rats to neuropathic pain in diabetic patients is not clear. A model of neuropathic pain after infection with varicella-zoster virus has also been reported recently.[35]

Ischemia constitutes an important factor in several human painful neuropathic conditions, such as diabetic neuropathy and carpal tunnel syndrome.[36,37] Several laboratories have successfully developed models of peripheral neuropathy of ischemic origin.[38-40] In our own laboratory, we have used a photochemical method to induce sciatic nerve ischemia that produced a well-characterized partial nerve injury involving both myelinated and unmyelinated fibers.[40] This was associated with the development of profound mechanical and cold allodynia lasting 1–2 months.[40] A major contralateral effect was also present (unpublished observations).

It has been reported that treatment of the sciatic nerve by applying chromic gut suture,[22] acidified saline,[41] or the proinflammatory cytokine tumor necrosis factor α[42] in its vicinity induced pain-related behaviors, probably as a result of nerve inflammation. These may be considered as models of inflammatory neuritis, although evidence for this is still lacking. Clinically, states of acute inflammatory polyneuritis, such as the Guillain–Barré syndrome, were usually associated with painful symptoms.[28,29] Although animal models of such conditions are well established in the form of, for example, the Lewis rat model of experimental allergic neuritis,[43] the presence of pain-like behaviors in these models is less well characterized and should be an interesting topic for further experimentation.

Agents used in chemotherapy, such as vincristine or taxol, frequently induce a peripheral neuropathy in patients that is accompanied by painful paresthesiae and dysesthesiae.[28] Models of these conditions have been recently developed in rats, with the reported presence of allodynia and hyperalgesia.[44,45] These models should be useful for defining mechanisms, treatments, and possibly prevention of these specific pain states.

ANIMAL MODELS OF CENTRAL PAIN

Central pain, defined as pain following a primary lesion or dysfunction in the CNS, is usually difficult to treat.[46] Many different types of lesions or disease processes involving the somatosensory system at various levels can lead to the development of central pain, with vascular lesions (infarcts or hemorrhages), demyelinating diseases (multiple sclerosis), and traumatic spinal cord injuries being the three major causes.[46] Until fairly recently, the mechanisms of central pain following spinal cord or brain injury had not been specifically addressed and no animal models were available. It has previously been reported that rats and monkeys exhibited autotomic behavior following spinal cord injury.[11,13] Moreover, application of an excitatory agonist such as tetanus toxin, alumina gel, or strychnine has been found to cause symptoms indicative of the presence of central pain, such as hyperalgesia and allodynia, in early[47] and more recent[48,49] studies. However, the relevance of these models to clinical central pain is questionable in terms of etiology and characteristics.

Our laboratory has been studying a model of ischemic spinal cord injury in rats using a photochemical method.[50-52] We have been able to show that rats subjected to such injury appear to develop pain-like behaviors acutely after the spinal injury[50,51] and also in a more chronic fashion.[52] The chronic phase of the pain-like behaviors – characterized by segmental allodynia and hyperalgesia to mechanical and cold stimulation, excessive scratching, and hindpaw autotomy – has many similarities to the clinical situation of central pain in patients with spinal cord injury.[53,54] The physiology and pharmacology of the model have been extensively explored and the model appears to be very useful in testing the effects of novel treatments for central pain.[53] Several other models of spinal cord injury-induced central pain have also become available.[54] These include the excitotoxic injury model,[55] the spinal contusion model,[56] and a hemisection model.[57] Despite differences in experimental settings, findings from these models appear to be consistent with our model of ischemic injury.

ON THE VARIABILITY OF THE EXPRESSION OF NEUROPATHIC PAIN-LIKE BEHAVIORS AFTER PERIPHERAL NERVE INJURY

The classes of sensory abnormalities in various models of neuropathic pain are not described here in detail as the type, magnitude, and duration of neuropathic pain-like behavior in the same animal model often differ among laboratories. Such variability can be partially, but not fully, explained by genetic factors, which are known to play important roles in determining the susceptibility to neuropathic pain as well as the pattern of responses.[58,59] Several other sources of variability can also be considered. Age and sex of the experimental animals used may play a role[60-62] and so do environment-related factors, such as seasonal, diurnal, social, and dietary effects.[63,64] Differences in testing methods and procedures, as well as in ways of producing injury, are also likely to have a major impact on the development of sensory abnormalities.[4] In this context, it is interesting to note that many attempts to replicate a model often yield results significantly different from the original report. Thus, minor differences in lesioning procedures might have a profound effect on the pattern, magnitude, and duration of the effect, again illustrating the complexity of disorders associated with neuropathic pain.

Another variability often overlooked in this area of research is that not all animals develop neuropathic pain-like behaviors under standard experimental conditions in the same laboratory. The animals which do not exhibit pain-like behaviors are often labeled as operative failures and these results are discarded. We have suggested that this may not be the case.[65,66] Thus, with our spinal cord injury model we were able to show that rats with or without allodynia have similar lesions in the spinal cord.[66] Moreover, systemic or intrathecal administration of the opioid receptor antagonist naloxone effectively triggered the appearance of pain-like behaviors in spinally injured rats with no pain-like symptoms.[65,66] Our data would therefore suggest that the activity of the endogenous opioid systems plays an important role in determining the development of neuropathic pain after spinal cord injury. Shi et al. have recently shown that the rates of the development of allodynia-like behaviors in several models of peripheral nerve injury seem to be determined by another endogenous inhibitory peptide, galanin, in sensory neurons.[67] It is well known clinically that only a minority of nerve-injured patients develop neuropathic pain,[1] and it would be interesting to determine whether similar underlying mechanisms are responsible.

WHAT ANIMAL MODELS HAVE TAUGHT US ABOUT THE MECHANISMS OF NEUROPATHIC PAIN

A great deal of research into the experimental models that address various aspects of the mechanisms of neuropathic pain has been carried out. This, together with improved clinical tools for examination and analysis, as well as more systematic clinical research, has greatly improved our understanding of the mechanisms of neuropathic pain.[3,68] In several areas, animal models have been particularly rewarding.

Jessel et al. were the first to report that peripheral axotomy is associated with a reduction in the levels of substance P (SP), a major excitatory peptide in sensory neurons, in the spinal cord.[69] This was followed by numerous studies showing that such reduction was due to reduced SP synthesis in sensory neurons,[70] and a similar decrease occurred for at least two other peptides, calcitonin gene-related peptide (CGRP) and somatostatin, which are normally expressed in moderate to high amounts in dorsal root ganglion (DRG) neurons.[71,72] In contrast, several other peptides, such as galanin, neuropeptide Y (NPY), vasoactive intestinal peptide (VIP), and pituitary adenylate cyclase-activating peptide (PACAP), which were expressed in low amounts in normal sensory neurons, were upregulated following nerve injury.[73-77] Thus, with regard to peptides, the phenotype of sensory neurons appears to be altered by injury to their axons.[5] Recent studies have indicated that such plastic changes also apply to many other substances, some of which may also have roles in sensory transmission. These include nitric oxide synthase,[78] cytokines,[79] and trophic factors.[80] Evidence has also been presented to indicate that some of the excitatory peptides upregulated in sensory neurons may be involved in the transmission or modulation of nociceptive information after nerve injury.[81,82] Such plasticity occurring in sensory neurons after nerve injury may underlie important differences between nociceptive and neuropathic pain. Although it is not known whether similar plasticity also occurs in patients with nerve injury, recent studies in monkeys has indicated that, for at least of some of changes, this may indeed be the case.[83,84]

The responses of DRG cells and neurons in the dorsal horn to pain-inducing and pain-inhibiting substances either released endogenously or administered exogenously are also altered following nerve injury. For example, there is a downregulation of μ-opioid receptors[85-87] and VR-1 vanilloid receptors[88] in sensory neurons, which may underlie changes in the effectiveness of opioid analgesics and capsaicin-like drugs after nerve injury. The expression of different types of sodium channels on sensory neurons is also altered in a complex fashion after nerve injury, which may be related to the documented effectiveness of systemically administered local anesthetics in neuropathic pain.[89-91] There are also complex

behavioral signs of neuropathic pain in an experimental rat model. *Neurosci Lett* 1995; **183:** 54–7.

62. Wagner R, DeLeo JA, Coombs DW, Myers RR. Gender differences in autotomy following sciatic cryoneurolysis in the rat. *Physiol Behav* 1995; **58:** 37–41.

63. Berman D, Rodin BE. The influence of housing conditions on autotomy following dorsal rhizotomy in rats. *Pain* 1982; **13:** 307–11.

64. Shir Y, Ratner A, Raja SN, *et al*. Neuropathic pain following partial nerve injury in rats is suppressed by dietary soy. *Neurosci Lett* 1998; **240:** 73–6.

65. Xu X-J, Hao J-X, Seiger Å, *et al*. Chronic pain-related behaviors in spinally injured rats: evidence for functional alterations of the endogenous cholecystokinin and opioid systems. *Pain* 1994; **56:** 271–8.

66. Hao J-X, Yu W, Xu X-J. Evidence that spinal endogenous opioidergic systems control the expression of chronic pain-related behaviors in spinally injured rats. *Exp Brain Res* 1998; **118:** 259–68.

67. Shi T-J, Cui J-G, Linderoth B, *et al*. Regulation of galanin and neuropeptide Y in dorsal root ganglia and dorsal horn in rat mononeuropathic models: possible relation to tactile sensitivity. *Neuroscience* 1999; **93:** 741–57.

● 68. Bridges SW, Thompson N, Rice ASC. Mechanisms of
◆ neuropathic pain. *Br J Anaesth* 2001; **87:** 12–26.

69. Jessell T, Tsunoo A, Kanazawa I, Otsuka M. Substance P: depletion in the dorsal horn of rat spinal cord after section of the peripheral processes of primary sensory neurons. *Brain Res* 1979; **168:** 247–59.

70. Nielsch U, Keen P. Reciprocal regulation of tachykinin- and vasoactive intestinal peptide-gene expression in rat sensory neurones following cut and crush injury. *Brain Res* 1989; **481:** 25–30.

71. Villar MJ, Cortes R, Theodorsson E, *et al*. Neuropeptide expression in rat dorsal root ganglion cells and spinal cord after peripheral nerve injury with special reference to galanin. *Neuroscience* 1989; **33:** 587–604.

72. Villar MJ, Wiesenfeld-Hallin Z, Xu X-J, *et al*. Further studies on galanin-, substance P-, and CGRP-like immunoreactivities in primary sensory neurons and spinal cord: effects of dorsal rhizotomies and sciatic nerve lesions. *Exp Neurol* 1990; **112:** 29–39.

73. McGregor GP, Gibson SJ, Sabate IM, *et al*. Effect of peripheral nerve section and nerve crush on spinal cord neuropeptides in the rat: increased VIP and PHI in the dorsal horn. *Neuroscience* 1984; **13:** 207–16.

74. Shehab SAS, Atkinson ME. Vasoactive intestinal polypeptide (VIP) increases in the spinal cord after peripheral axotomy of the sciatic nerve originates from primary afferent neurons. *Brain Res* 1986; **372:** 37–44.

75. Hökfelt T, Wiesenfeld-Hallin Z, Villar MJ, Melander T. Increase of galanin-like immunoreactivity in rat dorsal root ganglion cells after peripheral axotomy. *Neurosci Lett* 1987; **83:** 217–20.

76. Wakisaka S, Kajander KC, Bennett GJ. Increased neuropeptide Y (NPY)-like immunoreactivity in rat sensory neurons following peripheral axotomy. *Neurosci Lett* 1991; **124:** 200–3.

77. Zhang Q, Shi TJ, Ji RR, *et al*. Expression of pituitary adenylate cyclase-activating polypeptide in dorsal root ganglia following axotomy: time course and coexistence. *Brain Res* 1995; **705:** 149–58.

78. Verge VMK, Xu Z, Xu X-J, *et al*. Marked increase in nitric oxide synthase mRNA in rat dorsal root ganglia after peripheral axotomy: in situ hybridization and functional studies. *Proc Natl Acad Sci USA* 1992; **89:** 11617–21.

79. Murphy PG, Grondin J, Altares M, Richardson PM. Induction of interleukin-6 in axotomized sensory neurons. *J Neurosci* 1995; **15:** 5130–8.

80. McMahon SB, Bennett DLH, Michael GJ, Priestley JV. Neurotrophic factors and pain. In: Jensen JS, Turner JA, Wiesenfeld-Hallin Z eds. *Proceedings of the 8th World Congress on Pain. Progress in Pain Research and Management*, vol. 8. Seattle, WA: IASP Press, 1997: 353–80.

81. Wiesenfeld-Hallin Z, Xu X-J, Håkansson R, *et al*. Plasticity of the peptidergic mediation of spinal reflex facilitation. *Neurosci Lett* 1990; **116:** 293–8.

82. Dickinson T, Mitchell R, Robberecht P, Fleetwood-Walker SM. The role of VIP/PACAP receptor subtypes in spinal somatosensory processing in rats with an experimental peripheral mononeuropathy. *Neuropharmacology* 1999; **38:** 167–80.

83. Zhang X, Ju G, Elde R, Hökfelt T. Effect of peripheral nerve cut on neuropeptides in dorsal root ganglia and the spinal cord of monkeys with special reference to galanin. *J Neurocytol* 1993; **22:** 342–81.

● 84. Hökfelt T, Zhang X, Xu Z-Q, *et al*. Cellular and synaptic
◆ mechanisms in transition of pain from acute to chronic. In: Jensen TS, Turner JA, Wiesenfeld-Hallin Z eds. *Proceedings of the 8th World Congress on Pain. Progress in Pain Research and Management*, vol. 8. Seattle, WA: IASP Press, 1997: 133–53.

85. Besse D, Lombard MC, Perrot S, Besson JM. Regulation of opioid binding sites in the superficial dorsal horn of the rat spinal cord following loose ligation of the sciatic nerve: comparison with sciatic nerve section and lumbar dorsal rhizotomy. *Neuroscience* 1992; **50:** 921–33.

86. Zhang X, Bao L, Shi TJ, *et al*. Down-regulation of mu-opioid receptors in rat and monkey dorsal root ganglion neurons and spinal cord after peripheral axotomy. *Neuroscience* 1998; **82:** 223–40.

87. Porreca F, Tang QB, Bian D, *et al*. Spinal opioid mu receptor expression in lumbar spinal cord of rats following nerve injury. *Brain Res* 1998; **795:** 197–203.

88. Michael GJ, Priestley JV. Differential expression of the mRNA for the vanilloid receptor subtype I in cells of the adult rat dorsal root and nodise ganglia and its down-regulation by axotomy. *J Neurosci* 1999; **19:** 1844–54.

89. Cummins TR, Waxman SG. Downregulation of tetrodotoxin-resistant sodium currents and upregulation of a

rapidly repriming tetrodotoxin-sensitive sodium current in small spinal sensory neurons after nerve injury. *J Neurosci* 1997; **17**: 3503–14.

90. Okuse K, Chaplan SR, McMahon SB, *et al.* Regulation of expression of the sensory neuron-specific sodium channel SNS in inflammatory and neuropathic pain. *Mol Cell Neurosci* 1997; **10**: 196–207.

91. Dib-Hajj SD, Tyrrell L, Black JA, Waxman SG. NaN, a novel voltage-gated Na channel, is expressed preferentially in peripheral sensory neurons and down-regulated after axotomy. *Proc Natl Acad Sci USA* 1998; **95**: 8963–8.

92. Wall PD, Devor M. Sensory afferent impulses originate from dorsal root ganglia as well as from the periphery in normal and nerve injured rats. *Pain* 1983; **17**: 321–39.

93. Lombard MC, Besson JM. Attempts to gauge the relative importance of pre- and postsynaptic effects of morphine on the transmission of noxious messages in the dorsal horn of the rat spinal cord. *Pain* 1989; **37**: 335–45.

94. Guilbaud G, Benoist JM, Jazat F, Gautron M. Neuronal responsiveness in the ventrobasal thalamic complex of rats with an experimental peripheral mononeuropathy. *J Neurophysiol* 1990; **64**: 1537–54.

95. Nyström B, Hagbarth KE. Microelectrode recordings from transected nerves in amputees with phantom limb pain. *Neurosci Lett* 1981; **27**: 211–16.

96. Lenz FA, Kwan HC, Martin R, *et al.* Characteristics of somatotropic organization and spontaneous neuronal activity in the region of the thalamic principal sensory nucleus in patients with spinal cord transection. *J Neurophysiol* 1994; **72**: 1570–87.

97. Lenz FA, Garonzik IM, Zirh TA, Dougherty PM. Neuronal activity in the region of the thalamic principal sensory nucleus (ventralis caudalis) in patients with pain following amputations. *Neuroscience* 1998; **86**: 1065–81.

98. Hao J-X, Xu X-J, Yu Y-X, *et al.* Transient spinal cord ischemia induces a temporary hypersensitivity of dorsal horn wide dynamic range neurons to myelinated fiber input. *J Neurophysiol* 1992; **68**: 384–91.

99. Laird JM, Bennett GJ. An electrophysiological study of dorsal horn neurons in the spinal cord of rats with an experimental peripheral neuropathy. *J Neurophysiol* 1993; **69**: 2072–85.

100. Sotgiu ML, Biella G, Riva L. Poststimulus afterdischarges of spinal WDR and NS units in rats with chronic nerve constriction. *Neuroreport* 1995; **6**: 1021–4.

101. Kingery WS, Lu JD, Roffers JA, Kell DR. The resolution of neuropathic hyperalgesia following motor and sensory functional recovery in sciatic axonotometic mononeuropathies. *Pain* 1994; **58**: 157–68.

102. Tal M, Bennett GJ. Extra-territorial pain in rats with a peripheral mononeuropathy mechanical-hyperalgesia and mechano-allodynia in the territory of an uninjured nerve. *Pain* 1994; **57**: 375–82.

103. Woolf CJ, King AE. Dynamic alterations in the cutaneous mechanoreceptive fields of dorsal horn neurons in the rat spinal cord. *J Neurosci* 1990; **10**: 2717–26.

●104. Woolf CJ. Central mechanisms of acute pain. In: Bond
◆ MR, Charlton JE, Woolf CJ eds. *Proceedings of the VI World Congress on Pain, Pain Research and Clinical Management*, vol. 4. Amsterdam: Elsevier, 1991: 25–34.

105. Devor M, Wall PD, Catalan N. Systemic lidocaine silences ectopic neuroma and DRG discharge without blocking nerve conduction. *Pain* 1992; **48**: 261–8.

106. Mao J, Price DD, Hayes RL, *et al.* Intrathecal GM1 ganglioside and local nerve anesthesia reduce nociceptive behaviors in rats with experimental peripheral mononeuropathy. *Brain Res* 1992; **584**: 28–53.

107. Xu X-J, Hao J-X, Arnér S, *et al.* Systemic mexiletine relieves the chronic allodynia-like symptoms in spinally injured rats. *Anesth Analg* 1992; **74**: 648–52.

108. Hao J-X, Yu Y-X, Seiger Å, Wiesenfeld-Hallin Z. Systemic tocainide relieves mechanical hypersensitivity and normalizes the responses of hypersensitive dorsal horn wide dynamic range neurons after transient spinal cord ischemia in rats. *Exp Brain Res* 1992; **91**: 229–35.

109. Chaplan SR, Bach FW, Shafer SL, Yaksh TL. Prolonged alleviation of tactile allodynia by intravenous lidocaine in neuropathic rats. *Anesthesiology* 1995; **83**: 775–85.

110. Arner S, Lindblom U, Meyerson BA, Molander C. Prolonged relief of neuralgia after regional anesthetic blocks: a call for further experimental and systematic clinical studies. *Pain* 1990; **43**: 287–97.

111. Rowbotham MC, Reisner LM, Fields HL. Both intravenous lidocaine and morphine reduce pain of post-herpetic neuralgia. *Neurology* 1991; **41**: 1024–8.

112. Sangameswaran L, Fish LM, Koch BD, *et al.* A novel tetrodotoxin-sensitive, voltage-gated sodium channel expressed in rat and human dorsal root ganglia. *J Biol Chem* 1997; **272**: 14805–9.

113. Arnér S, Meyerson B. Lack of analgesic effect of opioids on neuropathic and idiopathic forms of pain. *Pain* 1988; **33**: 11–23.

114. Portenoy RK, Foley KM, Inturrisi CE. The nature of opioid responsiveness and its implications for neuropathic pain: new hypothesis derived from studies of opioid infusions. *Pain* 1991; **43**: 273–86.

115. Puke MJC, Wiesenfeld-Hallin Z. The differential effects of morphine and the a_2 adrenoceptor agonists clonidine and dexmedetomidine on the prevention and treatment of experimental neuropathic pain. *Anesth Analg* 1993; **77**: 104–9.

116. Bian D, Nichols ML, Ossipov MH, *et al.* Characterization of the antiallodynic efficacy of morphine in a model of neuropathic pain in rats. *Neuroreport* 1995; **6**: 1981–4.

117. Lee Y-W, Chaplan SR, Yaksh TL. Systemic and supraspinal, but not spinal, opiates suppress allodynia in a rat neuropathic pain model. *Neurosci Lett* 1995; **186**: 111–14.

15

Oral opioids and chronic noncancer pain

C ROGER GOUCKE AND PAUL J GRAZIOTTI

It is generally accepted that oral opioids are useful in a small proportion of patients with chronic pain. However, patients who develop problems with opioid therapy, particularly addictive behavior traits, are time-consuming and frustrating to manage, their manipulative behavior stressing even the most tolerant staff. The long-term effects of opioids are unknown, and their more widespread use in society almost certainly leads to a greater availability for illicit use and abuse. For these reasons proscriptive legal frameworks discourage opioid prescribing.

Despite this, the prescription of opioids in Western countries is escalating[1] and, as discussed below, evidence is accumulating for their efficacy and safety. As with all areas in medicine, patient selection is of prime importance, and therefore the procedures for this will form the bulk of this chapter. An analysis of the evidence of efficacy and the techniques used to reduce the incidence of problems and to improve our outcomes is also included.

Selecting patients who may benefit from more complicated routes of opioid administration, for example intrathecal pumps, is even more demanding. Consequently, in general, patients should never be considered for these alternative routes unless an adequate trial of oral opioids has demonstrated opioid sensitivity with unacceptable side-effects.

EVIDENCE FOR EFFICACY

There is ample evidence for the efficacy of opioids in certain pain models. Peripheral, spinal, and supraspinal modes of action have been proposed, modeled, studied, and confirmed.[2,3] These data support our rational prescribing for patients with cancer pain and acute pain in whom the painful source is usually clear and the major determinant of a patient's pain behavior.

Patients with chronic pain, however, present with a different paradigm. Many, if not all, have a significant painful source, but it may not be the predominant factor determining their pain behavior. Consequently, treatment with opioids, which may only reduce part of the pain process, may be inappropriate at best and detrimental at worst. Many countries and societies have developed guidelines[4–7] in an attempt to improve the success of opioid prescribing for this group of patients. These guidelines are published in the absence of any level 1 evidence of efficacy (a systematic review of relevant randomized controlled trials with meta-analysis where possible), of their impact on prescribing patterns, or of other outcomes, either positive or negative. An analysis of the clinical evidence supporting the use of opioids in chronic noncancer pain to date follows.

Arkinstall *et al.* demonstrated over a 3-week period that a new long-acting codeine preparation was a better analgesic than placebo in a double-blind study on patients with chronic pain.[8] Patients received 7 days' treatment each of twice daily, controlled release codeine (200–400 mg daily) or placebo. The codeine treatment was associated with significantly lower pain intensity scores on the visual analog scale (VAS), pain intensity category scores, pain scores by day of treatment, and time of day and rescue analgesic consumption regardless of which arm of the crossover they were on.[8**]

Jadad et al. reported a double-blind randomized crossover study with parenteral patient-controlled analgesia in patients with neuropathic pain and confirmed an analgesic response for the short duration of the trial.[9]**

Moulin et al.[10]** studied the use of oral morphine (in a slow-release preparation) versus benztropine (which has many of the side-effects of morphine – sedation, lightheadedness, nausea, dry mouth, constipation, and urinary hesitancy) in a double-blind randomized crossover trial over 9 weeks. Patients had stable noncancer pain of at least 6 months' duration. Average pain intensity of the previous week was classified as at least moderate on a category scale and at least 5 on a 0–10 VAS. The pain was of a myofascial, musculoskeletal, or rheumatic nature and had failed to respond to nonsteroidal anti-inflammatory drugs (NSAIDs) and at least one tricyclic antidepressant (TCA). Patients went through a treatment cycle that increased the dose of drug weekly for 3 weeks, followed by maintenance and evaluation for 6 weeks, then reducing the dose of drug in reverse order to the titration for 2 weeks. The cycle was then repeated with the other drug.

The doses of morphine were 15, 30, and 60 mg twice daily and the maintenance dose was the highest tolerated during the evaluation phase. Doses of benztropine were 0.25-, 0.5-, and 1.0-mg capsules twice daily. Matching placebos ensured the study remained blinded. Paracetamol 500 mg was available as rescue medication. The patients' psychological status, quality of life, and pain intensity were assessed using standard methods.

Forty-six patients completed the study; their mean dose of morphine was 83.5 mg and of benztropine was 1.5 mg. Patients showed a significant reduction in pain intensity (VAS) compared with placebo when the morphine was administered first. Morphine (regardless of whether it was given as the first or second drug) also significantly reduced the sum of differences in pain intensity from baseline. Further analysis confirmed that the analgesic response was independent of the side-effects. Significantly, morphine was not associated with any improvement in psychological state or level of function. Thus, the analgesic effect of morphine in this study was independent from any improvement in psychological state.[10]**

Jamison et al.[11]* studied 36 patients with back pain in a randomized, open, repeated dose comparison of an anti-inflammatory drug and two opioid regimens over a 28-week period. Patients were selected on the basis of pain of more than 6 months' duration, pain intensity of more than 40/100 on the VAS, and an unsuccessful response to traditional pain treatment. Patients underwent a 4-week washout period of no opioid medication before being randomly assigned to one of three treatment regimens for 16 weeks: (1) naproxen only, (2) fixed dose oxycodone, or (3) titrated dose oxycodone and sustained release morphine sulfate. All patients were then assigned to a titrated dose of opioids for 16 weeks and then gradually tapered off their medication for 12 weeks. Participants were monitored for a 1-month post-treatment washout period. Total period of observation was 1 year. During the trial, utilizing a number of standard questionnaires, diaries, and weekly telephone interviews, patients were monitored for pain, activity, mood, medication, hours awake, and adverse effects and were monitored for signs of abuse and noncompliance. Three of the 36 patients could not tolerate the opioids owing to side-effects. Two patients developed behavioral problems related to their opioid medication. One patient was noncompliant and lost to follow-up and one showed signs of over-reliance on medication (high doses of opioids with minimal effect on pain) and emotional distress. While, statistically, patients reported improved pain and mood during the study, there was no improvement in activity levels, and at the end of the 12-month follow-up no significant differences were found between subjects who believed they were better and those who believed they were either worse or the same. Patients who varied their medication dose from week to week reported less pain and better mood then those who did not. Even patients who were reporting an improvement in pain relief and mood still scored greater than 50/100 on the VAS.[11]*

This study suggests that opioids may improve mood and pain scores in certain patients but this is unlikely to translate to improved activity levels. Most benefit seems to occur when patients are allowed to titrate their dose rather than take the same dose every day. Despite two patients developing signs of abuse behavior (6%), the authors concluded that "opioid therapy for chronic back pain was used without significant risk of abuse." There was no long-term benefit once patients had been weaned off their opioid medication.

These studies have observed the effect of opioids prescribed over relatively short periods. Translating their results to the clinical setting where opioids are often prescribed over long periods, sometimes indefinitely, is questionable.

Most published evidence is in the form of retrospective analysis from single pain management centers. These involve small numbers (fewer than 200) and conclude that a proportion of patients benefit, but drug abuse, dependence, and addiction occur in 3.2%[12] to 18.9%.[13]*

PATIENT SELECTION

- Establish a diagnosis for the pain.
- Ensure psychological issues are addressed concurrently.
- Ensure an adequate trial of conservative treatment.

It is essential that all reasonable attempts are made to establish a cause for the pain behavior, this will include nociceptive, neuropathic, and psychological contributions. The demonstration of pathology commensurate with the degree of pain behavior is desirable. However, patients often have pathology which is difficult to interpret, e.g. degenerative changes on spinal radiographs. In some cases, the treating physician can be confident that these changes are relevant to the patient's pain behavior, but in others they can be the least important contributor. Investigations, for example the effects of local anesthetic blocks, must be taken into account along with other clinically relevant information to determine whether the nociceptive stimulus is the main cause of the patient's pain behavior. Opioids are not appropriate for patients whose main problem is loneliness, fear, anxiety, hypervigilance, or activity intolerance.

Certain conditions result in neuropathic pain, which is usually a clinical diagnosis and may not be reflected in investigations such as radiographs or nerve conduction studies. Examples include postherpetic neuralgia, trigeminal neuralgia, postlaminectomy syndrome, and painful peripheral neuropathies. Although the use of opioids in neuropathic pain syndromes has been deemed ineffective in the past, evidence is accumulating that they do have analgesic effects. Kupers et al. suggested that the efficacy of morphine in neuropathic pain was primarily an affective response resulting in an improvement in mood.[14*] Rowbotham et al., in a double-blind crossover study of 19 patients using i.v. morphine, lidocaine (lignocaine), or saline with postherpetic neuralgia, showed that the patients receiving morphine and lidocaine had significantly better analgesia than those receiving the placebo.[15**] Dellemijn and Vanneste, in a larger, similarly designed study with 50 patients using i.v. fentanyl, diazepam, or saline, demonstrated a significant improvement in "unpleasantness" and pain intensity with fentanyl over the other infusions. Sedation was controlled for by the diazepam, suggesting that it was not responsible for the perception of analgesia.[16**]

Patients for whom opioids are being considered should be psychologically stable, although it is recognized that this is difficult to define. It is not uncommon for patients in chronic pain to develop psychological problems, including depression and anxiety states, as a result of the pain, and therein lies a dilemma for the physician. Will treating the pain reverse some of the psychological abnormalities? Or are the psychological abnormalities a significant contributor to the overall pain behavior? Studies would suggest the former in most cases.[17] It is important, however, to avoid treating "distress" with opioids. Some patients' lives degenerate into chaos for reasons unrelated to their pain syndrome. Opioids may appear to help with their distress, but may make little impact on their pain behavior or level of function. Of course, it is not always easy to differentiate distress related to sociodomestic disintegration from that related to severe pain. It is important in this situation to manage the opioid therapy with a trial and with consent as outlined below. Otherwise, in our experience, well-intentioned but uncontrolled prescribing usually results in escalating doses with a negative overall outcome.

For certain groups of patients a formal psychological/psychiatric assessment is useful before prescribing opioids. This may include patients with poorly defined pathology, younger patients, those with high levels of distress, and those with previous or ongoing substance abuse. Such a formal assessment may lead to information related to personality disorders, identification of treatment-resistant depression, past history of sexual, physical, or emotional abuse, and may be essential in designing alternative or complementary management plans. Specific treatment aimed at reducing anxiety, improving coping mechanisms, and, where appropriate, cognitive behavioral therapy may potentiate the effect of opioid therapy. Consideration should be given to managing these more complex patients in a multidisciplinary pain center.

Having reached an appropriate diagnosis and identified significant psychological issues, it is important to determine that patients have had a thorough trial of previous conservative therapy before consideration is given to the medium- to long-term use of opioids. This may mean combined intervention with:

- active exercise programs;
- attention to improving coping mechanisms;
- a formalized multidisciplinary pain management program;
- attention to psychosocial stresses;
- the use of appropriate invasive physical treatments;
- drug therapy, which should include trials of:
  - nonopioid analgesics;
  - tricyclic antidepressants;
  - anticonvulsant and membrane-stabilizing medications (e.g. sodium valproate, gabapentin, carbamazepine).

It is important not to cease these additional management techniques with the institution of opioid therapy. Opioids should be seen as a means to an end, not the endpoint of treatment. The analgesia obtained should ideally allow an increased participation in these therapies.

CONTRAINDICATIONS

No specific painful condition is a contraindication to the use of opioids. As already mentioned, careful consideration should be given to certain patient groups who may have a higher chance of developing addictive behavior.

Patients with a past history of substance abuse, particularly opioid abuse, have already demonstrated an addictive personality trait. This will require a stricter adherence to protocols, e.g. written consent.

Young patients with obscure or minor pathology who demonstrate high levels of distress generally fail to improve their level of function with opioids.

Patients in acrimonious or protracted workers' compensation claims need to be clear about the objectives of opioid therapy. These objectives can also be included in a formal written consent. In the absence of these objectives being met, ongoing prescription of opioids will only increase the acrimony and reduce the chances of successfully rehabilitating the patient.

SIDE-EFFECTS AND THEIR MANAGEMENT

Side-effects of treatment with oral opioids are common. Nausea and sedation often occur early in the treatment regimen but can be minimized if the dose is reduced and then gradually increased again over time. Sometimes, regular oral antiemetics may be useful until the nausea settles. Dexamphetamines have been suggested as a treatment for severe sedation in cancer patients,[18]* but their use in chronic noncancer pain is not established. We would urge caution. Interaction with other sedatives, especially alcohol and benzodiazepines, is well recognized.

Cognitive dysfunction without overt sedation is more common early in treatment with opioids, but studies[19]***,[20]* suggest that regular use of opioids is much less likely to result in impairment of psychomotor or cognitive processes than in healthy volunteers. The cognitive dysfunction effects of pain alone are unknown. Haythornthwaite *et al.* measured cognitive function in patients with chronic pain, comparing those on long-term opioids with those having "usual care," and concluded that long-acting opioid medications do not impair cognitive functioning in patients with chronic noncancer pain.[21]*

With regard to driving, there is no evidence that regular use of opioids results in a significantly higher rate of accidents. In fact, Budd *et al.* examined body fluids from fatally injured drivers in Los Angeles and identified opioids in only one in 594 samples. He surmised that opioid users "either don't drive or don't crash if they do drive."[22]* However, patients must be cautioned when commencing opioid use, and also after dosage escalations. They should not drive until they have been on a stable dose for 1–2 weeks. Motor vehicle insurance companies may insist that clients declare information regarding prescribed opioids in order to honor their policy.

Constipation is a regular side-effect of opioid use and requires prophylactic treatment. For some patients, regular intake of fruits and other high-fiber foods is sufficient, but most require a regular laxative. It is advisable to commence with bowel stimulants, for example senna-containing compounds, and graduate to osmotic agents (sorbitol) if required.

The side-effect profile of opioids is often variable for different drugs in a particular patient. Consequently, changing from one opioid to another may be effective in reducing side-effects. Tolerance, constipation, and nausea, in particular, vary from patient to patient with different drugs. Kalso and Vainio[23]* demonstrated a difference between individual patients with different opioids. Although McQuay[24]* would argue against the rationale for changing drugs, it would seem to us that there is no difference between changing from one opioid to another in pain patients and changing from one NSAID to another. Apart from having different metabolites, the variations in the side-effect profiles of different opioids might be explained by variable receptor activity and asymmetry of cross-tolerance. To assess properly any advantage of the substituted drug, one should aim for an equi-analgesic effect.

Another option in patients with severe side-effects in the presence of established opioid sensitivity is to vary the route of administration of the opioid. Transdermal administration of fentanyl causes less constipation and drowsiness in cancer patients,[25]* and the same would be expected in the population with noncancer pain. Intrathecal administration of opioids allows a 10- to 100-fold reduction in the opioid dose, and therefore side-effects requiring treatment are less likely to be a problem. Unfortunately, intrathecal opioids are associated with a different profile of side-effects.

PHARMACEUTICAL CONSIDERATIONS

Given our current state of knowledge, how can we ensure the maximum benefit from the prescription of oral opioids for chronic noncancer pain?

Special consideration with regard to the use of opioids in the elderly is necessary; clinical practice guidelines have recently been published discussing these issues.[26]***

Sustained release morphine preparations are the drugs of choice for use in patients with chronic noncancer pain because of their single or twice daily usage and stable blood concentrations as a consequence of their more predictable pharmacokinetics. The regular administration of morphine will lead to a significant concentration of the active metabolite, morphine-6-glucuronide (M6G). This is more potent than morphine and may also contribute analgesic action through a separate receptor subtype.[27]*

Immediate release morphine as a morphine mixture (5–10 mg/ml) may be used for dose finding prior to establishing sustained release morphine, but it is generally unnecessary. However, it may be useful for breakthrough pain or exacerbations.

Methadone, another long-acting opioid, is widely used in the treatment of addiction. There has been increasing interest in its use for the management of cancer-related pain as well as in chronic noncancer pain. Methadone is well absorbed from the gastrointestinal tract, with peak plasma concentrations at 4 h.[28]*** There is, however, a wide range in its oral bioavailability. This may be due to differences in absorption, self-induction of metabolism, or previous alcohol exposure. Methadone is eliminated by oxidative biotransformation in the liver, is classified as a capacity-limited opioid,[29] and is found in urine and feces. Its two urinary metabolites lack pharmacological activity.

Plasma methadone concentrations decline in a biexponential manner after parenteral administration. The initial phase lasts 2–3 h and the terminal phase lasts 15–60 h (cf. morphine, which has a 2- to 4-h terminal half-life). Again, there are wide interindividual variations. These unpredictable pharmacokinetics may be responsible for its unpopularity in pain medicine. Prolongation of half-life correlates well with increasing age. Methadone clearance appears to be increased by concurrent use of phenytoin and decreased by concurrent use of amitriptyline and fluvoxamine through their effects on the functional cytochrome P_{450} 3A4 in the hepatocyte.[29]

Although the pharmaceutical preparation of methadone available in most countries is as a racemate, it has been known for some time that the L-enantiomer of methadone is the main opioid analgesic. It shows between 10 and 30 times greater affinity at the opioid receptor than the D-enantiomer, which was previously thought to be inert.[30] The D-enantiomer has shown functional *in vivo* N-methyl-D-aspartate (NMDA) receptor antagonist activity.[31] This may lead to an increasing role for methadone in treating neuropathic pain.

Single-dose studies with methadone show an analgesic effect of 4–6 h. However, with multiple dosing, the main determinant of the duration of action is the slow terminal elimination phase.

There is little in the literature on the use of methadone in chronic noncancer pain. However, there are abundant references to its use in addiction medicine and a few in cancer pain control. Initial reports suggested that morphine and methadone had analgesic equivalence, but more recent studies have recommended much lower doses of methadone if converting from morphine to methadone. Dose ratios ranged from 2.5:1 to 14.3:1 (median 7.75:1).[32]***

We are not aware of any studies establishing the appropriate dose ratio when changing from methadone to morphine, however we would start with milligram to milligram equivalence.

In opioid-naive patients, small (2.5–5 mg) 4- to 6-hourly doses of methadone have been suggested for the first 1–3 days, followed by a single daily dose. Ideally, dose changes should not be made more frequently than every 3 days, and careful monitoring must be made until a stable effective dose has been established. Because of the wide interindividual variability of methadone, a more specific dosing regime cannot be recommended.

Opioid toxicity is a potentially serious problem and may be particularly so in the chronic noncancer pain population. Deaths have been reported in the addiction literature when patients who were previously on a stable dose of methadone ceased their drug for a short period of time and then developed severe respiratory depression on restarting the same dose (apparently due to a rapid loss of tolerance). Deaths in the addiction/forensic literature often report concomitant high levels of benzodiazepines and occasionally alcohol in postmortem blood and liver samples. It is important that patients with chronic noncancer pain are warned of these risks if opioids are to be used.

If methadone is ceased for more than 2 days, we would recommend a conservative restarting dose at 30% of the previous dose.

The majority of chronic pain patients report pain that is present more or less continuously; however, some people report pain only on movement and others report a diurnal or seasonal variation to their pain.

For patients with chronic recurrent or noncontinuous pain patterns, controlled release or long-acting medications may not be necessary.

Opioids with shorter duration of action, such as immediate release morphine hydrochloride suspension or morphine sulfate tablets, codeine phosphate, oxycodone, dextroproxyphene, and tramadol, may be useful in these situations. We frequently see patients using controlled release opioids who cease these medications intermittently if their pain resolves and then recommence them if the pain deteriorates.

There is agreement internationally that intramuscular opioids should play no part in the treatment of chronic noncancer pain. In particular, intramuscular meperidine (pethidine) should be avoided. It has a short half-life, a possible increased risk of dependence due to its psychomimetic effects, and the potential for excitatory central nervous system effects from accumulated normeperidine (norpethidine) concentrations following repeated dosage.

PRACTICAL TIPS

While aberrant or addictive behavior is not common among patients with chronic pain who are taking opioids, even a 1% incidence can have significant implications for physicians and clinics, and perhaps society, given the number of patients with chronic pain. Patients who develop these behaviors can consume an inordinate amount of time and resources. Thus, it is preferable to have in place strategies to try to avoid the development of this scenario. These strategies can be varied depending on the "index of suspicion" of the doctors who are prescribing the treatment and would include a consent form and trial of opioids. Practical issues of opioid prescribing in chronic noncancer pain are also discussed in Chapter P7.

CONSENT

Patients prescribed opioids for the treatment of chronic noncancer pain should be fully informed of the potential consequences of this therapy.

Verbal consent may be sufficient for some patients, or the consent form can be presented in the form of a contract. Fishman et al.[33] and Gitlin,[34] who recently reviewed the possible contents of a consent form, observed that the "contract" is an attempt to improve care through the use of an educational vehicle and to facilitate a course of treatment that has been mutually endorsed. It also provides a mechanism for obtaining informed consent.

Most importantly, the consent form should clearly define the goals of therapy. These goals may need adjustment as treatment progresses, however the importance of unambiguous endpoints cannot be overstated particularly if problems with prescribing develop. An information leaflet can be usefully incorporated into a consent form.

Informed consent should include:

- Aims set for less pain rather than no pain.
- Realistic functional goals.
- Discussion regarding the likelihood of dependence and the risk of addictive behavior, i.e. that all patients will become dependent and are likely to experience withdrawal symptoms if opioids are suddenly ceased.
- Lack of data on the long-term outcome of the effects of medically prescribed opioids.
- The potential for cognitive impairment, including:
  - driving motor vehicles while commencing opioid therapy;
  - temporary worsening around the time of dose escalation;
  - the likelihood of increased sedation if benzodiazepines and/or alcohol are used.
- The possibility (for women) of physical dependence of children born to them if they continue to take opioids in late pregnancy.
- Indications for the cessation of treatment with opioids and an indication of unacceptable behavior. Included here could be practice rules about repeat prescriptions and amount of notice required.
- Patients must accept responsibility for:
  - ensuring that his or her supply of medication does not run out after hours;
  - the security of his or her medication;
  - keeping review appointments;
  - using only one doctor (or their nominee in case of leave) to supply this medication.
- Side-effects and their management should be discussed, e.g. constipation, nausea, sedation, dry mouth, urinary hesitancy, possible hormonal effects.
- If methadone is the drug to be prescribed, emphasis on the risks of cessation and restarting and unapproved dose escalations must be made.

In selected patients it may be appropriate to discuss the definitions of the following terms and to include them in the information/consent form in order to increase compliance and ensure a more thorough understanding of consent.

Tolerance refers to decreasing pain control with the same dose of opioid over a given time period. Tolerance to side-effects such as sedation and nausea appears earlier than it does to analgesia. It usually occurs in the first 6 months of dosing. Tolerance does not imply addiction.

Physical dependence refers to a constellation of physiological signs and symptoms seen on abrupt withdrawal of an opioid. The severity of symptoms varies between patients. They include coryza, tremor, sweating, abdominal cramps, arthralgia, myalgia, vomiting, and diarrhea. Patients can be reassured regarding this phenomenon. It is the same for opioids as it is for many other medications, e.g. antihypertensives, antiepileptics, or insulin.

Addiction is a psychosocial disorder characterized by the compulsive use of a substance and preoccupation with obtaining it. This is despite evidence that continued use results in physical, emotional, social, or economic harm.

A TRIAL OF ORAL OPIOIDS

Before prescribing opioids on a long-term basis, a trial should be undertaken. It must be stressed that one physician should institute and monitor the trial. Goals should be identified and the endpoints clearly stated. Goals may include restoration of function, improvement in the activities of daily living, return to work, psychological stability, improved family and social interactions, and decreased use of health care resources, including use of other analgesics. Once identified, these goals can be incorporated into an individualized consent form.

The trial should commence with the equivalent of sustained release morphine (10–50 mg b.i.d.) and assessed weekly.

At each review it is essential to assess analgesic effect, level of function (goal achievement), side-effects, and any aberrant behavior. The goals of therapy should be reinforced along with encouragement and appropriate adjuvant treatment.

The analgesic effect from the opioid should allow a significant reduction, if not cessation, of other analgesics.

Depending on the response, the dose could be increased or decreased. The trial should last for 4–6 weeks. The prescriber should be aware of the occasional difficulty in determining the appropriate dose when rapid tolerance appears to be occurring.

We would infer that, for opioid-naive patients, a rapid

dose escalation without any analgesic response is a trial failure.

In general, round-the-clock medication is the accepted regimen. However, as already discussed, patients with fluctuating pain conditions (chronic recurrent or non-continuous) may be more appropriately treated using a variable dosing regimen with shorter-acting drugs such as oxycodone or morphine elixir.

There is controversy regarding the expectation that patients will improve in function. Is it adequate for patients to achieve analgesia only? Is it adequate for patients to state that they feel better only? To some extent this is defined by the patient's clinical situation and, often, his or her age. Ideally, patients should demonstrate an improvement of function. Perception of improved analgesia and reduction of other analgesics should be the minimum requirement. Failure to achieve at least partial analgesia at a moderate dose should be considered a failure of the trial and any further long-term opioid treatment is contraindicated. Assessment with reports from significant others may be useful at this stage.

Most patients who experience minimal or no analgesic effect will cease the drug themselves prior to the end of the trial. Similarly, many patients who experience adverse side-effects, such as severe nausea or constipation, will determine that these outweigh the analgesic benefits and cease the drug.

At the end of the trial period, if the agreed outcomes have not been achieved, the drug should be tapered over a few days and ceased.

MONITORING

Once a decision has been made to prescribe opioids on an ongoing basis, patients should at first be reviewed fairly frequently (e.g. weekly) by the prescribing physician. The time interval between reviews can then be increased to monthly. A detailed review by a pain management center should be undertaken annually. At each review, analgesic efficacy, side-effects, evidence of aberrant behavior, and any improvement in the level of function should be assessed. In many countries, the responsible regulatory authorities must be notified.

Over time, some degree of tolerance often develops insidiously. The question then arises as to what is the maximum dose? While function is improved by the opioids and side-effects are tolerated, there is no need to restrict the dose.[35]

Evidence of aberrant behavior has been well characterized by Portenoy and should be assessed at each visit.[36] Aberrant behavior is variable in its importance and relevance. Table 15.1 indicates factors which Portenoy considered to be less indicative of the development of addictive behavior. They indicate a need to assess the dose of drug, the psychological factors of relevance, the patient's expectations, or the type of medication.

Table 15.2 suggests behaviors which are more indicative of addictive behavior and should result in a serious reassessment of the appropriateness of opioid prescription. In many cases, it will be necessary to reduce and then cease the opioid. In other cases, a more regulated supply, such as daily or weekly prescriptions, may be appropriate. An initial written consent form indicating those factors for which supply will be weaned and ceased will make this easier.

SUMMARY

There is growing evidence that a small group of patients with chronic noncancer pain may benefit from the use of oral opioids.

The challenge facing the medical profession rests with identifying this group and alleviating suffering without significantly increasing illicit use, addiction, or medication-induced suffering.

Having mechanisms in place for trialing opioids with clear endpoints together with mutually acceptable rules which all parties adhere to are essential. Best practice may mean a firm yet caring "no" where appropriate, rather than inappropriate prescribing of opioids.[37] It may be more useful to initiate nonopioid treatment options for loneliness, fear, depression, anxiety hypervigilance, or

Table 15.1 *Less predictive features of aberrant drug-related behavior*

Aggressive complaining about the need for more drug
Drug hoarding during periods of reduced symptoms
Requesting specific drugs
Openly acquiring similar drugs from other medical sources
Unsanctioned dose escalation
Unapproved use of the drug to treat other symptoms

Table 15.2 *More predictive features of aberrant drug-related behavior*

Selling prescription drugs
Prescription forgery
Stealing or borrowing drugs from others
Injecting oral formulations
Obtaining prescription drugs from nonmedical sources
Concurrent abuse of alcohol or illicit drugs
Multiple nonsanctioned dose escalations
Multiple episodes of prescription loss
Repeatedly seeking prescriptions from other physicians or emergency departments without informing the prescriber or after warnings to desist
Evidence of deterioration in function, at work, in the family, or socially, that appear to be drug related
Repeated resistance to therapy changes despite clear evidence of adverse physical or psychological effects from the drug

Table 15.3 *Questions to ask before prescribing opioids for chronic noncancer pain*

1 Has the patient tried opioids for this condition before?
2 Is the diagnosis established? (If not, are further investigations required?)
3 Does the patient have neuropathic (nerve damage) pain? If so, have nonopioids, membrane stabilizers, anticonvulsants, and antidepressants been tried?
4 Has the patient had a reasonable trial of nonpharmacological treatment, including assessment and treatment of psychosocial factors contributing to pain behavior?
5 Is the patient well known to me and psychologically stable?
6 Does the patient have a history of previous drug, alcohol, or substance abuse?
7 Does the patient understand the implications of long-term opioid therapy – is written consent necessary?
8 Do I have back-up resources (i.e. multidisciplinary support) when required?

activity intolerance. Table 15.3 summarizes the questions we believe a treating doctor should ask himself/herself before prescribing opioids for a patient with chronic noncancer pain.

We have provided a framework which is practical, is based on the evidence to date, and is combined with current clinical practice. Further research is required to identify the long-term outcomes, the cost–benefit ratios, and whether certain conditions will prove to be more responsive than others.

REFERENCES

1. International Narcotics Control Board. *Narcotic Drugs: Estimated World Requirements for 1999. Statistics for 1997*. New York, NY: United Nations, 1999.
2. Stein C, Comisel K, Haimel E, *et al*. Analgesic effect of intra-articular morphine after arthroscopic knee surgery. *New Engl J Med* 1991; **325:** 1123–6.
3. National Health and Medical Research Council. *Acute Pain Management: Scientific Evidence National Health and Medical Research Council*. Canberra: AGPS, 1999.
4. Schug SA, Merry AF, Acland RH. Treatment principles for the use of opioids in pain of non-malignant origin. *Drugs* 1999; **42:** 228–32.
5. Graziotti PJ, Goucke CR. The use of oral opioids in patients with chronic non-cancer pain: management strategies. *Med J Aust* 1997; **167:** 30–4.
♦ 6. Haddox JD, Joranson D, Angarola RT, *et al*. The use of opioids for the treatment of chronic pain (position statement of the American Academy of Pain Medicine and the American Pain Society). *Clin J Pain* 1997; **13:** 6–8.
7. Jovey RD, Ennis J, Gardner-Nix J, *et al*. The use of opioid

analgesics for the treatment of non-cancer pain: a consensus statement and guidelines from the Canadian Pain Society. *Pain Res Manage (J Can Pain Soc)* 1998; **3:** 197–208.
♦ 8. Arkinstall W, Sandler A, Goughnour B, *et al*. The efficacy of controlled release codeine in chronic non-malignant pain: a randomised placebo controlled trial. *Pain* 1995; **62:** 169–78.
♦ 9. Jadad R, Carroll D, Glynn CJ, *et al*. Morphine responsiveness of chronic pain: double blind randomised crossover study with patient controlled analgesia. *Lancet* 1992; **339:** 1367–71.
♦ 10. Moulin DE, Iezzi A, Amireh R, *et al*. A randomised trial of oral morphine for chronic non-cancer pain. *Lancet* 1996; **347:** 143–7.
11. Jamison RN, Raymond SA, Slawsby EA, *et al*. Opioid therapy for non-cancer back pain. *Spine* 1998; **23:** 259–60.
12. Taub A. Opioid analgesics in the treatment of chronic intractable pain of non-neoplastic origin. In: Kitahata LM, Collins D eds. *Narcotic Analgesics in Anesthesiology*. Baltimore, MD: Williams Wilkins, 1982: 199–208.
13. Tennant FS, Robinson D, Sagherian A, *et al*. Chronic opioid treatment of intractable, non-malignant pain. *NIDA Res Monogr* 1988; **81:** 174–80.
14. Kupers RC, Konings H, Adriaensen H, *et al*. Morphine differentially affects the sensory and affective ratings in neurogenic and idiopathic forms of pain. *Pain* 1991; **47:** 5–12.
15. Rowbotham MC, Reisner-Keller LA, Fields H. Both iv lignocaine and morphine reduce the pain of post-herpetic neuralgia. *Neurology* 1991; **41:** 1024–8.
16. Delemijn PL, Vanneste SA. Randomised double blind active placebo controlled cross-over trial of iv fentanyl in neuropathic pain. *Lancet* 1997; **349:** 753–8.
17. Waddell G, Pilowski I, Bond MR. Clinical assessment and interpretation of abnormal illness behaviour in low back pain. *Pain* 1989; **39:** 39–41.
18. Bruera E, Watanabe S. Psychostimulants as adjuvant analgesics. *J Pain Symptom Manage* 1994; **6:** 412–15.
19. Zacny JP. A review of the effects of opioids on psychomotor and cognitive function in humans. *Exp Chem Psycho Pharm* 1995; **3:** 43–4.
20. Vainio A, Ollila J, Matikainen E. Driving ability in cancer patients receiving long-term morphine analgesia. *Lancet* 1995; **346:** 667–70.
♦ 21. Haythornthwaite JA, Menefee LA, Quatrano-Piacentinial AL, *et al*. Outcome of chronic opioid therapy for non-cancer pain. *J Pain Symptom Manage* 1998; **15:** 185–94.
22. Budd RD, Mutto JJ, Wong JK. Drugs of abuse found in fatally injured drivers in Los Angeles County. *Drug Alcohol Depend* 1989; **23:** 153–8.
23. Kalso E, Vainio A. Morphine and oxycodone hydrochloride in the management of cancer pain. *Clin Pharmacol Ther* 1990; **47:** 639–46.

◆ 24. McQuay H. Opioids in pain management. *Lancet* 1999; **353:** 29–32.

25. Ahmedzai S, Brooks D. Transdermal fentanyl versus sustained release oral morphine in cancer pain: preference, efficacy and quality of life. *J Pain Symptom Manage* 1997; **13:** 254–61.

26. American Geriatrics Society Panel on Chronic Pain in Older Persons. The management of chronic pain in older persons. *J Am Geriatr* 1998; **46:** 635–51.

27. Rossi GC, Brown GT, Leventhal L. Novel receptor mechanisms for heroin and morphine 6 beta glucuronide analgesia. *Neurosci Lett* 1996; **216:** 1–4.

● 28. Fainsinger R, Schoeller T, Bruera E. Methadone in the management of cancer pain: a review. *Pain* 1992; **52:** 137–47.

29. Gourlay GK. Different opioids – same actions. in: opioid sensitivity in chronic non-cancer pain. In: Kalso E, McQuay HJ, Weisenfeld-Hallin Z eds. *Progress in Pain Research and Management*, vol. 14. Seattle, WA: IASP Press, 1991: 104.

30. Shimoyama N, Shimoyama M, Elliott KJ, *et al.* D-Methadone is anti-nociceptive in the rat formalin test. *J Pharmacol Exp Ther* 1997; **283:** 648–52.

31. Gorman AL, Elliott KJ, Inturrisi CE. The D- and L-isomers of methadone bind to the non competitive site on the NMDA receptor in rat forebrain and spinal cord. *Neurosci Lett* 1997; **223:** 5–8.

32. Ripamonti C, Groff L, Brunelli C, *et al.* Switching from morphine to oral methadone in treating cancer pain: what is the equianalgesic dose ratio? *J Clin Oncol* 1998; **10:** 3216–21.

◆ 33. Fishman SM, Baudman TB, Edward A, *et al.* The opioid contract in the management of chronic pain. *J Pain Symptom Manage* 1999; **18:** 27–37.

34. Gitlin MC. Contracts for opioid administration for the management of chronic pain: a re-appraisal. *J Pain Symptom Manage* 1999; **18:** 6–8.

35. Horning MR. Chronic opioids: a reassessment. *Alaska Med* 1997; **39:** 103–10.

● 36. Portenoy RK. Opioid therapy for chronic non malignant pain: a review of the critical issues. *J Pain Symptom Manage* 1996; **11:** 203–17.

● 37. Bendtsen P, Hensing G, Ebeling C, *et al.* What are the qualities of dilemmas experienced when prescribing opioids in general practice. *Pain* 1999; **82:** 89–96.

16

Topical analgesics for chronic pain

GLYN R TOWLERTON AND ANDREW S C RICE

The concept of direct application of an analgesic to a site of tissue injury is an enchanting prospect that is deeply engrained in many cultures. The attractive logic underpinning the development of topical preparations of analgesics is that direct drug delivery close to the site of action might reduce the side-effects associated with systemic routes of administration. However, few drugs readily penetrate intact skin as the epidermis forms an effective lipid barrier. Overcoming this pharmaceutical problem has proved a real challenge. The pharmaceutical industry has addressed this in a variety of ways. The aim of this chapter is to evaluate the progress in this area and any resultant clinical benefits.

TRANSCUTANEOUS DRUG DELIVERY

Several factors have to be addressed to achieve cutaneous penetration of drugs, including the lipid solubility of the molecule and the surface area over which it is applied. Formulation of compounds into a lipophilic medium enhances penetration through the stratum corneum. Hydrophilic properties aid subsequent diffusion through the epidermal layers. The state of epidermal hydration and local corial blood flow will also affect local and systemic uptake,[1] as may the extensive cutaneous first-pass metabolism of some nonsteroidals.[2] It is these superficial layers which contribute to the variability of drug delivery by different topical preparations. The dermis does not offer so great a barrier to penetration and therefore absorption is much greater if the integrity of the epidermis has been compromised, which could influence the potential for side-effects as well as efficacy. Evolving strategies to overcome these problems are being evaluated. Iontophoreis, phonophoresis, and, latterly, submi-

cron oil droplets and liposomes have all been employed to enhance drug delivery.

Precise dosing and maintaining agent contact with the skin have proved problematic for several compounds. The introduction of premedicated patches will go some way to overcoming this. The lack of rubefaction and attendant local circulatory changes may alter the delivery profiles of these agents. Continuing development and understanding of the molecular basis of peripheral pain may allow a more targeted approach.

The use of a variety of topical preparations of several different classes of analgesic has been reported for a range of conditions, but most success has been enjoyed with the nonsteroidal anti-inflammatory drugs (NSAIDs).

TOPICAL NONSTEROIDAL ANTI-INFLAMMATORY DRUGS

As a generic group, the NSAIDs form one of the most commonly prescribed groups of drugs in clinical practice, constituting in the UK about 5% of all National Health Service (NHS) prescriptions.[3] Naturally, such an extensively prescribed group of drugs is associated with appreciable side-effects, for instance the estimated attributable risk of attending hospital with gastrointestinal (GI) events is 1.3–1.6 per year for regular users of NSAIDs. In the USA, NSAID-induced adverse effects are estimated to represent over 30% of the overall cost of treating arthritis.

Many approaches to limit the extent of systemically administered NSAID-induced adverse events have been tried: prodrugs, enteric coating, suppositories, combinations with gastroprotective agents, and, lately, altering the relative cyclo-oxygenase 1 (COX-1)/COX-2 inhibition profile. Tramer et al.[4] compared the efficacy of NSAIDs by different routes (not including topical) and found no overall advantage in alternating other routes of introduction. Topical application provides an attractive alternative approach that could limit systemic side-effects and also aid drug penetration into relatively poorly vascularized target tissues, e.g. tendons. However, a lack of firm evidence supporting the efficacy and safety of topical nonsteroidal anti-inflammatory drugs (T/NSAIDs) has led some authorities to question their place in the present pharmacopeias.[5,6] Nevertheless, such preparations are already sufficiently well established to represent a cost of £33 million per annum in the UK alone,[7] and 26% of the total prescribed NSAIDs in some studies.[8]

Some authors claim the benefit arguments for T/NSAIDs are weak.[6] Certainly, based on their cost [over three times more expensive than oral NSAIDs (O/NSAIDs)], there is some credence to this. However, the overall cost–benefit analysis needs to encompass not only efficacy and cost but also any reduction in the costs of adverse effects.

Indications and contraindications

The use of T/NSAIDs has been advocated in a heterogeneous group of acute and chronic painful conditions, the majority of which represent acute insults to musculocutaneous or skeletal tissue. Anatomical sites evaluated cover the body literally from head to foot: jaw,[9*] shoulder,[10**] elbow,[11**] breast,[12*] lower back,[13*] knee,[14*,15] leg ulcers,[16*] and foot.[17*] Some T/NSAIDS have been granted regulatory approval in the UK for use in acute musculoskeletal conditions, such as soft-tissue injury and arthritis. Regulatory approval may be granted soon by the Food and Drug Administration (FDA) for T/NSAIDs in the USA. At present, there are several over-the-counter topical salicylate preparations available, as sole agents or in combination rubefacient preparations. These contain a variety of compounds, including adrenocortical extract, capsaicin, camphor, histamine, menthol, mucopolysaccharide polysulfuric acid esters, nicotinates, and salicylic acid. The evidence for efficacy of these proprietary combination preparations has not been extensively documented.[6] The view of some patients that topical preparations are somehow more benign and perhaps an alternative to mainstream pharmacological agents, combined with the high placebo effect attendant on emollients, has led some authors[6] to recommend the use of a rubefacient as first-line therapy before prescribing T/NSAIDs.[8]

The contraindications are essentially the same for any NSAID. Reports of systemic adverse effects are rare,[18] but are documented and include exacerbation of bronchospasm and renal, dermatological, and gastrointestinal effects. They are contraindicated in pregnancy and lactation, as are many classes of medications. They may interact with antihypertensive agents, but the chance is extremely remote for topical preparations (Table 16.1).

Dosage and treatment paradigms

There are many different preparations of T/NSAIDs in the form of gels, patches, sprays, suspensions, foams, and creams. Gel formulations are reputed to possess cooling and soothing properties, whereas creams have the advantage of emolliency and lubrication. The mode of application – massage, thermal changes, occlusive dressing, or repetitive application – may determine the uptake of active compound.

Single doses are subject to much greater interpatient variability than multiple dosing.[1] The average duration of clinical effect of the T/NSAIDs is between 2 and 6h, necessitating four or more applications per day and reaching steady-state tissue concentrations after 4–5days.[19,20] Several reports advocate the use of occlusive dressings to improve penetration, but these are advised against in various pharmacopeias and are found to be difficult to use.[21] Premedicated patches, such as flurbiprofen and diclofenac hydroxyethylpyrrolidine (DHEP) should obliviate the need for this. Recent reports of the use of patches claim to provide consistent release of the compound and do not appear, in these short-term studies, to be associated with a higher incidence of cutaneous adverse effects than other preparations.[22*]

Precise dosing is difficult, and, indeed, the majority of reports do not state how the subjects were instructed to apply the compounds. Pharmacopeias advise either to apply a certain length of cream, for example 3 cm (approximately 1 g) piroxicam gel, rubbed in three or four times daily until no residual is seen, or ibuprofen, for example 5% spray, applying 5–10 sprays (1–2 ml) with gentle massage after every one or two sprays. The increased availability of premedicated patches will allow for easier and more uniform delivery.

Side-effects and their management

Since the potential for systemic absorption exists following topical administration, the potential side-effects for the T/NSAIDs are the same as for NSAIDs administered by any other route. It is a reduction in incidence of dose-related systemic side-effects which is being sought, but this must be weighed against the potential for introducing a new set of cutaneous adverse events. The meta-analysis by Moore and colleagues[23***] of over 10,000 patients enrolled in 86 trials reported an incidence of systemic events in 0.5% of subjects and local reaction in 3.6%. Adverse effects were no more common than in the placebo groups. It is salient to note that the majority of trials have not reported any long-term follow-up analysis

intensity. Of those who did respond, a 50% reduction in pain intensity was reported.

Overall, although limited, there is emerging evidence of the efficacy of capsaicin for these conditions.

Complex regional pain syndrome and postamputation pain

The are a few anecdotal reports but there are no controlled trials that have examined the use of topical capsaicin in a range of other neuropathic pain conditions. Cases of complex regional pain syndrome (CRPS),[81]* notalgia paresthetica,[55]** and painful upper limb stumps following traumatic amputation[82]* have been reported to benefit from the application of capsaicin. Wallengren and Klinker[55]** reported a crossover trial in notalgia paresthetica (periscapular pruritus) with 0.025% cream five times a day; the NNT of this trial for 50% pain relief was 3.33. Wist and Risburg[83]* documented pain relief within only 2 days' application of 0.025% capsaicin t.i.d. to an infraclavicular malignant melanoma, the effects remained until the patient's death 4 weeks later.

Facial pain and headache

Fusco and Alessandri[84]* reported the cases of 12 trigeminal neuralgia sufferers who used 1 g capsaicin t.i.d. Six patients reported complete relief and four reported partial relief of maxillary and mandibular pain. Treatment terminated with the onset of desensitization. A further three-case series[85]* reported benefit when 0.075% cream was applied to the facial trigger points.

Hautkappe et al.[53] reported that capsaicin was better than placebo in an analysis of cluster headaches. Three studies were cited for cluster headaches and two randomized placebo-controlled trials were reported to show a significant response to intranasal capsaicin for cluster headaches; when combined, these gave an overall 53% improvement with capsaicin compared with 20% for placebo.

Evidence for capsaicin in diabetic neuropathy

There is evidence supporting the use of capsaicin in diabetic neuropathy, with an NNT of 4.2;*** however, the individual reports show mixed results. Its use as a monotherapy has been questioned.**

Evidence for capsaicin in arthritis

There is evidence to support its use in monoarthritides or oligoarthritic conditions, with an NNT of 3.3.*** There is also evidence for its use in rheumatoid arthritis,** and a suggested benefit in nonspecific conditions such as neck pain.*

Evidence for capsaicin in postherpetic neuralgia

Evidence is lacking to suggest that capsaicin is effective as a monotherapy,*** with studies being contradictory.**

Evidence for capsaicin in postsurgical pain

Evidence from pooled data does not support this therapy, but later studies have not been subjected to systematic analysis.*** There have been some later studies that have suggested an improvement.**

Evidence for capsaicin in complex regional pain syndrome, skin, and amputation

Anecdotal reports suggest its use in these conditions.*

Evidence for capsaicin in facial pain and cluster headaches

There is evidence to support the intranasal use of capsaicin in cluster headaches.*** Its use in facial pain is supported by anecdotal evidence only.*

The shift from the more traditional use of capsaicin, as a counter irritant, to producing desensitization has been demonstrated to be effective in a variety of disorders. Nevertheless, the problem of the unavoidable sensations associated with capsaicin application will have biased most trials and the evidence for efficacy should be viewed with this in mind. However, the small attendant benefits and the perceived large incidence of noncompliance often limit its use as a monotherapy in these conditions. Further research to reduce the initial excitatory phase and developments of novel capsaicin analogs may pave the way for the attractive goal of truly local selective analgesia.

POT POURRI

The use of a variety of miscellaneous analgesics delivered by the topical cutaneous route has been reported for a range of malignant and nonmalignant conditions. By and large, the evidence for efficacy is limited to anecdotal reporting. Those that have been subjected to randomized trials – clonidine and dimethylsulfoxide (DMSO) – have produced conflicting results. More consistent results have been seen in palliation of neuropathic pain with local anesthetic preparations.

Local anesthetics

The use of topical application of local anesthetics in chronic pain has been reported in postherpetic neuralgia and persistent surgical pain. The use of a eutectic mixture of local anesthetic (EMLA) has been shown to reduce both spontaneous and "evoked" pain associated with PHN.[86]*

A randomized double-blind trial carried out by Rowbotham et al.[87]** demonstrated the efficacy of 5% lidocaine gel (Lidoderm Gel) in PHN. Significant VAS pain relief was demonstrated that lasted from 30 min to 12 h. The same group[88]** went on to demonstrate the return of pain on double-blind withdrawal of therapy. There were minimal side-effects noted, although 28% of the active and 34% of the control group did develop skin redness or rash. They suggested that application using occlusive dressings was poorly tolerated. They also reported a similar trial with 5% lidocaine adhesive patches covering up to 420 cm[2].[87] This application did not lead to clinically significant plasma levels of lidocaine (0.1 µg/ml), with approximately 3% being absorbed systemically. Lidoderm is marketed in the USA as 10×14 cm patches.

Fassoulaki et al.[89] in a randomized double-blind trial reported that the application of a eutectic mixture of local anesthetic (EMLA) reduced the occurrence of persistent surgical pain after breast surgery. Forty-six patients were randomized to either placebo application or EMLA 20 g before surgery and for 4 days postoperatively. There were no reports of systemic toxicity during the trial and the use of EMLA was associated with significantly reduced incidence and intensity of persistent pain at 3 months (22% vs. 68%, $P = 0.004$).

Clonidine

The α_2-adrenoreceptor agonist clonidine has been shown to be a useful analgesic in a number of settings. Several studies have examined topical application in neuropathic and sympathetically maintained pain. It has been reported[90]* to reduce mechanical allodynia and thermal hyperalgesia in sympathetically maintained pain. However, in a randomized double-blind[91]** crossover study, including 24 patients with diabetic polyneuropathy, transdermal clonidine 0.3 mg/day failed to show significant differences from placebo. Nevertheless, nine patients who elected to continue the study did respond to withdrawal of treatment and subsequent rechallenge with clonidine. This prompted the authors to do a two-stage "enriched enrolment" design trial[92]** in which 12 responders were selected out of 41 patients. These were then entered into four 1-week crossover double-blind trials, which demonstrated a 20% reduction in pain intensity.

Epstein et al.[93]* used clonidine (0.2 mg/ml) cream q.d.s. for 4 weeks, applied at the site of facial neuralgia and neuropathic pain, in 17 patients. This open-label clinical trial showed an improvement in analog pain ratings of 36% mean reduction in burning. Sugai et al.[94]* reported the use of clonidine cream (60 µg/g) following sympathetic blockade; 30% of the patients in this trial experienced some reduction in pain scores.

Dimethylsulfoxide

The industrial solvent DMSO has been employed in a heterogeneous group of conditions. Experimental evidence testifies to a range of effects encompassing hydroxyl radical scavenger, nitric oxide release, and dose-dependent C-fibre neural blockade.[95] This may be pertinent as wide ranges of concentrations, between 5% and 90% DMSO, have been used. There are a large number of reports, mainly anecdotal, attesting to its efficacy. Overall, authors have found the evidence unconvincing.[96] Trials in chronic pain have shown effects compared with placebo in rheumatoid,[97]** osteoarthritis,[98]** and musculoskeletal[99]**conditions, but the effects do not appear to be consistent. An open-label study in CRPS demonstrated significant changes in VAS.[99] Two randomized trials of DMSO in CRPS that were carried out later failed to achieve significant changes in pain scores (VAS), but there was some reduction in the subjective parameters studied.[101]**,[102]**

Opioids

Topical opioids have been advocated for cutaneous malignant pain for several generations. There are several recent reports, although Heberden[103] advocated its use in pain caused by hemorrhoids in the eighteenth century. The evidence of topical opioid efficacy is limited to anecdotal reports only, but is supported by in vivo experimental evidence.[104] The use of transdermal fentanyl, as a preparation for systemic delivery, is not discussed here.

Poor transcutaneous absorption may be aided by local inflammation. Preferential uptake by inflamed tissue has also been suggested to limit potential side-effects. Back and Finlay[105]* reported three cases of patients, all receiving systemic opioids, who appeared to gain pain relief from the topical application of 10 mg diamorphine on a hydrogel wound dressing. Morphine (0.08%) on a 100-cm[2] hydrogel dressing was also documented by Kranajnik and Zylicz[106]* to produce pain relief. The same authors[107]* reported a series of six cancer patients who benefited (48% mean change in VAS) from topical opioids alone or as adjuvants to systemic therapy.

Evidence for topical clonidine

There is evidence to support the use of clonidine in a limited number of patients with neuropathic pain.**

Evidence for topical opioids

Anecdotal reports suggest a benefit in malignant cutaneous pathology.*

Evidence for local anesthetics

There is evidence to suggest that the use of premedicated patches of lidocaine is useful in PHN pain.**

Evidence for dimethylsulfoxide

Some studies have produced inconsistent results,** with anecdotal studies only suggesting a benefit in CRPS.*

CONCLUSIONS

The evidence for the use of topical therapies is mixed. Perhaps this is not surprising given the heterogeneous nature of the pathology they are employed to relieve. Topical NSAIDs are certainly better than placebo in arthritic and soft-tissue injury, but how much better is debatable. At present, the evidence suggests a better effect in musculoskeletal pathology than in the major arthropathies. The magnitude of effect of capsaicin in arthritis and neuropathy questions its use as a monotherapy in these conditions. Although there is a vast number of publications devoted to these agents, their use can only be justified on the present evidence as adjunct agents or where other drugs are not tolerated. However, their systemic side-effects are exceedingly low and their use in a targeted population may have great merits.

The use of local anesthetic and NSAIDs in neuropathic pain may become more widespread. Clonidine and opioids have yet to accumulate evidence of their efficacy to advocate wholesale use. Ongoing research into all the agents may provide a superior pharmacopeia with which to combat chronic pain, if other newer developments do not supersede them. The heterogeneity of most pain gives some credence to the lay public's devotion to simple proprietary combination therapies, and evidence would suggest that some of these are more efficacious. Perhaps it is these therapies that we need to concentrate on and not single-agent preparations.

REFERENCES

1. Muller M *et al.* Transdermal penetration of diclofenac after multiple epicutaneous administration. *J Rheumatol* 1998; **25:** 1833–6.
2. Cross S, Anderson C, *et al.* Is there tissue penetration after application of topical salicylate formulations? *Lancet* 1997; **350:** 636.
3. Wynne H, Campbell M. Pharmaco-economics of non-steroidal anti-inflammatory drugs (NSAIDs). *Pharmacoeconomics* 1993; **3:** 107–23.
4. Tramer M, *et al.* Comparing analgesic efficacy of non-steroidal anti-inflammatory drugs given by different routes in acute and chronic pain: a qualitative systematic. *Acta Anaesthesiol Scand* 1998; **42:** 71–9.
5. Anonymous. More topical NSAIDs: worth the rub? *Drugs Ther Bull* 1990; **28:** 27–8.
6. Anonymous. Topical NSAIDs: a gimmick or a godsend. *Lancet* 1989; **30:** 779–80.
7. Duerden M, *et al.* Topical NSAIDs are better than placebo: safety, efficacy, and therapeutic role of NSAIDs must be clarified. *Br Med J* 1998; **317:** 280–1.
8. Sift-Carter R, *et al.* Use of topical NSAIDs in patients receiving systemic NSAID treatment: a pharmacy based study in Germany. *J Clin Epidemiol* 1997; **50:** 217–18.
9. Svensson L, Houe P, Arendt-Nielsen L. Effect of systemic versus topical nonsteroidal anti-inflammatory drugs on postexercise jaw-muscle soreness: a placebo-controlled study. *J Orofac Pain* 1997; **11:** 353–62.
10. Burnham R, *et al.* The effectiveness of topical diclofenac for lateral epicondylitis. *Clin J Sport Med* 1998; **8:** 78–81.
11. Schapira D, Linn S, Scharf Y. A placebo-controlled evaluation of diclofenac diethylamine salt in the treatment of lateral epicondylitis of the elbow. *Curr Ther Res* 1991; **49:** 162–8.
12. Irving A, Morrison S. Effectiveness of topical non-steroidal anti-inflammatory drugs in the management of breast pain. *J R Coll Surg Edinburgh* 1998; **43:** 158–9.
13. Waikakul S, Danputipong P, Soparat K. Topical analgesics, indomethacin plaster and diclofenac emulgel for low back pain: a parallel study. *J Med Assoc Thai* 1996; **79:** 486–90.
14. Waikakul S, *et al.* Topical analgesics for knee arthrosis: a parallel study of ketoprofen gel and diclofenac emulgel. *J Med Assoc Thai* 1997; **80:** 593–7.
15. Algozzine G, *et al.* Trolamine salicylate cream in osteoarthritis of the knee. *JAMA* 1982; **247:** 1311–13.
16. Vowden K. Topical analgesics in leg ulcer patients. *J Wound Care* 1997; **6:** 239.
17. Diedsclag W. A double blind study of the efficacy of topical ketorolac tromethamine gel in the treatment of ankle sprain in comparison to placebo and etofenamate. *J Clin Pharmacol* 1990; **30:** 82–9.
18. Graham R. Transdermal non-steroidal anti-inflammatory agents. *Br J Clin Pract* 1995; **49:** 33–5.
19. Patel R, Leswell P. Comparison of ketoprofen, piroxicam, and diclofenac gels in the treatment of acute soft-tissue injury in general practice. General Practice Study Group. *Clin Ther* 1996; **18:** 497–507.
20. Taburet A, *et al.* Pharmacokinetic comparison of oral and local action transcutaneous flurbiprofen in healthy volunteers. *J Clin Pharm Ther* 1995; **20:** 101–7.
21. Rowbotham M. Topical analgesic agents. In: Fields HL, Liebeskind JC eds. *Progress in Pain Research and Management*. Seattle, WA: IASP Press, 1993: 211–27.
22. Muldon C, Earl R, Rees J. Safety and tolerability of flurbiprofen LAT. *Clin Rheumatol* 1994; **13:** 357.
23. Moore R, *et al.* Quantitative systematic review of topically applied non-steroidal anti-inflammatory drugs. *Br Med J* 1998; **316:** 333–8.
24. Joss JD, LeBlond RF. Potentiation of warfarin anticoagulation associated with topical methyl salicylate. *Ann Pharmacother* 2000; **34:** 729–33.
25. Sanely J, *et al.* Local NSAIDs gel (Eltenac) in the treatment of osteoarthritis of the knee: a double blind

study comparing eltenac with oral diclofenac and placebo gel. *Scand J Rheumatol* 1997; **26:** 287–92.

26. Dickenson D. A double blind evaluation of topical piroxicam gel with oral ibuprofen in osteoarthritis of the knee. *Curr Ther Res* 1991; **49:** 199–207.

27. Benedittis G, Lorenzetti A. Topical aspirin/diethyl ether mixture versus indomethacin and diclofenac/diethyl ether mixtures for acute herpetic neuralgia and postherpetic neuralgia: a double-blind crossover placebo controlled study. *Pain* 1996; **65:** 45–51.

28. Memeo A, *et al*. Evaluation and tolerability of a new topical formulation of flurbiprofen in acute soft tissue injuries. *Drug Invest* 1992; **4:** 441–9.

◆ 29. Evans J, *et al*. Topical non-steroidal anti-inflammatory drugs and admission to hospital for upper gastrointestinal bleeding and perforation: a record linkage case-controlled study. *Br Med J* 1995; **311:** 22–6.

30. Roth S. A controlled clinical investigation of 3% diclofenac/2.5% sodium hyaluronate topical gel in the treatment of uncontrolled pain in chronic oral NSAID users with osteoarthritis. *Int J Tissue React* 1995; **17:** 129–32.

31. Radermacher J, *et al*. Diclofenac concentration in synovial fluid and plasma after cutaneous application in inflammatory and degenerative joint disease. *Br J Clin Pharmacol* 1991; **31:** 537–41.

32. Dawson M, *et al*. The disposition of biphenylacetic acid following topical application. *Eur J Clin Pharmacol* 1988; **33:** 639–42.

33. McLatchie G. Soft tissue trauma: a randomised controlled trial of the topical application of feldinac, a new NSAID. *Br J Clin Pract* 1989; **43:** 277–8.

34. Rabinowitz J, *et al*. Comparative tissue absorption of oral 14C-asprin and topical triethanolamine 14C-salicylate in human and canine knee joints. *J Clin Pharmacol* 1982; **22:** 42–8.

35. Tegeder I, Lotsch J, Kinzig-Schippers M, *et al*. Comparison of tissue concentrations after intramuscular and topical administration of ketoprofen. *Pharm Res* 2001; **18:** 980–6.

● 36. Anonymous. Rational use of NSAIDS for musculoskeletal disorders. *Drugs Ther Bull* 1994; **32:** 91–5.

37. Barradell L, Whittington R, Benfield P. Mistoprostil pharmoeconomic of its use as prophylaxis against gastroduodenal damage induced by non-steroidal anti-inflammatory drugs. *Pharmoeconomics* 1999; **3:** 140–70.

38. Peacock M, Rapier C. The topical NSAID felbinac is a cost effective alternative to oral NSAIDs for the treatment of rheumatic conditions. *Br J Med Econ* 1993; **6:** 135–42.

39. El-Hadidi T, El-Garf A. Double-blind study comparing the use of Voltaren Emulgel versus regular gel during ultrasonic sessions in the treatment of localised traumatic and rheumatic painful conditions. *J Int Med Res* 1991; **19:** 219–27.

40. Bouchier-Hayes T, Rotman H, Darekar B. Comparison of the efficacy and tolerability of diclofenac gel (voltarol Emugel) and felbinac gel (Traxam) in the treatment of soft tissue injuries. *Br J Clin Pract* 1990; **44:** 319–20.

41. Galeazzi M, Marcolongo R. A placebo-controlled study of the efficacy and tolerability of a non-steroidal anti-inflammatory drug, DHEP plaster, in inflammatory peri- and extra-articulator rheumatological diseases. *Drugs Exp Clin Res* 1991; **19:** 131–6.

42. Akermark C, Forsskahl B. Topical indomethacin in overuse injuries in athletes: a randomised double-blind study comparing Elmetacin with oral indomethacin and placebo. *Int J Sports Med* 1990; **11:** 393–6.

● 43. Grahame R, *et al*. A meta-analysis to compare flurbiprofen LAT to placebo in the treatment of soft tissue rheumatism. *Clin Rheumatol* 1994; **13:** 357.

44. Ginsburgh F, Famaey J-P. Double blind, randomised crossover study of the percutaneous efficacy and tolerability of a topical indomethacin spray versus placebo in the treatment of tendinitis. *J Intern Med Res* 1991; **41:** 131–6.

45. Alexander J. Post herpetic neuralgia. *Anaesthesia* 1985; **40:** 1133–4.

46. McQuay H, *et al*. Benzydamine cream for the treatment of postherpetic neuralgia: minimum duration of treatment in a cross over trial. *Pain* 1990; **40:** 131–5.

47. Bareggi S, Pirola R, Benedittis GD. Skin and plasma levels of acetylsalicylic acid: a comparison between topical aspirin/diethyl ether mixture and oral aspirin in acute herpes zoster and postherpetic neuralgia. *Eur J Clin Pharm* 1998; **54:** 231–5.

48. Morimoto M, Inamori K, Hyodo M. The effect of indomethacin stupe for phn – particularly in comparison with chloroform–aspirin solution. *Pain* 1990; **5:** 59.

49. King R. Concerning the management and pain with herpes zoster and postherpetic neuralgia. *Pain* 1988; **33:** 73–8.

50. Tharion G, Bhattacharji S. Aspirin in chloroform as an effective adjuvant in the management of chronic neurogenic pain. *Arch Phys Med Rehabil* 1997; **78:** 437–9.

51. Kassirer M. Concerning the management and pain with herpes zoster and postherpetic neuralgia. *Pain* 1988; **35:** 368–9.

◆ 52. Caterina M, *et al*. The capsaicin receptor: a heat-activated ion channel in the pain pathway. *Nature* 1997; **389:** 816–24.

● 53. Hautkappe M, *et al*. Review of the effectiveness of capsaicin for painful cutaneous disorders and neural dysfunction. *Clin J Pain* 1998; **14:** 97–106.

54. Nolano M, *et al*. Topical capsaicin in humans: a parallel loss of epidermal nerve fibre and pain sensation. *Pain* 1999; **81:** 135–45.

55. Wallengren J, Klinker M. Successful treatment of notalgia paresthetica with topical capsaicin: vehicle controlled double blind crossover study. *J Am Acad Dermatol* 1995; **32:** 287–9.

56. Robbins W, *et al*. Treatment of intractable pain with topical large dose capsaicin: preliminary report. *Anesth Analg* 1998; **86:** 579–83.

57. Fuchs P, Pappagello M, Meyer R. Topical EMLA pretreatment fails to decrease the pain induced by 1% topical capsaicin. *Pain* 1999; **80:** 637–42.

● 58. Craft R, Porreca F. Therapeutic potential of capsaicin-like molecules: treatment parameters of desensitisation. *Life Sci* 1992; **51:** 1767–75.

59. Watson C, Evans R, Watt V. Post herpetic neuralgia and capsaicin. *Pain* 1988; **33:** 333–40.

60. McCleane G. The analgesic efficacy of topical capsaicin is enhanced by glyceryl trinitrate in painful osteoarthritis: a randomised, double blind, placebo-controlled study. *Eur J Pain* 2000; **4:** 355–60.

61. Jaggar S, *et al*. The capsaicin analogue EC665 prevents the hyper-reflexia and referred hyperalgesia associated with inflammation of the rat urinary bladder. *Pain* 2001; **89:** 229–35.

62. Urban L, Campbell E, Panesar M. In vivo pharmacology of SDZ 249-665, a novel, non-pungent capsaicin analogue. *Pain* 2000 **89**(1): 65–74.

63. The Capsaicin Study Group. Treatment of painful diabetic neuropathy with topical capsaicin. *Arch Intern Med* 1991;**151:** 2225–9.

● 64. Watson C. Topical capsaicin as an adjuvant analgesic. *J Pain Symptom Manage* 1994; **9:** 425–33.

◆ 65. Zhang WY, Li Wan Po A. The effectiveness of topically applied capsaicin. *Eur J Clin Pharmacol* 1994; **46:** 517–22.

◆ 66. McQuay H, Moore A. Topical capsaicin. In: McQuay H, Moore A, eds. *An Evidence-Based Resource for Pain Relief*. Oxford: Oxford University Press,1998: 249–50.

67. The Capsaicin Study Group. Effect of treatment with capsaicin on daily activity of patients with painful diabetic neuropathy. *Diabetes Care* 1992; **15:** 159–65.

68. Low P, *et al*. Double blind, placebo controlled study of the application of capsaicin cream in chronic distal painful polyneuropathy. *Pain* 1995; **62:** 163–8.

● 69. Rians C, Bryson H. Topical capsaicin: a review of its pharmacological properties and therapeutic potential in post-herpetic neuralgia, diabetic neuropathy and osteoarthritis. *Drugs Ageing* 1995; **7:** 317–28.

70. Biesbroeck R. A double blind comparison of topical capsaicin and oral amitryptiline in painful diabetic neuropathy. *Adv Ther* 1995; **12:** 111–20.

● 61. Matucci-Cerinic M, *et al*. Neurogenic influences in arthritis: potential modification by capsaicin. *J Rheumatol* 1995; **22:** 1447–9.

62. McCarthy G, McCarthy D. Effect of topical capsaicin in painful osteoarthritis of the hand. *J Rheumatol* 1992; **19:** 604–7.

73. Deal C, Schnitzer T, Lipstein E. Treatment of arthritis with topical capsaicin: a double blind trial. *Clin Ther* 1991; **13:** 383–95.

74. Altman R. Capsaicin cream 0.025% as monotherapy for osteoarthritis: a double blind study. *Semin Arthritis Rheum* 1994; **23:** 41–7.

75. Mathias B, *et al*. Topical capsaicin for chronic neck pain: a pilot study. *Am J Phys Med Rehabil* 1995; **74:** 39–44.

76. McCleane G. Topical application of doxepin hydrochloride, capsaicin and a combination of both produce analgesia in chronic human neuropathic pain: a randomized, double-blind, placebo-controlled study. *Br J Clin Pharmacol* 2000; **49:** 574–9.

77. Bernstein J, Korman N, Bickers D. Topical capsaicin treatment of chronic postherpetic neuralgia. *J Am Acad Derm* 1989; **21:** 265–70.

78. Drake H, *et al*. Randomised double blind study of topical capsaicin for the treatment of post herpetic neuralgia. *Pain* 1990; **5:** 58.

◆ 79. Ellison N, *et al*. Phase III placebo-controlled trial of capsaicin cream in the management of surgical neuropathic pain in cancer patients. *J Clin Oncol* 1997; **15:** 2974.

80. Watson C, Evans R. The postmastectomy pain syndrome and topical capsaicin: a randomised trial. *Pain* 1992; **51:** 375–9.

81. Cheshire W, Synder C. Treatment of reflex sympathetic dystrophy with topical capsaicin, case report. *Pain* 1990; **42:** 307–11.

82. Cannon D, Wu Y. Topical capsaicin as an adjuvant analgesic for the treatment of traumatic amputee neurogenic residual limb pain. *Arch Phys Med Rehabil* 1998; **79:** 591–3.

83. Wist E, Risberg T. Topical capsaicin in the treatment of hyperalgesia, allodynia and dysaesthetic pain caused by malignant tumour infiltration of the skin. *Acta Oncol* 1993; **32:** 343–7.

84. Fusco B, Alessandri M. Analgesic effect of capsaicin in idiopathic trigeminal neuralgia. *Anaesth Analg* 1992; **74:** 375–7.

85. Lincoff N, Rath P, Hirano M. The treatment of periocular and facial pain with topical capsaicin. *J Neuroophthalmol* 1998; **18:** 17–20.

86. Attal N, *et al*. Effects of single and repeated applications of a eutectic mixture of local anaesthetic (EMLA) cream on spontaneous and evoked pain in post-herpetic neuralgia. *Pain* 1999; **81:** 203–9.

◆ 87. Rowbotham M, *et al*. Lidocaine patch: double blind controlled study of a new treatment method for post herpetic neuralgia. *Pain* 1996; **65:** 39–44.

88. Galer B, *et al*. Topical lidocaine patch relives post herpetic neuralgia more effectively than a vehicle topical patch: results of an enriched enrolment study. *Pain* 1999; **80:** 533–8.

89. Fassoulaki A, Sarantopoulos C, Melemeni A, Hogan Q. EMLA reduced acute and chronic pain after breast surgery for cancer. *Reg Anaesth Pain Med* 2000; **25:** 337–9.

90. Davis K, *et al*. Topical application of clonidine relieves

hyperalgesia in patients with sympathetically maintained pain. *Pain* 1991; **47:** 309–18.

91. Zeilger D, *et al*. Transdermal clonidine versus placebo in painful diabetic neuropathy. *Pain* 1992; **48:** 403–8.

◆ 92. Byas-Smith M, *et al*. Transdermal clonidine compared to placebo in painful diabetic neuropathy using a two stage "enriched enrolment" design. *Pain* 1995; **60:** 267–74.

93. Epstein J, Grushka M, Le N. Topical clonidine for orofacial pain: a pilot study. *J Orofacial Pain* 1997; **11:** 346–51.

94. Sugai N, *et al*. Clonidine hydrochloride ointment for transdermal use in sympathetically maintained pain. In: *Proceedings of the 8th World Congress on Pain*. Seattle, WA: IASP Press, 1996: 250.

95. Evans M, Reid K, Sharp J. Dimethylsulfoxide (DMSO) blocks conduction in peripheral nerve C fibers: a possible mechanism of analgesia. *Neurosci Lett* 1993; **150:** 145–8.

● 96. Trice J, Pinals R. Dimethyl sulfoxide: a review of its use in the rheumatic disorders. *Semin Arthritis Rheum* 1985; **15:** 45–60.

97. Matsumoto J. Clinical trials of DMSO in rheumatoid arthritis patients in Japan. *NY Acad Sci* 1967; **141:** 560–8.

98. Vuopala U, Vesterinen E, Kaipainen W. The analgesic action of DMSO ointment in arthrosis: a double blind study. *Acta Rheumatol Scand* 1971; **17:** 57–60.

99. Percy E, Carson J. The use of DMSO in tennis elbow and rotator cuff tendonitis: a double-blind study. *Med Sci Sports Exerc* 1981; **23:** 215–19.

100. Langendijk P, *et al*. Good results of treatment of reflex sympathetic dystrophy with a 50% dimethylsulfoxide cream. *Ned Tijdschr Geneeskd* 1993; **137:** 500–3.

101. Geertzen J, *et al*. Reflex sympathetic dystrophy: early treatment and psychological approach. *Arch Phys Med Rehabil* 1994; **475:** 442–6.

102. Zuurmond W, *et al*. Treatment of acute reflex sympathetic dystrophy with DMSO 50% in a fatty cream. *Acta Anaesthesiol Scand* 1996; **40:** 364–7.

103. Heberden W. In: Hafner ed. *Commentaries on the History and Cure of Disease*. New York, NY: New York Academy of Medicine, 1962: 213.

104. Kolesnikov Y, Pasternak G. Topical opioids in mice: analgesia and reversal of tolerance by a topical *N*-methyl-ᴅ-aspartate antagonist. *J Pharmacol Exp Ther* 1999; **290:** 247–52.

105. Back I, Finlay I. Analgesic effect of topical opioids on painful skin ulcers. *J Pain Symptom Manage* 1995; **10:** 493

●106. Kranajnik M, Zylicz Z. Topical morphine for cutaneous cancer pain. *Palliative Med* 1997; **11:** 325.

107. Kranajnik M, *et al*. Potential uses of topical opioids in palliative care – report of 6 cases. *Pain* 1999; **80:** 121–5.

108. Morgenlander J, Hurwitz B, Marsey E. Capsaicin for the treatment of pain in the Guillain–Barré syndrome. *Ann Neurol* 1990; **28:** 199.

109. Tarng D, *et al*. Hemodialysis-related pruritus: a double-blind, placebo-controlled, crossover study of capsaicin 0.025% cream. *Nephron* 1996; **72:** 617–22.

110. Puig L, Alegre M, Moragas JD. Treatment of meralgia paraesthetica with topical capsaicin. *Dermatology* 1995; **191:** 73–4.

111. Sinoff S, Hart M. Topical capsaicin and burning pain. *Clin J Pain* 1993; **42:** 307–11.

112. Watson C, Bickers D, Millikan L. A randomised vehicle control trial of topical capsaicin in the treatment of post herpetic neuralgia. *Clin Ther* 1993; **15:** 510–26.

113. Ellis C, Berberian B, Sulca V. A double blind evaluation of topical capsaicin in pruritic psoriasis. *J Am Acad Dermatol* 1993; **29:** 438–42.

114. Hersh E, Pertes R, Ochs H. Topical capsaicin – pharmacology and potential role in the treatment of temporomandibular pain. *J Clin Dent* 1994; **5:** 54–9.

17

The use of nonsteroidal anti-inflammatory drugs and acetaminophen (paracetamol) in chronic pain

JOHN HUGHES AND AYMAN EISSA

The use of nonsteroidal anti-inflammatory drugs (NSAIDs) and acetaminophen (paracetamol) in chronic pain is discussed together because of their common convention of usage.

NONSTEROIDAL ANTI-INFLAMMATORY AGENTS

Nonsteroidal anti-inflammatory drugs have been used for over 100 years; they possess anti-inflammatory, anti-pyretic, and analgesic properties, and have been the mainstay for treating chronic inflammatory conditions.[1] There is, however, a lack of evidence for their relative efficacy in chronic and neuropathic pain.

This generic group of drugs is one of the most commonly prescribed in clinical practice. It is estimated that over 100 million people take NSAIDs regularly.[2] Over 20 million prescriptions for NSAIDs were dispensed in England alone during 1999.[3] In 1994, over $900 million was spent on over-the-counter analgesics in the USA, $100 million of which was for aspirin, which approximates to 20,000 tons of aspirin consumed each year, averaging 225 tablets per head of population.[4]

NSAIDs have well-recognized side-effects which themselves put a burden on health system budgets; annual estimates for UK expenditure in terms of acute hospital admissions and co-prescribing is £251 million.[5]

Assessing the real risks and benefits of NSAIDs is complicated by the fact that many agents are available without prescription. A Swedish survey from the general popula-tion of over 18-year-olds obtained 12,000 replies (79% response rate). It suggested that 7% of men and 12% of women used prescription analgesics, with 20% and 30%, respectively, using nonprescription analgesics. Only 2% of men and 4% of women reported using both prescription and nonprescription medication together. Nonprescription analgesic use was higher in the under 44-year age group and prescription analgesic use increased with age.[6] It would be reasonable to assume that a large proportion of the nonprescription analgesics would contain NSAIDs.

In a Canadian study, elderly patients who had been specially trained to present standard clinical scenarios were presented in a blinded fashion to clinicians. Their management was assessed and the results suggest that there is some unnecessary prescribing and poor complications management of NSAIDs . If these results are generalizable, then current prescribing habits contribute to avoidable complications.[7]* Elderly patients are at greater risk of side-effects and account for a significant proportion of prescriptions. These drugs are, however, safe and efficacious in the elderly if used with caution.[8]

A systematic review of NSAID efficacy concluded that these agents are effective analgesics for postoperative and acute musculoskeletal pain.[9]***

Mechanisms of action

NSAIDs work by inhibiting cyclo-oxygenase (COX), which was originally thought to be a single enzyme. More recently, it was discovered that there are several COX enzymes: COX-1 is predominantly involved with normal regulation of physiological function whereas COX-2 has a normally low expression and is upregulated during inflammation.[1] COX-2 is expressed within the central nervous system (CNS) under normal circumstances, but its precise role, at least in terms of analgesia, requires further elucidation. It is anticipated that selective inhibition of COX-2 will provide analgesia with fewer side-effects than the nonselective NSAIDs. Newer data from animal studies, however, suggest that both COX-1 and COX-2 are expressed under basal and stress conditions. They have been isolated from a variety of tissues, including ovary, brain, kidney, and bone.[10] This suggests a more complex relationship than initially thought. It should be remembered that the full picture of benefit and side-effect may not be apparent until a drug has been in routine clinical use for some time, as was the case following the release of phenylbutazone some years ago.

Indications and contraindications

In general terms, these agents are prescribed for the treatment of pain associated with the inflammatory arthritides (e.g. rheumatoid arthritis), osteoarthritis, musculoskeletal disorders, dysmenorrhea, and mild to moderate pain. The indications are licensed specifically for each agent and are found in the general pharmacopoeia for each country. The contraindications are also specified in the license for each agent, but some general principles apply. These include a history of hypersensitivity to aspirin or other NSAIDs, pregnancy, breast feeding, and those with coagulation disturbances. Caution should be used when prescribing for the elderly and for those with renal, hepatic, or cardiac impairment. The other common caution is in those with a history of gastrointestinal ulceration or bleeding.

Some specific indications and contraindications are mentioned in Table 17.1. These are not exhaustive and local licensing limitations should be considered.

Apazone (azapropazone) has a restricted use in the UK for ankylosing spondylitis, rheumatoid arthritis, and acute gout, only after other agents have failed to be effective.[11] It is contraindicated in patients with a history of peptic ulceration, inflammatory bowel disease, blood disorders, porphyria, and renal impairment. A systematic review assessing gastrointestinal risk put apazone into a high-risk category and questioned its routine use.[12***]

Phenylbutazone also has prescribing restrictions[11] limited to ankylosing spondylitis only when other treatments are unsuitable. Regular blood counts are required; specific contraindications include those listed above as well as blood and coagulation disorders, porphyria, Sjogren syndrome, thyroid disease, and children under 14 years of age.

Administration and dosage

From a systematic review[9***] there is little evidence that parenteral administration of NSAIDs has any advantage over the oral route. Other reviews[13***,14***] suggest that current studies comparing analgesia and safety between NSAIDs may mislead if they only examine single doses, do not span the dose–response range, or do not use equianalgesic dosing. The ceiling effect for analgesia with NSAIDs is frequently not reached because toxicity prevents further dose escalation.

Patients vary in their response to these agents with regard to efficacy and side-effects. A systematic rotation of drug and dose titration may allow the minimum effective dose to be reached while minimizing the risk of side-effects. The formulation and dosing schedules for each agent vary. The smallest effective dose should be the aim in each individual case. In some instances, slow-release preparations may be more effective than intermittent standard release.

Table 17.1 *Some specific indications and contraindications*[11]

Generic name	Specific indications	Specific contraindications
Aspirin	Juvenile arthritis	Under 12 years except juvenile arthritis
Apazone[a]	Restricted use (see text)	
Diclofenac	Juvenile arthritis	Porphyria, concomitant NSAID use, or anticoagulant
Ibuprofen	Juvenile arthritis, migraine, fever in children	
Ketorolac	Short-term management	
Meloxicam	Ankylosing spondylitis	Renal failure
Mefenamic acid	Juvenile arthritis	Inflammatory bowel disease
Naproxen	Juvenile arthritis	
Phenylbutazone	See text	
Piroxicam	Juvenile arthritis	Porphyria

a. Apazone (azapropazone).
NSAID, nonsteroidal anti-inflammatory drug.

Table 17.2 lists some of the common NSAIDs available. Not all preparations are available in every country. Many of these agents are also found in "over-the-counter" remedies as compound preparations and are not included in this chapter. There are slow-release formulations available for some agents. Where possible, the selectivity for COX is reported, as is the relative toxicity for gastrointestinal complications relative to ibuprofen.

NSAIDs are often classified by chemical structure. In reality, there are several chemical classifications possible. When rotating NSAIDs it is often suggested to try a representative from each class. This approach is pragmatic rather than scientific and lack of efficacy of one member of a class does not exclude other members of the same class from being effective, but clinically a failed trial of one member often results in a trial from a different class.[15]

Side-effects and their management

Overall, NSAIDs have a good safety record, but, owing to the enormous quantities prescribed, they account for a large proportion of serious adverse drug events (Table 17.3). In 1985, of all reported adverse drug reactions, NSAIDs accounted for 25% in men and 30% in women.[16] The elderly account for approximately 40% of NSAID prescriptions[17] and are at greater risk of side-effects, as are women. The Committee on Safety of Medicines in the UK reported on seven NSAIDs and their relative risk of serious adverse reactions.[18] It concluded that ibuprofen was the safest; ketoprofen, indomethacin, naproxen, and diclofenac had intermediate risk; piroxicam may have a higher risk; and apazone has the highest risk; they were unable to comment on other agents.

Table 17.2 *Commonly available NSAIDs*

Generic name	Proprietary name[11,78]	Selectivity for COX-2 activity (ratio COX-2/COX-1)[41]	Availability	Relative risk of GI toxicity[12***]
Aspirin	Disprin, Anadin, Aspro	Nil (0.26)	OTC, PoM	1.6
Apazone[a]	Rheumox		PoM	
Celecoxib	Celebrex	High (9.10)	PoM	
Choline magnesium trisalicylate	Trilisate			
Diclofenac	Voltarol, Diclomax, Novo-Difenac, Voltaren	Nil (4.4)	PoM	1.8
Etodolac	Dolobid, Lodine, Novo-Diflunisal	High (23.3)	PoM	1.6
Fenbufen	Lederfen		PoM	
Fenoprofen	Motrin, Nuprin, Nalfon	Nil (1.00)	OTC, PoM	
Ibuprofen	Advil, Brufen, Fenbid, Motrin, Nuprin, Rufen, Trendar, Novo-Profen	Nil (0.38)	OTC, PoM	1.0
Indomethacin	Indocid, Indocin, Indomax	Nil (0.23)	PoM	2.4
Ketoprofen	Actron, Apo-Keto, Orudis, Oruvail, Rhodis	Nil (0.17)	OTC, PoM	4.2
Ketorolac	Toradol	Nil (0.003)		
COX-1 specific	PoM			
Meloxicam	Mobic	High (11.00)	PoM	
Mefenamic acid	Meclomen, Nu-Diclo, Ponstan, Ponstel, Dysman		PoM	
Nabumetone	Relifex, Relafen		PoM	
Naproxen	Anaprox, Naprelan, Naprosyn, Naxen, Nycopren, Synflex	Nil (0.33)	OTC, PoM	2.2
Nimesulide		High (5.90)		
Oxaprozin	Daypro			
Phenylbutazone	Butacote, Butazolidin, Cotylbutazone		PoM	
Piroxicam	Feldene, Nu-Pirox		PoM	3.8
Rofecoxib	Vioxx	High (> 20)		2.1
Sulindac	Clinoril, Novo-Sundac		PoM	
Tenoxicam	Mobiflex		PoM	
Tolmetin	Tolectin	Nil (2.70)		3.0

Not all agents are available in all countries.
Relative risk of toxicity is for gastrointestinal complications relative to ibuprofen (data from various sources).
a. Apazone (azapropazone).
PoM, prescription only medicine; OTC, over-the-counter medicine.

Table 17.3 *Commonly reported side-effects[9]***,[11]*

Gastrointestinal discomfort	Dizziness
Nausea	Vertigo
Diarrhea	Tinnitus
Vomiting	Photosensitivity
Drowsiness	Hematuria
Headache	Blood disorders
Hypersensitivity reactions (rashes, bronchospasm, angioedema)	Anxiety

Side-effects may present with a life-threatening event. There are groups of patients at higher risk of this and it is important to recognize them. They include the elderly, hypovolemic patients, immunocompromised patients, or those taking corticosteroids, and patients who have concomitant anticoagulant use, renal impairment, a past history of NSAID intolerance, or asthma.

COX-2 inhibitors

There has been considerable interest in the development of COX-2 inhibitors in the hope that they may be associated with an improved side-effect profile. Meloxicam was introduced first and preferentially inhibits COX-2, but at therapeutic doses it may also inhibit COX-1.[19] It does show a trend for reduced gastrointestinal side-effects.[20]** Rofecoxib was launched in the UK in June 1999. The voluntary reporting scheme for possible adverse reactions had received 1,120 reports by May 2000.[21] There were an estimated 557,100 prescriptions dispensed by that date. Approximately half of the reports (554) were for gastrointestinal complications, with 177 for cardiovascular reactions. Other reactions included psychiatric (53), angioedema (35), renal failure (26), respiratory (25), and liver failure (12). In Australia there have been 31 reported cases of serious gastrointestinal complications out of 919 reported adverse reactions for celecoxib during the first 6 months of marketing.[22] These are suspected reactions only and were voluntarily reported. They may not be directly due to the agents but may be due to other factors relating to the individual cases. Relative risk cannot be derived from this information, but it reminds practitioners that new drugs must be monitored for reactions and remain under review following their launch.

There is evidence that these agents may induce fewer gastrointestinal side-effects. A randomized control trial comparing celecoxib with naproxen or placebo in rheumatoid arthritis demonstrated similar efficacy, treatment failure, and withdrawal rates, but endoscopic evidence of ulcers was greater in the naproxen group.[23]** A further trial comparing celecoxib with diclofenac, again in rheumatoid arthritis, reported adverse events occurring in approximately 70% of subjects in both groups; again, there was significantly higher endoscopic ulcer rates reported in the diclofenac group.[24]** A 12-week randomized control trial comparing celecoxib with placebo or naproxen in osteoarthritis of the knee demonstrated the efficacy of celecoxib to be similar to naproxen with similar treatment failure rates. The side-effects and withdrawal rates were similar in all groups.[25]** A 6-month double-blind trial comparing meloxicam with naproxen in patients with rheumatoid arthritis demonstrated fewer gastrointestinal side-effects but there was a statistically higher withdrawal rate because of lack of efficacy. Adverse events were reported in approximately 60% of patients in each group.[26]** A similar 6-month trial in osteoarthritis demonstrated no real difference between meloxicam and diclofenac.[20]** A recent review examining rofecoxib and the more recently launched celecoxib concluded that although there are theoretical advantages with regard to side-effects for these agents they remain unproven in clinical practice and require further evaluation.[19]

Gastric complications

Patients taking long-term NSAIDs have a point prevalence for gastric or duodenal ulcers of up to 20%.[27] Estimates from the USA suggest serious gastrointestinal (GI) hemorrhage occurs in 80,000 people per year with a death rate of 6,000. Precise figures are not available as patients often have associated risk factors such as smoking, alcohol, and concomitant drug use.[2] The risk of fatal adverse reactions to NSAIDs may be higher; in the USA, NSAIDs carry a warning label stating a 2–4% risk of serious gastrointestinal reactions.[16] A more recent model for estimating rare adverse events, namely death, following NSAID use has been postulated.[28]*** This quantitative estimation combines data from controlled trials and observational studies. The authors estimate that approximately 1 in 1,200 patients will die from gastrointestinal complications following NSAID use of at least 2 months' duration. This equates to 2,000 deaths per year in the UK.

A cohort study[29]* examined 52,000 patients over 50 years old who had been prescribed one or more NSAID prescriptions over a 2-year period compared with 74,000 controls. Follow-up was for 3 years looking at hospital admissions for gastrointestinal complaints. The risk of admission was 2% for treated patients compared with 1.4% for controls. A meta-analysis[12]*** of gastrointestinal complications of NSAIDs was used to produce a table of relative risk. It showed ibuprofen to have the lowest risk and used it as the comparator (see Table 17.2). The authors commented that ibuprofen is generally used in a low-dose regimen (up to 1,600 mg/day) and demonstrated a dose–response curve. Higher daily doses of ibuprofen increase the relative risk towards that of the other NSAIDs. Many patients who take these agents will terminate therapy because of upper abdominal pain irrespective of proven gastrointestinal complications. Further evidence of this is seen in the drop-out rate of many trials and in clinical practice.

The concomitant use of gastro-protective agents may

be effective in reducing gastric complications. Commonly used groups include H$_2$ antagonists (e.g. ranitidine), prostaglandin analogs (e.g. misoprostol) or proton pump inhibitors (e.g. omeprazole). A recent review suggests that double-dose H$_2$ antagonists and the proton pump inhibitors are effective prophylactic agents at preventing chronic NSAID-related endoscopic gastric and duodenal ulcers. Misoprostol has been shown to reduce the relative risk of endoscopic ulcer complications by 75% compared with placebo, which corresponds to a 10% absolute risk reduction; it is, however, associated with troublesome side-effects in up to 27% of patients. Double-dose H$_2$ antagonists compared with placebo have a relative risk reduction of 56%, which corresponds to a 12% absolute risk reduction without a corresponding problem with side-effects. The authors also comment that the development of COX-2 inhibitors may lead to a change in current practice.[30]***

Respiratory

NSAIDs may aggravate asthma and reversible airway disease.[31] A subset of asthma sufferers are intolerant to aspirin. Approximately half of this group are steroid dependant.[32]* The commission on safety of medicines in the UK specifically warns of the risk to asthma sufferers.[11] Other respiratory risk factors include nasal polyps and rhinitis.[16] The NSAIDs are therefore relatively contraindicated in this group of patients.

Renal complications

The risk to healthy individuals with normal renal function and no risk factors is minimal as their renal perfusion is less dependent on renal prostaglandin mechanisms.[33] NSAIDs are the commonest cause of drug-induced renal damage in clinical practice, but the overall proportion of patients on renal replacement therapy owing to analgesic nephropathy has fallen from 5% in the 1970s to 0.6% in 1998.[34] Inhibition of intrarenal prostaglandin production has been hypothesized to cause a critical reduction in renal blood flow and glomerular filtration rate, especially in patients with concomitant renal impairment, cardiac failure, sepsis, or hypovolemia. The elderly and those undergoing surgery are also at higher risk. Most NSAIDs at full dose have the potential to cause acute renal failure within 24–48 h of initiating treatment; this is usually reversible.[35]

Other complications include sodium retention and elevated potassium, which cause hypertension and edema particularly in the elderly. Other drugs that reduce renal blood flow when used with NSAIDs increase the risk of renal failure (e.g. diuretics, angiotensin converting enzyme inhibitors, or receptor antagonists and cyclosporins).[34] Sulindac and nabumetone may pose less risk than other NSAIDs.[36]*

Nephrotoxic effects may occur but are less frequent. These may not relate to prostaglandin synthesis and the risk factors are not clear. Resolution occurs following withdrawal of the drug but may not be complete.[35]

Liver

NSAIDs tend to be plasma protein bound with low volumes of distribution and are hepatically metabolized. Mild elevations in liver enzymes are common, with the elderly being at greatest risk. Toxic hepatitis is rare.

Platelets

Aspirin irreversibly inhibits cyclo-oxygenase and inhibits prostaglandin synthesis for the 7- to 10-day lifespan of platelets. The non-aspirin NSAIDs reversibly block cyclo-oxygenase, so only need to be withdrawn 2 or 3 days before surgical intervention for platelet function to return to normal. The risk of bleeding will be increased in those who are coprescribed anticoagulants such as warfarin. The COX-2 inhibitors may have less effect on platelet inhibition and not have the potential benefit for those with ischemic heart disease.[37,38]

Cardiac

A recent matched case–control study has looked at the risk of developing congestive cardiac failure (CCF) following recent NSAID use. They suggest that NSAID use other than low-dose aspirin doubles the risk of admission with CCF and this rises to 10-fold if there is a history of heart disease. There also appeared to be a relationship to the dose of NSAID used. If confirmed, these findings suggest that up to 19% of hospital admissions of patients with CCF are related to NSAIDs.[39]*

Other side-effects

Agranulocytosis and aplastic anemia are rare complications. Phenylbutazone has a greater association with this complication.[40] The risk of marrow suppression is 1 in 3,000 patient–years of treatment but has a 50% mortality associated with it.[16]

Hypersensitivity reactions are common with all NSAIDs. Rarely, more serious reactions occur, such as Stevens–Johnson syndrome.

Other rarely reported complications include alveolitis, pulmonary eosinophilia, pancreatitis, eye changes, toxic epidermal necrolysis, and aseptic meningitis.[11]

Pharmaceutical and pharmacological issues

Many preparations have been developed in an attempt to circumvent the side-effects of NSAIDs. A systematic review comparing routes of administration suggests that the oral route should be used when patients can swallow. The intramuscular and rectal routes are associated with higher adverse effect rates, including pain on injection, rectal irritation, and diarrhea.[9***]

A large *in vitro* analysis of COX-1 and COX-2 selectivity for NSAIDs has been performed for a wide range of agents.[41] This demonstrates the relative specificities for COX-1 against COX-2 and also demonstrates the level of COX-1 inhibition when COX-2 is inhibited by 80% (see Table 17.2). The postulate is that this is the level of COX-2 inhibition required for a therapeutic benefit. The analysis suggests that the agents with greatest COX-1 selectivity correlate with those that have higher GI side-effects.

Evidence of effectiveness

An outline of effectiveness can be seen in Table 17.4.

Musculoskeletal pain

Analgesics are commonly prescribed for musculoskeletal pain in the general population.[6] Many of the prescription and nonprescription agents commonly used are likely to contain NSAIDs. There is some good evidence for the beneficial role of NSAIDs in low back pain compared with placebo, but it becomes limited when compared with acetaminophen. When considering chronic

low back pain separately, there is insufficient evidence to perform subgroup analysis and the authors suggest further research into this area.[42***] A series of *N*-of-1 which examined the efficacy of NSAIDs for chronic musculoskeletal pain demonstrated the difficulties encountered with research in this area. There was no benefit for NSAIDs, but there was a high incidence of side-effects and high drop-out rates that resulted in small numbers of patients completing the trial.[43**]

Arthritic pain

Rheumatoid arthritis patients are frequently prescribed NSAIDs. A double-blind placebo-controlled trial comparing naproxen, celecoxib, and placebo demonstrated that the active agents were significantly more efficacious than placebo. There were fewer treatment failures in the active groups (approximately 25%) than in the placebo groups (45%). Adverse events were common in all groups but few led to withdrawal from the study.[23**] A further double-blind randomized trial comparing celecoxib with diclofenac over 24 weeks in patients with rheumatoid arthritis reached a similar conclusion.[24**] However, it should be noted that although NSAIDs are useful in treating rheumatoid arthritis, other agents are often more effective.[44***]

In a survey assessing global preferences (effectiveness and side-effects) between acetaminophen and NSAIDs in patients with osteoarthritis, rheumatoid arthritis, and

Table 17.4 *Review of evidence of effectiveness*

Condition	Comment	Agents	Outcome	Reference
Low back pain	Acute and chronic	NSAIDs vs. placebo	Statistical improvement for NSAID	42***
	Acute	NSAIDs vs. acetaminophen[a]	No difference	
Chronic back pain	Subgroup assessment	NSAIDs vs. placebo	Unable to assess	
		NSAIDs vs. acetaminophen[a]	Limited evidence of NSAID advantage	
		Acetaminophen[a]/codeine vs. tramadol	Similar efficacy with combination being better tolerated	76**
Rheumatoid arthritis	Response to treatment	NSAIDs, COX-2 inhibitors and placebo	Significant improvement compared with placebo; no difference between active agents	23**, 24**
		Steroids vs. NSAIDs	Steroids show advantage in low-dose, short-term use	44***
Rheumatic disease	Survey of patient preference for benefit and side-effects	NSAIDs and acetaminophen[a]	Preference for NSAIDs 60%, acetaminophen[a] 14%, and no preference 25%	45
Osteoarthritis	Long-term comparison	Naproxen vs. acetaminophen[a]	Similar efficacy with high drop-out rate suggesting neither is satisfactory	46**
		Ibuprofen vs. acetaminophen[a]	Similar effects both better than placebo	71**
	Systematic review of relative efficacy	NSAIDs	Relative efficacy data not yet available	13, 14
Neuropathic pain	Review	NSAIDs	Probably no role to play	48

a. Acetaminophen (paracetamol).

NSAID, nonsteroidal anti-inflammatory drug.

fibromyalgia, 60% had a general preference for NSAIDs. However, the authors of this survey point out that this demonstrates a perception of effectiveness which may differ from actual effectiveness. The results may be biased by the beliefs and perceptions of patients and their physicians.[45]

NSAIDs are commonly used in osteoarthritis (OA). A 2-year double-blind comparison of naproxen and acetaminophen using a model of OA of the knee showed little difference between treatments for those completing the trial, with the withdrawal rates being high (65%). The reasons for withdrawal were not significantly different between groups, although gastrointestinal reactions were higher in the naproxen group.[46**] The Cochrane collaboration has reviewed the use of NSAIDs in OA of the knee.[13***] The reviewers concluded that, despite a large number of publications, few are random control trials and many have substantial design faults. The authors were unable to demonstrate a difference in efficacy between agents or for withdrawal rates and suggested that prescribing should be based on relative safety, patient acceptability, and cost. Similar comments were made in a review which used OA of the hip as the model.[14***] Pain can follow hip arthroplasty as can heterotopic bone formation in the soft tissues surrounding the joint. A systematic review confirms that perioperative NSAIDs reduce the risk of heterotopic bone formation. The significance of the short-term side-effects is less clear, and the long-term effect on pain and clinical outcome has not been fully elucidated.[47***] This further supports the need for additional properly controlled long-term studies.

Neuropathic pain often proves difficult to manage and the evidence suggests that NSAIDs are probably ineffective.[48***]

Chronic pain in the elderly is particularly difficult to manage. The population is aging and the elderly have a significantly higher incidence of chronic pain. Estimates from the USA suggest 70 million older people are prescribed regular analgesics, the majority of which are NSAIDs. It is suggested that all NSAIDs should be used with caution and that high doses should be avoided.[49] There is a large individual variation with regard to minimal effective dose and toxic dose. Dose titration is very valuable in this group and it is suggested that side-effects are regularly monitored in patients using NSAIDs in the long term.

ACETAMINOPHEN AND ITS COMMON COMBINATIONS

Acetaminophen has been available worldwide "over the counter" for 40 years.[50] Today, it is an ingredient in a large number of prescription and nonprescription formulations and is one of the most commonly used drugs. In 1999, over 10 million prescriptions for acetaminophen alone were filled in England.[3]

Mechanism of action and metabolism

Acetaminophen is an effective analgesic with antipyretic but not anti-inflammatory activity.[46**] The mechanism of its analgesic action is not fully understood, but the antipyretic effects appear to be mediated by inhibition of prostaglandin synthesis in the hypothalamus.[51,52] At therapeutic dosages, it does not inhibit COX in peripheral tissues, which explains its lack of anti-inflammatory activity.[53]

Administration and dosage

The proper use of acetaminophen is crucial to optimizing its effectiveness and achieving pain relief. Patients may conclude that acetaminophen is ineffective after taking only one or two tablets a day for short periods of time and subsequently terminate treatment; this is an inadequate trial period for chronic pain conditions, which require up to 4 g/day in divided doses for at least a week.[53] The oral route is preferable, with suspensions and dispersible preparations being available. Rectal and parenteral preparations are available (in some countries).

Acetaminophen/codeine combinations versus acetaminophen alone

Most, but not all, of the trials included in the systematic reviews on combination preparations are based on acute pain; chronic pain patients are included, but in much smaller numbers. Interpretation has to be made with caution.

A systematic review[54***] concluded that codeine added to the analgesic efficacy of acetaminophen by using derived outcome measures of pain relief such as the sum of the pain intensity difference. This meta-analysis of six head-to-head comparison trials using pooled data estimated a significant 6.7-point difference in the sum of the pain intensity (95% confidence interval 3.2–10.3) between the acetaminophen/codeine combination and acetaminophen alone; this was not translated into a significant increase in the proportion of patients obtaining moderate to excellent pain relief [response rate ratio 1.14 (0.97 to 1.34)]. In this meta-analysis, caffeine (a common additive in many proprietary products that combine analgesics) did not add to the efficacy of acetaminophen, as measured by either the sum of the pain intensity difference or the response rate ratio.

A separate systematic review[55***] assessed the efficacy and safety of acetaminophen/codeine combinations versus acetaminophen alone and concluded that most trials were of good to very good quality, that only the single-dose studies could be combined for analysis of analgesic efficacy, and that pooled efficacy results indicated that acetaminophen/codeine combinations added a 5% increase in analgesia using the sum pain intensity difference measure. This effect was small but statistically significant and was similar to the difference in analgesic effect between codeine and placebo. The cumulative incidence of side-effects with each treatment was similar in the single-dose trials. In the multidose studies a significantly higher proportion of side-effects occurred with acetaminophen/codeine preparations. They concluded that for occasional pain relief the acetaminophen/codeine combination might be appropriate, but repeated use increases the occurrence of side-effects.

There are many preparations available that combine acetaminophen with other analgesics. A list of some of the more common combinations is given in Table 17.5. This is in no way exhaustive and is, in the main, limited to analgesic combinations. Many over-the-counter remedies contain acetaminophen with a wide variety of other agents and these have not been addressed in this chapter.

Side-effects and their management

Acetaminophen is generally well tolerated. Skin rashes and other allergic reactions occur occasionally. The rash is usually erythematous or urticarial, but may be more serious and accompanied by a drug fever and mucosal lesions.

In a few isolated cases, the use of acetaminophen has been associated with neutropenia, pancytopenia, and leukopenia. The most serious adverse effect of acute overdosage of acetaminophen is a dose-dependant, potentially fatal, hepatic necrosis. Renal tubular necrosis and hypoglycemic coma may also occur.[56]

Gastric

Acetaminophen causes little or no gastrointestinal irritation and is not associated with ulcer formation.[57]

Renal

The effect of acetaminophen on renal function is minimal because it does not influence renal prostaglandin synthesis. There is negligible evidence for its involvement in the development of classic analgesic nephropathy (papillary necrosis, chronic interstitial nephritis) when used alone and it has not been conclusively associated with any evidence of end-stage renal disease.

Renal toxicity has been documented with acetaminophen only in overdose and is thought to be secondary to acute hepatic failure.[53] In a 1996 position paper, the National Kidney Foundation (UK) recommended acetaminophen as the non-narcotic analgesic of choice "for episodic use in patients with underlying renal disease." Both experimental and epidemiological data have found an association between combinations of aspirin, acetaminophen, caffeine, and/or codeine and increased renal toxicity.[58]

Hepatic

Acetaminophen has been associated with liver toxicity in combination with massive overdose or chronic alcohol abuse. Patients consuming more than three units of alcohol per day should consult with their physician before taking analgesics.[53,59,60*,61]

Table 17.5 *Some common acetaminophen (paracetamol) combinations*

Combination name	Acetaminophen	Other agent
Acetaminophen/**hydrocodone**, Hyco-pap, Lorcet HD, Vicodin	500 mg	Hydrocodone 5 mg
Acetaminophen/oxycodone, Pendocet, Percocet	325 mg	Oxycodone 5 mg
Acetaminophen/propoxyphene	325 or 650 mg	Propoxyphene 50, 65 or 100 mg
Darvocet-N	650 mg	Propoxyphene 100 mg
Benoral (salicylate/acetaminophen ester)	970 mg	Aspirin 1.15 g equivalent
Co-codamol 8/500	500 mg	Codeine phosphate 8 mg
Co-codamol 30/500, Solpadol, Tylex, Kapake	500 mg	Codeine phosphate 30 mg
Co-dydramol	500 mg	Dihydrocodeine tartrate 10 mg
Remedeine	500 mg	Dihydrocodeine tartrate 20 mg
Co-proxamol, Distalgesic	325 mg	Dextropropoxyphene hydrochloride 32.5 mg
Domepramol	500 mg	Domepridone 10 mg
Excedrin Migraine	250 mg	Aspirin 250 mg/caffeine 65 mg
Fortagesic	500 mg	Pentazocine 15 mg
Midrid	325 mg	Isometheptene mucate 65 mg
Migraleve	500 mg	Buclizine hydrochloride 6.25 mg
Paradote	500 mg	Methionine 100 mg
Paramax	500 mg	Metaclopromide hydrochloride 5 mg

Bold, nonproprietary name.

Acetaminophen in patients with chronic liver disease

There is no evidence that preexisting chronic liver disease increases the risk of hepatotoxicity after administration of acetaminophen in therapeutic doses for short periods of time (up to 5 days). Cytochrome P_{450} enzyme levels are not increased and excretion of various conjugates (including cysteine and mercapturic acid conjugates) remain unchanged in the presence of liver disease.[62*,63*,64*,65,66] The elimination half-life of acetaminophen is statistically prolonged, but clinically unimportant. In a double-blind, two-period crossover of acetaminophen or placebo, each given for 2 weeks to patients with chronic liver disease, no changes in liver function were seen with either acetaminophen or placebo.[62*,65*,67*,68,69]

Pharmaceutical and pharmacological issues

Acetaminophen is rapidly absorbed, with peak plasma concentrations occurring within 1 h. If taken with food, peak concentrations may be delayed until 4 h after ingestion.

Acetaminophen is metabolized and eliminated via three pathways:

1 Approximately 90% is conjugated with sulfate or glucuronide. Although the sulfate is less important in adults, it has been proposed as a more active pathway in children, which could account for their greater tolerance to higher doses.
2 Between 5% and 10% is metabolized by a cytochrome P_{450} mixed-function oxidase system. The intermediate metabolite of this pathway, N-acetyl-p-benzoquinoneimine (NAPQI), is detoxified by the addition of sulfhydryl groups. NAPQI has a half-life $(t_{1/2})$ that is three times longer than that of acetaminophen (36 h vs. 12 h respectively). This is responsible for the hepatic injury associated with acetaminophen toxicity. Normally, glutathione acts as the sulfhydryl group. In nutritionally depleted patients or in the presence of overdose, there may be insufficient glutathione to protect the liver. Renal injury is thought to occur via the same mechanism.
3 Less than 5% is eliminated unchanged in the urine.

The volume of distribution of acetaminophen is 0.75–1.0 l/kg, with protein binding of 35–50%.[70]

Evidence of effectiveness

Arthritic pain

In osteoarthritis acetaminophen is as effective as NSAIDs for the management of mild to moderate OA pain and is the recommended first-line therapy by the American College of Rheumatology (ACR) for OA of the hip or knee.[53] A randomized, double-blind trial in OA of the hip or knee demonstrated that 4.0 g acetaminophen daily was more effective than placebo and as effective as commonly used NSAIDs for the relief of joint pain and improvement of function in patients.[71**] Additionally, the majority of patients with OA were elderly and were at increased risk of NSAID-related GI and renal adverse effects. A prospective, double-blind control study over 2 years for the treatment of OA concluded that the efficacy of acetaminophen and naproxen were similar.[46**] There have also been concerns that NSAIDs may have deleterious effects on articular cartilage metabolism and joint loading.[72–75]

Although acetaminophen and NSAIDs are both effective for the relief of mild to moderate pain, NSAIDs may be necessary for treating pain resulting from inflammatory conditions. When treating a largely noninflammatory condition such as OA, acetaminophen may be a more appropriate therapeutic option because of its lack of GI and renal adverse events compared with those seen with NSAIDs.[53]

In a survey of 1,799 patients with three types of rheumatic disease – rheumatoid arthritis, osteoarthritis, or fibromyalgia – Wolfe et al.[45] concluded that there was a statistically significant preference for NSAIDs compared with acetaminophen among the three groups. This preference decreased with age and was less pronounced in OA patients. In the over 65 years age group, overall satisfaction was the same for acetaminophen and NSAIDs in 33% of patients compared with 15% in the under 50 years age group.

Chronic back pain

A double-blind, multiple dose, randomized, crossover study comparing a fixed dose capsule preparation of acetaminophen/codeine with tramadol in patients with refractory chronic back pain found that they were both efficacious but that the acetaminophen combination was better tolerated.[76**]

Headache

Three double-blind, randomized, placebo-controlled trials concluded that the nonprescription combination of acetaminophen, aspirin, and caffeine was highly effective for the treatment of migraine headache. It also alleviated the nausea, photophobia, and functional disability associated with migraine attacks, with an excellent safety profile and tolerability.[77**]

There are no good data to support or refute a role for acetaminophen in the management of neuropathic pain.

CONCLUSIONS

- Acetaminophen is well tolerated and safe except in overdose.
- Acetaminophen is a first-line agent in mild to moderate pain of OA.
- Combinations of acetaminophen with other agents offer little real benefit and have increased risk of side-effects. They may be of benefit in short-term use.
- There is good evidence for the benefit of NSAIDs in acute and chronic inflammatory pain with minimal evidence in neuropathic pain.
- NSAIDs are widely used by prescription and as over-the-counter medicines. The side-effects of NSAIDs are potentially life-threatening, but this must be viewed in the context of the enormous scale of usage of this class of drugs.
- New research into the specific cyclo-oxygenase antagonists holds potential for improved safety. As yet, this has not been fully realized and further evaluation is required.
- Clinically, NSAIDs with lower risk should be tried first, but studies comparing efficacy and side-effects may mislead. The efficacy of acetaminophen should be assessed first.
- Parenteral NSAID administration has no benefit over the oral route.
- Trialing several agents and drug rotation may be beneficial with some patients.
- Elderly patients are at greater risk of side-effects than the young.
- Further high-quality systematic review or new research has to be done to evaluate:
  - relative efficacies between agents;
  - long-term effects in terms of risk and benefit;
  - the effects of common combinations in chronic pain;
  - what role, if any, there is in neuropathic pain for these agents.

REFERENCES

1. Talley JJ. Selective inhibitors of cyclooxygenase-2 (COX-2). *Prog Med Chem* 1999; **36**: 201–34.
2. Berd CB, Sundel R. COX-2 inhibitors: a status report. In: *IASP Newsletter: Technical Corner*. Seattle, WA: IASP, 1998.
3. Department of Health. NSAIDs and aspirin as an analgesic. Summary of prescription items dispensed according to British National Formulary classification. In: *UK Prescription Cost Analysis Data*. London: Department of Health, 1999.
4. Latham J, Davis BD. The socioeconomic impact of chronic pain. *Disability Rehabil* 1994; **16**: 39–44.
5. Moore RA, Phillips CJ. Cost of NSAID adverse effects to the UK National Health Service. *J Med Econ* 1999; **2**: 45–55.
6. Antonov KIM, Isacson DGL. Prescription and nonprescription analgesic use in Sweden. *Ann Pharmacother* 1998; **32**: 485–9.
7. Tamblyn R, Berkson L, Dauphinee WD, *et al*. Unnecessary prescribing of NSAIDs and the management of NSAID-related gastropathy in medical practice. *Ann Intern Med* 1997; **127**: 429–38.
8. Sager DS, Bennett RM. Individualizing the risk/benefit ratio of NSAIDs in older patients. *Geriatrics* 1992; 47 (8): 24–31.
9. Tranmer MR, Williams JE, Carroll D, *et al*. Comparing analgesic efficacy of non-steroidal anti-inflammatory drugs given by different routes in acute and chronic pain: a qualitative systematic review. *Acta Anaesthesiol Scand* 1998; **42**: 71–9.
10. Lipsky LP, Abramson SB, Crofford L, *et al*. The classification of cyclooxygenase inhibitors. *J Rheumatol* 1998; **25**: 2298–303.
11. British Medical Association and Royal Pharmaceutical Society of Great Britain. Non-steroidal anti-inflammatory drugs. In: *British National Formulary (BNF)*. Bath: British Medical Association and Royal Pharmaceutical Society of Great Britain, 2000: 10.1.1.446.
12. Henry D, Lim LLY, Rodriguez LAG, *et al*. Variability in risk of gastrointestinal complications with individual non-steroidal anti-inflammatory drugs: results of a collaborative meta-analysis. *Br Med J* 1996; **312**: 1563–66.
13. Watson MC, Brookes ST, Kirwan JR, Faulkner A. Non-aspirin, non-steroidal anti-inflammatory drugs for osteoarthritis of the knee (Cochrane Review). In: *The Cochrane Library, Oxford, Update Software*, issue 3. Oxford: Cochrane Library, 2000.
14. Towheed T, Shea B, Wells G, Hochberg M. Analgesia and non-aspirin, non-steroidal anti-inflammatory drugs for osteoarthritis of the hip (Cochrane Review). In: *The Cochrane Library, Oxford, Update Software*, issue 3. Oxford: Cochrane Library, 2000.
15. Flynn BL. Rheumatoid arthritis and osteoarthritis: current and future therapies. *Am Pharm* 1994; 34 (11): 31–42.
16. Nuki G. Pain control and the use of non-steroidal analgesic anti-inflammatory drugs. *Br Med Bull* 1990; **46**: 262–78.
17. Shimp LA. Safety issues in the pharmacologic management of chronic pain in the elderly. *Pharmacotherapy* 1998; **18**: 1313–22.
18. Relative safety of oral non-aspirin NSAIDs. *Curr Probl Pharmacovigilance* 1994; **20**: 9–11.
19. Are Rofecoxib and Celecoxib safer NSAIDS? *Drug Ther Bull* 2000; 38 (11): 81–6.
20. Hosie J, Distel M, Bluhmki E. Meloxicam in osteoarthritis: a 6-month, double-blind comparison with

diclofenac sodium. *Br J Rheumatol* 1996; 35 (Suppl. 1): 39–43.

21. In focus: Rofecoxib (Vioxx). *Curr Probl Pharmacovigilance* 2000; **26:** 13.

22. Celecoxib: early Australian reporting experience. *Aust Adverse Drug React Bull* 2000; **19:** 6–7.

23. Simon LS, Weaver AL, Graham DY, *et al*. Anti-inflammatory and upper gastrointestinal effects of celecoxib in rheumatoid arthritis. *JAMA* 1999; 282 (20): 1921–8.

24. Emery P, Zeidler H, Kvien TK, *et al*. Celecoxib versus diclofenac in long-term management of rheumatoid arthritis: randomised double-blind comparison. *Lancet* 1999; **354:** 2106–11.

25. Bensen WG, Fiechtner JJ, McMillen JI, *et al*. Treatment of osteoarthritis with celecoxib, a cyclooxygenase-2 inhibitor: a randomized controlled trial. *Mayo Clinic Proc* 1999; **74:** 1095–105.

26. Wojtulewski JA, Schattenkirchner M, Barcelo P, *et al*. A six-month double-blind trial to compare the efficacy and safety of meloxicam 7.5 mg daily and naproxen 750 mg daily in patients with rheumatoid arthritis. *Br J Rheumatol* 1996; 35 (Suppl. 1): 22–8.

27. Hawkey CJ. The gastroenterologist's caseload: contribution of the rheumatologist. *Semin Arthritis Rheum* 1997; 26 (6): 11–15.

● 28. Tramer MR, Moore RA, Reynolds DJM, McQuay HJ. Quantitative estimation of rare adverse events which follow a biological progression: a new model applied to chronic NSAID use. *Pain* 2000; **85:** 169–82.

29. MacDonald TM, Morant SV, Robinson GC, *et al*. Association of upper gastrointestinal toxicity of non-steroidal anti-inflammatory drugs with continued exposure: cohort study. *Br Med J* 1997; **315:** 1333–7.

● 30. Rostom A, Wells G, Tugwell P, *et al*. Prevention of NSAID-induced gastroduodenal ulcers (Cochrane Review). In: *The Cochrane Library, Oxford, Update Software*, issue 4. Oxford: Cochrane Library, 2000.

31. Sturtevant J. NSAID-induced bronchospasm – a common and serious problem. A report from MEDSAFE, the New Zealand Medicines and Medical Devices Safety Authority. *NZ Dent J* 1999; 95 (421): 84.

32. Szczeklik A, Nizankowska E, Duplaga M. Natural history of aspirin-induced asthma. AIANE Investigators. European Network on Aspirin-Induced Asthma. *Eur Respir J* 2000; **16:** 432–6.

● 33. Murray MD, Brater DC. Effects of NSAIDs on the kidney. *Prog Drug Res* 1997; **49:** 155–71.

34. Stuart R, Rodger C. Analgesic-induced renal damage. *Prescribers J* 2000; 40 (2): 151–64.

35. Pugliese F, Cinotti GA. Nonsteroidal anti-inflammatory drugs (NSAIDs) and the kidney. *Nephrol Dial Transplantation* 1997; **12:** 386–8.

36. Cangiano JL, Figuerao J, Palmer R. Renal hemodynamic effects of nabumetone, sulindac and placebo in patients with osteoarthritis. *Clin Ther* 1999; **21:** 503–12.

37. Bombardier C, Laine L, Reicin A, *et al*. Comparison of upper gastrointestinal toxicity of rofecoxib and naproxen in patients with rheumatoid arthritis. *N Engl J Med* 2000; **343:** 1520–8.

38. Cox-2 selective NSAIDs lack anti-platelet activity. *Curr Probl Pharmacovigilance* 2001; **27:** 7.

39. Page J, Henry D. Consumption of NSAIDs and the development of congestive heart failure in elderly patients: an underrecognized public health problem. *Arch Intern Med* 2000; **160:** 777–84.

40. Fowler PD. Marrow toxicity of the pyrazoles. *Ann Rheumatol Dis* 1967; **26:** 344–5.

41. Warner TD, Giuliano F, Vojnovic I, *et al*. Nonsteroid drug selectivities for cyclo-oxygenase-1 rather than cyclo-oxygenase-2 are associated with human gastrointestinal toxicity: a full in vitro analysis. *Pharmacology* 1999; **96:** 7563–8.

● 42. van Tulder MW, Scholten RJPM, Koes BW, Deyo RA. Nonsteroidal anti-inflammatory drugs for low back pain (Cochrane Review). In: *The Cochrane Library, Oxford, Update Software*, issue 3. Oxford: Cochrane Library, 2000.

43. Sheather-Reid RB, Cohen ML. Efficacy of analgesics in chronic pain: a series of N-of-1 studies. *J Pain Symptom Manage* 1998; **15:** 244–52.

● 44. Gotzsche PC, Johansen HK. Short-term low-dose corticosteroids vs placebo and nonsteroidal antiinflammatory drugs in rheumatoid arthritis (Cochrane Review). In: *The Cochrane Library, Oxford, Update Software*, issue 3. Oxford: Cochrane Library, 2000.

45. Wolfe F, Zhao S, Lane N. Preference for nonsteroidal antiinflammatory drugs over acetaminophen by rheumatic disease patients: a survey of 1,799 patients with osteoarthritis, rheumatoid arthritis, and fibromyalgia. *Arthritis Rheum* 2000; **43:** 378–85.

◆ 46. Williams JH, Ward JR, Egger MJ, *et al*. Comparison of naproxen and acetaminophen in a two-year study of treatment of osteoarthritis of the knee. *Arthritis Rheum* 1993; **36:** 1196–1206.

● 47. Neal B, Rodgers A, Dunn L, Fransen M. Non-steroidal anti-inflammatory drugs for preventing heterotopic bone formation after hip arthroplasty (Cochrane Review). In: *The Cochrane Library, Oxford, Update Software*, issue 3. Oxford: Cochrane Library, 2000.

● 48. Kingery WS. A critical review of controlled clinical trials for peripheral neuropathic pain and complex regional pain syndromes. *Pain* 1997; **73:** 123–9.

49. Ferrell BR, Ferrell BA. Management of chronic pain in the elderly: pharmacology of opioids and other analgesic drugs. In: Ferrell BR, Ferrell BA eds. *Pain in the Elderly*. Seattle, WA: IASP Press, 1996: 21–34.

50. D'Arcy PF. Paracetamol. *Adverse Drug React Toxicol Rev* 1997; **16:** 9–14.

51. Flower RJ, Vane JR. Inhibition of prostaglandin synthetase in brain explains the anti-pyretic activity of paracetamol. *Nature* 1972; **240:** 410–11.

52. *Physician's Desk Reference,* 51st edn. Montvale, NJ: Medical Economics Company, 1997.

53. Schnitzer TJ. Non-NSAID pharmacologic treatment options for the management of chronic pain. *Am J Med* 1998; **105:** 45S–52S.

● 54. Zhang WY, Li Wan Po A. Analgesic efficacy of paracetamol and its combination with codeine and caffeine in surgical pain – a meta-analysis. *J Clin Pharm Ther* 1996; **21:** 261–82.

● 55. De Craen AJM, Di Guilio G, Lampe-Schoenmaeckers AJEM, *et al.* Analgesic efficacy and safety of paracetamol–codeine combinations versus paracetamol alone: a systemic review. *Br Med J* 1996; **313:** 321–5.

56. Insel PA. Analgesic–antipyretics and antiinflammatory agents: drugs employed in the treatment of rheumatoid arthritis and gout. In: Gilman AG, Rail TW, Niles AS, Taylor P, eds. *Goodman and Gilman's The Pharmacological Basis Of Therapeutics,* 8th edn. McGraw-Hill, 1990.

57. Vickers FN. Mucosal effects of aspirin and acetaminophen: report of a controlled gastroscopic study. *Gastrointest Endosc* 1967; 14 (2): 94–9.

58. Henrich WL, Agodoa LE, Barrett B. Analgesics and the kidney: summary and recommendations to the scientific advisory board of the National Kidney Foundation. *Am J Kidney Dis* 1996; **27:** 162–5.

● 59. Nelson SD. Molecular mechanism of the hepatotoxicity caused by acetaminophen. *Semin Liver Dis* 1990; 10 (4): 267–78.

● 60. Johnston SC, Pelletier LLJ. Enhanced hepatotoxicity of acetaminophen in the alcoholic patient: two case reports and a review of the literature. *Medicine* 1997; **76:** 185–91.

61. Schiodt FV, Rochling FA, Casey DL, *et al.* Acetaminophen toxicity in an urban county hospital. *N Engl J Med* 1997; **337:** 1112–17.

62. Benson GD. Hepatotoxicity following the therapeutic use of antipyretic analgesics. *Am J Med* 1983; 75 (5A): 85–93.

63. Forrest JA, Adriaenssens P, Finlayson NDC, *et al.* Paracetamol metabolism in chronic liver disease. *Eur J Clin Pharmacol* 1979; **15:** 427–31.

64. Andreasen PB, Hutters L. Paracetamol (acetaminophen) clearance in patients with cirrhosis of the liver. *Acta Med Scand* 1979; 624 (Suppl.): 99–105.

65. Gabrielle L, Leterrier F, Molinie C, *et al.* Determination of human liver cytochrome P-450 by a micromethod using electron paramagnetic resonance: study of 141 liver biopsies. *Gastroenterol Clin Biol* 1977; **1:** 775–82.

66. Farrell GC, Cooksley WGE, Powell LW. Drug metabolism in liver disease: activity of hepatic microzomal metabolizing enzymes. *Clin Pharmacol Ther* 1979; **26:** 483–92.

67. Forrest JA, Finlayson ND, Adjepon-Yamoah KK, *et al.* Antipyrine, paracetamol, and lignocaine elimination in chronic liver disease. *Br Med J* 1977; **1:** 1384–7.

68. Shamszad M, Soloman H, Mobarhan S, *et al.* Abnormal metabolism of acetaminophen in patients with alcoholic liver disease. *Gastroenterology* 1975; A-65: 865.

69. Amman R, Olsson R. Elimination of paracetamol in chronic liver disease. *Acta Hepatogastroenterol* 1978; **25:** 283–6.

70. James B, Mowry R, Furbee B, Chyka PA. Poisoning. In: Chernow B ed. *The Pharmacological Approach To The Critically Ill Patient,* 3rd edn. Baltimore, MD: Williams & Wilkins, 1994.

71. Bradley JD, Brandt KD, Katz BP, *et al.* Treatment of knee osteoarthritis: relationship of clinical features of joint inflammation to the response to a nonsteroidal antiinflammatory drug or pure analgesic. *J Rheumatol* 1992; **19:** 1950–4.

72. Hochberg MC, Altman RD, Brandt KD, *et al.* Guidelines for the medical management of osteoarthritis. Part I. Osteoarthritis of the hip. American College of Rheumatology. *Arthritis Rheum* 1995; **38:** 1535–40.

73. Schnitzer TJ. Osteoarthritis treatment update: minimizing pain while limiting patient risk. *Postgrad Med* 1993; **93:** 89–92.

74. Schnitzer TJ, Anderiachhi TP, Fedder D, *et al.* Effect of NSAIDs on knee loading on patients with osteoarthritis. *Arthritis Rheum* 1990; **33:** 592.

● 75. Ghosh P. Anti-rheumatic drugs and cartilage. *Bailliere's Clin Rheumatol* 1988; **2:** 309–38.

76. Muller FO, Odendaal CL, Muller FR, *et al.* Comparison of the efficacy and tolerability of a paracetamol/codeine fixed-dose combination with tramadol in patients with refractory chronic back pain. *Arzneimittelforschung* 1998; **48:** 675–9.

77. Lipton RB, Stewart WF, Ryan REJ, *et al.* Efficacy and safety of acetaminophen, aspirin, and caffeine in alleviating migraine headache pain. *Arch Neurol* 1998; **55:** 210–17.

78. Anti-inflammatory drugs, nonsteroidal (systemic). In: *US National Library of Medicine.* Micromedex, 2000. www.n/m.nih.gov/medlineplus/druginfo.

18

Antidepressants and chronic pain

SØREN H SINDRUP

Tricyclic antidepressants were introduced to treat depression nearly 40 years ago. At the same time, it was suggested that these drugs had an analgesic effect, but their use in clinical pain was actually prompted by empiric observations of pain relief in diabetic neuropathy around 20 years ago.[1,2] Now, the benefits of tricyclic antidepressants in various pain conditions have been confirmed by numerous controlled clinical trials, and some of the new antidepressants, such as the selective serotonin (5-hydroxytryptamine) reuptake inhibitors, appear also to relieve pain.[3***,4***,5***] The antidepressants are mainly used in neuropathic pains for which other analgesics are either ineffective or not suitable. At the present time, antidepressants are the mainstay in the treatment of painful polyneuropathies, postherpetic neuralgia, and central poststroke pain. Some of the initial trials in neuropathic pain used a combination of a tricyclic antidepressant and an antipsychotic drug (phenothiazine), but in the numerous later trials the tricyclic alone was sufficient to produce an analgesic effect.

Use of antidepressants in pain treatment requires, of course, a knowledge of the pain conditions that these drugs have been shown to relieve in adequately designed clinical trials. However, equally important for successful use of antidepressants is a basic understanding of their pharmacological effects and pharmacokinetics in order to choose the right drug and dosage schedule.

BASIC PHARMACOLOGY

The tricyclic antidepressants are named according to their basic tricyclic structure, as shown in Fig. 18.1. The tricyclics share this structure with, for example, the anticonvulsant drug carbamazepine.

The pharmacological actions of the tricyclic antidepressants at membrane and receptor level include their unique ability to inhibit presynaptic reuptake of serotonin and norepinephrine (noradrenaline), postsynaptic receptor blocking, and stimulating effects and interaction with ion channels (Table 18.1).[5-12] There are interdrug differences among the tricyclics and the new antidepressants are characterized by their distinct profiles (Table 18.1).

Some of the classical tricyclic drugs, such as amitriptyline and imipramine, mainly inhibit the reuptake of serotonin. However, when they are used clinically, they will provide a balanced inhibition of serotonin and norepinephrine since they are metabolized to substances (nortriptyline and desipramine respectively) that mainly act as norepinephrine reuptake inhibitors. The metabolites themselves have been developed as drugs which therefore must be regarded as relatively selective norepinephrine reuptake inhibitors. All the tricyclics more or less act the same way on postsynaptic receptors and probably also on ion channels, although minor differences in receptor affinity have been claimed to be responsible for differences in side-effects between the drugs. The more pronounced sedation seen with amitriptyline as compared with imipramine and clomipramine thus may be explained by the higher affinity of amitriptyline for H_1-histamine receptors. Likewise, the less pronounced orthostatic hypotension reported with nortriptyline may be related to its lower affinity for α_1-adrenergic receptors, and the impression that desipramine may generally have fewer side-effects may be a result of a generally lower affinity for the postsynaptic receptors.

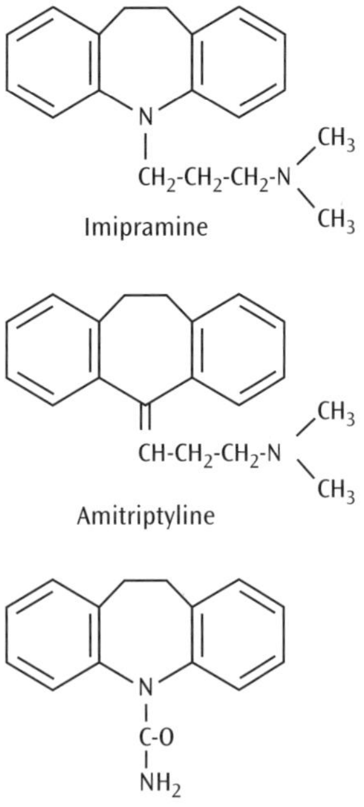

Imipramine

Amitriptyline

Carbamazepine

Figure 18.1 *The chemical structures of imipramine, amitriptyline, and carbamazepine.*

Many of the basic pharmacological actions of tricyclics have been described within the first decade after their introduction as antidepressants, but only during the last 10 years have the N-methyl-D-aspartate (NMDA)-antagonistic and ion channel-blocking effects been found and appreciated.[6–13] This opens the possibility that, as yet, unknown pharmacological actions may still appear for these old drugs.

It is important to have in mind that the selective serotonin reuptake inhibitors differ from the classical tricyclic antidepressants not only with respect to the presynaptic reuptake mechanism with which they interact, but also by being devoid of postsynaptic receptor-blocking effects and probably also devoid of action on ion channels. Balanced serotonin norepinephrine reuptake inhibitors without postsynaptic effects (Table 18.1) and, most recently, also selective norepinephrine reuptake inhibitors are pharmacologically interesting new compounds introduced within the last few years.

Monoamine oxidase inhibitor antidepressants such as the irreversible inhibitor phenylazine and the reversible moclobemide have been tried very little in pain treatment. These drugs will enhance serotonin and norepinephrine action by inhibiting the degradation of these monoamines.

Table 18.1 *Basic pharmacology of some antidepressant drugs*

	Tricyclic antidepressants		Selective serotonin reuptake inhibitors	Serotonin norepinephrine reuptake inhibitors	Tetracyclic antidepressant
	Imipramine Amitriptyline Clomipramine	Desipramine Nortriptyline Maprotiline	Paroxetine Citalopram Fluoxetine	Venlafaxine Milnacipran	Mianserin
Reuptake inhibition					
Serotonin	+	(+)	+	+	−
Norepinephrine	+[a]	+	−	+	(+)
Receptor blockade					
α-Adrenergic	+	+	−	−	+[b]
H_1-Histaminergic	+	+	−	−	++
Muscarin cholinergic	+	+	−	−	+
Serotonergic	−	−	−	−	+
NMDA[c]	+	+	−/?	?	?
Receptor stimulation					
Opioid	(+)	(+)	((+))/?	?	((+))
Ion channel blockade					
Sodium	+	+	(+)/?	−[d]	−[d]
Calcium	+	+	?	?	(+)

a. Mainly through the metabolites desipramine, nortriptyline, and desmethylclomipramine respectively.
b. Relatively potent blockade of α_2-adrenergic receptors causing norepinephrine release.
c. Should probably be regarded as an N-methyl-D-aspartate antagonist-"like" effect, since it appears not to be a direct receptor blockade.
d. As judged by no changes in electrocardiogram during treatment.
Norepinephrine (noradrenaline).
( ) Weak action; (( )) very weak action; ? unknown.

CLINICAL PHARMACOLOGY

The antidepressant drugs covered by this text are all well absorbed from the gastrointestinal tract and they can therefore be used orally.

The drugs undergo hepatic metabolism via the P_{450} system before excretion via the kidneys. There is a pronounced interindividual variation in pharmacokinetics of the tricyclic antidepressants, with up to a 30-fold difference in steady-state serum concentration on the same dose.[14] The extremes of this variation are due to genetic polymorphism of the P_{450} enzyme CYP2D6 (Fig. 18.2), which is one of the major enzymes in the metabolism of the tricyclics.[15,16] About 10% of the white population has a nonfunctional variant of the gene that codes for CYP2D6 and therefore lacks the enzyme. These individuals are called poor metabolizers of the probe drugs sparteine, debrisoquine, or dextromethorphan, which are used in phenotype tests for this genetic polymorphism. The remaining 90% of individuals with at least one functional *CYP2D6* gene are called extensive metabolizers. As mentioned, the poor metabolizers can be identified before treatment by a phenotype test with one of the probe drugs,[17] by a gene test employing polymerase chain reaction (PCR) technique,[18] or simply by monitoring steady-state serum concentrations during treatment. However, the phenotype test may be troublesome since it requires collection of urine 12 h after dosing of the probe drug, whereas genotyping is performed on leukocytes from a blood sample.

Some of the drugs from the other antidepressant drug classes are also partially metabolized via the CYP2D6, but the variation in steady-state pharmacokinetics is much less pronounced.[19–21] The pharmacokinetic variation of the other drug classes is also less important, since they have a more favorable therapeutic index. Dosing once or twice daily is usually sufficient for the antidepressant drugs, since plasma half-lives are not less than about 12 h.

The tricyclics and some of the other drugs show non-linear pharmacokinetics.[16,19,22,23] This means that there is no linear relationship between drug dose and steady-state serum concentration. Therefore, dose increments may result in disproportionately higher increments in serum concentration. Again, this is most important for the classical tricyclic compounds with the less favorable therapeutic index.

MECHANISM OF ACTION

The first controlled trial of tricyclic antidepressants in painful diabetic neuropathy reported that all the patients had a substantial degree of depression before treatment and that relief of pain was paralleled by relief of depression.[24**] It was therefore suggested that depression was masquerading as painful neuropathy and that the analgesic effect *per se* depended on the antidepressant effect. It is now accepted that tricyclic antidepressants have a genuine analgesic effect independent of the antidepressant effect and the key arguments for this are:

- antidepressants work faster in pain than in depression;[25**]
- antidepressant work at lower concentrations in pain than in depression;[26**,27**,28**,29**,30**]
- pain is relieved in patients with both depressed and normal mood;[29**]
- antidepressants act as analgesics in acute experimental pain.[31**,32**,33**]

This, however, does not preclude that depression and pain are basically relieved by the same pharmacological mechanisms of these drugs and that pain patients with concurrent depression (independent or secondary to the pain condition) will benefit additionally by the relief of depression, which has in fact been indicated in some trials.

A number of possible modes of analgesic action are inherited with the many known basic pharmacological effects (Table 18.2). For obvious reasons, the μ-opioid receptor interaction has attracted some attention. Animal experiments did in fact show that the acute analgesic effect was partially reversible by the opioid receptor antagonist naloxone.[34] However, this could also be seen if the tricyclics activated opioid neurons primarily via other types of receptors, and it is now generally held that, in comparison with opioid analgesics, the affinity of the

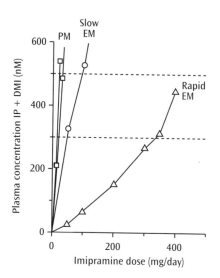

Figure 18.2 *The relationship between imipramine dose and plasma concentration of imipramine (IP) plus its active metabolite desipramine (DMI) in two poor metabolizers (PM) and the range of extensive metabolizers (EM) of sparteine/debrisoquine/dextromethorphan. The suggested therapeutic range for the treatment of neuropathic pain is shown by dashed lines (data from Sindrup et al.[16]).*

Table 18.2 *Possible links between pharmacological action and analgesic effect of antidepressants*

Pharmacological action	Link to pain relief
Reuptake inhibition of serotonin and norepinephrine	Serotonin and norepinephrine are neurotransmitters in diffuse noxious inhibitory control probably at both spinal and supraspinal levels. Reuptake inhibition will enhance/prolong the effect of otherwise released biogenic amines
α_1-Adrenergic receptor blockade	Blockade of highly sensitive adrenergic receptors on sprouting peripheral nerves (polyneuropathy, postherpetic neuralgia, post-traumatic peripheral nerve lesion) otherwise stimulated by norepinephrine from nearby sympathetic nerve fibers
α_2-Adrenergic receptor blockade	Release of norepinephrine and effect via diffuse noxious inhibitory control. Mode of action of clonidine
H_1-Histaminergic receptor blockade	Older antihistamines such as diphenhydramine have analgesic effect in clinical and experimental pain
NMDA receptor antagonist-"like" effect	Reduction of neuronal hyperexcitability at the spinal level. NMDA antagonists such as ketamine and dextromethorphan relieve some neuropathic pain conditions
Sodium channel blockade	Reduction of impulse generation in diseased peripheral nerves by membrane stabilization and probably also stabilization of neurons in the spinal cord. Suggested mode of action of antiarrhythmics and anticonvulsants in neuropathic pain
Calcium channel blockade	Inhibition of presynaptic transmitter release and postsynaptic impulse generation. Possible mechanism of action of gabapentin in neuropathic pain

NMDA, *N*-methyl-D-aspartate.
Norepinephrine (noradrenaline).

antidepressants for the μ-opioid receptors is far too low to be clinically significant.[35] Especially, this will hold for neuropathic pain that is the primary indication of the antidepressants and is known to respond relatively less adequately to opioids.[36**] The other pharmacological actions of interest in relation to analgesia with a relevant link to pain relief are highlighted in Table 18.2. The actual mechanism of action has not been settled and may vary from pain condition to pain condition, as well as between different patients with the same pain etiology but a different pain mechanism. Such interpatient differences in response have in fact been found in patients with the same pain condition.

Clinical trials in diabetic neuropathy have suggested that the reuptake inhibition of both serotonin and norepinephrine are of major importance.[37] It is probably impossible to sort out the contribution of each pharmacological action in detail owing to the extensive list of possible mechanisms (Table 18.2) and the lack of knowledge on the details of the basic pharmacology for all the compounds. The finding of a NMDA-antagonistic effect of tricyclic antidepressants was followed by experimental studies in animals supporting that this was the most likely mechanism of action,[13] but more recently it has been observed that there appears to be a clear correlation between the ability of different antidepressants to block sodium channels and their pain-relieving effect.

It is not unlikely that the tricyclic antidepressants have a multimodal mechanism of action and that their multiple pharmacological effects are the primary explanation for their efficacy in most patients with neuropathic types of pain and the reason why they are the current mainstay of treatment.

EFFICACY IN VARIOUS PAIN CONDITIONS

The efficacy of antidepressants in various chronic pain conditions has been evidenced in controlled trials and has already been extensively reviewed (Table 18.3).[3***,4***,5***,38***,39***] Additional controlled trials keep appearing,[40**,41**,42**] and numerous studies have been performed in neuropathic pain.[4***,38***,39***]

Numbers needed to treat (NNT) to obtain one patient with ≥ 50% pain relief (NNT ≥ 50%)[38***,39***,43] for different neuropathic pain conditions and for different antidepressants are shown in Table 18.4. The NNT ≥ 50% for tricyclic antidepressants is uniformly around 2.5 across various neuropathic pain conditions. The selective serotonin reuptake inhibitors appear to be less effective than the tricyclics with somewhat higher NNT ≥ 50% values. Several trials have shown that, in direct comparisons, tricyclics with a balanced inhibition of serotonin and norepinephrine (imipramine, amitriptyline, clomipramine) are more effective than tricyclics with relative selective norepinephrine reuptake inhibition (desipramine, nortriptyline, maprotiline)[42**,44**,45**,46**] and more effective than selective serotonin reuptake inhibitors.[25**,47**] Results from studies with the serotonin norepinephrine

Table 18.3 *Pain conditions in which tricyclic antidepressants have analgesic effect and corresponding evidence scoring*

Neuropathic pain conditions
    Painful diabetic neuropathy***
    Postherpetic neuralgia***
    Mixed patient groups with peripheral neuropathic
      pain (post-traumatic, postherpetic neuralgia,
      postinfectious neuropathy)**
    Central poststroke pain**

Headaches
    Chronic tension-type headache**
    Migraine prophylaxis**

Others
    Chronic pain of different etiology (probably both
      nociceptive and neuropathic pains)**

***Evidenced in systematic reviews.
**Evidenced in controlled trial(s).

reuptake inhibitor venlafaxine have still not been published, but preliminary data from one study in painful diabetic polyneuropathy show a significant effect, and from the data an NNT of 4.4 can be calculated.[48] Thus, the effect of this drug class seems to lie in between the effect of the selective serotonin reuptake inhibitors and the classical tricyclic antidepressants, with the full-scale reuptake inhibition, postsynaptic effects, and ion channel blockade.

Data from many of the controlled studies in neuropathic pain indicate that the tricyclics have an effect on all the different features of neuropathic pain, i.e. pain paroxysms, ongoing pain (deep aching, superficial burning, etc.), and touch-evoked pain.[25**,29**,45**,49**] However, it is an inherited problem with the present data that none of the studies addressed the issue of an effect on different types of pain.

Trials in nociceptive pain, such as pain in arthrosis and rheumatoid arthritis, and low back pain have generally failed to find an effect with tricyclic antidepressants.[3***,50***] In patients with chronic pain of different etiology attending an outpatient pain service, it has been found that adding a small dose of amitriptyline provides modest additional pain relief, and a clear dose–effect relation has also been reported in such settings.[51**,52**,53**] This kind of pain population must be anticipated to include also patients with primarily nociceptive pain.

Finally, tricyclic antidepressants are also effective in the treatment of chronic tension-type headache[41**,54**,55**] and in the prophylaxis of migraine attacks.[56**,57**] In chronic tension-type headache, it is currently one of the only treatments with an effect evidenced by controlled trials. The selective serotonin reuptake inhibitor citalopram does not have the potential for relief of tension-type headache,[41**] whereas the noradrenergic tricyclic drug maprotiline does.[55**] Tricyclics appear to be slightly less effective than β-blockers in migraine prophylaxis,[57**] but they are superior to placebo and may therefore still be an alternative for patients who cannot use β-blockers because of side-effects or contraindications.

SIDE-EFFECTS

The side-effects of the tricyclic antidepressants are mainly attributed to the postsynaptic receptor blocking effects, but the other pharmacological effects will also contribute to the side-effects (Table 18.5). Nearly all patients treated with tricyclics will experience a dry mouth and some of the other minor side-effects. The amount and intensity will vary from negligible to intolerable side-effects, and it is impossible in advance to determine which patient will suffer intolerable side-effects. In controlled trials in neuropathic pain, often around 25% of the patients will drop out as a result of side-effects. Elderly patients are generally more susceptible to the side-effects and it may be wise to choose tricyclics with less potent postsynaptic effects. It has been shown that nortriptyline is less prone to cause orthostatic hypotension[58] because of its lower affinity for α-adrenergic receptors. Amitriptyline is probably the compound that causes most sedation because of its higher affinity for H_1-histaminergic receptors. Most of the minor side-effects become less pronounced when treatment is continued.

The cardiac side-effects of the tricyclics are the most important, since they may be a contraindication to their use. These drugs can cause slowing of atrioventricular and intraventricular impulse conduction as well as cardiac decompensation.[59,60] Therefore, tricyclics should not be prescribed to patients with cardiac conduction disturbances or incompensation, or for at least 6 months after an acute myocardial infarction. An electrocardiogram is mandatory before treatment commences.

Table 18.4 *Numbers needed to treat to obtain one patient with more than 50% pain relief (95% confidence interval)*

	TCA	TCA optimal dose[a]	SNRI	SSRI
Painful diabetic neuropathy	2.4 (2.0–3.0)	1.4 (1.1–1.9)	4.4 (2.7–13)	6.7 (3.4–435)
Postherpetic neuralgia	2.3 (1.7–3.3)	ND	ND	ND
Nerve injury pain	2.5 (1.4–10.6)	ND	ND	ND
Poststroke pain	1.7 (1.1–3)	ND	ND	NA

a. Dose adjusted according to plasma concentration.
TCA, tricyclic antidepressant; SNRI, serotonin norepinephrine (noradrenaline) reuptake inhibitor; SSRI, selective serotonin reuptake inhibitor. ND, no data.

Tricyclics		
Anticholinergic	Dry mouth	
	Problems with accommodation	
	Tachycardia/palpitation	
	Constipation	
	Micturition difficulties/urine retention	
Antihistaminergic	Sedation	
α-Adrenergic blockade	Orthostatic hypotension	
Membrane stabilization	Atrioventricular conduction disturbance	
(sodium/calcium channel blockade)	Interventricular conduction disturbance	
	Negative inotrophic effect	
Various	Sweating	
	Nausea	
	Dizziness	
Selective serotonin reuptake inhibitors	Nausea	
	Gastric upset	
	Insomnia	
	Nervousness	
	Headache	
Serotonin norepinephrine reuptake inhibitors	Nausea	
	Sweating	
	Dizziness	
	Headache	
	Hypertension	
	Sedation	

Table 18.5 *Side-effects of antidepressants used in pain treatment*

Norepinephrine (noradrenaline).

Tricyclic antidepressants are also contraindicated in patients with convulsive disorders, since they may increase the tendency to seizures. Glaucoma may be precipitated because of the anticholinergic effect, but tricyclics can be used in patients with adequately treated glaucoma.

The selective serotonin reuptake inhibitors are better tolerated than the tricyclics. However, they still cause side-effects and in clinical trials some patients drop out because of the side-effects of these compounds. The norepinephrine serotonin reuptake inhibitors also have fewer side-effects than the tricyclics. The side-effect profile for these drug classes is different from the profile seen with tricyclics (Table 18.5) and the serotonergic effect may be responsible for the prominent gastrointestinal side-effects.

DOSING

Dosing of tricyclic antidepressants deserves special attention in order to obtain the optimal effect and avoid toxicity in the individual patient. The treatment needs to be tailored for each patient. The reason for this is the combination of a relatively low therapeutic index and the large interindividual pharmacokinetic variability described above.

Dose–effect and serum concentration–effect relations have been found in several studies. In a group of chronic pain patients, there was a significantly better response with a daily amitriptyline dose of 75 mg than of 25 mg

or 50 mg in a trial specifically designed to study dose–effect relations.[53**] The same tendency was seen in studies with fixed dose titration of imipramine from 50 mg to 100 mg daily and amitriptyline from 25 mg to 100 mg daily in painful diabetic neuropathy[26**] and nerve injury pain.[40**] Further, a linear relationship between the final amitriptyline dose achieved and pain relief in diabetic neuropathy and postherpetic neuralgia has been found for the dose range 25–150 mg/day.[29**,49**]

Concentration–effect relations seem to be more appropriate owing to the large interindividual variation in pharmacokinetics. In one of the first controlled trials of tricyclics in diabetic neuropathy, it was found that patients with a notable improvement with imipramine had higher serum concentrations of imipramine plus its active metabolite desipramine than patients with no or only some improvement.[26**] Apparently, serum concentrations above around 400 nM separated patients with good and poor response. This lower effective level in painful diabetic neuropathy was supported by a later single-blind dose-titration study (Fig. 18.3).[27**] It was found that nearly all the patients who had a response with imipramine had achieved an individual maximal response at serum concentrations of imipramine plus its active metabolite above 400 nM. However, it must be emphasized that some patients actually achieved their maximal effect at much lower serum levels, i.e. at concentrations around 200 nM. Concentration–effect relations have also been found in a few trials with amitriptyline. In central poststroke pain, responders generally had serum concentrations of amitriptyline above 300 nM and non-

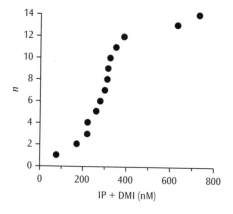

Figure 18.3 *Cumulated number of patients with individual maximal response by plasma concentration of imipramine (IP) plus desipramine (DMI) during a single-blinded imipramine dose-titration study in patients with chronic painful diabetic neuropathy (data from Sindrup et al.[27]).*

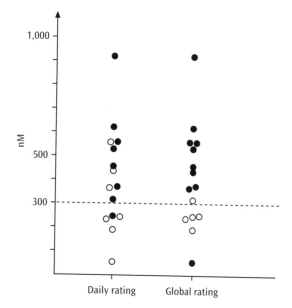

Figure 18.4 *Relationship between the serum concentration of amitriptyline plus its active metabolite nortriptyline and response to treatment as measured by daily pain rating and global rating of effect in patients treated with amitriptyline for central poststroke pain (from Leijon and Boivie[28]).* ●, *Responders;* ○, *nonresponders.*

responders below this level (Fig. 18.4).[28]** A similar relation was found in patients with diabetic neuropathy[29]** and postherpetic neuralgia.[30]** There are also studies that fail to give a relation between plasma concentration and effect for tricyclic antidepressants, but in many of these trials the dose was titrated according to effect and side-effects, as has been the case for some of the trials showing a relationship. With this procedure, it will be much less likely to detect concentration–effect relations than in trials employing fixed drug doses.

It is thus indicated that the lower effective drug level is 400 nM for imipramine and 300 nM for amitriptyline when these drugs are used to treat neuropathic pain. This is lower than the corresponding levels for treatment of depression, i.e. 700 nM and 500 nM. The lower level for the toxic effects of these drugs is variable but is probably around 2.2 mM and 1.25 mM respectively. Therefore, it must be concluded that the therapeutic index for imipramine and amitriptyline is also rather low when these drugs are used to treat neuropathic pain. When these facts are linked to the large person-to-person pharmacokinetic variability, it is obvious that standard dosing cannot be recommended. Thus, a dose of 100 mg imipramine will in some patients result in clearly toxic serum concentrations of imipramine, and in others it will result in drug levels that will probably be ineffective (Fig. 18.2). It is also highly inappropriate to increase drug dose to obtain drug levels over the so-called lower effective level in all patients, as some patients achieve maximal and sufficient response at much lower levels.

The most feasible way to handle the initial phase of treatment is:

- Start with imipramine or amitriptyline 25 mg in the evening and double this evening dose after 2 days.
- After 2 weeks measure plasma drug level (sample 12 h after dosing).
- If the response on 50 mg is insufficient, increase the

dose by 25 mg every other week until adequate pain relief is achieved or to a dose expected to give rise to a plasma drug level above 400 nM (imipramine) or 300 nM (amitriptyline).

- A second measurement of plasma drug level may be appropriate in nonresponders to this regimen.
- In case of insufficient response in spite of adequate drug level, another treatment option should be tried.

A therapeutic window for amitriptyline in postherpetic neuralgia has been indicated by empiric observations.[61] Although this has only been reported once for amitriptyline and not for any of the other tricyclics, it seems wise to withdraw the treatment if a drug level as given above does not produce any analgesic effect at all.

With other tricyclic antidepressants, a similar plasma level-monitored drug dose titration can be used, although the relationship between concentration and effect remains unknown. The important thing here is to avoid increasing the dose to one that results in toxic plasma concentrations. The selective serotonin reuptake inhibitors can be dosed without monitoring of drug levels. The dose can, if necessary, be increased until a sufficient response is achieved or until the maximal dose recommended for each drug is reached.

DRUG CHOICE

For the choice of antidepressant drugs for neuropathic pain, see Table 18.6.

Based on theoretical considerations and clinical trials, the drugs of first choice for treatment of neuropathic pain should be the classical tricyclic antidepressants with a balanced reuptake inhibition, i.e. imipramine, amitriptyline, or clomipramine. Numerous trials with direct drug-to-drug comparison have shown superiority of the balanced reuptake inhibitors over the noradrenergic tricyclics[42**,44**,45**,46**] and the selective serotonergic drugs.[25**,49**,62] One trial that failed to find a difference between amitriptyline (balanced) and desipramine (noradrenergic) may have done so because the drugs were dosed according to effects and side-effects, favoring the drug with fewer side-effects, i.e. desipramine.[47**] In studies with direct comparison, the NNT ≥ 50% was 2.1 for clomipramine compared with 3.1 for desipramine[45**] and 1.4 for imipramine compared with 6.7 for paroxetine.[25**] In pain treatment, amitriptyline is the most extensively studied of the balanced tricyclics, but imipramine and clomipramine may still be preferable as they may have less sedation than amitriptyline.

If treatment with the balanced tricyclics produces intolerable side-effects, one of the noradrenergic tricyclics with fewer side-effects should be tried. This is also worthwhile for patients with no effect on the balanced tricyclics, since some studies have shown that patients not responding on the balanced compounds may actually respond to the noradrenergic tricyclics and, of course, vice versa.[25**,45**,46**] With the recent data on venlafaxine this drug may be tried as the drug of third choice; the selective serotonin reuptake inhibitors rank as drugs of fourth choice because of their relatively low efficacy. These two drug groups may be used as first-line drugs in patients in whom contraindications to the use of tricyclics are present, e.g. elderly subjects with cardiac disease.

Knowledge about which antidepressant to choose for the non-neuropathic pain condition is scarce. Most trials have been performed with the classical, balanced tricyclics and there appears to be an effect with the relatively noradrenergic compounds.[55**] In a trial in chronic tension-type headache, the selective serotonin reuptake inhibitor citalopram had no effect, whereas amitriptyline was clearly effective.[41**] Probably, the rank order for antidepressants in neuropathic pain also holds for other pain conditions and the schedule suggested above could be used.

EFFICACY OF ANTIDEPRESSANTS COMPARED WITH OTHER DRUG CLASSES

The efficacy of antidepressants can be compared with the efficacy of other drug classes in neuropathic pain. Such comparisons have, however, not been carried out in direct drug-to-drug trials, but must rely on NNT values from different trials (Fig. 18.5). The efficacy of tricyclics is generally better than or similar to the efficacy of anticonvulsants[63**] and opioids,[64**,65**,66**] and is clearly better than antiarrhythmics.[67**] It is important to have in mind that in one of the trials of an opioid in neuropathic pain, the opioid was used as add-on therapy for one-third of the patients. Further, for the antiarrhythmic drug mexiletine, the primary positive study did not give dichoto-

---

Table 18.6 *Choice of antidepressant drug in pain treatment*

Drugs of first choice
Balanced tricyclic antidepressants with postsynaptic effects
   Imipramine
   Clomipramine
   Amitriptyline
   Contraindications: Cardiac conduction disturbance or decompensation, orthostatic hypotension, convulsive disorders

Drugs of second choice
Relative noradrenergic tricyclic antidepressants with postsynaptic effects
   Desipramine
   Nortriptyline
   Maprotiline
   Contraindications: Cardiac conduction disturbance or decompensation, convulsive disorders

Drugs of third choice
Serotonin norepinephrine reuptake inhibitor (SNRI)
   Venlafaxine

Drugs of fourth choice
Selective serotonin reuptake inhibitors (SSRI)
   Paroxetine
   Citalopram
   Other SSRIs?

Norepinephrine (noradrenaline).

43. Pud D, Eisenberg E, Spitzer A, *et al*. The NMDA receptor antagonist amantadine reduces surgical neuropathic pain in cancer patients: a double blind, randomized, placebo controlled trial. *Pain* 1998; **75:** 349–54.

● 44. Sawynok J. Adenosine receptor activation and nociception. *Eur J Pharmacol* 1998; **347:** 1–11.

45. Choca JI, Green RD, Proudfit HK. Adenosine A1 and A2 receptors of the substantia gelatinosa are located predominantly on intrinsic neurons: an autoradiography study. *J Pharmacol Exp Ther* 1988; **247:** 757–64.

46. Li J, Perl ER. ATP modulation of synaptic transmission in the spinal substantia gelatinosa. *J Neurosci* 1995; **15** (5 Pt 1): 3357–65.

47. Karlsten R, Gordh T, Hartvig P, Post C. Effects of intrathecal injection of the adenosine receptor agonists R-phenylisopropyl-adenosine and *N*-ethylcarboxamide-adenosine on nociception and motor function in the rat. Anesth Analg 1990; **71:** 60–4.

● 48. Cronstein BN. A novel approach to the development of anti-inflammatory agents: adenosine release at inflamed sites. *J Invest Med* 1995; **43:** 50–7.

49. Keil GJ, DeLander GE. Adenosine kinase and adenosine deaminase inhibition modulate spinal adenosine- and opioid agonist-induced antinociception in mice. *Eur J Pharmacol* 1994; **271:** 37–46.

50. Karlsten R, Gordh T, Svensson BA. A neurotoxicologic evaluation of the spinal cord after chronic intrathecal injection of R-phenylisopropyl adenosine (R-PIA) in the rat. *Anesth Analg* 1993; **77:** 731–6.

51. Rane K, Karlsten R, Sollevi A, *et al*. Spinal Cord morphology after chronic intrathecal administration of adenosine in the rat. *Acta Anaesthesiol Scand* 1999; **43:** 1035–40.

52. Rane K, Segerdahl M, Goiny M, Sollevi A. Intrathecal adenosine administration: a phase 1 clinical safety study in healthy volunteers, with additional evaluation of its influence on sensory thresholds and experimental pain. *Anesthesiology* 1998; **89:** 1108–15.

53. Sylvén C, Eriksson B, Jensen J, *et al*. Analgesic effects of adenosine during exercise-provoked myocardial ischaemia. *Neuroreport* 1996; **7:** 1521–5.

54. Segerdahl M, Ekblom A, Sjölund KF, *et al*. Systemic adenosine attenuates touch evoked allodynia induced by mustard oil in humans. *Neuroreport* 1995; **6:** 753–6.

55. Sjölund KF, Segerdahl M, Sollevi A. Adenosine reduces secondary hyperalgesia in two human models of cutaneous inflammatory pain. *Anesth Analg* 1999; **88:** 605–10.

56. Segerdahl M, Irestedt L, Sollevi A. Antinociceptive effect of perioperative adenosine infusion in abdominal hysterectomy. *Acta Anaesthesiol Scand* 1997; **41:** 473–9.

57. Belfrage M, Sollevi A, Segerdahl M, *et al*. Systemic adenosine infusion alleviates spontaneous and stimulus evoked pain in patients with peripheral neuropathic pain. *Anesth Analg* 1995; **81:** 713–17.

58. Belfrage M, Segerdahl M, Arner S, Sollevi A. The safety and efficacy of intrathecal adenosine in patients with chronic neuropathic pain. *Anesth Analg* 1999; **89:** 136–42.

59. Sawynok J. The 1988 Merck Frosst Award. The role of ascending and descending noradrenergic and serotonergic pathways in opioid and non-opioid antinociception as revealed by lesion studies. *Can J Physiol Pharmacol* 1989; **67:** 975–88.

60. Ono H, Mishima A, Ono S, *et al*. Inhibitory effects of clonidine and tizanidine on release of substance P from slices of rat spinal cord and antagonism by alpha-adrenergic receptor antagonists. *Neuropharmacology* 1991; **30:** 585–9.

61. Davis KD, Treede RD, Raja SN, *et al*. Topical application of clonidine relieves hyperalgesia in patients with sympathetically maintained pain. *Pain* 1991; **47:** 309–17.

62. Stone LSBC, Vulchanova L, Wilcox GL, *et al*. Differential distribution of alpha2A and alpha2C adrenergic receptor immunoreactivity in the rat spinal cord. *J Neurosci* 1998; **18:** 5928–37.

63. Eisenach JC, Hood DD, Curry R. Intrathecal, but not intravenous, clonidine reduces experimental thermal or capsaicin-induces pain and hyperalgesia in normal volunteers. *Anesth Analg* 1998; **87:** 591–6.

64. Eisenach JC, Hood DD, Curry R. Relative potency of epidural to intrathecal clonidine differs between acute thermal pain and capsaicin-induced allodynia. *Pain* 2000; **84:** 57–64.

65. Max MB, Schafer SC, Culnane M, *et al*. Association of pain relief with drug side effects in postherpetic neuralgia: a single-dose study of clonidine, codeine, ibuprofen, and placebo. *Clin Pharm Ther* 1988; **43:** 363–71.

66. Byas-Smith MG, Max MB, Muir J, Kingman A. Transdermal clonidine compared to placebo in painful diabetic neuropathy using a two-stage "enriched enrollment" design. *Pain* 1995; **60:** 267–74.

67. Kirkpatrick AF, Derasari M, Glodek JA, Piazza PA. Postherpetic neuralgia: a possible application for topical clonidine. *Anesthesiology* 1992; **76:** 1065–6.

68. Carabine UA, Milligan KR, Moore J. Extradural clonidine and bupivacaine for postoperative analgesia. *Br J Anaesth* 1992; **68:** 132–5.

69. Tamsen A, Gordh T. Epidural clonidine produces analgesia. *Lancet* 1984; **2:** 231–2.

70. Caterina MJ, Rosen TA, Tominaga M, *et al*. A capsaicin-receptor homologue with a high threshold for noxious heat. *Nature* 1999; **398:** 436–41.

71. Zhang WY, Li Wan Po A. The effectiveness of topically applied capsaicin. A meta-analysis. *Eur J Clin Pharmacol* 1994; **46:** 517–22.

72. McMahon SB. NGF as a mediator of inflammatory pain. *Biol Sci* 1996; **351:** 431–40.

73. Heumann R, Korsching S, Bandtlow C, Thoenen H. Changes of nerve growth factor synthesis in nonneuronal cells in response to sciatic nerve transection. *J Cell Biol* 1987; **104:** 1623–31.

74. Laudiero LB, Aloe L, Levi-Montalcini R, *et al*. Multiple

sclerosis patients express increased levels of beta-nerve growth factor in cerebrospinal fluid. *Neurosci Lett* 1992; **147:** 9–12.

75. Weskamp G, Otten U. An enzyme-linked immunoassay for nerve growth factor (NGF): a tool for studying regulatory mechanisms involved in NGF production in brain and in peripheral tissues. *J Neurochem* 1987; **48:** 1779–86.

76. Woolf CJ, Safieh-Garabedian B, Ma QP, Crilly PWJ. Nerve growth factor contributes to the generation of inflammatory sensory hypersensitivity. *Neuroscience* 1994; **62:** 327–31.

77. Lindholm D, Heumann R, Meyer M, Thoenen H. Interleukin-1 regulates synthesis of nerve growth factor in non-neuronal cells of rat sciatic nerve. *Nature* 1987; **330:** 658–9.

78. Averill S, Mac Mahon SB, Clary DO, *et al.* Immunocytochemical localisation of trkA receptors in chemically identified subgroup of adult rat sensory neurones. *Eur J Neurosci* 1995; **7:** 1484–94.

79. Petty BG, Cornblath DR, Adornato BT, *et al.* The effect of systemically administered recombinant human nerve growth factor in healthy human subjects. *Ann Neurol* 1994; **36:** 244–6.

80. Lowe EM, Anand P, Terenghi G, *et al.* Increased nerve growth factor levels in the urinary bladder of women with idiopathic sensory urgency and interstitial cystitis. *Br J Urol* 1997; **79:** 572–7.

81. Buxbaum DM. Analgesic activity of D9 tetrahydrocannabiol in the rat and mouse. *Psychopharmacologia* 1972; **25:** 275–80.

82. Martin BR. Characterisation of the antinociceptive activity of intravenously administered delta-9-tetrahydrocannabinol in mice. In: Harvey DJ ed. *Marihuana 84*. Oxford: IRL Press, **1985:** 685–91.

83. Poster DS, Penta BS, MacDonald JS. Delta-9-tetrahydrocannabinol in clinical oncology. *JAMA* 1981; **245:** 2047–51.

84. Compton DR, Aceto MD, Lowe J, Martin BR. In vivo characterization of a specific cannabinoid receptor antagonist (SR141716A): Inhibition of delta-9tetrahydrocannabinol induced responses and apparent agonist activity. *J Pharmacol Exp Ther* 1996; **277:** 586–94.

85. Rinaldi-Carmona M, Barth F, Heaulme M, *et al.* SR141716A a potent and selective antagonist of the brain cannabinoid receptor. *FEBS Lett* 1994; **350:** 240–4.

86. Tsou KBS, Brown S, Sanudo-Pena MC, *et al.* Immunohistochemical distribution of cannabinoid CBI receptors in the rat central nervous system. *Neuroscience* 1998; **83:** 392–411.

87. Herzberg U, Eliav E, Bennett GJ, Kopin IJ. The analgesic effects of R(+)-WIN 55,212–2 mesylate, a high affinity cannabinoid agonist, in a rat model of neuropathic pain. *Neurosci Lett* 1997; **221:** 157–60.

88. Carey MP, Burish TG, Brenner DE. Delta-9-tetrahydro-

cannabinol in cancer chemotherapy: research problems and issues. *Ann Intern Med* 1983; **99:** 106–14.

89. Levitt M. Cannabinoids as antiemetics in cancer chemotherapy. In: Mechoulam R ed. *Cannabinoids as Therapeutic Agents*. Boca Raton, FL: CRC Press, 1986.

90. Voth EA, Schwartz RH. Medical application of delta-9-tetrahydrocannabinol and marijuana. *Am Coll Phys* 1997; **126:** 791–8.

91. Sallan SE, Zinberg NE, Frei E. Antiemetic effect of delta-9-tetrahydrocannabinol in patients receiving cancer chemotherapy. *N Engl J Med* 1975; **293:** 795–7.

92. Noyes R, Burn KF, Avery DH, Canter A. The Analgesic properties of delta-9-tetrahydrocannabimol and codeine. *Clin Pharmacol Ther* 1975; **18:** 84–9.

● 93. Burnstock G, Wood JN. Purinergic receptors: their role in nociception and primary afferent neurotransmission. *Curr Opin Neurobiol* 1996; **6:** 526–32.

94. Holton P. The liberation of adenosine triphosphate on antidromic stimulation of sensory nerves. *J Physiol* 1959; **145:** 494–504.

95. Sawynok J, Downie JW, Reid AR, *et al.* ATP release from dorsal spinal cord synaptosomes: characterization and neural origin. *Brain Res* 1993; **610:** 32–8.

96. Bean BP. ATP-activated channels in rat and bullfrog sensory neurones. Concentration dependence and kinetics. *J Neurosci* 1990; **10:** 1–10.

97. Cook SP, Vulchanova L, Hargreaves KM, *et al.* Distinct ATP receptors on pain-sensing and stretch-sensing neurons. *Nature* 1997; **387:** 505–8.

98. Lewis C, Neldhart S, Holy C, *et al.* Coexpression of P2X2 and P2X3 receptor subunits can account for ATP-gated currents in sensory neurons. *Nature* 1995; **377:** 432–5.

99. Ho BT, Huo YY, Lu JG, *et al.* Analgesic activity of anticancer agent suramin. *Anticancer Drugs* 1992; **3:** 914.

100. Gehlert DR, Schober DA, Hipskind PA, *et al.* (3H) LY303870; a novel nonpeptide radioligand for the NK-1 receptor. *J Neurochem* 1996; **66:** 1095–102.

101. Cao YQ, Manthy PW, Carlson EJ, *et al.* Primary afferent tachykinin are required to experience moderate to intense pain. *Nature* 1998; **392:** 390–4.

102. Neumann S, Doubell TP, Leslie T, Woolf CJ. Inflammatory pain hypersensitivity mediated by phenotypic switch in myelinated primary sensory neurons. *Nature* 1996; **384:** 360–4.

103. Campbell EA, Gentry CT, Patel S, *et al.* Selective neurokinin-1 receptor antagonists are anti-hyperalgesic in a model of neuropathic pain in the guinea-pig. *Neuroscience* 1998; **87:** 527–32.

104. Goldstein DJ, Offen WW, Klein EG. Lanepitant, an NK-1 antagonist, in migraine prophylaxis. *Clin Pharmacol Ther* 1999; **65:** 119.

105. Xiao WH, Bennett GJ. Synthetic omega-conopeptides applied to the site of nerve injury suppress neuropathic pains in rats. *J Pharmacol Exp Ther* 1995; **274:** 666–72.

106. Sluka KA. Blockade of calcium channels can prevent

the onset of secondary hyperalgesia and allodynia induced by intradermal injection of capsaicin in rats. *Pain* 1997; **71:** 157–64.

107. Gurdal H, Sara Y, Tulunay FC. Effects of calcium channel blockers on formalin-induced nociception and inflammation in rats. *Pharmacology* 1992; **44:** 290–6.

108. Bowersox SS, Luther R. Pharmacotherapeutic potential of omega-conotoxin MVIIA (SNX-111), an N-type neuronal calcium channel blocker found in the venom of Conus magus. *Toxicon* 1998; **36:** 1651–8.

109. Tenorio E, Wadsworth A, Luther RR, *et al.* Ziconotide (SNX-111) a specific, selective N-type calcium channel blocker suppresses capsaicin-induced heat and mechanical hyperalgesia. *Soc Neurosci Abst* 1998; **24:** Abst 495.3.

110. Jain KK. An evaluation of intrathecal ziconotide for the treatment of chronic pain. *Expert Opin Invest Drugs* 2000; **9:** 2403–10.

and open operations. Mesencephalotomy is an alternative operation and is probably more appropriate when the pain involves more diffuse areas of the head and neck.[47]

It appears from limited published reports that about 75–85% of patients with head and neck cancer will experience good pain relief with either the open or percutaneous technique. The pain relief can be very impressive and can last for many months, but not often for years.[48]* Also, some patients have experienced sensory changes in the area of the pain but not had any diminution of the pain itself. The most significant complications, usually temporary, include ipsilateral arm incoordination, contralateral leg hypesthesia or anesthesia, and ipsilateral arm (rarely leg) decreased proprioception. Less frequent complications include Horner syndrome, dysarthria, gait changes, hiccups, and death, estimated to be 5–10% in patients with advanced cancer. Trigeminal tractotomy has been reported in combinations with other nerve and/or root sections in the same area.

Lesions in the descending trigeminal tract and the adjacent nucleus caudalis are important since they usually affect pain and temperature, but not touch sensation.[49] This observation is generally attributed to the nucleus caudalis, which functions as a relay station for pain and temperature transmission from cranial nerves II, V, IX, and X. The nucleus lies on the surface of the medulla, posterior to the dorsal spinocerebellar tract, lateral to the fasciculus cuneatus, and inferior to the restiform body.[48]

Trigeminal tractotomy can be performed by either a percutaneous or an open surgical technique. The percutaneous technique involves stereotactic placement of an electrode needle at the C1–foramen magnum.[50,51] The electrode has a 0.5- to 0.6-mm diameter, is placed 6 mm lateral to the midline, and is angled 30° cephalad. Electrical stimulation (50 Hz, low voltage) when the electrode tip is placed 4 mm into the spinal cord should result in facial stimulation. Stimulation of the spinothalamic tract (abnormal sensations in the contralateral body) will result if the electrode is placed too ventral. If the placement is too dorsal, stimulation will be felt in ipsilateral areas via the fasciculus cuneatus.

The open operation is based on the description by Sjoqvist.[49] Bone is removed from the occiput and C1 unilaterally with the patient in a prone position. To create the nucleus caudalis lesion, the dura is opened and a transverse knife incision is made at a depth of 3–5 mm below the surface of the cervicomedullary junction, starting 4–8 mm inferior to the obex. The incision extends medially from the fasciculus cuneatus to the rootlets of the spinal accessory nerve. An oblique incision angling from superior–posterior to inferior–anterior is useful to avoid injury to the restiform body but still place the lesion as superior as possible. For coverage of oral areas, the lesion can be extended to involve part of the spinothalamic tract and its associated fasciculus.

Intraventricular infusion of opioid

The intraventricular route for analgesic delivery appears to be utilized best in the treatment of head and neck cancer pain. There is also a rare indication in patients who initially respond well to the intraspinal infusions of opioids but subsequently develop an apparent tolerance and have a very limited (1–3 months) remaining survival time. Intraventricular injections or infusions have a very similar safety and side-effect profile to that of intraspinal infusions. The one exception is an increased risk of respiratory depression, but this is almost always only seen in the first 3 days of the intraventricular delivery.[52,53]

Although this route of opioid infusion is a well-described augmentative technique at the intracranial level, it is normally a last resort option.[54] Supraspinal pathways are presumed to be involved in the analgesic effect.[52,55,56] As with intraspinal delivery, morphine sulfate is the usual agent, although the potency with intraventricular delivery appears to be as much as 1,000 times greater than intrathecal infusions (daily dose range from 50–700 μg/day). The length of action of an opioid after intraventricular injection appears to be significantly longer than with intraspinal delivery.[53]

The use of this route is closely related to the observation that hydrophilic compounds, such as morphine, have been observed to have a rapid spread in cerebrospinal fluid (CSF) after lumbar intrathecal injections. Also, the hydrophilic nature of these compounds makes it more difficult for them to attach to the desired receptors. Thus, in most patients intrathecal infusion or injection of morphine will provide a concentration gradient sufficient to reach high cervical spinal cord levels. In a similar manner with intraventricular injection, the extent of diffusion and concentration in the brain are dependent on the lipophilicity of the opioid.[57] With morphine ventricular injection, brain concentrations persist for a few hours, although the drug is unevenly dispersed in the tissue. It would appear that passive diffusion, rather than active transport, controls the movement of morphine, which is hydrophilic, through the ventricular system. In contrast, fentanyl, sufentanil, and etorphine, all of which are lipophilic opioids, are cleared in the CSF after 1 h as they bind better to lipophilic receptors.[57]

As supported by the above observation, the lipophilicity of the opioid must be considered in intraventricular opioid delivery. For example, in sheep, certain drugs, particularly lipophilic opioids, appear to have difficulty diffusing through the cerebrospinal fluid pathways to reach distant receptors. A study by Payne and Inturris[57] examined drugs such as hydromorphone, morphine, methadone, naloxone, and sucrose to test the effects. About 90 min after intraventricular injection in the sheep, morphine, hydromorphone, and sucrose were identified in the lumbar CSF. Methadone was never found in the CSF, presumably because the ventricular injection of lipophilic opioids creates distinctly different CSF distributions from those created by hydrophilic drugs, such as morphine.[57]

Important factors in the choice of intraventricular morphine delivery are the location of the pain, age of the patient, and the history of opioid usage. In one study, lumbar subarachnoid administration of morphine appeared to provide better pain relief for the lower limbs whereas craniofacial or diffuse pain was more responsive to intracerebroventricular delivery.[58] Seiwald and Kofler[59] have provided a useful clinical description of a series of 20 patients (18 patients suffering from cancer) treated with ventricular morphine injections between 1990 and 1993. It is clear that the ventricular injection through a catheter-reservoir system was nondestructive and effective for the treatment of nociceptive pain.[59] Analgesia onset occurred within minutes and very low dosages were required. Somatic-type pain was ameliorated in 95% of the patients. Neuropathic pain, however, appeared to respond minimally to this form of morphine delivery.[59]*

From a technical viewpoint, the opioids can be delivered either as an infusion or an injection. For infusion, an implanted infusion pump is placed subcutaneously in the anterior abdominal wall and connected by subcutaneous tubing to an implanted ventricular catheter. Other patients can be treated adequately via an implanted ventricular catheter connected to a subcutaneous Ommaya reservoir-type device with only one or two injections per day.[53]

Deep brain stimulation

Electrical stimulation to the spinal cord or peripheral nerves is the traditional form of nervous system stimulation and has been used clinically for over 40 years. Stimulation of deep brain structures, however, is specifically indicated for intractable central pain from almost any cause, e.g. from lesions in the spinal cord. As a last resort option, it is also indicated for patients who have failed to experience adequate pain relief with spinal cord or peripheral nerve stimulation.

Effective pain relief can be achieved with deep brain stimulation in most patients in these categories.[60] The most common causes for lack of pain relief are anatomic variations in individual patients and presumed physiological changes in the usual pain transmission pathways in chronic pain patients. Complications can occur in both cancer and noncancer patients and are related to the placement of the deep brain stimulator electrode. It appears that the complication rate is lower when the intracranial target for electrode placement is the periventricular gray (PVG) region than when it is the periaqueductal gray (PAG) region.

Although not a typical indication, deep brain stimulation can be used in cancer pain patients. In a series of 31 patients with cancer pain who had been treated with deep brain stimulation, 87% experienced satisfactory relief, with 55% of these experiencing lasting relief until death.[61]* Again, this is a last resort option, but can be effective for pain that is not well treated by common neurosurgical ablative procedures. Examples include pain from diffuse bone metastases, recurrent pain from head and neck cancer, midline or bilateral pain (especially of the lower body), and brachial or lumbosacral plexopathy.[61]

The more typical use of deep brain stimulation is for the relief of chronic noncancer pain. Many studies suggest that the degree of pain relief is equal to or better than that with spinal stimulation techniques.[60]* Deep brain stimulation of either the PAG region or thalamic sensory nuclei has been reported as acutely effective in 61–80% of noncancer patients with an overall success rate of 50–63%.[62-65] Another series indicated a 90% postoperative success with lower long-term success rates ranging from 65% to 80%.[60] Overall, permanent complications occur in 1–2% of patients and include hemiparesis, intracranial hemorrhage, and death.[66] Transient complications include infection, hardware malfunction, implantation site pain, and mild reversible neurologic deficits.

Technically, the electrode implantation is performed under local anesthesia using a burr hole located over the coronal suture and 3 cm from the midline. CT or MRI stereotactic guidance is used to place accurately the stimulation electrode in the desired intracranial target location.[60] The initial targets include the PVG, PAG, or ventral posterior lateral thalamus.[60] For best results, some surgeons will place electrodes in multiple areas in the same patient. Others will use preliminary intraoperative stimulation to determine the best electrode target location. The choice of target can also be based upon the type and severity of the pain.

OTHER INTRACRANIAL PROCEDURES

Cingulotomy

Creation of lesions in the cingulate gyrus dates back to 1948, when Hugh Cairns at Oxford removed a portion of the anterior cingulate gyrus in an open operation.[9] The use of the open cingulotomy in the 1940s and 1950s produced significant improvements in psychiatric symptoms in most patients.[8] In 1962, Foltz first described the application of stereotaxy to bilateral anterior cingulate lesions for pain relief. At about the same time, Ballantine began to use ventriculogram-guided stereotaxy to create smaller anterior cingulate gyrus lesions. The mechanism for pain relief, however, remains unclear, although it probably relates to interruption of the limbic system.

The most common application of a cingulotomy is for patients with affective disorders. There are numerous reports, however, of its application to patients with severe pain.[1-3,67-70] In several series of patients undergoing cingulotomy, up to 30% of patients suffered from severe pain of cancer or noncancer causes.

Perhaps the best cancer pain indication is for diffuse or multiply located cancer pain, mainly nociceptive in character.[14*,15*] A typical indication is severe pain from diffuse bone metastases. Moderate, marked, or complete pain relief (at 3 months postprocedure) was experienced in approximately 51% of patients with cancer pain.

A similar follow-up in noncancer patients showed 45% with moderate, marked, or complete pain relief after 3 months. For noncancer patients, the procedure appears to be less effective for neuropathic pain or survival times that are longer than 8 months.[14,15]

Using ventricular or stereotactic guidance, the main cingulotomy complications have been controllable seizures (9% incidence), transient mania (6% incidence), decreased memory (3% incidence), hemiplegia from intracerebral hematoma (0.3% incidence), and a low but measurable mortality rate (0.9%).[71,72] The only abnormalities in detailed neuropsychiatric examinations have been rare difficulties in memory on an organized serial learning test, and occasional difficulties in performing two tapping tests and in copying complex figures.[67,73,74]

The cingulotomy target is located in the coronal plane, 20–30 mm posterior to the anterior tip of the lateral ventricles.[13] On that coronal slice, the specific target is 1.5 mm lateral to the midline and 15 mm superior to the roof of the lateral ventricles.[71,75] With the advent of stereotactic guidance and closed cingulotomy techniques, there really is no present role for the open surgical techniques. For the closed technique, radiofrequency is used most commonly and lesions are created at 75°C for 60–90 s. These radiofrequency lesions are cylindrical in shape, approximately 10–20 mm long and 5–7 mm in diameter, and centered in each cingulate gyrus.

Mesencephalotomy

One of the newer intracranial pain relief procedures is an ablative lesion in the midbrain, namely mesencephalic tractotomy (mesencephalotomy), especially in the treatment of head and neck cancer. Bosch, in his studies with 40 patients suffering from deafferentation pain and cancer pain, utilized this operation for the treatment of thalamic pain, trigeminal neuralgia, postherpetic neuralgia, and phantom limb pain of the arm.[76] Although nociceptive pain is often sensitive to opioids, mesencephalic surgery and electrical stimulation of gray matter is a successful and viable alternative. Because of neuropathic side-effects, the operation is usually limited to patients with short life expectancy and lateralized nociceptive pain.

The results of this operation vary because of the nature of the particular diseases. With a well-defined target, the operation can produce pain relief similar to other pain relief operations, such as open anterior cordotomy,

midline myelotomy, and dorsal root entry zone (DREZ) lesions.[76] Significant pain relief with this procedure has been reported in 65–75% of patients on both short-term and long-term (2–4 year) follow-up. The longest duration of pain relief in cancer patients is in the extremities, whereas pain in the chest and abdomen do not respond adequately.[76*]

The major side-effect appears to be a difficulty with ocular movement and binocular vision. Mortality rates vary from 1% to 7%.[22,77] With large mesencephalic lesions, postoperative dysesthesiae have also been reported.[78,79] It appears that these side-effects are reduced with the use of a smaller electrode, intraoperative neural recording, and more precise electrical stimulation.[78]

The area of evoked pain is limited to a very small range (about 2–3 mm of target) and requires the use of a bipolar concentric electrode for extremely precise localized stimulation.

The usual stereotactic technique is performed under general anesthesia to further standardize the procedure. The target is the midbrain at the superior colliculus or inferior colliculus level. In the studies carried out by Bosch, the target was identified based on stereotaxis using intraoperative ventriculography with water-soluble medium via a frontal burr hole route.[76] The accuracy of the stereotactic trajectory to the rostral midbrain reduces morbidity and other risks.[78] Lesions at the inferior colliculus level appear to provide a lower incidence of ocular problems but with a lower success rate (50–70%).

Hypothalamotomy

Hypothalamic lesions have been reported for psychoaffective disorders since 1962 and for cancer pain since 1971. Indications for hypothalamotomy are similar to cingulotomy in terms of cancer pain from rather diffuse sites, especially where there is an emotional or visceral component.[80] Cancer pain appears to respond better than noncancer pain.

Twenty-eight patients are reported to have undergone the procedure for pain control between 1971 and 1982.[81*,82] In one series of the hypothalamotomy procedure, "good" results were reported in 62% of patients; the procedure was bilateral in 15 of the 21 patients.[80,83] Although the published reports are very limited, there appears to be no significant complication.

Initial reports suggested that the target is 2 mm below the AC–PC line midpoint and 2 mm lateral to the lateral wall of the third ventricle. Recent reports have suggested that more posterior lesions might have increased effectiveness.[84]

As with most of the intracranial procedures, the exact mechanism of action remains unclear. Electrical stimulation of the hypothalamotomy target prior to actual ablation of the area has been shown to result in elevated ventricular cerebrospinal fluid concentrations of β-endorphin. These concentrations remain elevated for at least 2 days after the hypothalamotomy ablation.[83] Although the indirect effects on other brain areas are not clear, degenerated axon fibers are found after hypothalamotomy in the ipsilateral reticular formation, pallidum, somatosensory cortices, nucleus ventrocaudalis parvocellularis of Hassler (Vcpc), and nucleus parafascicularis. No degenerated fibers have been found in the dorsomedial nucleus of the thalamus.[84]

Pulvinotomy

Lesions in the pulvinar of the thalamus were first described for pain relief in 1966.[27] Thirty patients were reported to have undergone pulvinotomy by 1975. Intractable cancer pain is the main indication for pulvinotomy. The qualities and involved areas of pain that best respond to pulvinotomy appear to be similar to those for cingulotomy or hypothalamotomy.[85] There is no loss of somatic sensation from pulvinotomy, and existing pain is most affected by this procedure.[21] The pulvinar lesions might be especially effective for cancer patients with longer expected survival times because the procedure appears to provide pain relief for as long as 24 months.

Pulvinotomy has been reported for patients with thalamic pain (10 patients), phantom pain (10 patients), peripheral neuropathy (six patients), herpetic neuralgia (five patients), anesthesia dolorosa (five patients), and cancer pain (five patients).[39] Moderate to excellent pain relief has been reported in as many as 25% of patients for periods ranging from 1 to 2.5 years.[85*,86*] The main side-effect of pulvinotomy has been a temporary change in emotions, such as lachrymoseness, childishness, excessive excitability, and euphoria. No apparent changes in speech, intelligence quotient (IQ), or vision have been noted.[39,87]

Thalamotomy lesions, when they have been extended backward to involve the anterior pulvinar, have been found more effective than a centrum medianum thalamotomy alone.[86,88]

The oral and medial parts of the pulvinar are involved in pain appreciation.[89] Electrophysiological studies in cats have demonstrated that the pulvinar is involved in an indirect route for afferent stimuli.[27] From the pulvinar, afferent transmission connections have been traced to the temporal lobe and, from there, to the posterior sensory cortex.[86]

The lesions in the pulvinar have been created in one hemisphere, contralateral to the site of pain, but appear to be more effective with bilateral lesions. Lesions have been reported in the medial or in both the medial and lateral areas of pulvinar.[21,39,85] Pulvinotomy coordinates for pulvinar lesions have been 4 mm superior to the AC–PC line, 5 mm posterior to the AC–PC line, and lateral to the AC–PC line by either 10–11 mm for a medial target or 15–16 mm for a lateral target.[85] Ultrasonic probes, using a setting of 75 W and 2.5 MHz for 30 s at two to six separate sites, are used to create lesions which are 5–6 mm in diameter.[85]

Combined procedures

Possible combinations of the above-mentioned procedures are being examined as the intracranial procedures become technically easier to perform, especially with the increased use of stereotactic methods. With a rather large amount of psychosurgery literature as a basis, many of these combinations are now being tested for pain relief when they have been shown to be psychoactive. The simultaneous use of cingulotomy and anterior capsulotomy, in which lesions are created in both the cingulate gyrus and the anterior limb of the internal capsule, is one of the most common combinations. This combination has been used in the treatment of severe cancer-related pain and appears to provide better relief for neuropathic pain than cingulotomy alone.[90] Pulvinotomy lesions have been combined with the various thalamotomy targets in an effort to provide better pain relief than is seen with a single thalamotomy site.[88] One of the greatest research challenges in this area is to find a scientific basis for the best combinations of these procedures in pain control.

SPINAL PROCEDURES

Cordotomy

Despite a variety of intracranial procedures, spinal cordotomy is an example of an old operation being "rediscovered" with improved technology. The application of percutaneous techniques and CT guidance to cordotomy has made this procedure safer, easier to apply, and possibly more effective. It remains a standard option for pain relief in a selected set of patients. The most important aspect of cordotomy now is to carefully evaluate the patient's pain. Patients with unilateral cancer pain, especially in one limb (e.g. one leg) appear to be the best candidates for cordotomy. Also important in patient selection is a complete preoperative evaluation of pulmonary function because mortality is frequently related to respiratory problems.

In one of the largest reported cordotomy series,[91*] long-term success with no pain was found in 33% of patients and partial pain relief in 12%. Persistent pain was noted in 6% and a dysesthetic pain in 34%, whereas 2.6% required a repeat cordotomy for continued pain relief. A decrease in the degree of pain relief over time has been noted, with 37% of patients having satisfactory analgesia even after 5–10 years.[92] One of the main causes for a failure to obtain postoperative pain relief is a lack of adequate anatomic localization of pain sites during the surgery. After cordotomy, some patients do experience new burning dysesthetic sensations in the area of the previous pain or new sensations of frank pain in similar and/or different locations, often just above the level of the previous pain.

One of the main sequelae of this operation is the possible loss of the sensation of temperature on the contralateral side to the cordotomy. In many evaluations, this loss has been considered a desired outcome since it correlates with the degree of pain relief. Complications included persistent paresis (2%), bladder dysfunction (2%), temporary respiratory failure (0.5%), and death (0.5%). Other postoperative changes include contralateral limb weakness from lesioning too deep, transient Horner syndrome, and respiratory problems. It has been suggested that cordotomy affects more than just C-fibers because, as noted above, pain relief coincides with a lessened skin sensation of temperature and painful pinch.[93]

The traditional open surgical technique for a cordotomy is performed by having the patient in an upright sitting position. The anterolateral surface of the spinal cord is exposed and an avascular area found for the incision. A surgical scalpel blade is projected 6 mm through the cervical area and 4–5 mm in the thoracic area. The blade is used to cut ventrally to transect the ventral quadrant of the spinal cord but spare the medial funiculus. The open operation, because it carries greater risks than the percutaneous technique, is usually considered a less effective surgical option.

In the percutaneous method, radiographic fluoroscopy is used to position a radiofrequency electrode needle at the level of the C1–2 interspace. The cordotomy needle is advanced into the side of the neck contralateral to the pain. The target for the needle tip is the lateral spinothalamic tract; the needle tip is specifically positioned to correlate with the area of pain.[67] For proper positioning in the tract, intraoperative stimulation testing is used with the electrode needle and the patient is questioned about sensory changes and twitching. CT has facilitated the insertion of the electrodes into the spinal cord and has made the operation more accurate (Fig. 23.2A and B).

Dorsal root entry zone lesions

The surgical creation of lesions in the dorsal root entry zone (DREZ) of the spinal cord is a procedure best applied to patients who are experiencing pain secondary to nerve root avulsion from, for example, brachial plexus injury.[60] Other good patient candidates have painful paraplegia, phantom limb or stump pain, and postherpetic pain syndromes.[60,94] Like the other neurosurgical operations, it is usually considered for chronic pain that cannot be adequately treated by noninvasive medical options. Patients with high emotional tendencies are rarely good candidates for this surgery.

For brachial plexus avulsion pain, acceptable pain relief was achieved in 65–80% of patients at follow-up intervals of 12–48 months. With a longer follow-up period, however, the success rate is more typically 60–65%[94*] The success rates are lower (50–60%) with follow-up periods of 5–7 years in the treatment of phantom limb or stump pain. Other, less successful indications include pain from trauma to the cauda equina or conus medullaris. The degree of pain relief in these patients is more variable, although as many as 74% of patients, with a mean follow-up of 3 years, experienced adequate pain relief.[94] Although DREZ lesioning has been reported in the treatment of intercostal postherpetic neuralgia, the success rates are significantly lower.

The DREZ operation has been used for the radicular or segmental ("endzone") pain that occurs at or just below the level of spinal cord injury. Success rates of 70–75% have been reported for this type of pain.[95*,96*] DREZ lesioning, however, does not appear to be effective for the diffuse, burning lower body or phantom pain that occurs after spinal cord injury. Although the success rate is significantly lower, these spinal cord lesions can be used in the treatment of central pain from an injury or other damage to the spinal cord.

Complications include permanent sensory or motor changes in about 15–20% of patients. Another 5% of patients will experience transient sensory or motor changes. Infection or cerebrospinal fluid leak has also been reported in approximately 5–7% of patients.

The procedure was first performed by Nashold in 1976 in a patient with severe pain secondary to brachial plexis avulsion. That patient remains completely pain free.[97]

The procedure is intended to treat deafferentation pain arising from abnormally active secondary nociceptive neurons in the dorsal horn of the spinal cord.[60] Lesions are created in the spinal cord to reduce or eliminate this cellular hyperactivity seen after deafferentation in central pain syndromes. The operation involves ablation of Lissauer's tract and laminae I–V in the spinal cord on the side of the pain. This, in turn, leads to lesions that destroy overactive neurons in the central nuclear groups of the dorsal horn at the affected spinal cord levels.[60] These lesions can lead to peripheral anesthetic areas but, in these conditions, such anesthetic areas usually already exist.

The DREZ operation involves making a series of lesions directed at the substantia gelantinosa and adjoining fiber tracts (Fig. 23.3). A laminectomy, either unilateral or bilateral, is performed at the dermatomal level of the area of the pain.[98,99] After the dura mater is opened, the entry area of the dorsal rootlets into the spinal cord (the dorsal root entry zone) is visualized. An electrode (0.25-mm diameter, 2-mm exposed metal tip) is inserted about 2–3 mm into this zone. Radiofrequency thermal technique is usually employed to make the lesions. The radiofrequency settings use a tip temperature of 75°C for 15–20 s. A series of such small lesions is made along the

A

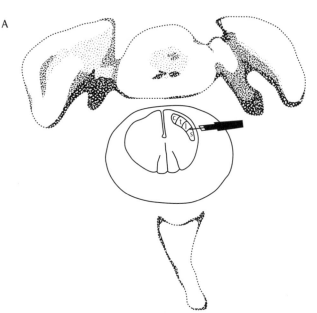

Figure 23.2 *(A) Drawing of placement of electrode in the posterolateral section of the spinothalamic tract for percutaneous cordotomy using CT-guidance (From Kanpolat, Caglar, and Bilgic 1993). (B) Actual placement of percutaneous cordotomy electrode. (From Kanpolat, Caglar, and Bilgic 1993.)*

B

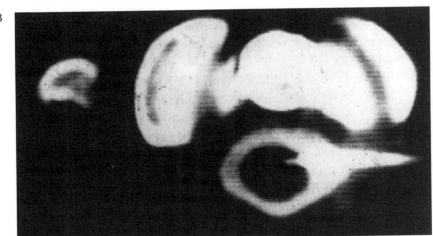

vertical line of the rootlets, spanning at least two or three dermatomal levels (Fig. 23.4). Depending upon the number of dermatomes involved, approximately 20–50 such lesions (separated by about 1 mm each) are created in a typical patient. The longest series of lesions can extend over 5 cm in length. Laser and ultrasound have also been reported in the creation of these DREZ lesions.[66,100]

Midline myelotomy

In 1934, Putnam performed the first midline myelotomy, although it had been conceptualized in 1927 by Armour as a possible treatment for a patient affected by tabetic abdominal pain.[101,102] Since its first use, the procedure has undergone many technical adjustments for new applications. It appears to be most effective for lower body pain, especially midline or bilateral. Myelotomy, therefore, complements the applications for cordotomy, which is not as useful for midline or bilateral pain. An advantage

of midline myelotomy is that it can provide relief from hyperpathia and background pain without sensory loss or loss of ability to localize and discriminate between sharp and dull stimuli.[103]

Moderate to marked pain relief has been observed in approximately 70% of patients, with only rare complications or side-effects.[103]* The goal is the interruption of all decussating second-order spinothalamic pain fibers in the anterior commissure of the spinal cord. Because it severs all decussating fibers, the pain relief is bilateral. With the increasing use of long-term spinal infusions of opioids, the application of this procedure has been decreasing over the past 15 years. Only 425 total cases have been reported in the neurosurgical literature.[103–116]

The mechanism of pain relief remains unclear, although many methods for the procedure have been described over many decades. It might affect a putative paleospinothalamic tract in the posterior half of the spinal cord. This operation might also cut tracts in the anterior part of the medial borders of the posterior columns.

110. Lippert RG, HY, Nielsen SL. Spinal commissurotomy. *Surg Neurol* 1974; **2**: 373.

111. Papo I, LA. High cervical commissural myelotomy in the treatment of pain. *J Neurol Neurosurg Psychiatry* 1976; **39**: 105.

112. King RB. Anterior commissurotomy for intractable pain. *J Neurosurg* 1977; **47**: 7.

113. Payne NS. Dorsal longitudinal myelotomy for the control of perineal and lower body pain. *Pain* 1984; **2** (Suppl.): S320.

114. Fink RA. Neurosurgical treatment of non-malignant intractable rectal pain: microsurgical commissural myelotomy with the carbon dioxide laser. *Neurosurgery* 1984; **14**: 64.

●115. Sweet WH, PCE. Operations in the brain stem and spinal canal, with an appendix on open cordotomy. In: Melzack R, Wall PD eds. *Textbook of Pain*. Edinburgh: Churchill Livingstone, 1984: 615–31.

●116. Adams JE, LR, Hosobuchi Y. Commissural myelotomy. In: SH, Sweet WH eds. *Current Techniques in Operative Neurosurgery*. New York, NY: Grune & Stratton, 1988: 1185–9.

117. Hirshberg RM, A-CN, Lawand NB, *et al*. Is there a pathway in the posterior funiculus that signals visceral pain? *Pain* 1996; **67**: 291–305.

118. Al-Chaer ED, LN, Westlund KN, Willis WD. Visceral nociceptive input into the ventral posterolateral nucleus of the thalamus: a new function for the dorsal column pathway. *J Neurophysiol* 1996; **76**: 2661–74.

119. Al-Chaer ED, LN, Westlund KN, Willis WD. Pelvic visceral input into the nucleus gracillis is largely mediated by the postsynaptic dorsal column pathway. *J Neurophysiol* 1996; **76**: 2675–90.

◆120. Feng Y, Cui M, Al-Chaer ED, Willis WD. Epigastric pain relief by cervical dorsal column lesion in rats. *Anesthesiology* 1998; **89**: 411–20.

the elderly population. It is associated with pain, weakness, and disability.[19] Physical therapy measures have been shown to improve multiple outcome variables in this population. The FAST (Fitness Arthritis and Seniors Trial) study showed that both aerobic fitness and strengthening programs are effective in improving pain and function in patients with osteoarthritis.[24**] This was a randomized, controlled trial of 365 adults over 60 years of age with radiographically documented knee osteoarthritis. Self-reported disability, knee pain scores, time to climb/descend stairs, and time to get in and out of a car all declined while distance walked in 12 min increased post-treatment. Fisher showed that increases in strength, endurance, and speed correlated with reductions in dependency and pain in patients with knee osteoarthritis.[19] However, small numbers limited this study. Pain, disability, and medication use decreased in 119 patients with chronic neck pain treated with any of three approaches.[25*] These included intensive strengthening, active and passive physical therapy, or manipulation. All three groups showed improvement compared with controls, but no significant differences were seen between groups. Benefits were maintained through 12-month follow-up. Utilization of patient-based passive modalities can also be of symptomatic benefit in the osteoarthritis population. Instruction in the use of heat prior to activity and ice massage or packs for an inflamed joint can provide significant short-term relief. Education in joint-care principles and moderation of activity can help patients avoid pain flares.

Chronic pain due to osteoporotic compression fractures and the secondary musculoskeletal deformities is treated with spine stabilization exercises and increasing back extensor strength.[26*,27*,28*] Spine extensor muscle strengthening is performed in an attempt to off-weight the anterior spinal column and has been shown to correlate with reduced number of compression fractures. Appropriate use of bracing can also be beneficial. Bracing options range from a posture training support or Velcro-elastic lumbosacral corset to a rigid bivalved thoracolumbosacral orthosis in cases with severe pain or deformity. The benefits of bracing must be weighed against the difficulties and limitations associated with donning and doffing the orthosis and the potential for further deconditioning. A vital aspect of osteoporosis rehabilitation is instruction in lifting and reaching biomechanics to avoid spine compressive forces, which can result in further fracture and disability.[28]

Complex regional pain syndromes (CRPS I and II; previously known as reflex sympathetic dystrophy and causalgia) are challenging entities to treat successfully. Most reviews of complex regional pain syndrome advocate physical therapeutic interventions in treatment.[29***,30***,31***,32***] These include instruction in the use of desensitization techniques such as warm/cold baths, whirlpool, and desensitization massage. Compression garments on the affected extremity can help both with desensitization and the edema that commonly accompanies CRPS. A transcutaneous electrical nerve stimulation trial can be carried out to determine possible benefit. This generally includes two instructional sessions with a therapist and a multiweek rental period to ensure an adequate trial has taken place. Multiple electrode positions and stimulation parameters can be utilized. Active range of motion, stretching, and strengthening are heavily emphasized in order to maintain function of the involved extremity. These measures are commonly combined with therapeutic injections to increase tolerance of activity.

Several other chronic pain problems are commonly treated in part with physical therapy. Medial and lateral epicondylitis of the elbow is treated with the appropriate use of thermal modalities, stretching with an extended elbow and strengthening with variable resistance.[33*] Dines et al. have outlined an extensive, progressive physical therapy program for the rehabilitation of the unstable shoulder.[34*] This involves a step-wise progression from immobilization through work-related activities. Gonzales advocates the use of physical therapy as part of a treatment program for central pain disorders.[35***] He states that increasing peripheral sensory input and frontal orbital brain activity exerts inhibitory effects on pain pathways and can provide a distracting influence. While the above are based on sound concepts, most have not been studied in a randomized, controlled manner.

CHRONIC LOW BACK PAIN AND DIAGNOSTIC LIMITATIONS

Chronic low back pain is one of the most frequent causes of chronic pain and disability in the world. The immense financial impact of this problem is well documented and functional restoration for chronic low back pain has been extensively studied. A common limitation of this literature is lack of a specifically defined pain generator. Multiple structures in the spine are known to be primary pain generators or to contribute to abnormalities that result in pain. These include the annulus fibrosis, nerve roots (compression or chemical irritation from disk injury, foraminal, lateral recess or central stenosis), osseous pain secondary to spondylolysis/listhesis, or the zygapophysial joints.

It is widely accepted that far too frequently a specific cause for low back pain is not established. Unfortunately, history and physical examination have been shown to be of limited value in establishing a specific pain generator in patients with chronic low back pain.[36–42] Although radiographs, computed tomography, and MRI can give detailed information on normal and abnormal anatomy, these abnormalities do not necessarily establish a pain generator.[38,43] One must be cautious of asymptomatic radiographic abnormalities.

Efficacy of nonspecific treatments for nonspecific low back pain is significantly limited by the fact that generalized treatments are not likely to help all specific painful spine conditions. Nonspecific treatment of a nonspecific problem dooms an investigator to nonspecific outcome. Therapy for diskogenic pain should differ from therapy for zygapophysial joint pain or other specific condition. This limitation of diagnostic specificity has only recently begun to be addressed through utilization of diagnostic blocks prior to initiating rehabilitation. Once chronic low back pain patients are divided into specific diagnostic groups, we should be able to determine and design the most effective therapies. Until this first step is taken, "mechanical low back pain" or "failed back syndrome" will continue to prove frustrating to treat and study. This interaction between specific diagnoses and specific therapeutic programs represents a growing field of spine rehabilitation and is based to some extent on previously developed concepts.

SPINE REHABILITATION PROGRAMS

Current spine rehabilitation programs represent an evolution from previously developed concepts. In the 1930s, an isometric flexion program for back pain was popularized.[20*] Flexion exercises were thought to open zygapophysial (facet) joints and intervertebral foramina. This theoretically resulted in decreased nerve compression and pain. The program combined stretching of hip flexors and back extensors with abdominal and gluteal muscle strengthening. While likely beneficial in reducing loading of the facet joints,[44*] there is significant concern that these exercises increase pressure in the intervertebral disk[45*] and potentially increase diskal pain.

McKenzie later encouraged a program utilizing primarily extension principles.[20*] These programs have included extension postures both standing and prone, prone trunk extension, and prone leg lifting. The goal of the program was to centralize pain. Centralization entails bringing about a reduction of distal radiating or radicular pain. This program was thought to be most beneficial for diskal pain, while possibly aggravating central or foraminal stenotic pain or zygapophysial joint pain. Manniche et al. studied 62 patients with chronic low back pain and compared intensive exercise programs with and without hyperextension components.[46] Although spinal mobility was significantly increased in the hyperextension group, there were no functional differences between groups. In a similar study, intensive extension-based exercise was shown to be superior to reduced intensity exercises or passive therapy.[47] From these earlier programs, concepts and exercises have continued to be refined and expanded. New concepts in neutral spine mechanics have emerged and shaped current physical therapy treatment programs.

DYNAMIC LUMBAR STABILIZATION

Dynamic lumbar stabilization is an individual-based physical therapy program for patients with low back pain well described by Jull et al.[48***] Instruction in neutral spine mechanics and back protection principles are followed by a series of progressively more challenging exercises performed in a neutral spine position. The concept of "neutral spine" is a balance in spine position between flexion and extension that is pain free. The patient is taught to maintain this position during strengthening exercises and later in functional activities. These exercises are initially performed in a supine position with later progression to prone, quadruped, and standing exercises. Emphasis is placed on strengthening those muscles thought to be active in dynamically stabilizing the spine. These are commonly the same muscles shown to be selectively deconditioned in chronic low back pain.[11] The goal is to strengthen dynamic spine-stabilizing musculature and incorporate this stabilization into functional activities (engrams) so that it becomes second nature.

O'Sullivan et al.[49**] studied 44 patients with chronic low back pain presumed secondary to radiographically documented spondylolysis or spondylolisthesis. The intervention group underwent specific strengthening of deep abdominal muscles with coactivation of lumbar multifidi proximal to the pars defect. This activation was then incorporated into previously aggravating static postures and activities. The control group underwent treatment directed by their primary practitioner. Following the 10-week program, the treatment group showed a significant reduction in pain and functional disability relative to the control group. This was maintained at 30-month follow-up. The authors felt a specific treatment approach to be more effective than a general conservative program.

In a prospective, randomized, controlled study of 69 nurses and nurses' aids, back strengthening exercises were performed for 20 min six times a month in the treatment group. This group showed a decrease in the frequency and intensity of low back pain episodes as well as decreased days off work from low back pain relative to a control group with no interventions.[50**] Other similar studies have shown functional exercises to increase return to work[51*] and reduce sick-listing for low back pain patients.[22*]

EVOLUTION OF COMPREHENSIVE PAIN REHABILITATION PROGRAMS

It is naive to assume that all complex chronic pain can be rectified with exercise alone. Chronic pain can be a multidimensional problem with many related psychosocial issues. Bigos et al. have shown that reporting of low back injury as most significantly related to job satisfaction and recent evaluations by superiors.[52] Furthermore, the employee's impression of the physical intensity of job demands is predictive of low back injury, apart from objective lifting requirements.[15] The degree of disability compensation also appears to directly affect disability rates.[53]

Fordyce has described the utilization of operant conditioning techniques for chronic pain treatment.[54***] Extensive discussion of these methods is beyond the scope of this chapter. Operant conditioning methods are employed to extinguish pain behaviors and positively reinforce a patient's improving physical abilities. Prior environmental reinforcers such as rest, breaks from activity, and increased family attention because of pain behavior are replaced by verbal encouragement for completed tasks and neutral responses to pain behaviors. This is not a straightforward or simple task. It requires specially trained and motivated therapists. In a survey of 119 orthopedic physical therapists, 75% felt that physical therapy was not beneficial for chronic pain. Ninety-five percent preferred not to work with chronic pain patients, and the majority did not meet the accepted minimum on pain knowledge scores.[55] The fact that 75% of therapists felt physical therapy to be ineffective for chronic pain is significant. This is in sharp contrast to the 93% of physicians who felt physical therapy was the most effective mode of treatment for chronic pain.[1] This discrepancy in underlying beliefs would undoubtedly have an impact on treatment outcome. Physicians and therapists alike should have special training in the treatment of chronic pain patients and a belief that their therapeutic interventions can be effective.

With recognition of the psychological and social contributions to chronic pain and disability, and the challenges of treating chronic pain in a standard medical environment, comprehensive interdisciplinary pain rehabilitation programs have been created. These programs attempt to deal with the individual as a whole, with regard for their individual work environment. The programs take on multiple forms, but are commonly based in functional restoration through physical exercise via an operant conditioning approach.[56***] An overview of functional restoration is shown in Fig. 24.2.

COMPREHENSIVE PAIN REHABILITATION TEAM

Comprehensive rehabilitation teams (Table 24.3) commonly consist of a physician trained in musculoskeletal disorders, a physical therapist, occupational therapist, psychiatrist or psychologist, nurse, and a vocational specialist. The success of such an interdisciplinary intervention stems from a unified approach to the patient. It is

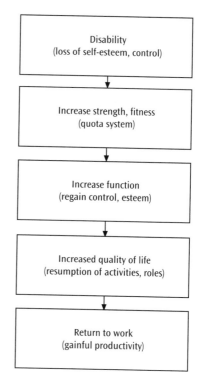

Figure 24.2 *Functional restoration.*

very important that the patient be treated consistently by all team members.[17]

The rehabilitation team physician (physiatrist, psychiatrist, neurologist, orthopedist, anesthesiologist) must be trained in musculoskeletal medicine and be familiar with the use of diagnostic imaging and testing. They ensure that the medical workup has been completed, and monitor the need for further diagnostic or surgical interventions. He or she also addresses ongoing disability and legal issues.

The physical therapists oversee and instruct daily exercise, strengthening, and mobilization. They must be trained in utilization of operant conditioning techniques to successfully deal with pain behaviors and the difficulties mobilizing deconditioned individuals.[56***] Therapy is initially focused on retraining "weak links" in the kinetic chain. These represent the most obvious strength or coordination deficits contributing to the patient's pain. Emphasis is placed on quantification of daily function to follow progress. Occupational therapists assist with job-

Table 24.3 *Comprehensive pain rehabilitation program staff composition*

Patient
Physician
Physical therapist
Occupational therapist
Psychologist
Nurse
Vocational specialist

specific activity simulation/work hardening and in evaluation and improvements in worksite ergonomics.[57]

The psychologist's role is multifaceted. They provide counseling for the patient and family with respect to disability and positive/negative reinforcement concepts. Stress management principles, addictive medication use and withdrawal, and appropriate antidepressant treatment are other areas where the psychologist can assist in guiding treatment. When problems arise with the treatment team relating to a specific individual, the psychologist can often provide insight into these difficulties.

Nurses can function as extensions of the physician as well as liaisons to the community and employers together with the vocational specialist. Nurses are also an excellent source of education and information for the patient and family. The vocational specialist assists in finding gainful employment that is consistent with the patient's documented functional abilities.

The patient must be motivated to take an active role in their restoration. Certain views and behaviors can be altered with comprehensive interventions, but the patient with disincentives for improvement (financial or other secondary gains) or expectations of passive pain relief will prove recalcitrant to any treatment. Patients must feel that they are active, contributing members of the rehabilitation team, rather than the passive subject of interventions.

COMPREHENSIVE PAIN REHABILITATION PROGRAM DESCRIPTION

The initial step in a comprehensive pain rehabilitation program (CPRP) treatment is functional capacity evaluation (FCE) of the patient/candidate. This can be a brief and simple evaluation of walking, sitting, and daily activities. A full functional capacity evaluation generally includes a 2- to 8-h, 2-day, systematic and detailed quantification of ability to sit, stand, lift, push, pull, squat, carry, etc.[58] Attention is paid to pain behaviors, effort, consistency, heart rate, breathing, and sweating. Quantification of the candidate's physical abilities sets a baseline from which improvements can be objectively documented. Following initial evaluation, some programs utilize a preparticipation outpatient physical therapy program in preparation for the more intense core functional restoration program. This allows some degree of acclimatization and development of more appropriate expectations of participation in functional restoration.

The primary functional restoration takes place on multiple fronts. Participants engage in cardiovascular endurance exercise, strengthening, relaxation, stretching, education, and cognitive–behavioral retraining.[59] Most commonly, a quota system is used. From the previously established functional baseline (initial FCE), participants are given progressive goals that they must meet each day before the reward of rest is given. This may include a certain number of lifting repetitions or distance to pedal on a stationary bicycle. Initially, the increments in goals are small to ensure success.[22] Pain behavior is ignored or responded to in a neutral manner whereas successful completion of a requirement is rewarded with praise. Improvements in function can be graphed and displayed for the patient to reinforce gains made in therapy.[60] Successful completion of progressive physical demands improves patients' sense of control over their ability to function.[3,61] This empowers the patient and improves self-esteem, beginning to reverse the learned helplessness of the pain-to-disability cascade.

As the patient's general abilities improve, a transition to work simulation takes place. These are tasks chosen to reproduce critical job demands. They are reproduced as accurately as possible and the quota system is once again used to measure progress. Successful completion of these tasks further increases the patient's esteem and confidence for return to work.[62] At completion of the core program, the patient is given an individual maintenance therapy program to be carried out long term.

Cognitive–behavioral interventions take place throughout the program. Anxiety about program participation or medication withdrawal can be managed with the assistance of psychologists. From individual psychotherapy meetings to the day-to-day interactions with all members of the team, a consistent reinforcement is given to the patient.[63] Patients are taught relaxation therapy as a coping strategy to break the muscle–tension–pain cycle that commonly exists.[64] Family counseling is utilized to encourage active participation in the rehabilitation process and educate family members about the philosophy of the CPRP approach.[17] They are taught to reinforce wellness, reduce reinforcement of illness behavior, and allow the patient to assume responsibility for their recovery.[65] The vocational specialist or social services representative eases the transition into the workplace and ensures any necessary workplace ergonomic alterations are carried out.

Throughout the program, the rehabilitation team members meet regularly to ensure communication, consistent expectations of the patient, and to make individual program alterations as needed.[62,63] Unanticipated or individual problems can be addressed and dealt with as a team. This open, unified team approach is thought to be one of the keys to treatment success.

EFFICACY OF COMPREHENSIVE REHABILITATION PROGRAMS

There is a significant body of literature supporting the efficacy of CPRPs. Multiple outcome parameters, including pain, strength, range of motion, disability, return to work, and injury recurrence rates, have been evaluated (Table 24.4). Comparison with less comprehensive treatments has also been performed.

with TC. As the studies also used more than one potential control group, some studies contributed data to both comparisons. The results of the analyses are shown in Figs 25.1 and 25.2. Figure 25.1 shows the ES values for all the measurement domains when active CBT is compared with waiting list controls. The average effect size is shown with the 95% confidence intervals. In no case does the lower confidence interval cross the *x*-axis of the graph where the ES scale = 0. In other words, receiving CBT is reliably more effective than the effect of waiting for treatment, and it therefore seems that the treatment gains cannot simply be explained by the passage of time.

Figure 25.2 shows the results when CBT is compared with other active treatments. In this figure, the range bars representing the 95% confidence intervals for the mean ES either embrace the horizontal dashed line, which represents no difference between treatments, or in the case of three comparisons shows that CBT is superior. The overall conclusion is that as a class of treatment CBT is at least as good as other active treatments for chronic pain.

While this work concluded that CBT is an effective treatment, careful review and analysis of all the papers revealed a range of issues where improvement to the design and conduct of treatment trials can be made:

1 For example, we concluded that most trials were statistically underpowered, and that some trials were overcomplex with multiple treatment and control groups.
2 We also observed that the content and differentiation of control groups from treatment requires more consideration.[21] Patients assigned to a waiting list in

one trial may continue to receive existing treatments (such as physical therapy or pharmacotherapy) that may be equivalent to the treatment control in another trial. The distinction between the content of active treatment and control condition can also be a fine one. Being allocated to a control condition will have different psychological consequences to being allocated to an active treatment, even though that treatment is based on predominantly nonpsychological principles, e.g. physical therapy.
3 There was variation in quality and quantity of treatment given. Some authors gave explicit accounts of the treatment procedures with reference to manualized interventions which were appropriately monitored, but this was not universally so.
4 Our analysis also revealed that there is a paucity of information about the impact of CBT on economically important outcomes, such as return to work and the use of the health services (drug costs, etc.).

FUTURE DEVELOPMENTS IN TREATMENT EFFECTIVENESS

The common goal of pain specialists is to provide more effective treatments. We define this as an improvement in treatment outcomes, an increase in the number of patients treated, and an overall reduction in cost. There are two frequent suggestions of how to increase the treatment effectiveness. The first suggestion is to select patients more carefully for treatments. The argument for

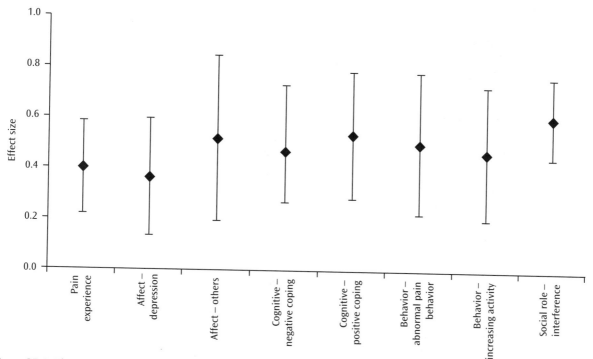

Figure 25.1 *The ES values for all the measurement domains when active cognitive–behavior therapy is compared with waiting list controls.*

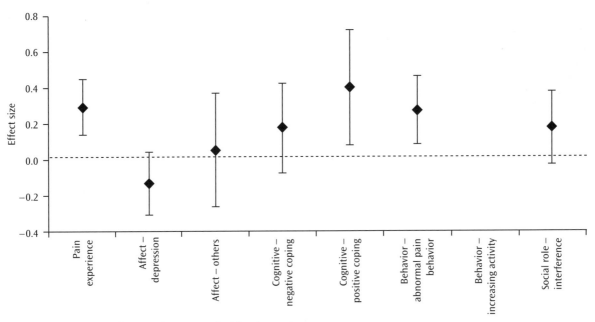

Figure 25.2 *The results when CBT is compared with other active treatments.*

this approach is that given a heterogeneous patient population such as adult chronic pain patients, there is no reason why treatment gains should be expected with all patients. Therefore, prediction by demographic, medical, diagnostic, psychological, or social variables should identify those to be excluded and those who are most likely to gain from treatment.

The second suggestion of how to increase the treatment effectiveness is to attempt to specify treatments better. Because CBT is a compound treatment applied to the complex problem of chronic pain, there is often the suggestion that treatment should or could be refined down to its "critical ingredients." The implication is that, after refining the core, the remainder of treatment programs can be abandoned. If a refined program can be delivered to well-selected patients then surely we will have excellent outcomes and a cost-effective return on investment in treatment resources?

These ideas accord with principles of management, but assume that reliable data are available on patient characteristics as predictors and on specific treatment-outcome associations. These assumptions are unfortunately without sufficient basis:

1 First, no patient characteristics have reliably emerged from prospective studies. This may in part be caused by poor hypotheses, poor operationalization of constructs, or low power of studies. But it is not easily remedied: given the many candidate variables, possible interactions among them, and the modest reliability of many measures, the necessary studies are of a size beyond any feasibility. Meanwhile, "clinical wisdom" and judgment of motivation for treatment tends to disenfranchise the most disabled and distressed patients and those with poor education or language skills.

2 Second, the implicit model is of components of therapy that are distinct and separable, and that the process of therapy is an additive one. The description of therapy given above makes it clear that this model does not accord with theory or practice of CBT for pain management. We should consider that in some cases the delivery of particular treatment components might actually detract from gains made by other components. Also, some components (e.g. relaxation) may only serve to allow other components (e.g. attention management) to be attempted.

Improvements in chronic pain management in general, including CBT, require a professional recognition that the imperative to make treatment more efficient carries the very real risk of throwing the baby out with the bath water. The poor record of audit or evaluation of many treatment programs exacerbates this risk. Improvement will follow the use of a more evidence-based approach in scrutinizing each treatment component and of empirical and experimental work to identify the processes by which particular outcomes are improved: an excellent example is the work by Johan Vlaeyen and colleagues on pain-related fear and avoidance of activity (see Chapter P14).

Perhaps the real challenge comes from the identification and specification of a successful and desired outcome of CBT for chronic pain. For some people, this is an easy issue (e.g. to reduce pain or to return to paid employment), but for many it is complex. We should recognize that there are different stakeholders in patient change: the patient, the patient's physicians, employer or potential employer, third-party payers, government support agencies, and taxpayers at large. These stakeholders may have different and even conflicting goals and priorities. Within each outcome, more careful consideration needs to be given to what would be a realistic gain, and to what extent this meets the expectations of stakeholders. Success is a slippery concept.

We can foresee a time when CBT for chronic pain is understood as a broad categorization of perhaps 20 different well-specified therapies that can be targeted at perhaps 20 different well-specified patient groups. At present, this is not the case. The first step in reaching a broader and more comprehensive collection of specific therapies is to first recognize that the outcomes from compound and programmatic CBT are positive and among the most effective treatments in the chronic pain clinic. A substantial amount of work has already been done to define treatments and to build the evidence base. The next step will be to develop treatment components from a theoretical and empirical base and to better understand the needs of specific populations. Excluding patients from treatments and reducing treatment content may produce good short-term data on a limited set of outcomes, but will not lead to long-term effectiveness. Research effort should perhaps be spent instead on understanding how patients individualize their own path through a complex treatment.

CONCLUSION

Psychological therapy and, in particular, cognitive–behavior therapy for adults with chronic pain are effective treatments for helping patients to manage the deleterious effects of chronic pain. Multidisciplinary CBT has been established practice for over 30 years, and the evidence base is now sufficiently robust to allow the research and development of critical aspects of treatment.

REFERENCES

1. Loeser JD. Mitigating the dangers of pursuing care. In: Cohen JM, Campbell JN eds. *Pain Treatment Centers at a Crossroads: A Practical and Conceptual Reappraisal.* Seattle, WA: IASP Press, **1996:** 101–8.
● 2. Morley S, Eccleston C, Williams ACdeC. Systematic
◆ review and meta-analysis of randomized controlled trials of cognitive behaviour therapy for chronic pain in adults, excluding headache. *Pain* 1999; **80:** 1–13.
3. Fordyce WE, Fowler RS, Lehmann JF, *et al.* Operant conditioning in the treatment of chronic pain. *Arch Phys Med Rehabil* 1973; **54:** 399–408.
4. Sharpe M, Mayou R, Seagroatt V, *et al.* Why do Doctors Find Some Patients Difficult to Help? *Q J Med* 1994; **87:** 187–93.
5. Jensen MP, Karoly P, Harris P. Assessing the affective component of chronic pain: development of the pain discomfort scale. *J Psychosom Res* 1991; **35:**149–54.
6. McCracken LM. Learning to live with the pain: acceptance of pain predicts adjustment in persons with chronic pain. *Behav Res Ther* 1998; **74:** 21–8.
7. Turk DC, Okifuji A, Scharff L. Chronic pain and depression – role of perceived impact and perceived control in different age cohorts. *Pain* 1995; **61:** 93–101.
8. Fernandez E, Turk, DC. The scope and significance of anger in the experience of chronic pain. *Pain* 1995; **61:** 165–75.
9. Wade JB, Price DD, Hamer RM, *et al.* An emotional component analysis of chronic pain. *Pain* 1990; **40:** 303–10.
10. Pincus T, Williams ACdeC. Models and measurements of depression in chronic pain. *J Psychosom Res* 1999; **47:** 211–19.
11. Banks SM, Kerns RD. Explaining high rates of depression in chronic pain: a diathesis-stress framework. *Psychol Bull* 1996; **95:** 95–110.
12. Clyde Z, Williams ACdeC. Depression and mood. In: Linton SJ ed. *New Avenues for the Prevention of Chronic Musculoskeletal Pain and Disability.* Amsterdam: Elsevier Science, in press.
13. Hotopf M, Lewis G, Normand C. Putting trials on trial – the costs and consequences of small trials in depression: a systematic review of methodology. *J Epidemiol Community Health* 1997; **51:** 354–8.
14. Wells A. *Emotional Disorders and Metacognition: Innovative Cognitive Therapy.* Chichester: Wiley Press, 2000.
15. Barnard PJ, Teasdale JD. Interacting cognitive subsystems: a systemic approach to cognitive–affective interaction and change. *Cogn Emotion* 1991; **5:** 1–39.
16. Van den Hout JHC, Vlaeyen JWS, Houben RMA, *et al.* The effects of failure feedback and pain-related fear on pain report, pain tolerance, and pain avoidance in chronic low back pain patients. *Pain* 2001; **92:** 247–57.
17. Turk DC, Rudy TE. Neglected topics in the treatment of chronic pain patients – relapse, noncompliance, and adherence enhancement. *Pain* 1991; **44:** 5–28.
18. Chalmers I Altman DG. *Systematic Reviews.* London: BMJ Publishing, 1995.
19. McQuay HJ, Moore RA. *An Evidence-based Resource for Pain Relief.* Oxford: Oxford University Press, 1998.
20. Malone MD, Strube MJ. Meta-analysis of non-medical treatments for chronic pain. *Pain* 1988; **34:** 231–44.
● 21. Flor H, Fydrich T, Turk DC. Efficacy of multidisciplinary
◆ pain treatment centers: a meta-analytic review. *Pain* 1992; **49:** 221–30.

Alternative and complementary therapies

MILES J BELGRADE

Acupuncture, chiropractic, homeopathy, herbal medicine, traditional Chinese medicine. These practices are often described as alternative medicine or complementary medicine because they lie outside the dominant health system of a Western industrialized society. Yet, in many cultures these techniques may be mainstream. Indeed, world health practices are so varied and culturally based that allopathic medicine is a subordinate and foreign alternative to the indigenous medicine of many societies. A chapter such as this discussing alternative and complementary medicine must be written from a regional point of view. This chapter is written from the perspective of a Western industrialized society in which allopathic medicine dominates health care, where a biological model of health and disease dictates the approach to healing.

Mainstream medicine relies on pathophysiologic diagnoses derived from history and laboratory investigations and on treatment using pharmaceutical agents, surgery, physical rehabilitation, and radiation therapies. To a lesser extent, a restricted set of behavioral and psychological therapies is also part of this tradition. The axiomatic foundations of this medicine are the scientific method and the biological sciences that evolve from it. Although many, if not most, therapies in this system are empirically derived, those therapies that are scientifically derived or validated are the most valued. Those disease states in which the pathophysiology is undetermined or vague tend to be poorly served by this system of medicine, which depends so heavily on well-defined pathophysiologic causes of disease.

WHY DO PAIN PATIENTS SEEK ALTERNATIVE AND COMPLEMENTARY THERAPIES?

Pain management is an excellent example of where the biomedical model falls short. First, pain management is by definition an experience that is subjective[1] and cannot be measured directly. Second, the pathophysiologic processes that produce clinical pain problems are still incompletely understood. We can only infer what the pathology is in broad generalities, e.g. inflammatory, neuropathic, or mechanical. Complex social and psychological factors play such an important role in chronic pain problems that attempts to treat chronic pain exclusively using scientific principles are doomed to fail under our current state of scientific knowledge. Pain has a motivational component, i.e. it is accompanied by a drive to eliminate it. The result is that patients continually seek alternative treatments to eliminate their pain.

All of the following conditions lead patients to seek alternative or complementary therapies for pain: incomplete pathophysiologic characterization, lack of scientifically derived treatments, inability of allopathic treatments to control the social and psychological components of complex chronic pain, high motivation for symptom elimination, and lack of physician enthusiasm for treatment. In fact, chronic pain may be the affliction that physicians are most loath to treat. Many physicians shun the chronic pain patient because they feel powerless to help these individuals who often have unrealistic expectations and require large amounts of time during and after office hours. It is no wonder that these patients look elsewhere for help.

Astin identified chronic pain as a predictor of alternative medicine use.[2] Other predictors include poorer health status, more education, anxiety, back problems, urinary tract problems, interest in spirituality and personal growth psychology, and having had a transformation in world view. Interestingly, dissatisfaction with conventional medicine did not predict use of alternative medicine. In fact, only about 4% of individuals report relying exclusively on alternative therapies.[2,3]

The discomfort of allopathic treatments is often a deterrent for patients. Surgical treatments carry inevitable discomfort and recovery periods of varying degrees. Pharmaceuticals' side-effects frequently interfere with normal functioning. The public's perception of these agents as foreign substances can even result in avoidance of medicines that are usually well tolerated. These "costs" of allopathic treatment also fuel the flight to "natural" alternatives.

Patients seeking treatment for pain want physicians to listen to them and to believe them. These elements of the physician–patient relationship are as important as successful pain reduction.[4] Yet, time constraints and productivity expectations on physicians by disinterested third parties may reduce the listening time to 10 min or less. The solo practitioner of an alternative therapy may offer 30–60 min of unhurried time to listen to his or her patients and satisfy that essential ingredient of success.

PREVALENCE

Several large surveys in the USA, Europe, and Australia have demonstrated the extent of alternative and complementary medicine use by the public. Eisenberg and colleagues showed that the use of alternative therapies in the USA increased from 34% to 42% between 1990 and 1997.[3] Use of these therapies was most prominent in chronic conditions such as back pain and headache, but individuals also sought alternative therapies for health maintenance even when asymptomatic. Millar estimated that 15% of Canadians had visited an alternative health care practitioner in the previous 12 months.[5] In Australia, the estimated prevalence of alternative medicine use was 49%.[6] In Europe, participation in alternative therapies ranges from 23% in Denmark to 49% in France.[7] Estimates of prevalence may vary widely depending on the study methods used. The choice of study population and the scope of what is considered alternative medicine (e.g. use of prayer or local heat and ice are such common practices that it would be misleading to include these in survey data), for example, will greatly impact prevalence estimates.

In the USA, the high rates of alternative medicine use crosses socioeconomic, racial, and geographic boundaries, but use was higher among whites, females, those who were college educated, and those living in the west of the USA.[3] The types of therapies that patients use will depend on many factors besides patient preference, such as availability and cost. Table 26.1 summarizes the relative use among 16 different alternative health practices as reported in the 1997 survey carried out by Eisenberg et al.[3] The most common therapies were relaxation techniques (16.3%), herbal medicine (12.1%), massage (11.1%), and chiropractic (11.0%), while acupuncture was used by 1% of the population. The number of visits to an alternative medicine practitioner varies depending on the nature of the therapy. Thus, chiropractic, acupuncture, and massage therapy will require more visits to a practitioner in a given time period than herbal medicine or homeopathy.

COST

A conservative estimate of out-of-pocket costs to consumers for alternative therapies in the USA is $27 billion. This compares with out-of-pocket expenses of $9.1 billion for hospitalizations and $29.3 billion for physician services.[3] Payment by insurers for alternative and complementary therapies has become a greater issue as the popularity and demand has increased. Yet, insurance reimbursement in the USA did not significantly change for most alternative therapies between 1990 and 1997.[3] Complete or partial coverage is greatest for biofeedback (74%), chiropractic (56%), megavitamins (56%), and imagery (55%). It is lowest for folk remedies (0%), homeopathy (0%), and hypnosis (5%). In Britain, Pal and Morris surveyed 20 private medical insurers regarding payment for complementary treatment.[8] Most of the responders indicated that they paid for chiropractic, osteopathy, homeopathy, and the Alexander technique – sometimes only with a consultant referral.

PHYSICIAN ATTITUDES

Acceptance of alternative and complementary therapies by physicians is not uniform. Many physicians themselves are practitioners of one or more complementary therapies. Others are skeptical, misinformed, and oppositional. All physicians share a culture that respects logical thinking, responsibility, and evidence-based treatment. Physicians as a whole abhor magical thinking and pandering, particularly in regard to patients with serious illness. Many physicians have seen patients die as a result of cancer after being led to alternative therapies by alternative practitioners who pandered to vulnerable patients. These practitioners often exploit patients' fear of medical treatment and its side-effects by promising "natural" cures.

For chronic conditions that are not life threatening, physicians tend to be more forgiving of alternative

Table 26.1 *Relative use of alternative therapies in the USA*

Type of therapy	Used in past 12 months (%)	Mean number visits per user in past 12 months
Relaxation	16.3	20.9
Herbal medicine	12.1	2.9
Massage	11.1	8.4
Chiropractic	11.0	9.8
Spiritual healing	7.0	–
Megavitamins	5.5	8.6
Self-help group	4.8	18.9
Imagery	4.5	11.0
Commercial diet	4.4	7.3
Folk remedies	4.2	1.0
Lifestyle diet	4.0	2.8
Energy healing	3.8	20.2
Homeopathy	3.4	1.6
Hypnosis	1.2	2.8
Biofeedback	1.0	3.6
Acupuncture	1.0	3.1

Adapted from Eisenberg *et al.*[3]

treatments and less rigid about their lack of scientific foundation. In a meta-analysis of 12 surveys of physicians' perceptions regarding complementary medicine, Ernst and coworkers concluded that most of the surveys implied that physicians perceived complementary therapies as moderately useful and/or effective.[9] Manipulative therapies (osteopathy or chiropractic), acupuncture, and homeopathy were deemed most useful or effective in the majority of these surveys. All but one of the 12 surveys was of physicians in general practice in the UK, Europe, New Zealand, and Israel.

A survey of rheumatologists in the UK revealed that they regarded acupuncture and osteopathy as the most desirable complementary treatments. They felt that these therapies should be available on the National Health Service and supported the suggestion that these disciplines be taught in medical schools.[8] Another survey of rheumatologists in the Netherlands indicated a favorable attitude toward manipulation among 49%, whereas 37% were favorable toward acupuncture and 23% toward homeopathy.[10] Rheumatologists provide specialty care to a large number of chronic pain patients with fibromyalgia, arthritis, and other connective tissue disorders. Their views on alternative treatments have an impact on the role these treatments play in the lives of patients.

Medical schools in the USA are responding to the new awareness of alternative medicine's pervasiveness. A survey of family practice residency program directors and US medical school family medicine department chairs revealed that nearly 30% were currently teaching some form of alternative medicine.[11] Another 12% were either starting to teach or considering teaching such a course. Most of these courses were elective. Daly listed 51 alternative medicine courses at 44 medical schools in the USA.[12] These courses had titles such as "Complementary Medicine," "Public Health Perspectives on Alternative Health Care," "Chinese QiGong I & II," "The Program

of Mind–Body Studies," and "Complementary Medicine – An integrated 1st, 2nd and 4th year program." Among the schools listed were Harvard Medical School, Cornell Medical College, Mayo Medical School, and University of California, Los Angeles School of Medicine.

The US congress showed its support of research into alternative medicine by establishing the Office of Alternative Medicine (OAM) at the National Institutes of Health in 1992, and by designating that office as the National Center for Complementary and Alternative Medicine with an annual budget of $50 million.[13] This organization has started a number of large clinical trials that are expected to stimulate further research. In addition, the OAM has funded 13 research centers at institutions across the USA that are carrying out a research agenda in various broad clinical areas. These areas include pain, human immunodeficiency/acquired immune deficiency syndrome (HIV/AIDS), addiction, aging, cancer, women's health issues, general medical conditions, pediatric conditions, neurological disorders, cardiovascular diseases, chiropractic, and asthma, allergy and immunology (Table 26.2).

DEFINITIONS

In 1993, Eisenberg *et al.* utilized a working definition of alternative medical therapies as interventions neither taught widely in medical schools nor generally available in US hospitals.[14] As we have seen, these alternative therapies are becoming more available in conventional medical settings and are being taught in medical schools.[11,12] A broader definition of complementary and alternative medicine is those medical systems, practices, interventions, applications, theories, or claims that are currently not part of the dominant or conventional medical sys-

Table 26.2 *Institution-affiliated centers of research in the USA on alternative medicine sponsored by the Office of Alternative Medicine at the National Institutes of Health*

Institution and location	Name of center	Specialty of center
Bastyr University, Bethel, WA	Bastyr University AIDS Research Center	HIV/AIDS
Columbia University, New York, NY	Center for Complementary and Alternative Medicine Research in Women's Health	Women's health issues
Harvard Medical School, Beth Israel Hospital, Deaconess Medical Center	Center for Alternative Medicine Research	General medical conditions
Kessler Institute for Rehabilitation, West Orange, NJ	Center for Research in Complementary and Alternative Medicine for Stroke and Neurological Disorders	Stroke and neurological conditions
Palmer Center for Chiropractic Research, Davenport, IA	Consortial Center for Chiropractic Research	Chiropractic
Stanford University, Palo Alto, CA	Complementary and Alternative Medicine Program at Stanford	Aging
University of Arizona, Health Sciences Center, Tucson, AZ	Program in Integrative Medicine	Pediatric conditions
University of California, Davis, CA	Center for Alternative Medicine Research in Asthma and Immunology	Asthma, allergy, and immunology
University of Maryland, School of Medicine, Baltimore, MD	Center for Alternative Medicine Pain Research and Evaluation	Pain
University of Michigan, Ann Arbor, MI	University of Michigan Complementary and Alternative Medicine Research Center for Cardiovascular diseases	Cardiovascular diseases
University of Minnesota Medical School, Minneapolis, MN	Center for Addiction and Alternative Medicine Research	Addiction
University of Texas Health Science Center, Houston, TX	University of Texas Center for Alternative Medicine	Cancer
University of Virginia, Charlottesville, VA	University of Virginia Center for the Study of Complementary and Alternative Therapies	Pain

HIV, human immunodeficiency virus; AIDS, acquired immune deficiency syndrome. From Marwick.[13]

tem in a society.[15] Under this definition, the list of practices that are considered alternative or complementary medicine will continually change as society changes and as those practices supported by research become incorporated into mainstream medicine. Eskinazi proposed a refined definition of alternative medicine as a broad set of health care practices that are not readily integrated into the dominant health care model because they pose challenges to diverse societal beliefs and practices.[16] The idea of a challenge to conventional practice is important. It highlights the difference between what is called "alternative" and what is called "complementary."

The terminology used to describe the broad scope of practices that are considered "alternative" or "complementary" to mainstream medical practice is diverse and often confusing. *Alternative medicine, complementary medicine, holistic medicine, integrative therapies, natural medicine*, and *traditional medicine* are all terms that have been used nearly synonymously to represent an approach to health that is different from the biomedical system that is so entrenched in the Western industrialized world. Each of the adjectives alternative, holistic, complementary integrative, etc. has slightly different connotations which define a relationship with mainstream

medicine. The term *alternative* implies "instead of" or "apart from" conventional medicine, whereas *complementary* connotes "in addition to" as a way of completing an approach to healing. *Integrative* medicine suggests multiple approaches that are applied "together" or "in concert" with one another. *Holistic* is an older term which was used to emphasize an "all-encompassing" approach to the person rather than the disease, illness, or symptom. Traditional medicines usually refer to a culturally based system such as traditional Chinese medicine, traditional Native American healing practices, and Ayurvedic medicine. In industrialized Western societies, the term *traditional medicine* is sometimes used misleadingly to refer to the allopathic or biomedical model. Perhaps a more suitable term for those systems of healing that arise from one of the world's cultures is *world medicine*.

Even more problematic is the term *natural* as in *natural healing, natural medicine*, or *naturopathy*. The term generally implies techniques that rely only on botanicals and substances that are used in their natural form, i.e. they are not modified by chemical or physical processes. The scope of what natural healing means has expanded to include techniques such as massage and acupuncture and other approaches that purport to promote the body's own power to heal itself by correcting mechanical or energy imbalances.[17]

UNDERSTANDING THE SCOPE OF ALTERNATIVE AND COMPLEMENTARY THERAPIES

The definition of alternative and complementary medicine developed above is almost equivalent to defining it as everything except conventional medicine. This creates a challenge to categorize and classify countless therapies and systems of healing in a way that makes sense and provides an intellectual handle on a large and disparate field.

We can broadly separate all of alternative and complementary medicine into three main classifications: world medicine systems, other comprehensive systems of medicine that are not culturally based, and individual therapies (Fig. 26.1). Unlike individual therapies, a *system* of medicine provides treatment for a whole spectrum of symptoms, illnesses, or diseases. It is generally a complete system of medicine with its own philosophy, or science of health and disease, and its own diagnostic approach. A world medicine system evolves from the belief system and cultural practices of a society. Examples of world medicine are traditional Chinese medicine and Ayurvedic medicine, which originates from India. Other systems of medicine, such as homeopathy, may evolve from a philosophical construct of health and disease, but are not part of a world cultural tradition. Individual therapies treat a narrower range of conditions with a specific type of intervention, but they do not by themselves provide a model of health and illness. Hypnosis, massage, vitamin therapy, and relaxation techniques are examples of individual therapies.

To classify individual therapies further, it is useful to think of them as falling into one or more of seven functional categories of treatment:

1 Mindful.
2 Spiritual.
3 Energy based.
4 Stimulation based.
5 Movement based.
6 Mechanical or manipulative.
7 Nutriceutical.

These are shown in Table 26.3 with examples in each category. Mindful therapies utilize the mind to produce changes in physical and emotional status. Meditation, hypnosis, and yoga fall into this category. Spiritual therapies imply a letting go of the mind, giving up control to a higher power as with prayer. Energy-based techniques rely on a construct of a vital energy or energy field that exists in living systems. When the flow of energy is out of balance or obstructed, disease can occur. The goal of energy-based treatments is to restore the optimal energy balance to achieve health. Therapeutic touch and acupuncture use this concept as their foundation. Note that yoga can be considered as mindful, spiritual, energy based, and movement based. Acupuncture is a stimulation-based technique, but it is part of a world medicine system – traditional Chinese medicine – which uses the concept of a vital energy (qi). Aromatherapy is also a stimulation-based approach to healing. It consists of inhaled essences of plants or topically applied essential oils. The absorption of micromolecules through the skin or respiratory mucosa is believed to produce favorable chemical changes, thus aromatherapy may also be a form of nutriceutical treatment. Vitamins, herbs, and diets are also examples of nutriceutical therapies which involve the absorption and assimilation of substances into the body to produce a change in state that is favorable to the living system.

Movement-based therapies include dance therapy, t'ai chi ch'uan, exercise, yoga, and other techniques that rely on movement and posture to promote health. Many of these movement-based therapies also rely on concepts of energy medicine as part of their foundation. Mechanical or manipulative therapies include chiropractic, osteopathic, craniosacral therapy, and massage. These approaches usually apply external forces to cor-

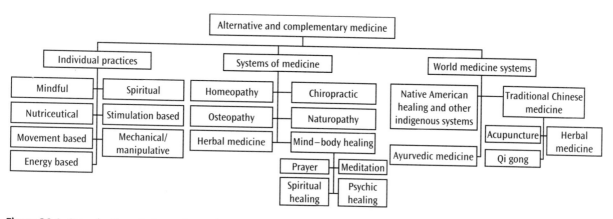

Figure 26.1 *Organization of alternative and complementary therapies.*

Table 26.3 *Categories of individual alternative and complementary therapies with examples*

Mindful	Spiritual	Energy based	Stimulation based	Movement based	Mechanical/ manipulative	Nutriceutical
Hypnosis	Prayer	Massage	TENS	Exercise	Chiropractic	Vitamins
Imagery	Spiritual	Therapeutic	Acupuncture	Dance	Osteopathy	Diet
Meditation	healing	touch	Massage	Alexander	therapy	Herbal
Relaxation	Psychic	Homeopathy	Aromatherapy	technique	Massage	medicine
Biofeedback	healing	Acupuncture	Therapeutic	T'ai chi	Craniosacral	Homeopathy
Yoga	Yoga	Qi gong	touch	Qi Gong	therapy	Aromatherapy
		Yoga	Music	Yoga	Rolfing	

TENS, transcutaneous electrical nerve stimulation.

rect a mechanical problem of the spine, bones, muscle, or other soft tissues.

Organizing the universe of alternative treatments into these seven functional categories helps the clinician to plan a treatment strategy. When a patient is not having success achieving pain control, and has tried several therapies within one or two categories, suggesting choices from a different category makes sense. When faced with a vulnerable patient, certain types of treatment may pose challenges that are best avoided. The abuse victim may have difficulty with mindful and spiritual therapies that require a process of letting go. They also may not tolerate the vigorous physical contact inherent in some of the manipulative therapies. If they are seeking complementary treatment, the clinician should discuss these issues and may recommend less threatening types of treatment from the nutriceutical or movement-based groups.

In the following sections we will describe selected alternative and complementary treatments that span the three main groups (world medicine systems, other complete systems, and individual therapies) and most of the seven functional categories of alternative treatments.

ACUPUNCTURE AND TRADITIONAL CHINESE MEDICINE

In our classification scheme, acupuncture is part of a world medicine system (traditional Chinese medicine) and is categorized as both a stimulation-based and an energy-based technique. Its origin dates to at least 600 BC, preceding the availability of iron and steel for fashioning needles.[18] Acupuncture theory postulates a system of channels or meridians on the body named after organs or bodily systems, and a vital energy called *qi* that flows through the channels. Acupuncture points lie along the channels. Good health and well-being occur when the flow of energy is balanced. Illness occurs when the energy flow is out of balance. It may be depleted from a channel or it may accumulate within a channel at a point of obstruction. By needling acupuncture points, the flow of qi can be restored to its proper balance.

Acupuncture technique and theory are embedded in traditional Chinese medicine, which in turn springs from Taoist philosophy. Taoism emphasizes the inextricable relationship between humans and the natural world, drawing upon three fundamental concepts: *yin* and *yang*, the system of five phases or elements, and the vital energy qi.[18] Yin and yang conceptualize the dualistic nature of the universe and living systems in particular. Cold (yin) and heat (yang), internal (yin) and external (yang), deficiency (yin) and excess (yang) help to characterize the balance of nature and the processes leading to disease. Another way to characterize the properties of matter or of processes that occur in the universe is with the system of five phases or five elements: wood, fire, earth, metal, and water. These are not elements in the same way we think of the more than 100 universal elements of modern science. The five elements of traditional Chinese medicine are metaphors describing different properties or behavior of things in nature. Unlike yin and yang and the five elements, which pertain to both living and nonliving things in the universe, the concept of qi defines living systems. It is created and replenished by breathing and eating. It flows through the 12 pairs of meridians throughout a 24-h day, so it takes about 2 h to traverse from one channel to the next.

The traditional acupuncturist will access information about the balance of qi in the various organs through a systematic diagnostic process that relies on history and some unique physical assessments such as the appearance of the tongue and a complex analysis of the characteristics of the radial pulse. Pain indicates stagnation of qi in one or more of the channels or invasion of the channel by wind, heat, or cold. All of these concepts are crystallized in the world's first medical text titled *Huang Ti Nei Ching*, translated as *The Yellow Emperor's Classic of Internal Medicine*, which dates at least as early as 200 BC.[19]

Brief history of acupuncture

During the fourth to the tenth centuries, acupuncture became ingrained in Chinese medicine and was officially recognized as an independent specialty of the Imperial Medical Academy of the Tang government in AD 618. During this same period, acupuncture, together with other branches of Chinese medicine, was introduced in other countries such as Japan.[20] Throughout the eleventh to the early twentieth century, volumes of written material came out on acupuncture prescriptions. Acupuncture training programs became established in China, which allowed the growth of clinical experience with acupuncture and refinement in techniques. Complications of acupuncture were documented, lists of dangerous points appeared, and indications for acupuncture were identified.

As Western medicine was introduced in China in the eighteenth century, acupuncture began to lose official favor. It was banned from the imperial court in 1822, but it was still practiced widely and its use spread in Europe and other countries even as Western medicine was making its way into China. In the 1940s, Mao Tse Tung revived the status of acupuncture practice as he found it a useful, inexpensive, and expedient alternative to Western medicine, which was expensive and difficult to access during his quest for power against Chiang Kai Shek. Chairman Mao encouraged the development of acupuncture and fostered simplification of acupuncture practice so that large numbers of nonphysicians (*barefoot doctors*) could use it in their communities together with herbal remedies.

In 1971, *New York Times* journalist James Reston wrote about his experience with acupuncture for postoperative pain while covering the American–Chinese ping-pong games. His report heralded a new beginning for acupuncture in the West. National magazines ran stories on acupuncture. Teams of medical investigators from the USA flocked to China to find out more about this mysterious and apparently wondrous treatment that was so different from pharmaceutical or surgical therapies familiar to the Western mind. The initial frenzy of excitement settled down as some of the unrealistic expectations were not met, but acupuncture continued to be an important part of the alternative medicine arena in the USA.

The National Institutes of Health (NIH) of the USA sponsored a consensus conference in November 1997 to determine the status and role of acupuncture in American medicine.[21]*** The objectives of the conference were (1) to form conclusions about the efficacy of acupuncture, its role in various conditions, its biological mechanisms, and what remaining issues must be addressed to incorporate acupuncture into today's health care system, and (2) to identify directions for future research. The 12-member panel represented a wide spectrum of interests and expertise from public citizens to medical specialists to acupuncturists. They concluded that:

1 Acupuncture is widely practiced in the USA.
2 Sufficient evidence exists to support the use of acupuncture as primary therapy for adult postoperative and chemotherapy-induced nausea and vomiting and for postoperative dental pain.
3 Sufficient evidence exists to support adjunctive use of acupuncture for various other conditions such as addiction, stroke rehabilitation, headache, menstrual cramps, tennis elbow, fibromyalgia, myofascial

pain, osteoarthritis, low back pain, carpal tunnel syndrome, and asthma.
4 Findings from basic research have begun to elucidate the mechanisms of acupuncture, including the release of opioids and other peptides in the central and peripheral nervous system and changes in neuroendocrine function.
5 Issues of training, licensure, and reimbursement remain to be clarified.
6 There is sufficient evidence of acupuncture's potential value to encourage further studies and to expand its use into conventional medicine.

These conclusions from an authoritative agency of the US government help to legitimize acupuncture practice and development.

Acupuncture technique

Needles are generally made of stainless steel, but are sometimes gold or silver to achieve energizing or sedating effects. Twenty-eight- to 32-gauge solid needles are used. The length of the needle and depth of penetration depends on the thickness of the underlying soft tissue. Many acupuncture points overlie muscle and the depth of needle insertion is usually to the center of the muscle belly. Needles may be inserted perpendicularly, obliquely, or tangentially. The acupuncturist usually tries to elicit a special needling sensation called *deqi*, which refers to a deep, heavy, warm, spreading, or aching sensation that is felt to be crucial to achieve a therapeutic effect.

Stimulation of the acupuncture points is a necessary part of treatment. Needles may be stimulated in a variety of ways, e.g. manually by thrusting up and down or twisting back and forth or by tapping or scraping the handle of the needle. Electrical current can be applied to pairs of needles at frequencies of 3–5 Hz or at higher frequencies in the 100- or 1,000-Hz range (Fig. 26.2). The amplitude of stimulation is adjusted to patient tolerance. Needles and acupuncture points may also be heated in various ways, including the use of moxa, a plant that is burned near the acupuncture point or on the needle.

The duration of an acupuncture session is about 20–45 min. The frequency of sessions is variable, depending on the clinical problem, its chronicity, and availability of resources. Typically, treatments are carried out once to three times per week. Sometimes, treatments are offered daily or as infrequently as once or twice a month. A course of treatment consists of 10–20 sessions, but for intractable chronic conditions periodic maintenance therapy may be offered. Ultimately, the intervals between treatments and the duration of a course of acupuncture remain empiric.[22]

Points are chosen for acupuncture either through traditional Chinese diagnostic analysis or by a formula approach, which utilizes a limited number of basic rules for point selection:

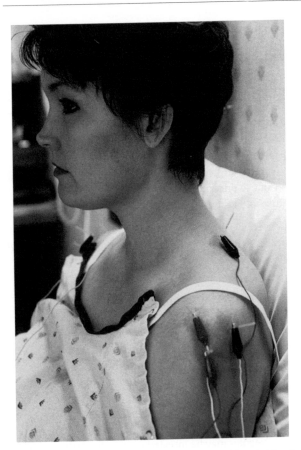

Figure 26.2 *Electroacupuncture for rheumatoid arthritis of the shoulder.*

1 For localized symptoms, needle points in that same region on any meridian, e.g. for shoulder pain, needle points on or near the shoulder.
2 Tender points are considered acupuncture points and can often be chosen for therapy.
3 Points on a meridian will influence symptoms or disorders along the entire meridian.
4 Six important distal points on the upper and lower limbs have effects on specific regions of the head, neck, and trunk. For example, the point Hoku (large intestine – 4) in the first dorsal interosseous muscle between the thumb and first finger affects the head and neck.
5 There are subsets of points that have certain general effects, such as sedation, tonification (energizing), and immune system regulation, or that influence certain tissues, such as muscle and tendons, bone, and cartilage.
6 There is a somatotopic organization on the surface of the ear, so that points on the ear can be chosen to influence any other part of the body.

Acupuncture risks

Common side-effects of acupuncture include syncope or near-syncope in about 1% of patients, bruising around the needle site in less than 1% of needle sticks, and persistent soreness from needling that outlasts the treatment by hours to days. Contact dermatitis has been reported and attributed to the nickel content in most stainless-steel needles.[23] Acupuncture should be avoided during pregnancy or used with caution because of the apparent effect of uterine muscle contraction and cervical dilation that has been produced by stimulating certain points.[24,25] Other risks of acupuncture can be divided into organ or tissue damage and infections. The lung is the organ most likely to be injured during acupuncture. Several reports of unilateral and bilateral pneumothorax have emerged.[22,26-28] Cases of spinal cord and peripheral nerve injuries have been associated with acupuncture owing to migration of a broken needle fragment or a purposefully retained needle.[29-32] Boxall reported 29 cases of serologically proven hepatitis B that was traced to an acupuncture clinic in Birmingham, UK.[33] Four cases of hepatitis B were reported and traced to acupuncture treatment received at a chiropractic clinic in Florida in 1980.[34] In both clinics, poor needle management was used, i.e. reusable needles, use of hollow syringe-type needles, and unsterilized needles.

The documentation of serious complications of acupuncture is an argument in favor of state regulation. This would help insure that practitioners meet certain standards of knowledge and practice that would limit public harm.

Scientific basis

Acupuncture, more than any other alternative medicine, has been studied scientifically. The discovery of opioid receptors and endorphins has led to a large number of investigations into the role these receptors and ligands play in experimental acupuncture analgesia. Few of these studies contradict the involvement of the endorphin system, and several lines of evidence demonstrate that the endogenous opioid system is part of acupuncture analgesia: acupuncture analgesia can be reversed with opioid antagonists such as naloxone;[35-38] increased endogenous opioid production has been measured directly after acupuncture;[39,40] antiserum to opioid receptors has been shown to block acupuncture analgesia.

By 1982, biogenic amines had been implicated in acupuncture analgesia in numerous studies reviewed by Han and Terenius.[41] Ablating the descending inhibitory pathway for pain at the dorsal and medial raphe nuclei blunted acupuncture analgesia. Blocking serotonin (5-hydroxytryptamine) receptors in rabbits and rats also diminished acupuncture analgesia. Administration of a serotonin precursor potentiates acupuncture analgesia. Measurements of serotonin and its byproducts showed increased levels in the lower brain stem during acupuncture analgesia.

Other neurochemical mediators have been implicated

in experimental acupuncture analgesia, including substance P, calcitonin gene-related peptide (CGRP), cholecystokinin (CCK), and *c-fos*, but these investigations represent more preliminary individual findings.[22]

Evidence of clinical benefit

The NIH consensus statement is a good source for a review of clinical evidence.[21] In the field of addiction medicine, Bullock *et al.* published a well-conceived, randomized, blinded, placebo-controlled trial of acupuncture for severe recidivist alcoholism.[42]** Their study demonstrated a persistent treatment effect of reduced desire for alcohol, fewer detoxification unit admissions, and fewer self-reported drinking episodes compared with a sham treatment. Several controlled trials for headache have shown benefit from acupuncture for both migraine and tension-type headache.[43,44]** A recent multicenter, randomized, clinical trial was undertaken to test the efficacy of acupuncture compared with sham acupuncture in the prevention of episodic tension-type headache.[45]** No differences were found between the two groups throughout the 3-month study period. In a systematic review of randomized controlled trials, Melchart and coworkers evaluated the role of acupuncture in recurrent headache disorders.[46]*** These authors concluded that acupuncture has a role in the treatment of recurrent headaches, but the quality and amount of evidence was not fully convincing. Fibromyalgia has been studied in controlled trials of acupuncture and shown to be effective with a durable benefit.[47]** Ezzo *et al.* carried out a recent systematic review of acupuncture studies for osteoarthritis of the knee.[48]*** The authors concluded that there is sufficient evidence that acupuncture may be effective in the treatment of knee osteoarthritis. In the management of low back pain, evidence is conflicting on the use of acupuncture. The Cochrane database review concluded that there is insufficient evidence for acupuncture's benefit in the management of nonspecific lower back pain.[49]*** On the other hand, a prospective randomized study comparing acupuncture with physiotherapy for low back and pelvic pain in pregnancy showed superiority of acupuncture in all measures.[50]**

HOMEOPATHY

Homeopathy is classified as a comprehensive healing system that is not embedded in a world culture. The techniques of homeopathy are both nutriceutical and energy based.

Homeopathy originated primarily as the discovery of one man – Samuel Hahnemann, a German physician who lived during the late eighteenth and early nineteenth centuries and who rejected the conventional medical practices of his time, such as bloodletting and the medicinal use of various toxic agents. Curious about the curative properties of cinchona bark for malaria, he experimented with it on himself and discovered that it produced a malaria-like illness in him. He concluded that such symptoms represented resistance to disease and that substances producing certain symptoms or effects in normal individuals would be effective in treating diseases that caused those same symptoms.[51] This led to the *doctrine of similars* or *like cures like*. Hahnemann carried out innumerable *provings* on himself and others using hundreds of substances, including botanical, animal, and mineral extracts. He developed the *Materia Medica*, a text of remedies that identified the substances and their associated effects. Many remedies were noxious and themselves toxic. Repeated dilutions would reduce the toxicity and apparently preserved and even increased the curative effect. This concept, called *potentization by dilution*, is central to homeopathic practice and puzzling to the scientific mind. Typical dilutions of remedies are designated 2X, 6X, 12X, 30c, 200c, 1000c, 10,000c, and 50,000c: 2X refers to a dilution of $1:10^2$, 6X is a dilution of $1:10^6$, and so on; 30c is a $1:100^{30}$ dilution. Substances that are diluted beyond $1:10^{24}$ result in a liquid without a single molecule of the original substance since the number of dilutions exceeds Avogadro's number. Such dilutions are common in homeopathy and impart some confidence in the safety and tolerability of the remedy. How such a liquid can exert a healing property forms the basis of homeopathy theory.

Substances are believed to contain an essential energetic property that is not diluted out, but that increases with successive dilutions. It is this energy or essence that strengthens the body's defenses against an illness. The preparation of remedies involves dilution and *succussion*, or shaking the diluent vigorously, to release or increase its energy. The potency of a remedy is determined by both the number of dilutions and the number of succussions.[52]

The homeopathic physician must take a different kind of history from the patient from the one that an allopathic physician would take. The homeopathic history is a detailed inquiry into the symptom complex and the environment and mind of the patient with respect to the symptoms. The purpose of this is to individualize the selection of remedies to match the symptoms. Classification of diseases and pathophysiology are not as important as the nature of the symptoms. Thus, diabetic neuropathy is not as relevant to a homeopathic assessment as burning, sensitive skin, interference with sleep, etc. This construct becomes useful to the allopathic practitioner particularly when the pathophysiology of symptoms such as chronic pain may be obscure.

Homeopathy is widely practiced in Europe, India, and Asia. It has a growing popularity in the USA as an alternative medicine, but was systematically excluded and obstructed by the American Medical Association in the early 1900s.[53] Forty percent of general practitioners in the

Netherlands practice homeopathy and 42% of general practitioners in Britain refer patients to homeopaths.[54]

Research

There have been many reports of the efficacy of homeopathic remedies, but few well-designed clinical trials. Kleijnen and coworkers did a meta-analytic review of 105 clinical trials of homeopathy up to 1990.[55]*** Although most of the studies were flawed methodologically, 75% showed a positive result. A randomized, double-blind study of 60 migraine sufferers demonstrated significant reductions in the number and intensity of monthly attacks in the homeopathy group compared with the placebo group. This response held for at least 2 months after treatments were discontinued.[56]** A randomized, double-blind, placebo-controlled trial of arnica 30X for muscle soreness in 519 long-distance runners found the remedy to be no more effective than placebo.[57]** Ernst and Pittler systematically reviewed the published controlled trials on *Arnica montana* and concluded that, on balance, the studies did not support the notion that arnica is more efficacious than placebo.[58]*** A controversial study of the concept of biological effects of ultrahigh dilutions was published in *Nature* in 1988.[59]** In this study, human basophils were found to release histamine when exposed to homeopathic dilutions of immunoglobulin E antiserum.

Patients seek out homeopathic treatment for a large array of mostly chronic conditions. In the USA, one survey reported that patients tended to be highly educated but uninformed about homeopathy. More than 70% reported getting some improvement in their primary symptom and nearly all were satisfied with the treatment regardless of the outcome.[60]

Risks

The extremely high dilutions of homeopathic remedies suggest the absence of risk. However, the use of toxic agents such as heavy metals, arsenic, and bromide combined with improper handling can result in adverse effects.[61] The reliability of the manufacturer is therefore an important safety factor. Avoiding remedies that use heavy metals such as mercury or cadmium may also be a warranted safety measure.

CHIROPRACTIC AND MANUAL THERAPIES

Chiropractic literally means "hand work" or "manual therapy." It can be classified as a comprehensive system of medicine or as an individual therapy in the mechanical–manipulative category. How one classifies chiropractic depends on how broadly one defines its scope. There is the school that sees chiropractic as a complete system of medicine applicable to a wide range of ailments from musculoskeletal pain to asthma and diabetes. On the other side, many chiropractors profess a narrower scope that primarily addresses neuromusculoskeletal symptoms.

History

The origination of chiropractic medicine is attributed to D. D. Palmer in the midwest of the USA in the late nineteenth century. The story goes that on September 18, 1895, Palmer cured a janitor in Iowa of deafness by manipulating a single cervical vertebra. Palmer developed a system of manual medicine techniques based on the folk medicine tradition of bonesetters and drawing on the philosophical constructs of mesmerism and vital energy, which he termed *innate intelligence*. Illness was explained by a blockage of flow of vital energy, which in turn was caused by *subluxations* of the vertebrae. Chiropractic manipulation corrects those subluxations and restores the energy flow.

In the USA there has been a long-standing battle between the institution of conventional medicine (embodied by the American Medical Association) and chiropractic. The AMA was largely successful at suppressing the legitimization of chiropractic in the first quarter of the twentieth century. By the mid-1970s every state had come to recognize chiropractic as a legitimate healing art by providing for licensing. The federal government of the USA then covered chiropractic treatment through its health care programs for the poor, the elderly, and workers' compensation. Finally, in 1990, the US Supreme Court upheld a lower court's ruling against the AMA and allied organizations for conspiring against chiropractors by prohibiting members from referring to a chiropractor.[62] More recently, the Agency for Health Care Policy and Research, a division of the Department of Health and Human Services of the US Government, approved chiropractic for the management of acute low back pain in its 1994 guidelines for acute low back problems in adults.[63]

Scope of practice

Many chiropractors do not adhere to the vitalistic view of innate intelligence, preferring a more mechanical interpretation of what goes wrong in the spine to cause disease. All schools of chiropractic rely on a construct of the *subluxation complex*, which is the target of their treatment. Other differences that distinguish various practitioners lie in the scope of techniques used. Many chiropractors employ techniques of conventional physical therapy such as the application of heat, ice, ultrasound, or electrical stimulation to the soft tissues as supplementary treatment. Some chiropractors are also trained in and prac-

23. Arner S, Meyerson BA. Lack of analgesic effect of opioids on neuropathic and idiopathic forms of pain. *Pain* 1988; **33**: 11–23.

● 24. McQuay HJ, Tramer M, Nye BA, *et al*. A systematic review of antidepressants in neuropathic pain. *Pain* 1996; **68**: 217–27.

● 25. McQuay H, Carroll D, Jadad AR, *et al*. Anticonvulsant drugs for management of pain: a systematic review. *Br Med J* 1995; **311**: 1047–52.

26. Khan OA. Gabapentin relieves trigeminal neuralgia in multiple sclerosis patients. *Neurology* 1998; **51**: 611–14.

27. Solaro C, Lunardi GL, Capello E, *et al*. An open-label trial of gabapentin treatment of paroxysmal symptoms in multiple sclerosis patients. *Neurology* 1998; **51**: 609–11.

28. Houtchens MK, Richert JR, Sami A, Rose JW. Open-label gabapentin treatment for pain in multiple sclerosis. *Multiple Sclerosis* 1997; **3**: 250–3.

29. Samkoff LM, Daras M, Tuchman AJ, Koppel BS. Amelioration of refractory dysesthetic limb pain in multiple sclerosis by gabapentin. *Neurology* 1997; **49**: 304–5.

30. Cianchetti C, Zuddas A, Randazzo AP, *et al*. Lamotrigine adjunctive therapy in painful phenomena in MS: preliminary observations. *Neurology* 1999; **53**: 433.

● 31. Kalso E, Tramer MR, McQuay HJ, Moore RA. Systemic local anaesthetic-type drugs in chronic pain: a systematic review. *Eur J Pain* 1998; **2**: 3–14.

32. Sakurai M, Kanazawa I. Positive symptoms in multiple sclerosis: their treatment with sodium channel blockers, lidocaine and mexiletine. *J Neurol Sci* 1999; **162**: 162–8.

33. United Kingdom Tizanidine Trial Group. A double blind, placebo-controlled trial of tizanidine in the treatment of spasticity caused by multiple sclerosis. *Neurology* 1994; **44** (Suppl. 9): S70–8.

34. Eide PK, Jorum E, Stubhaug A, *et al*. Relief of postherpetic neuralgia with the *N*-methyl-ᴅ-aspartic acid receptor antagonist ketamine: a double-blind, crossover comparison with morphine and placebo. *Pain* 1994; **58**: 347–54.

35. Nelson KA, Park KM, Robinovitz RN, *et al*. High-dose oral dextromethorphan versus placebo in painful diabetic neuropathy and postherpetic neuralgia. *Neurology* 1997; **48**: 1212–18.

36. Pud D, Eisenberg E, Spitzer A, *et al*. The NMDA receptor antagonist amantadine reduces surgical neuropathic pain in cancer patients: a double-blind, randomized, placebo-controlled trial. *Pain* 1998; **75**: 349–54.

● 37. McQuay HJ, Moore RA. Transcutaneous electrical nerve stimulation (TENS) in chronic pain. In: McQuay HJ, Moore RA eds. *An Evidence-based Resource for Pain Relief*. Oxford: Oxford University Press, 1998: 207–11.

38. Kidd D, Howard RS, Losseff NA, Thompson AJ. The benefit of inpatient neurorehabilitation in multiple sclerosis. *Clin Rehabil* 1995; **9**: 198–203.

39. Arner S, Lindblom U, Meyerson BA, Molander C. Prolonged relief of neuralgia after regional anesthetic blocks: a call for further experimental and systematic clinic studies. *Pain* 1990; **43**: 287–97.

40. Herman RM, Luzansky SCD, Ippolito R. Intrathecal baclofen suppresses central pain in patients with spinal lesions. *Clin J Pain* 1992; **8**: 338–45.

41. Taira T, Tanikawa T, Kawamura H, *et al*. Spinal intrathecal baclofen suppresses central pain after stroke. *J Neurol Neurosurg Psychiatry* 1994; **57**: 381–2.

42. Glynn CJ, Jamous MA, Teddy PJ, *et al*. Role of spinal noradrenergic system in transmission of pain in patients with spinal cord injury. *Lancet* 1986; **ii**: 1249–50.

43. Eisenach JC, DuPen S, Dubois M, *et al*. Epidural clonidine analgesia for intractable cancer pain. The Epidural Clonidine Study Group. *Pain* 1995; **61**: 391–9.

44. Nathan PW. Intrathecal phenol to relieve spasticity in paraplegia. *Lancet* 1959; 1099–102.

45. Hitchcock E. Hypothermic subarachnoid irrigation for intractable pain. *Lancet* 1967; **i**: 1133–5.

46. Lloyd JW. Treatment of intractable pain with cerebrospinal fluid barbotage. In: Morley TP ed. *Current Controversies in Neurosurgery*. Philadelphia, PA: WB Saunders, 1976: 520–5.

Peripheral neuropathies

PRAFULLA SHEMBALKAR AND PRAVEEN ANAND

The peripheral nervous system (PNS) is defined anatomically as the part of the nervous system in which neurons or their processes are related to Schwann cells. It includes the cranial nerves (with exception of the optic nerve), spinal nerve roots, dorsal root ganglia, peripheral nerve trunks, and nerve terminals. Any disorder of motor, sensory, or autonomic nerve fibers within the PNS could be classified as a neuropathy. The pathological processes that affect peripheral nerves may involve different sites and components of the PNS.

Peripheral neuropathies are described in different ways, based on: (1) the pattern of neurological signs and symptoms as sensory, motor, autonomic or mixed; (2) the distribution of affected nerves, as symmetrical versus asymmetrical, and distal or proximal; (3) the fiber type involved, as large versus small fiber; (4) the nature and brunt of the pathological process as axonal versus demyelinating; and (5) the time-course, as acute, subacute, or chronic. For example, multiple spinal roots are involved acutely in the Guillain–Barré syndrome, and in most cases preferentially affect the myelin sheath. The condition is thus described as an acute demyelinating inflammatory polyradiculopathy. The classification of the neuropathy narrows down the diagnostic possibilities. To illustrate, an acute onset suggests an inflammatory, immunologic, toxic, or vascular etiology. A polyneuropathy evolving subacutely over weeks and months is indicative of toxic, nutritional, or systemic diseases, whereas evolution over many years is indicative of a hereditary or metabolic disease. The dysfunction of an individual peripheral nerve is termed a mononeuropathy. The syndrome of peripheral neuropathy, however, has many causes. Therefore, it is essential to first attempt to find the cause (which is not possible always) so that the patient can be informed about prognosis and receive specific treatment. The diagnostic process can also help with choice of symptomatic treatment, as for pain, based on the understanding of pathophysiological mechanisms in different conditions.

DIAGNOSTIC POINTS IN PERIPHERAL NEUROPATHIES

1 Pathological process
  Axonal
  Demyelinating
2 Fiber type
  Large fiber
  Small fiber
  Mixed
3 Distribution of symptoms
  Symmetrical
  Asymmetrical
4 Onset of symptoms
  Acute
  Subacute
  Chronic

GENERAL CLINICAL DESCRIPTION OF NEUROPATHIC SYNDROMES

Polyneuropathies

Symptoms and signs are symmetrical and distal in most polyneuropathies.

Motor function

The feet and legs are usually affected earlier and more severely than the upper limbs. Truncal and cranial regions are the last to be affected, and are only involved in severe cases. Most of the common metabolic, toxic, and nutritional neuropathies show this predominantly distal pattern. An exception is seen in acute inflammatory neuropathies, where cranial nerve, respiratory, and upper limb involvement can occur early in the course of the disease. Facial and other cranial nerve paralyses can occur with sarcoidosis, Lyme disease, Sjögren syndrome, neoplastic invasion of meninges and nerve root infiltrations, or in rare metabolic neuropathies (Refsum, Tangier, and Riley–Day). Predominant involvement of upper limbs is unusual but may be seen in Sjögren syndrome, the chronic immune neuropathies, porphyric, lead, and amyloid polyneuropathy, and some inherited neuropathies.

Tendon reflexes

Deep tendon reflexes are diminished or lost in peripheral neuropathies as a rule. Reflexes may be diminished early in the course of neuropathy, but not absent. Reflexes may, however, be retained in small-fiber neuropathies.

Sensory loss

Like motor function, sensation is affected symmetrically and in distal segments in polyneuropathies. As the neuropathy worsens, sensory loss may spread from distal to proximal parts. In most polyneuropathies, all sensory modalities are impaired (pain and temperature, indicating small-fiber involvement; joint position and vibration sense, suggesting large-fiber dysfunction). Occasionally, selective damage to large or small fibers predominates. In polyneuropathy affecting mainly small nerve fibers, patients often present with burning, painful dysesthesiae, alteration of pinprick and temperature sensation, and autonomic dysfunction. Motor function, balance, and tendon jerks may be preserved. Some cases of amyloid and early distal diabetic polyneuropathies fall into this group. Large-fiber neuropathy, in contrast, is characterized by loss of joint position and vibration sense, ataxia, areflexia, and variable but often severe loss of motor function. In sensory neuronopathies (primary involvement of dorsal root ganglion), there is usually no motor loss.

POSITIVE SYMPTOMS IN PERIPHERAL NEUROPATHIES

Dysesthesiae, paresthesiae, and pain

Paresthesiae tend to be specially marked in the feet and hands in polyneuropathies, and localized to the affected part in other neuropathies. "Pins and needles," stabbing, pricking, tingling, electric, and band-like sensations are some of the terms used to describe these symptoms. Positive symptoms or numbness may be the only features in some neuropathies, with no objective sensory loss on clinical examination. Certain types of diabetic, nutritional, and alcohol-related neuropathies may present as "burning feet," which may be hypersensitive to touch and pin-prick.

Peripheral neuropathic pain may manifest as spontaneous pain (stimulus-independent pain), often in a numb region, or pain and hypersensitivity elicited by a stimulus (stimulus-evoked pain). Hyperalgesia is an increased response to a stimulus that is normally painful and is due to abnormal processing of nociceptor inputs. Allodynia is a pain elicited by a stimulus that does not normally provoke pain. Stimulus-evoked pain is common after peripheral nerve injury, and early small-fiber polyneuropathies. Many patients with neuropathic pain suffer from spontaneous and paroxysmal pain, with different mechanisms operating in the same subject.

MECHANISMS OF PAIN IN PERIPHERAL NEUROPATHY

Normally, impulses are generated at sensory nerve terminals or in cell bodies. In pathological states, impulses may arise from the damaged part of the axon and propagate toward both the central nervous system and the periphery. Such ectopic discharges may also arise from local patches of demyelination, neuromas, and soma in the dorsal root ganglia. The mechanisms underlying neuropathic pain have been reviewed elsewhere.[1-3] Persistent primary pain is attributed to activity in nociceptor C-fibers, which in turn leads to central changes. Similar activity in large myelinated A-fibers may produce paresthesiae, and they mediate secondary allodynia and hyperalgesia in the setting of central changes. The mechanism of ectopic discharges is attributed to changes in the expression and distribution of membrane ion channels, especially sodium channels. Two types of sodium channel are found in sensory neurons. The first are sensitive to a neurotoxin derived from the puffer fish – tetrodotoxin (TTX) – and are found in all sensory neurons. The second types are resistant to tetrodotoxin, and are found predominantly in nociceptor sensory neurons. The TTX-resistant channels have much slower activation and inactivation kinetics than TTX-sensitive channels and are implicated in pathological pain states. Channel proteins are synthesized in the cell body and transported by axoplasmic mechanisms to their peripheral targets, which include nodes of Ranvier and axon terminals. Accumulation of sodium channels at sites of ectopic impulse generation has been postulated to play a role in the ectopic discharges.[4] Recently, changes in the distribution of two TTX-resistant channels – Na_v 1.8 (SNS/PN3) and Na_v 1.9

associated with Sudeck's atrophy after injury. *Br Med J (Clin Res edn)* 1984; **288:** 173–6.

39. Veldman PH, Goris RJ. Multiple reflex sympathetic dystrophy: which patients are at risk for developing a recurrence of reflex sympathetic dystrophy in the same or another limb. *Pain* 1996; **64:** 463–6.

40. Wilhelm A. Stenosis of the subclavian vein: an unknown cause of resistant reflex sympathetic dystrophy. *Hand Clin* 1997; **13:** 387–411.

41. Mailis A, Wade J. Profile of Caucasian women with possible genetic predisposition to reflex sympathetic dystrophy: a pilot study. *Clin J Pain* 1994; **10:** 210–17.

42. Wilder RT. Reflex sympathetic dystrophy in children and adolescents: differences from adults. In: Jänig W, Stanton-Hicks M eds. *Progress in Pain Research Management.* Seattle, WA: IASP Press, 1996: 67–78.

● 43. Dietz FR, Mathews KD, Montgomery WJ. Reflex sympathetic dystrophy in children. *Clin Orthop* 1990; **258:** 225–31.

44. Kavanagh R, Crisp AJ, Hazelman BL, Coughlan RJ. Reflex sympathetic dystrophy in children: dystrophic changes are less likely [letter]. *Br Med J* 1995; **311:** 1503.

45. Beattie TF. Reflex sympathetic dystrophy in children: active early physiotherapy is the key to prevention. *Br Med J* 1995; **311:** 1503–4.

46. Stanton RP, Malcolm JR, Wesdock KA, Singsen BH. Reflex sympathetic dystrophy in children: in orthopedic perspective. *Orthopedics* 1993; **16:** 773–9.

◆ 47. Wilder RT, Berde CB, Wolohan M, *et al.* Reflex sympathetic dystrophy in children: clinical characteristics and follow-up of seventy patients. *J Bone Joint Surg Am* 1992; **74:** 910–19.

48. Geertzen JH, Dijkstra PU, Groothoff JW, *et al.* Reflex sympathetic dystrophy of the upper extremity – a 5.5-year follow-up. I. Impairments and perceived disability. *Acta Orthop Scand Suppl* 1998; **279:** 12–18.

49. Geertzen JH, Dijkstra PU, Groothoff JW, *et al.* Reflex sympathetic dystrophy of the upper extremity – a 5.5-year follow-up. II. Social life events, general health and changes in occupation. *Acta Orthop Scand Suppl* 1998; **279:** 19–23.

50. Zyluk A. The natural history of post-traumatic reflex sympathetic dystrophy. *J Hand Surg* 1998; **23:** 20–3.

● 51. Baron R. The influence of sympathetic nerve activity and catecholamines on primary afferent neurons. *IASP Newsletter* 1998: May/June: 3–7.

52. McMahon SB. Mechanisms of sympathetic pain. *Br Med Bull* 1991; **47:** 584–600.

53. Zochodne DW. Epineurial peptides: a role in neuropathic pain? *Can J Neurol Sci* 1993; **20:** 69–72.

54. Sommer C, Galbraith JA, Heckman HM, Myers RR. Pathology of experimental compression neuropathy producing hyperalgesia. *J Neuropathol Exp Neurol* 1993; **52:** 223–33.

55. Sorkin LS, Xiao WH, Wagner R, Myers RR. Tumour necrosis factor-alpha induces ectopic activity in noci-

ceptive primary afferent fibres. *Neuroscience* 1997; **81:** 255–62.

56. Wagner R, Janjigian M, Myers RR. Anti-inflammatory interleukin-10 therapy in CCI neuropathy decreases thermal hyperalgesia, macrophage recruitment, and endoneurial TNF-alpha expression. *Pain* 1998; **74:** 35–42.

◆ 57. Drummond PD, Skipworth S, Finch PM. Alpha 1-adrenoceptors in normal and hyperalgesic human skin. *Clin Sci* 1996; **91:** 73–7.

58. Novakovic SD, Tzoumaka E, McGivern JG, *et al.* Distribution of the tetrodotoxin-resistant sodium channel PN3 in rat sensory neurons in normal and neuropathic conditions. *J Neurosci* 1998; **18:** 2174–87.

59. Cummins TR, Waxman SG. Downregulation of tetrodotoxin-resistant sodium currents and upregulation of a rapidly repriming tetrodotoxin-sensitive sodium current in small spinal sensory neurons after nerve injury. *J Neurosci* 1997; **17:** 3503–14.

◆ 60. Levine JD, Fields HL, Basbaum AI. Peptides and the primary afferent nociceptor. *J Neurosci* 1993; **13:** 2273–86.

◆ 61. Chabal C, Jacobson L, Russell LC, Burchiel KJ. Pain response to perineuromal injection of normal saline, epinephrine, and lidocaine in humans. *Pain* 1992; **49:** 9–12.

62. Choi B, Rowbotham MC. Effect of adrenergic receptor activation on post-herpetic neuralgia pain and sensory disturbances. *Pain* 1997; **69:** 55–63.

63. Kurvers H, Daemen M, Slaaf D, *et al.* Partial peripheral neuropathy and denervation induced adrenoceptor supersensitivity: functional studies in an experimental model. *Acta Orthop Belg* 1998; **64:** 64–70.

◆ 64. Jänig W, Levine JD, Michaelis M. Interactions of sympathetic and primary afferent neurons following nerve injury and tissue trauma. *Prog Brain Res* 1996; **113:** 161–84.

65. Sato J, Perl ER. Adrenergic excitation of cutaneous pain receptors induced by peripheral nerve injury. *Science* 1991; **251:** 1608–10.

66. Chen Y, Michaelis M, Jänig W, Devor M. Adrenoreceptor subtype mediating sympathetic-sensory coupling in injured sensory neurons. *J Neurophysiol* 1996; **76:** 3721–30.

67. Gonzales R, Goldyne ME, Taiwo YO, Levine JD. Production of hyperalgesic prostaglandins by sympathetic postganglionic neurons. *J Neurochem* 1989; **53:** 1595–8.

68. Taiwo YO, Levine JD. Prostaglandin effects after elimination of indirect hyperalgesic mechanisms in the skin of the rat. *Brain Res* 1989; **492:** 397–9.

69. Taiwo YO, Bjerknes LK, Goetzl EJ, Levine JD. Mediation of primary afferent peripheral hyperalgesia by the cAMP second messenger system. *Neuroscience* 1989; **32:** 577–80.

70. Buritova J, Chapman V, Honore P, Besson JM. Interactions between NMDA- and prostaglandin receptor-

mediated events in a model of inflammatory nociception. *Eur J Pharmacol* 1996; **303:** 91–100.

71. Chapman V, Honore P, Buritova J, Besson JM. The contribution of NMDA receptor activation to spinal c-Fos expression in a model of inflammatory pain. *Br J Pharmacol* 1995; **116:** 1628–34.

72. Chapman V, Buritova J, Honore P, Besson JM. Physiological contributions of neurokinin 1 receptor activation, and interactions with NMDA receptors, to inflammatory-evoked spinal c-Fos expression. *J Neurophysiol* 1996; **76:** 1817–27.

73. Aguayo AJ, Bray GM. Pathology and pathophysiology of unmyelinated nerve fibers. In: Dyck PJ, Thomas PK, Lambert EH eds. *Peripheral Neuropathy*. Philadelphia, PA: W. B. Saunders, 1975: 363–78.

74. Belenky M, Devor M. Association of postganglionic sympathetic neurons with primary afferents in sympathetic-sensory co-cultures. *J Neurocytol* 1997; **26:** 715–31.

75. Melzack R, Wall PD. Pain mechanisms: a new theory. *Science* 1965; **150:** 971–9.

76. Cho HJ, Kim DS, Lee NH, *et al.* Changes in the alpha 2-adrenergic receptor subtypes gene expression in rat dorsal root ganglion in an experimental model of neuropathic pain. *Neuroreport* 1997; **8:** 3119–22.

77. Chung K, Lee BH, Yoon YW, Chung JM. Sympathetic sprouting in the dorsal root ganglia of the injured peripheral nerve in a rat neuropathic pain model. *J Comp Neurol* 1996; **376:** 241–52.

◆ 78. McLachlan EM, Jänig W, Devor M, Michaelis M. Peripheral nerve injury triggers noradrenergic sprouting within dorsal root ganglia. *Nature* 1993; **363:** 543–6.

79. Ramer MS, French GD, Bisby MA. Wallerian degeneration is required for both neuropathic pain and sympathetic sprouting into the DRG. *Pain* 1997; **72:** 71–8.

80. Petersen M, Zhang J, Zhang JM, LaMotte RH. Abnormal spontaneous activity and responses to norepinephrine in dissociated dorsal root ganglion cells after chronic nerve constriction. *Pain* 1996; **67:** 391–7.

81. McMahon SB. NGF as a mediator of inflammatory pain. *Philos Trans R Soc Lond (Biol)* 1996; **351:** 431–40.

82. Woolf CJ. Phenotypic modification of primary sensory neurons: the role of nerve growth factor in the production of persistent pain. *Philos Trans R Soc Lond (Biol)* 1996; **351:** 441–8.

83. Ascher P, Nowak L. The role of divalent cations in the N-methyl-D-aspartate responses of mouse central neurones in culture. *J Physiol* 1988; **399:** 247–66.

84. Nowak L, Bregestovski P, Ascher P, *et al.* Magnesium gates glutamate-activated channels in mouse central neurones. *Nature* 1984; **307:** 462–5.

◆ 85. Woolf CJ, Shortland P, Coggeshall RE. Peripheral nerve injury triggers central sprouting of myelinated afferents. *Nature* 1992; **355:** 75–8.

86. Kim HJ, Na HS, Sung B, Hong SK. Amount of sympathetic sprouting in the dorsal root ganglia is not correlated to the level of sympathetic dependence of

neuropathic pain in a rat model. *Neurosci Lett* 1998; **245:** 21–4.

◆ 87. Oyen WJ, Arntz IE, Claessens RM, *et al.* Reflex sympathetic dystrophy of the hand: an excessive inflammatory response? *Pain* 1993; **55:** 151–7.

88. van der Laan L, Goris RJ. Reflex sympathetic dystrophy: an exaggerated regional inflammatory response? *Hand Clin* 1997; **13:** 373–85.

89. Ramirez JM, French AS. Phentolamine selectively affects the fast sodium component of sensory adaptation in an insect mechanoreceptor. *J Neurobiol* 1990; **21:** 893–9.

90. Downing OA, Juul P. The effect of guanethidine pretreatment on transmission in the superior cervical ganglion. *Acta Pharmacol Toxicol (Copenhagen)* 1973; **32:** 369–81.

91. Brock JA, Cunnane TC. Studies on the mode of action of bretylium and guanethidine in post-ganglionic sympathetic nerve fibres. *Naunyn Schmiedebergs Arch Pharmacol* 1988; **338:** 504–9.

92. Walker AE, Nulson F. Electrical stimulation of the upper thoracic portion of the sympathetic chain in man. *Arch Neurol Psychiatry* 1948; **59:** 559–60.

◆ 93. Torebjork E, Wahren L, Wallin G, *et al.* Noradrenaline-evoked pain in neuralgia. *Pain* 1995; **63:** 11–20.

94. Tracey DJ, Cunningham JE, Romm MA. Peripheral hyperalgesia in experimental neuropathy: mediation by α_2-adrenoreceptors on postganglionic sympathetic terminals. *Pain* 1995; **60:** 317–27.

◆ 95. Drummond PD, Finch PM, Gibbins I. Innervation of hyperalgesic skin in patients with complex regional pain syndrome. *Clin J Pain* 1996; **12:** 222–31.

◆ 96. Drummond PD, Finch PM, Smythe GA. Reflex sympathetic dystrophy: the significance of differing plasma catecholamine concentrations in affected and unaffected limbs. *Brain* 1991; **114:** 2025–36.

97. Harden RN, Duc TA, Williams TR, *et al.* Norepinephrine and epinephrine levels in affected versus unaffected limbs in sympathetically maintained pain. *Clin J Pain* 1994; **10:** 324–30.

98. Wasner G, Schattschneider J, Heckmann K, *et al.* Vascular abnormalities in reflex sympathetic dystrophy (CRPS I): mechanisms and diagnostic value. *Brain* 2001; **124:** 587–99.

◆ 99. van der Laan L, ter Laak HJ, Gabreels-Festen A, *et al.* Complex regional pain syndrome type I (RSD): pathology of skeletal muscle and peripheral nerve. *Neurology* 1998; **51:** 20–5.

100. Bruehl S, Husfeldt B, Lubenow TR, *et al.* Psychological differences between reflex sympathetic dystrophy and non-RSD chronic pain patients. *Pain* 1996; **67:** 107–14.

101. DeGood DE, Cundiff GW, Adams LE, Shutty Jr MS. A psychosocial and behavioral comparison of reflex sympathetic dystrophy, low back pain, and headache patients. *Pain* 1993; **54:** 317–22.

●102. Lynch ME. Psychological aspects of reflex sympathetic

dystrophy: a review of the adult and paediatric literature. *Pain* 1992; **49:** 337–47.

103. Ciccone DS, Bandilla EB, Wu W. Psychological dysfunction in patients with reflex sympathetic dystrophy. *Pain* 1997; **71:** 323–33.

●104. Bruehl S, Carlson CR. Predisposing psychological factors in the development of reflex sympathetic dystrophy: a review of the empirical evidence. *Clin J Pain* 1992; **8:** 287–99.

●105. Van Houdenhove B, Vasquez G, Onghena P, *et al*. Etiopathogenesis of reflex sympathetic dystrophy: a review and biopsychosocial hypothesis. *Clin J Pain* 1992; **8:** 300–6.

106. Covington EC. Psychological issues in reflex sympathetic dystrophy. In: Jänig W, Stanton-Hicks M eds. *Progress in Pain Research Management*. Seattle, WA: IASP Press, 1996: 191–216.

107. Geertzen JH, de Bruijn-Kofman AT, deBruijn HP, *et al*. Stressful life events and psychological dysfunction in complex regional pain syndrome type I. *Clin J Pain* 1998; **14:** 143–7.

◆108. Kubler-Ross E, Wessler S, Avioli LV. On death and dying. *JAMA* 1972; **221:** 174–9.

109. Hardin KN. Chronic pain management. In: Camic P, Knight S eds. *Clinical Handbook of Health Psychology*. Seattle, WA: Hogrefe & Huber, 1998: 123–65.

◆110. Wilson PR, Low PA, Bedder MD, *et al*. Diagnostic algorithm for complex regional pain syndromes. In: Jänig W, Stanton-Hicks M eds. *Progress in Pain Research Management*. Seattle, WA: IASP Press, 1996: 93–106.

111. Simon DL. Algorithm for timely recognition and treatment of complex regional pain syndrome (CRPS): a new approach for objective assessment [letter]. *Clin J Pain* 1997; **13:** 264–72.

112. Galer BS, Bruehl S, Harden RN. IASP diagnostic criteria for complex regional pain syndrome: a preliminary empirical validation study. International Association for the Study of Pain. *Clin J Pain* 1998; **14:** 48–54.

●113. Fournier RS, Holder LE. Reflex sympathetic dystrophy: diagnostic controversies. *Semin Nucl Med* 1998; **28:** 116–23.

114. Gibbons JJ, Wilson PR. RSD score: criteria for the diagnosis of reflex sympathetic dystrophy and causalgia. *Clin J Pain* 1992; **8:** 260–3.

◆115. Chelimsky TC, Low PA, Naessens JM, *et al*. Value of autonomic testing in reflex sympathetic dystrophy. *Mayo Clin Proc* 1995; **70:** 1029–40.

116. Willner C, Low PA. Laboratory evaluation of complex regional pain syndrome. In: Low PA ed. *Clinical Autonomic Disorders: Evaluation and Management*, 2nd edn. Philadelphia, PA: Lippincott-Raven, 1997: 209–20.

117. Birklein F, Riedl B, Claus D, Neundorfer B. Pattern of autonomic dysfunction in time course of complex regional pain syndrome. *Clin Auton Res* 1998; **8:** 79–85.

118. Birklein F, Sittl R, Spitzer A, *et al*. Sudomotor function in sympathetic reflex dystrophy. *Pain* 1997; **69:** 49–54.

119. Low PA. Autonomic nervous system function. *J Clin Neurophysiol* 1993; **10:** 14–27.

120. Thimineur MA, Saberski L. Complex regional pain syndrome type I (RSD) or peripheral mononeuropathy? A discussion of three cases. *Clin J Pain* 1996; **12:** 145–50.

◆121. Baron R, Maier C. Reflex sympathetic dystrophy: skin blood flow, sympathetic vasoconstrictor reflexes and pain before and after surgical sympathectomy. *Pain* 1996; **67:** 317–26.

◆122. Dellemijn PL, Fields HL, Allen RR, *et al*. The interpretation of pain relief and sensory changes following sympathetic blockade. *Brain* 1994; **117:** 1475–87.

123. Kurvers HA, Jacobs MJ, Beuk RJ, *et al*. Reflex sympathetic dystrophy: evolution of microcirculatory disturbances in time. *Pain* 1995; **60:** 333–40.

124. Birklein F, Riedl B, Neundorfer B, Handwerker HO. Sympathetic vasoconstrictor reflex pattern in patients with complex regional pain syndrome. *Pain* 1998; **75:** 93–100.

125. Baron R, Wasner GL, Borgstedt R. Interaction of sympathetic nerve activity and capsaicin evoked spontaneous pain and vasodilatation in humans. *Neurology* 1998; **50:** 45.

126. Arnold JM, Teasell RW, MacLeod AP, *et al*. Increased venous alpha-adrenoceptor responsiveness in patients with reflex sympathetic dystrophy. *Ann Intern Med* 1993; **118:** 619–21.

127. Bruehl S, Lubenow TR, Nath H, Ivankovich O. Validation of thermography in the diagnosis of reflex sympathetic dystrophy. *Clin J Pain* 1996; **12:** 316–25.

128. Gulevich SJ, Conwell TD, Lane J, *et al*. Stress infrared telethermography is useful in the diagnosis of complex regional pain syndrome, type I (formerly reflex sympathetic dystrophy). *Clin J Pain* 1997; **13:** 50–9.

129. Heerschap A, den Hollander JA, Reynen H, Goris RJ. Metabolic changes in reflex sympathetic dystrophy: a 31P NMR spectroscopy study. *Muscle Nerve* 1993; **16:** 367–73.

●130. Sintzoff S, Sintzoff Jr S, Stallenberg B, Matos C. Imaging in reflex sympathetic dystrophy. *Hand Clin* 1997; **13:** 431–42.

131. Hohmann EL, Elde RP, Rysavy JA, *et al*. Innervation of periosteum and bone by sympathetic vasoactive intestinal peptide-containing nerve fibers. *Science* 1986; **232:** 868–71.

132. Cepollaro C, Gonnelli S, Pondrelli C, *et al*. Usefulness of ultrasound in Sudeck's atrophy of the foot. *Calcif Tissue Int* 1998; **62:** 538–41.

133. Lee GW, Weeks PM. The role of bone scintigraphy in diagnosing reflex sympathetic dystrophy. *J Hand Surg* 1995; **20:** 458–63.

134. Hoffman J, Phillips W, Blum M, *et al*. Effect of sympathetic block demonstrated by triple-phase bone scan. *J Hand Surg* 1993; **18:** 860–4.

135. Weiss L, Alfano A, Bardfeld P, *et al*. Prognostic value of triple phase bone scanning for reflex sympathetic dys-

trophy in hemiplegia. *Arch Phys Med Rehabil* 1993; **74:** 716–19.

136. Schweitzer ME, Mandel S, Schwartzman RJ, *et al*. Reflex sympathetic dystrophy revisited: MR imaging findings before and after infusion of contrast material. *Radiology* 1995; **195:** 211–14.

137. Lechevalier D, Dubayle P, Crozes P, *et al*. Magnetic resonance imaging in the warm and cold forms of algodystrophy of the foot. *J Radiol* 1996; **77:** 411–17.

◆138. Vallbo AB, Hagbarth KE, Torebjork HE, Wallin BG. Somatosensory, proprioceptive, and sympathetic activity in human peripheral nerves. *Physiol Rev* 1979; **59:** 919–57.

139. Torebjork E. Human microneurography and intraneural microstimulation in the study of neuropathic pain. *Muscle Nerve* 1993; **16:** 1063–5.

140. Cline MA, Ochoa J, Torebjork HE. Chronic hyperalgesia and skin warming caused by sensitized C nociceptors. *Brain* 1989; **112:** 621–47.

141. Torebjork HE, Lundberg LE, LaMotte RH. Central changes in processing of mechanoreceptive input in capsaicin-induced secondary hyperalgesia in humans. *J Physiol* 1992; **448:** 765–80.

142. Schmidt R, Schmelz M, Forster C, *et al*. Novel classes of responsive and unresponsive C nociceptors in human skin. *J Neurosci* 1995; **15:** 333–41.

●143. Roberts WJ. A hypothesis on the physiological basis for causalgia and related pains. *Pain* 1986; **24:** 297–311.

144. Dotson R, Ochoa J, Cline M, *et al*. Sympathetic effects on human low threshold mechanoreceptors. *Soc Neurosci Abs* 1990; **16:** 1280.

145. Sato J, Suzuki S, Iseki T, Kumazawa T. Adrenergic excitation of cutaneous nociceptors in chronically inflamed rats. *Neurosci Lett* 1993; **164:** 225–8.

146. Gold MS, White DM, Ahlgren SC, *et al*. Catecholamine-induced mechanical sensitization of cutaneous nociceptors in the rat. *Neurosci Lett* 1994; **175:** 166–70.

147. Dotson R, Ochoa J, Cline M, *et al*. Intraneuronal microstimulation of low threshold mechanoreceptors in patients with causalgia/RSD/SMP. *Soc Neurosci Abs* 1992; **18:** 290.

148. Casale R, Elam M. Normal sympathetic nerve activity in a reflex sympathetic dystrophy with marked skin vasoconstriction. *J Auton Nerv Syst* 1992; **41:** 215–19.

149. Clinchot DM, Lorch F. Sympathetic skin response in patients with reflex sympathetic dystrophy. *Am J Phys Med Rehabil* 1996; **75:** 252–6.

150. Low PA, Wilson PR, Sandroni P, *et al*. Clinical characteristics of patients with reflex sympathetic dystrophy (sympathetically maintained pain) in the USA. In: Jänig W, Stanton-Hicks M eds. *Progress in Pain Research Management*. Seattle, WA: IASP Press, 1996: 49–66.

●151. Boas RA. Sympathetic nerve blocks: in search of a role. *Reg Anesth Pain Med* 1998; **23:** 292–305.

●152. Kingery WS. A critical review of controlled clinical trials for peripheral neuropathic pain and complex regional pain syndromes. *Pain* 1997; **73:** 123–39.

●153. MacFarlane BV, Wright A, O'Callaghan J, Benson HA. Chronic neuropathic pain and its control by drugs. *Pharmacol Ther* 1997; **75:** 1–19.

154. Viel E, Pelissier J, Draussin G, *et al*. Algodystrophies of the limbs: physiopathology, preventive aspects. *Cah Anesthesiol* 1993; **41:** 163–8.

155. Ribbers GM, Geurts AC, Rijken RA, Kerkkamp HE. Axillary brachial plexus blockade for the reflex sympathetic dystrophy syndrome. *Int J Rehabil Res* 1997; **20:** 371–80.

156. Price DD, Long S, Wilsey B, Rafii A. Analysis of peak magnitude and duration of analgesia produced by local anesthetics injected into sympathetic ganglia of complex regional pain syndrome patients. *Clin J Pain* 1998; **14:** 216–26.

◆157. Rocco AG, Kaul AF, Reisman RM, *et al*. A comparison of regional intravenous guanethidine and reserpine in reflex sympathetic dystrophy: a controlled, randomized, double-blind crossover study. *Clin J Pain* 1989; **5:** 205–9.

158. Valentin N. Reflex sympathetic dystrophy treated with guanethidine: time for a change of name and strategy. *Acta Anaesthesiol Scand* 1996; **40:** 1171–2.

159. Kaplan R, Claudio M, Kepes E, Gu XF. Intravenous guanethidine in patients with reflex sympathetic dystrophy. *Acta Anaesthesiol Scand* 1996; **40:** 1216–22.

◆160. Jadad AR, Carroll D, Glynn CJ, McQuay HJ. Intravenous regional sympathetic blockade for pain relief in reflex sympathetic dystrophy: a systematic review and a randomized, double-blind crossover study. *J Pain Sympt Manage* 1995; **10:** 13–20.

161. Galer BS. Peak pain relief is delayed and duration of relief is extended following intravenous phentolamine infusion: preliminary report. *Reg Anesth* 1995; **20:** 444–7.

162. Hord AH, Rooks MD, Stephens BO, *et al*. Intravenous regional bretylium and lidocaine for treatment of reflex sympathetic dystrophy: a randomized, double-blind study. *Anesth Analg* 1992; **74:** 818–21.

163. Davis KD, Treede RD, Raja SN, *et al*. Topical application of clonidine relieves hyperalgesia in patients with sympathetically maintained pain. *Pain* 1991; **47:** 309–17.

164. Reuben SS, Steinberg RB, Madabhushi L, Rosenthal E. Intravenous regional clonidine in the management of sympathetically maintained pain. *Anesthesiology* 1998; **89:** 527–30.

165. Rauck RL, Eisenach JC, Jackson K, *et al*. Epidural clonidine treatment for refractory reflex sympathetic dystrophy. *Anesthesiology* 1993; **79:** 1163–9.

166. Bragstad A, Blikra G. Evaluation of a new skeletal muscle relaxant in the treatment of low back pain. *Curr Ther Res* 1979; **26:** 39–43.

167. Damulin IV. The use of sirdalud in painful muscle tonic syndromes. *Ter Arkh* 1997; **69:** 68–72.

168. Malik VK, Inchiosa Jr MA, Mustafa K, *et al*. Intravenous regional phenoxybenzamine in the treatment of reflex

sympathetic dystrophy. *Anesthesiology* 1998; **88:** 823–7.

169. Muizelaar JP, Kleyer M, Hertogs IA, DeLange DC. Complex regional pain syndrome (reflex sympathetic dystrophy and causalgia): management with the calcium channel blocker nifedipine and/or the alpha-sympathetic blocker phenoxybenzamine in 59 patients. *Clin Neurol Neurosurg* 1997; **99:** 26–30.

170. Stevens DS, Robins VF, Price HM. Treatment of sympathetically maintained pain with terazosin. *Reg Anesth* 1993; **18:** 318–21.

171. Schwartzman RJ, Liu JE, Smullens SN, *et al*. Long-term outcome following sympathectomy for complex regional pain syndrome type 1 (RSD). *J Neurol Sci* 1997; **150:** 149–52.

◆172. Valley MA, Rogers JN, Gale DW. Relief of recurrent upper extremity sympathetically-maintained pain with contralateral sympathetic blocks: evidence for cross-over sympathetic innervation. *J Pain Symptom Manage* 1995; **10:** 396–400.

173. Rocco AG. Radiofrequency lumbar sympatholysis: the evolution of a technique for managing sympathetically maintained pain. *Reg Anesth* 1995; **20:** 3–12.

174. Raja SN, Treede RD, Davis KD, Campbell JN. Systemic alpha-adrenergic blockade with phentolamine: a diagnostic test for sympathetically maintained pain. *Anesthesiology* 1991; **74:** 691–8.

175. Farah BA. Ketorolac in reflex sympathetic dystrophy. *Clin Neuropharmacol* 1993; **16:** 88–9.

176. Grundberg AB. Reflex sympathetic dystrophy: treatment with long-acting intramuscular corticosteroids. *J Hand Surg* 1996; **21:** 667–70.

177. Manahan AP, Burkman KA, Malesker MA, Benecke GW. Clinical observation on the use of topical nitroglycerin in the management of severe shoulder-hand syndrome. *Nebr Med J* 1993; **78:** 87–9.

178. Rosenberg JM, Harrell C, Ristic H, *et al*. The effect of gabapentin on neuropathic pain. *Clin J Pain* 1997; **13:** 251–5.

179. Mellick GA, Mellicy LB, Mellick LB. Gabapentin in the management of reflex sympathetic dystrophy [letter]. *J Pain Sympt Manage* 1995; **10:** 265–6.

180. Linchitz RM, Raheb JC. Subcutaneous infusion of lidocaine provides effective pain relief for CRPS patients. *Clin J Pain* 1999; **15:** 67–72.

181. Takahashi H, Miyazaki M, Nanbu T, *et al*. The NMDA-receptor antagonist ketamine abolishes neuropathic

pain after epidural administration in a clinical case. *Pain* 1998; **75:** 391–4.

182. Crowley KL, Flores JA, Hughes CN, Iacono RP. Clinical application of ketamine ointment in the treatment of sympathetically maintained pain. *Int J Pharm Compounding* 1998; **2:** 122–7.

183. van Hilten BJ, van de Beek WJ, Hoff JI, *et al*. Intrathecal baclofen for the treatment of dystonia in patients with reflex sympathetic dystrophy. *N Engl J Med* 2000; **343:** 625–30.

184. Fraioli F, Fabbri A, Gnessi L, *et al*. Subarachnoid injection of salmon calcitonin induces analgesia in man. *Eur J Pharmacol* 1982; **78:** 381–2.

185. Bickerstaff DR, Kanis JA. The use of nasal calcitonin in the treatment of post-traumatic algodystrophy. *Br J Rheumatol* 1991; **30:** 291–4.

186. Gobelet C, Meier JL, Schaffner W, *et al*. Calcitonin and reflex sympathetic dystrophy syndrome. *Clin Rheumatol* 1986; **5:** 382–8.

187. Hassenbusch SJ, Stanton-Hicks M, Schoppa D, *et al*. Long-term results of peripheral nerve stimulation for reflex sympathetic dystrophy. *J Neurosurg* 1996; **84:** 415–23.

188. Robaina FJ, Rodriguez JL, de Vera JA, Martin MA. Transcutaneous electrical nerve stimulation and spinal cord stimulation for pain relief in reflex sympathetic dystrophy. *Stereotact Funct Neurosurg* 1989; **52:** 53–62.

189. Kemler MA, Barendse GA, van Kleef M, *et al*. Spinal cord stimulation in patients with chronic reflex sympathetic dystrophy. *N Engl J Med* 2000; **343:** 618–24.

190. Dielissen PW, Claassen AT, Veldman PH, Goris RJ. Amputation for reflex sympathetic dystrophy. *J Bone Joint Surg Br* 1995; **77:** 270–3.

191. Bengtson K. Physical modalities for complex regional pain syndrome. *Hand Clin* 1997; **13:** 443–54.

192. Fialka V, Resch KL, Ritter-Dietrich D, *et al*. Acupuncture for reflex sympathetic dystrophy [letter]. *Arch Intern Med* 1993; **153:** 661–5.

193. Price DD, Gracely RH, Bennett GJ. The challenge and the problem of placebo in assessment of sympathetically maintained pain. In: Jänig W, Stanton-Hicks M eds. *Progress in Pain Research Management*. Seattle, WA: IASP Press, 1996: 173–90.

◆194. Verdugo RJ, Ochoa JL. Reversal of hypoaesthesia by nerve block, or placebo: a psychologically mediated sign in chronic pseudoneuropathic pain patients. *J Neurol Neurosurg Psychiatry* 1998; **65:** 196–203.

Central pain syndromes

GILBERT R GONZALES AND KENNETH L CASEY

Central pain (CP) refers to pain that results from a lesion within the central nervous system (CNS). The lesion – or, more specifically, the pathology – can be within the spinal cord, the brainstem, the thalamus, or the suprathalamic regions of the brain. The definition provided by the taxonomy committee of the International Association for the Study of Pain describes CP as regional pain usually associated with abnormal sensibility to temperature and to noxious stimulation.[1] Historically, as early as the eighteenth century, cases of severe pain associated with cerebrovascular lesions as well as with ischemic injuries of the brainstem were reported by neurologists.[2] In addition to this, Wallenberg syndrome, or lateral medullary stroke, was described as being associated with painful manifestations; later, in the nineteenth century, pain arising from lesions in the CNS, including the thalamus, was described in case and pathology reports.[3–5] An emerging picture of the role of the thalamus in CP was described in 1903 by Dejerine and Egger.[6] In 1906, Dejerine and Roussy described the specific CP syndrome known as thalamic syndrome (Table 30.1).[7]

The current definition of CP includes a variety of subtypes of CP, including Dejerine–Roussy syndrome (also known as thalamic syndrome), spinal cord CP, and CP from a number of locations within the CNS, with the common pathway of involvement being the spinothalamocortical tracts. The original definition by Riddoch, proposed in 1938, remains the most descriptive and applicable definition given so far.[8] Riddoch's description is that "by central pain is meant spontaneous pain and painful overreaction to objective stimulation resulting from lesions confined to the substance of the central nervous system including dysesthesia of a disagreeable kind."

A number of definitions that relate to CP are listed in Table 30.2.

ETIOLOGY

As previously stated, all levels of the central somatosensory nervous system pathways have been implicated as sites for the origin of CP when these sites are injured. Previous descriptions have focused on the pathoanatomic characteristics of lesions producing CP (see Table 30.3). Recently, Pagni[2] defined lesions causing CP according to their being either spontaneous or iatrogenic. The spontaneous lesions of the parietal cortex, the subcortical white matter, the suprathalamic white matter, the internal capsule, and the thalamus are predominantly poststroke injuries to the pathways leading to the cortex from the thalamus. Other lesions besides ischemic lesions have led to CP, including those caused by trauma, metastases, hemorrhage, arteriovenous malformation, and aneurysms and those caused by infections, including tuberculosis and toxoplasmosis abscesses. At the brainstem

Table 30.1 *Symptoms and findings in Dejerine–Roussy syndrome*[7]

Hemiparesis that regresses rapidly and does not include spasticity[a]
Decreased sensitivity to touch, pain, and temperature, with a disturbance of deep sensation and sometimes replaced by cutaneous hyperalgesia[a]
Ataxia on the affected side with astereognosis[a]
Severe and paroxysmal pain on the hemiparetic side
Choreoathetoid movements of paretic limbs

a. Consistent findings.

Table 30.2 *Definition of terms found in the central pain literature*

Acuesthesia	Ability to distinguish between sharp and blunt
Allachesthesia (allochiria)	Contralateral pain after stimulating an affected hypoesthetic area in paraplegia
Allodynia	Pain due to stimulus which does not normally provoke pain
Anesthesia	Absence of pain in response to stimulation which would normally be painful
Anesthesia dolorosa	Pain in an area which is anesthetic
Dysesthesia	An unpleasant abnormal sensation, whether spontaneous or evoked
Epicritic	Sharp pain associated with pathways involved with light touch, two-point discrimination, and small differences in temperature; lemniscal pathways
Hyperalgesia	An increased response to a stimulus which is normally painful
Hyperesthesia	Increased sensitivity to stimulation, excluding the special senses
Hyperpathia	A painful syndrome characterized by an abnormally painful reaction to a stimulus, especially a repetitive stimulus, as well as an increased threshold
Hypoalgesia	Diminished pain in response to a normally painful stimulus
Hypoesthesia	Decreased sensitivity to stimulation, excluding the special senses
Isothermognosis	All stimuli applied to the territory affected by procedures such as cordotomy are perceived as heat
Mitempfindung	"With sympathy;" a tactile sensation is referred to a point other than that which the stimulus has affected, including displaced tactile sensations such as graphesthesia
Neuralgia	Pain in the distribution of a nerve or nerves
Neurogenic pain	Pain initiated or caused by a primary lesion, dysfunction, or transitory perturbation in the peripheral or central nervous system
Neuropathic pain	Pain initiated or caused by a primary lesion or dysfunction in the nervous system
Neuropathy	A disturbance of function or pathological change in a nerve
Paresthesia	An abnormal sensation, whether spontaneous or evoked
Protopathic	Slow burning associated with pain and temperature pathways; reticular pathways
Remote pain	Spinal cord pain referred below the level of injury
Synesthesalgesia	Stimulation of the normal side gives rise to excruciating pain

Table 30.3 *Pathoanatomic characteristics of lesions resulting in central pain*

Location in CNS	Type of lesion	References
Parietal cortex	Trauma, cerebrovascular accident, metastatic tumor	9
Subcortical white matter	Infarct, hemorrhage, metastasis, AVM, aneurysm	9, 10
Suprathalamic white matter	Lacune, hemorrhage, tumor, AVM	9, 11
Internal capsule	Lacune, hemorrhage	12
Thalamus	Trauma, infarct, AVM, primary tumor, metastasis, thalamic extension of syringobulbia, vasculitis with infarct, tuberculosis, stereotactic lesion (VPL/VPM), hemorrhage, abscess	Tuberculosis, 13; hemorrhage, 13–17; abscess 18, 19
Brain stem	Syringobulbia, extra-axial mass (tuberculosis), ischemic lateral bulbar syndrome, bulbopontine multiple sclerosis	20–22
Spinal cord	Syringomyelia, multiple sclerosis, vascular lesion of cord, traumatic hematomyelia of cervical cord, traumatic hemisection of cord, anterolateral cordotomy in a patient operated on for relief of pain of peripheral origin, syphilitic myelitis	8, 23, 12

CNS, central nervous system; AVM, arteriovenous malformation; VPL/VPM, ventral posterolateral nucleus/ventral posteromedial nucleus.
Source: Gonzales GR. Central pain. *Semin Neurol* 1994; **14**: 255–62.

level, again ischemic lesions such as the lateral medullary or Wallenberg syndrome are the most common causes of CP, although multiple sclerosis and syringobulbia along with extra-axial compressive masses can also produce CP at this level. Spinal cord lesions producing CP are predominantly traumatic, although multiple sclerosis, syringomyelia, and vascular lesions of the cord can also produce spinal cord CP.

Iatrogenic lesions, which are much less common, include surgical lesions that have been produced primarily to treat other painful syndromes but that have resulted in CP as a direct consequence of the surgical procedure.

Iatrogenic lesions include parietal cortectomy, hemispherectomy, thalamotomies, mesencephalotomies, and bulbar tractotomies, including bulbar trigeminal tractotomy of Sjöqvist. Anterolateral cordotomies, both open and percutaneously performed, have resulted in spinal cord CP. Also, commissural myelotomy, section of the tract of Lissauer, posterior radiculotomy, dorsal root entry zone coagulation, cordectomy, and pyramidotomies and extrapyramidotomies of the spinal cord have all been reported to result in iatrogenic CP.

Supraspinal CP is predominantly caused by strokes: more than 90% of CP cases result from strokes and 78%

As aging progresses, normal changes in the body which affect residual limb pain include decreased perfusion of the distal end of the residual limb corresponding to generally decreased blood flow, thinning skin, shrinking muscles, and thinning fat pads. All of these changes affect the way the prosthesis fits and how much physical stress the residual limb can take. This means that a residual limb which has been pain free for decades may gradually become painful whereas a "tried and trusted" prosthesis may begin causing problems.

Pain also results from disuse – either just after amputation or years later! If the residual limb is not used, it will get progressively weaker from lack of exercise. Circulation will decrease and the bones will get softer and easier to damage. This leads to easy bruising as well as pain from the muscles and bones. The tendons and ligaments shrink and tighten with disuse. This interferes with both standing and moving. These can be very real problems and there is no quick cure for pain resulting from damage to weakened bones and shortened ligaments. Prevention is the best approach. The limb should be kept in good physical shape to avoid most of the pain problems and disabilities that come with disuse.[13]

PHANTOM SENSATIONS

Virtually everybody who has an amputation after very early childhood experiences sensations which seem to come from the amputated portion of the limb. This "shadow limb" is called the "phantom" and the feelings coming from it are called phantom sensations. Just after the amputation, the phantom usually feels as though it is the same size and shape as the amputated portion of the limb. Most people report that it feels as though they can move and control the phantom as well as they could control the actual limb. The sensations are so real and normal that many young, traumatic, lower limb amputees frequently try to get up and walk away a day or so after their amputations.[14,15] Phantom sensations normally include all of the sensations you would feel in an attached limb, including a sense of position, temperature, itching, and, very occasionally, a ring or other item worn for many years. The phantom frequently rests in the last position the limb was in before it was amputated. These sensations are normally not painful and should not be confused with phantom pain.

As time passes, the limb's shape becomes less vivid and control gradually slips away. For example, a typical below-knee amputee can initially feel the calf, ankle, and foot. Gradually, the foot "telescopes" into the end of the residual limb so the calf seems to have disappeared. Eventually, the ankle may disappear as well. For nearly everyone, telescoping does not happen if phantom pain is present. If phantom pain occurs years after the limb was amputated, the phantom usually grows to its original shape and vividness.

Nearly all amputees continue to sense the phantom all of their lives. In addition to the sense of shape, virtually all amputees report various feelings such as itching, warmth, twisting, etc. which seem to come from the limb. Occasionally, the missing limb feels as though it is in a very uncomfortable position. These feelings may change with time of day, fatigue, weather, and other factors. The great majority of amputees report that these feelings are painful at least occasionally.[16,17]

Central nervous system and peripheral mechanisms underlying the perception of the phantom have been elucidated over the last few decades[12,18] and have been thoroughly discussed elsewhere.[1] The great plasticity of the homunculus combined with changes in receptivity of spinal interneurons responding to receptive fields adjacent to the amputation site produce an ever-changing phantom which responds to changes in the residual limb as any referred sensation would. Interest in central neural plasticity has led to studies of the relationships between amputation, phantom pain, and the homunculus.[19,20]

PHANTOM PAIN

Painful feelings which appear to come from the amputated portion of the limb are called phantom pains. These referred pain sensations may be burning, stinging, cramping, shooting, twisting, or other unpleasant sensations. They are frequently stronger versions of the painless phantom sensations. Each amputee usually has one or a few descriptive types of phantom pain. The pain typically does not move around randomly. If burning pain is felt in the ankle, it may come and go, but that is where is seems to come from. The same amputee may also have cramping pain in the calf, but the two are usually not related. Factors which cause one to change do not usually change the other. This implies that they are likely to be caused by different physical problems.

There is no reason to think that those amputees who report phantom pain are either exaggerating normal phantom sensations or have anything wrong with their minds. In over 7,000 questionnaire responses, noted above, over 80% of the respondents said that they had enough phantom pain to cause them real problems for at least 1 week every year. Most reported episodes of pain which lasted anywhere from a few seconds per year to several weeks at a time, with several to many episodes per year. Some people had continuous pain which varied in amount from almost none to excruciating over the course of the year. For most, the pain interfered with work, sleep, hobbies, and desired social activities.

About half of the amputees who report phantom pain seem to be able to associate changes or onset of their pain with some change in themselves (such as residual limb irritation, exhaustion, back pain, or stress)[21] or outside themselves (such as changes in humidity). It is important to note that two amputees who describe their phantom pain as being identical in frequency, severity, and type of feelings may report entirely different events which change the pain. For most amputees, phantom pain is worst just after amputation while the residual limb is healing. However, it is not likely to go away permanently. A few amputees reported that the severity did not decrease after residual limb healing, but, rather, persisted throughout life. Almost none of the respondents to the surveys reported that their phantom pain went away completely with the years after amputation.

Many amputees are afraid to talk about their phantom pain with their health care providers for fear of being thought to be crazy. Some reported that their health care providers either told them outright or strongly indicated that anyone who felt pain in a limb no longer present had mental problems and should see a psychiatrist. This should no longer be the case! There is no evidence or indication that amputees are any crazier (or more sane) than people who have not had amputations.[22] Most health care providers have learned that referred pain is a very common problem and that phantom pain is one example of it, and they should be aware that phantom pain has a very real physical basis.

The physiological correlates of several descriptive types of phantom pain are known. For example, burning and tingling phantom pain are caused by decreased blood flow in the end of the residual limb, while cramping–squeezing phantom pain is caused by spasms in the residual limb.[22,23] Unfortunately, as yet, no physiological correlates have been found for shocking–shooting phantom pain.

Treatment of chronic phantom limb pain

History of treatment attempts

Sherman et al.[1] stated that:

> The literature on treatment of phantom pain is highly contradictory as it is largely based on short-term studies of small groups of patients. The lack of a year long follow-up as a part of routine clinical practice tends to prevent providers from realizing that treatments have not been effective. Numerous medical, psychiatric, and surgical treatments have been randomly applied to those amputees requesting treatment for phantom limb pain. An update of an analysis of the literature originally done by Sherman[24] combined with a survey of practitioners treating phantom pain[25] showed that sixty-eight unrelated treatments for phantom pain were in recent or current use. Both practitioners and the published literature universally reported them to be successful. They ranged from highly invasive intervention such as lobotomies, through spinal surgery and reamputation, to more innocuous treatments such as "phantom exer-

cises" (in which a sufferer is told to reach into himself and control the movements of his phantom – or even just recognize its existence), injection of the residual limb with local anesthetics, and relaxation training. Almost all of the research consisted of clinical, single group studies with follow-ups of less than six months. Reviews by senior clinicians based on their extensive clinical experience have stated that none of the treatments in the authors' areas of expertise were successful.[26] The survey of practitioners showed that all felt that they could successfully treat phantom pain using one or several of fifty treatments reported. Each "successful" treatment was included among the unsuccessful prior attempts by numerous other respondents.

The most promising of the recent treatments was transcutaneous electrical stimulation (TENS). Finsen et al.[27**] carried out a controlled study which showed that TENS is frequently effective initially. However, there was no difference between placebo and treatment groups by the end of the first year. Finsen et al.'s study is one of the only placebo controlled, long term follow-up studies in the field. Its negative result was published only after years of positive reports from short term, single group clinical trials. These trials were interpreted by many clinicians as indicating that an effective treatment was available and that phantom pain was no longer a major treatment problem. This typifies the failure of the literature on management of phantom limb pain and emphasizes the need for a change in editorial policy so that short-term, small group reports are not misinterpreted as having more than very limited clinical applicability.

The combined results of Sherman et al.'s studies shows that the overall success rate for treatment was dismal. When treatments provided by the medical community are considered, only 1.1% of the respondents received lasting important benefits (0.7% large permanent change and 0.4% cure); 8.9% reported minor permanent improvements; 7.3% reported major temporary help from their treatments; 5.5% reported some very minor help; and 27.4% reported no change at all. Thus, at most 8.4% of the respondents treated could be said to have been helped to any real extent. Many popular treatments such as acupuncture are not yet widely available in U.S. military and Veterans hospitals, so Sherman et al.'s respondents are not as likely to have tried these novel treatments as are civilian amputees. Clinicians trying to use the information in this chapter will find themselves attempting to juxtapose the potential validity of the reports from a few veterans reporting failure of a rarely reported technique, such as hypnosis, with the generalizability of single case studies such as Siegel's[28*] report of short term success (one month follow-up) using hypnosis. They will also need to decide if the lack of recent reports of success of a technique mean that earlier reports of success have not been confirmed. For example, Nashold et al.'s[29] report of success with five patients treated with DREZ [dorsal root entry zone] lesions is quoted in the literature but has rarely been replicated. Other groups have been unable to replicate studies such as Nielson *et al.*'s[30*] report of success using dorsal column stimulation with five of six amputees. Follow-up periods ranged from 7 to 25 months so one might conclude that the technique had proved to be effective. However, numerous others are emphatic that the technique's effectiveness for phantom pain is lost after several years.

The only invasive interventions which produced lasting effects were those which reduced sympathetic nerve activity among amputees having burning descriptions of phantom pain. For example, both multiple sympathetic blocks and sympathectomy frequently helped these amputees but not amputees with other descriptions of phantom pain. The results of sympathectomy seem to last for about one year. This is probably because burning phantom pain is related to decreased blood flow in the residual limb and increased sympathetic tone results in decreased peripheral blood flow. Both sympathetic blocks and sympathectomy result in at least temporarily decreased sympathetic tone which results in increased peripheral blood flow, which, in turn, reduces the burning pain.[1*]

There is no evidence that any surgical procedure performed on the residual limb or spinal cord has any lasting positive effect when done solely for relief of phantom pain. There is also no evidence that psychotherapy or major tranquilizers will cure the pain.[31*] Thus, most widely used treatments do not work and heroic efforts are doomed to failure. It is also important to note that these treatments have not stopped being used. They continue to resurface as practitioners are confronted with amputees requesting treatment for phantom limb pain. Some practitioners attempt to use treatments that normally form part of their treatment plan without checking the literature to ascertain that what sounds like a potential solution has, in fact, been tried and failed. This would not be so critical if such treatments were in the realm of the harmless but ineffective or briefly effective "phantom exercises" which keep being rediscovered and, thus, keep reappearing in newspaper stories.[32] Unfortunately, many of the highly invasive treatments causing permanent damage and disability continue to be used even though they are known to have no lasting effect.

Assessment of subchronic and chronic phantom limb pain[1]

Good treatment usually begins with good assessment. Phantom pain is no exception to this dictum.

a. Search for sources of referred pain: In order to optimize the chances that the initial treatment will work it is crucial to (1) listen to the patient's description of the pain and the factors that affect it, and (2) get a home log of pain and related factors. The one week home log is needed to permit changes in phantom pain to be correlated with changes in diet items (e.g. onions), excretion, changes in weather, physical or mental stress, and use of the prosthesis. Patients frequently miss relationships due to time lags of hours to days.

Phantom pain is almost always exacerbated by episodes of residual limb pain. Evaluate and treat the residual limb pain as appropriate before proceeding very much further with treatments aimed only at phantom pain. If the log indicates that phantom pain is related to use of the prosthesis [especially duration of use), carefully evaluate its fit and effect on gait. Dr. Daniel Shapiro is a physiatrist whose specialty is amputee care. He (personal communication, 1995] states that "An ill-fitting prosthetic device is one of the most easily treatable causes of phantom pain, yet inexplicably, it is often overlooked. Pain, numbness, or paresthesia related to prosthetic use is a red flag. The symptoms are usually not as unpleasant as other phantoms and are in a dermatomal distribution. The clinician should obtain a history of phantom phenomena related to sitting, standing, or ambulating in the prosthesis or starting shortly after the prosthesis is removed. The dermatomal distribution suggests a local nerve root compression. Palpation of the suspected nerve reproduces the symptoms. Percussion sign is usually positive.[33] Palpation of the nerve with the prosthesis donned provides further confirmation. Prosthetic pressure and shearing usually cause redness, hyperpigmentation, blistering, abscess, ulceration, or callosities over the involved area. Xeroradiography will further demonstrate abnormal compression by the prosthesis or migration of the distal fibula–tibia articulation. Prosthetic adjustment is curative. Compression of the common peroneal nerve during ambulation can be corrected by fusion of the fibula–tibia at the distal end to prevent migration. In the unilateral upper extremity amputee, the prosthetic harness may cause phantom pain on the amputated side or referred pain on the contralateral side. In the bilateral upper extremity amputee, in addition, the prosthetic harness may cause phantom pain in the contralateral side by compressing the brachial plexus. Compression by the prosthetic socket is analogous to that of the lower extremity prosthesis.

Normal referral patterns are still operative even if the limb to which pain is referred has been amputated, so look for referral of pain into the phantom from the back, bladder, etc. When relationships between activity or residual limb swelling and phantom pain are evident, a radical change in the way the residual limb is wrapped may be helpful. Interestingly, one of the only double-blind, crossover studies done in the treatment of phantom pain was performed by Conine *et al.*[34**] with 34 amputees who wore a special metal stranded fabric when episodes of phantom pain began. Twenty-one of their subjects reported the most decrease in pain when wearing the experimental garment as opposed to the placebo. Only two showed nearly complete pain relief and average differences in pain intensity between the groups were very small so the clinical importance of the device is still open to question.

Environmental factors may also be important in initiating and intensifying episodes of phantom pain. If changes in weather are related to changes in phantom pain, a trial of anti-inflammatories and/or other medications, which you might use when attempting to ameliorate the effects of changes in the weather upon pain due to arthritis is appropriate. If phantom pain changes with physical stress, have the patient reduce physical activity levels, check the prosthesis, and check for changes in blood flow in the residual limb with activity.

b. Be aware of psychological factors that may exacerbate the pain: Ensure that the subject understands (1) that phantom pain is not likely to be of psychological origin and (2) how it is possible to continue to feel body parts that have been amputated. A psychological screen (including the MMPI [Minnesota Multiple Personality Inventory]) is not always necessary but is appropriate for identifying masked depression, situational anxiety, and hysterical reaction to loss of a limb. Both anxiety and depression magnify pain. If the log shows a change in phantom pain with changes in stress and anxiety, treat these latter symptoms appropriately (reduction through increased understanding, relaxation training, etc.). Major psychological disorders can exacerbate the pain. If the patient is isolated from other amputees, referral to a local amputee support group can be helpful. If the patient has an overwhelming need for pain (pain games within the family, somatization of problems, etc.), treat them appropriately before attempting other interventions aimed solely at relieving phantom pain.

As noted earlier, Flor[35] and her team have shown that the distribution of limb representations is different in the sensory homunculus of amputees with and without phantom pain. This group has recently[36**] performed a small controlled trial in which they taught amputees without phantom pain. This was accomplished by teaching amputees to increase their two-point discrimination in areas associated with the amputation site. They found that phantom pain decreased when the homunculus normalized. If these findings are substantiated in larger studies, an entirely new approach to treating not only phantom pain, but many other types of chronic pain as will, will have been born.

Recommended procedure for evaluating and treating patients with chronic phantom pain

Rational/background

As early as 1979, it became apparent that different descriptions of phantom pain responded to different treatments.[37***] Our initial attempts to treat phantom limb pain with a combination of biofeedback and relaxation techniques showed excellent success for up to 6 months to 3 years of follow-up with 14 of 16 successive phantom pain patients. The major difference between those patients who succeeded in learning to control their pain and those who did not was the ability to relax in any measurable way. Our two failures neither demonstrated the ability to relax nor reported subjective feelings which would be associated with learning to relax or to control their muscle tensions.

In an attempt to align behavioral and medical treatments of phantom pain with underlying physiological correlates, amputees who showed increased burning phantom limb pain in response to decreased blood flow in the residual limb were treated with peripheral vasodilators and temperature biofeedback. When increased muscle tension and spasms in the residual limb were related to episodes of cramping phantom pain, muscle relaxants and muscle tension biofeedback were used to control the pain.[1*] There are reports of other, newer interventions, but without controls. Success has been reported with thermal/electromyograph (EMG) biofeedback,[38] electroconvulsive therapy,[39] ketamine,[40] and gabapentin.[41]

Among the most recent cases, EMG biofeedback was effective for 13 of 14 trials for cramping phantom pain. EMG biofeedback had minimal success with two and no success with 10 of 12 trials for burning phantom pain. It had no success with eight trials of shocking phantom pain. Temperature biofeedback was ineffective for four trials of cramping phantom pain, was effective for six of seven trials with burning phantom pain, and had no success with three trials for shocking phantom pain. Nitroglycerine ointment (a topical vasodilator) was ineffective for one trial of cramping phantom pain and one of shocking phantom pain, but successful for two trials of burning phantom pain. Pentoxifylline (Trental) (a blood viscosity enhancer) was ineffective for two trials of cramping phantom pain and one of shocking phantom pain. Nifedipine (a systemic vasodilator) was effective for three trials of burning phantom pain but ineffective for one trial of cramping and two trials of shocking phantom pain. Cyclobenzaprine (Flexeril) (a muscle relaxant) was effective for two trials of cramping phantom pain but ineffective for one of shocking phantom pain. Indomethacin (Indocin) (an anti-inflammatory agent) was ineffective for two trials of cramping phantom pain. These medications have potential side-effects and cannot be used with many patients who have a variety of medical problems. Thus, the use of "self-control-oriented" strategies is encouraged to avoid these limitations.

It is clear that burning phantom pain responds to interventions which increase blood flow to the residual limb whereas cramping phantom pain responds to interventions which decrease tension and spasms in major muscles of the residual limb. Shocking–shooting phantom pain responds neither well nor consistently to either type of intervention. The physiological bases for these changes are discussed elsewhere.

It is strongly recommended that biofeedback of appropriate parameters be used in conjunction with other self-control training strategies to treat cramping–squeezing and burning–tingling phantom limb pain. It is important for clinicians to recognize that biofeedback as utilized for control of phantom limb pain is not some kind of black box psychomagic. Rather, it is simply the process of recording the physiological parameters (such as muscle tension in the residual limb) which precede changes in phantom pain, and showing the signals to patients. The patient uses the information to change the signal. The patient also learns to associate sensations related to onset of phantom pain with tension in the muscle, decreased blood flow, etc. and to use the learned ability to control the parameter to prevent the onset of pain or to stop it if it has already begun.

Burning phantom pain

If the patient reports burning phantom pain (including tingling and similar descriptions), increased phantom pain with decreased atmospheric temperature, or decreased residual limb temperature before increased phantom pain, first give a trial of temperature biofeedback from the residual limb in conjunction with relaxation training containing warming exercises. If this is not effective, try peripheral vasodilators (such as nitroglycerine paste applied to the distal end of the residual limb) and, if necessary, multiple sympathetic blocks (single blocks tend to be of short duration and ineffective as a treatment, but may be a useful diagnostic tool).

Cramping phantom pain

If the patient reports cramping phantom pain (including twisting, gripping, etc.) or the residual limb shows spikes in the EMG and/or spasms during phantom pain, give a trial of muscle tension biofeedback from the residual limb in conjunction with muscle tension awareness and control training. If this is not effective, give a long trial of muscle relaxants.

Other descriptions of phantom pain

Luckily, cramping and burning descriptors and their close relatives are the most commonly encountered. The others, such as shocking–shooting and twisting, are relatively rare. Their mechanisms are not known and no treatments have been shown to consistently provide significant relief for more than a few months for the vast majority of amputees. Thus, there is no way to predict which treatments, if any, will provide lasting benefits. The guideline below can be followed for the best chance of relieving the pain.

Bartusch et al.[42*] reported that two patients with chronic shocking–shooting phantom limb pain who were unresponsive to other treatment modalities responded very well to clonazepam and that the effects were maintained for at least 6 months. Sherman et al.[5*]

reported one patient who successfully treated himself for shocking–shooting phantom pain by not permitting the limb to change temperature quickly (as would happen when going outside on a cold winter day or getting out of a warm bath). Tsushima[43*] reported one patient who had at least 2 months of relief from shooting phantom pain after temperature biofeedback but not after muscle tension biofeedback. McKechnie[44*] reported one case of sharp phantom pain (which Sherman et al.[1] included with their reports of shocking–shooting pain) being responsive to progressive muscle relaxation training for at least 6 months. The training included relaxing the muscles of the residual limb and imagining relaxing the muscles of the phantom. A comment at the end of the article indicates that distraction training did not help this patient. Although not commented on by the author, readers should be aware that progressive muscle relaxation exercises have been shown to increase blood flow to the extremities. Thus, the observed changes could be due to many factors ranging from changes in muscle tension and blood flow in the residual limb to exercising the phantom.

What to do if initial attempts are unsuccessful or if the mechanism for the description given is unknown

The following treatments have shown fair success with short-term follow-up and have not been reported as useless in amputee surveys. They should be tried for cases of cramping and burning phantom pain which do not respond to the treatments recommended above as well as for other descriptions of phantom pain. A 6- to 8-week trial of relaxation training for pain control can be followed by TENS. Try many locations on the residual limb with many intensities and wave forms. It must be emphasized that a long-term, controlled study showed that TENS is ineffective upon follow-up. However, other studies have indicated at least temporary relief which could be used to disrupt the pain cycle long enough for healing to take place on its own or for other treatments to work. For example, Katz and Melzack[45**] performed a controlled study which showed that auricular TENS can make small but statistically significant reductions in phantom pain for a brief period. We are not aware of long-term follow-up for any of these studies. If these trials are ineffective, an active range of motion exercises along with phantom exercises may help. Next, try ultrasound at the residual limb. If it is initially successful, add steroids. The last attempt would be a trial of sedative hypnotics followed by tricyclic antidepressants.

Reports of several treatments having sufficient information and follow-up to permit evaluation have appeared in the clinical literature in the years since the surveys upon which these recommendations are based were conducted. Davis[46*] found mexiletine to give good to excellent results in reducing chronic phantom pain in 18 of 31 patients. Eleven of the 31 showed a "favorable response" when clonidine was added. Only two did not respond at all. For the combined group, 12 were defined as having excellent results, 16 had a good result, and 13 did not show a clinically significant change. Unfortunately, the descriptions of phantom pain are not included in the report. All of the patients were followed for 1 year and maintained their decreases in pain. As far as can be determined from the report, none was actually cured, but, according to their visual analog pain scales, were significantly helped.

Jaeger and Maiger[47]** treated 21 patients having acute just-postamputation phantom pain with calcitonin. They gave each patient the drug or placebo infusions and found that only the drug reduced reports of phantom pain. Pain was reduced from a median of 7 to 4 on a visual analog scale regardless of whether placebo or the real drug was given first. One week after treatment, 19 of the 21 had more than 50% relief of pain. Of these, 16 were pain free. After 1 year, eight of the 13 surviving patients had more than 75% pain relief. There was a second year of follow-up but the results are difficult to understand. The authors state that they were the same as after 1 year. The value of this treatment is difficult to determine because many amputees show a similar decrease in phantom pain intensity and frequency during the years following amputation, as reported in this study.

Both of these studies meet the criteria for reasonable studies with reasonable follow-up periods. They need to be replicated with larger numbers of subjects and better descriptions of the phantom pain before they can be accepted into the recommended armamentarium for phantom pain – but they are certainly worth a try if the mechanism-based treatments do not work.

Gross[48]* reported four cases in which local anesthesia to hyperalgesic points on the intact limb reduced or abolished phantom pain in four amputees. Patients were followed for between 6 months and 2 years with continuing relief. Monga and Jaksic[49] report using acupuncture with one patient who had received a number of previously unsuccessful treatment attempts, including the use of β-blockers and tranquilizers. Hypnotherapy did help this patient for a half hour or so after each session. Acupuncture was by both needle and electric stimulation to the residual limb and reduced the pain sufficiently for the patient to use a prosthesis. No long-term follow-up is reported. Thus, there is no way to tell whether this is another currently popular treatment that will fall by the wayside after failing to stand the test of time or whether it really works. The authors can only encourage further testing and long-term follow-up of the above and numerous other techniques being tried on a few patients. Of course, any treatment that relieves otherwise intractable pain for a given period may be worth using if only to provide temporary relief. It may be more useful if it is sufficiently free of side-effects that it can be repeated as needed.

If the above treatments do not work, other interventions (such as major tranquilizers, revision of a normal residual limb, sympathectomy, and surgical invasion of the spinal cord and brain) are even less likely to produce lasting results. It is probably best to tell the patient that current treatments are not likely to succeed. The best option may be referral to a comprehensive pain rehabilitation program to optimize the patient's ability to manage the complex social, physical, and psychological deconditioning that inevitably occurs after amputation.

REFERENCES

● 1. Sherman R, Devor M, Jones C, *et al. Phantom Pain.* New York, NY: Plenum Press, 1997.

2. Lambert AW, Dashfield AK, Cosgrove C, *et al.* Randomized prospective study comparing preoperative epidural and intraoperative perineural analgesia for the prevention of postoperative stump and phantom pain following major amputation. *Reg Anesth Pain Med* 2001; **26**: 316–21.

3. Elizaga AM, Smith DG, Sharar SR, *et al.* Continuous regional analgesia by intraneural block: effect on postoperative opioid requirements and phantom limb pain following amputation. *J Rehabil Res Dev* 1994; **31**: 179–87.

4. Schwenkreis P, Witscher K, Janssen F, *et al.* Assessment of reorganization of the sensorimotor cortex after upper limb amputation. *Clin Neurophysiol* 2001; **112**: 627–35.

5. Sherman R., Jones C, Shannon S. *The Amputee's Guide.* London: British Limbless Ex-serviceperson's Association, 1993 (revised, March 1995).

6. Machin P, Williams AC. Stiff upper lip: coping strategies of World War II veterans with phantom limb pain. *Clin J Pain* 1998; **14**: 290–4.

7. Nicolajsen I, Ilkjaer S, Jensen TS. Relationship between mechanical sensitivity and postamputation pain: a prospective study. *Eur J Pain* 2000; **4**: 327–34.

8. Weiss SA, Lindell B. Phantom limb pain and etiology of amputation in unilateral lower extremity amputees. *J Pain Symptom Manage* 1996; **11**: 3–17.

9. Sherman R, Barja R. Treatment of post-amputation and phantom limb pain. In: Foley K, Payne R eds. *Current Therapy of Pain.* Ontario: BC Decker, 1989.

◆ 10. Sherman R, Sherman C, Parker L. Chronic phantom and stump pain among American veterans: results of a survey. *Pain* 1984; **18**: 83–95.

11. Sherman R. Sherman C. A comparison of phantom sensations among amputees whose amputations were of civilian and military origins. *Pain* 1985; **2**: 91–7.

12. Devor M. In: Sherman R, Devor M, Jones C, *et al. Phantom Pain.* New York, NY: Plenum Press, 1997.

13. Dillingham TR, Pezzin LE, MacKenzie EJ, *et al.* Use and satisfaction with prosthetic devices among persons with trauma-related amputations: a long-term outcome study. *Am J Phys Med Rehabil* 2001; **80**: 563–71.

14. Boonstra AM, Rijnders LJ, Groothoff JW, *et al.* Children

with congenital deficiencies or acquired amputations of the lower limbs: functional aspects. *Prosthetics Orthotics Int* 2000; **24:** 19–27.

15. Wilkins KL, McGrath PJ, Finley GA, *et al.* Phantom limb sensations and phantom limb pain in child and adolescent amputees. *Pain* 1998; **78:** 7–12.

● 16. Finnoff J. Differentiation and treatment of phantom sensation, phantom pain, and residual-limb pain. *J Am Podiatr Assoc* 2001; **91:** 23–33.

17. Ehde DM, Czerniecke JM, Smith DG, *et al.* Chronic phantom sensations, phantom pain, residual limb pain, and other regional pain after lower limb amputation. *Arch Phys Med Rehabil* 2000; **81:** 1039–44.

18. Melzack R. Phantom limbs, the self, and the brain (The D.O. Hebb memorial lecture). *Can Psychol* 1989; **30:** 1–16.

19. Flor H, Elbert T, Knecht S, *et al.* Phantom-limb pain as a perceptual correlate of cortical reorganization following are amputation. *Nature* 1995; **375:** 482–4.

20. Liaw MY, You DL, Cheng PT, *et al.* Central representation of phantom limb phenomenon in amputees studied with single photon emission computerized tomography. *Am J Phys Med Rehabil* 1998; **77:** 368–75.

21. Angrilli A, Koster U. Psychophysiological stress responses in amputees with and without phantom limb pain. *Physiol Behav* 2000; **68:** 699–706.

22. Sherman R, Sherman C, Bruno G. Psychological factors influencing chronic phantom limb pain: an analysis of the literature. *Pain* 1987; **28:** 285–95.

23. Sherman R, Griffin R, Evans C, Grana A. Temporal relationships between changes in phantom limb pain intensity and changes in surface electromyogram of the residual limb. *Int J Psychophysiol* 1992; **13:** 71–7.

24. Sherman R. Special review: published treatments of phantom limb pain. *Am J Phys Med* 1980; **59:** 232–44.

◆ 25. Sherman R, Sherman C, Gall N. Survey of current treatment of phantom limb pain in the United States. *Pain* 1980; **8:** 85–99.

26. Sherman R, Arena JG, Bruno G, Smith J. Precursor relationships between stress, physical activity, meteorological factors, and phantom limb pain. In: *Proceedings of the Annual Meeting of the American Pain Society, Toronto Canada*. Seattle, WA: American Pain Society, 1988.

27. Finsen V, Persen L, Lovlien M, *et al.* Transcutaneous electrical nerve stimulation after major amputation. *Br J Bone Joint Surg* 1988; **70(B):** 109–12.

28. Siegel EF. Control of phantom limb pain by hypnosis. *Am J Clin Hypn* 1979; **21:** 285–6.

29. Nashold B, Ostdahl R, Bullitt E, *et al.* Dorsal root entry zone lesions: a new neurosurgical therapy for deafferentation pain. In: Bonica J ed. *Advances in Pain Research and Therapy*. New York, NY: Raven Press, 1983.

30. Nielson K, Adams J, Hosobuchi Y. Phantom limb pain: treatment with dorsal column stimulation. *J Neurosurg* 1975; **42:** 301–7.

31. Melzack R, Wall P. *The Challenge of Pain*. New York, NY: Basic Books, 1982.

32. *New York Times*. Phantom exercises for phantom pain. January 22, 1995.

33. Christopher RP, Koepke GH. Peripheral nerve entrapment as a cause of phantom sensation and stump pain in lower extremity amputees. *Arch Phys Med Rehabil* 1963; **44:** 631–4.

34. Conine T, Hershler C, Alexander S, Crisp R. The efficacy of farabloc in the treatment of phantom limb pain. *Can J Rehabil* 1993; **6:** 151–61.

35. Flor H, Birbaumer N, Sherman R. Phantom limb pain. *Pain: Clinical Updates* 2000; **8:** 1–4.

36. Flor H, Denke C, Schaefer M, Grusser S. Effect of sensory discrimination training on cortical reorganization and phantom limb pain. *Lancet* 2001; **357:** 1763–4.

37. Sherman R, Gall N, Gormly J. Treatment of phantom limb pain with muscular relaxation training to disrupt the pain-anxiety-tension cycle. *Pain* 1979; **6:** 47–55.

38. Belleggia G, Birbaumer N. Treatment of phantom limb pain with combined EMG and thermal biofeedback: a case report. *Appl Psychophysiol Biofeedback* 2001; **26:** 141–6.

39. Rasmussen KG, Rummans TA. Electroconvulsive therapy for phantom limb pain. *Pain* 2000; **85:** 297–9.

40. Nikolajsen L, Hansen CL, Nielsen J *et al.* The effect of ketamine on phantom pain: a central neuropathic disorder maintained by peripheral input. *Pain* 1996; **67:** 69–77.

41. Rosenberg JM, Harrell C, Ristic H *et al.* The effect of gabapentin on neuropathic pain. *Clin J Pain* 1997; **13:** 251–5.

42. Bartusch SL, Sanders BJ, D'Alessio JG, Jernigan JR. Clonazepam for the treatment of phantom limb pain. *Clin J Pain* 1996; **12**(1): 59–62.

43. Tsushima W. Treatment of phantom limb pain with EMG and temperature biofeedback: a case study. *Am J Clin Biofeedback* 1982; **5:** 150–3.

44. McKechnie R. Relief from phantom limb pain by relaxation exercises. *J Behav Ther Exp Psychiatry* 1975; **6:** 262–3.

45. Katz J, Melzack R. Auricular TENS reduces phantom limb pain. *J Pain Symptom Manage* 1991; **6:** 73–83.

46. Davis R. Successful treatment for phantom pain. *Orthopedics* 1993; **16:** 691–5.

47. Jaeger H, Maiger C. Calcitonin in phantom limb pain: a double-blind study. *Pain* 1992; **48:** 21–7.

48. Gross D. Contralateral local anesthesia in the treatment of phantom limb and stump pain. *Pain* 1982; **13:** 313–20.

49. Monga T, Jaksie T. Acupuncture in phantom limb pain. *Arch Phys Med Rehabil* 1981; **62:** 229–31.

Acute herpes zoster pain

JANINE PERNAK DE GAST AND ANNA SPACEK

Pain is frequently the most distressing symptom of herpes zoster (HZ) infection.[1] The pain mechanism is not clarified yet. Pain during the acute phase of HZ infection is due to the peripheral nerve and ganglion lesion, whereas pain occurring in postherpetic neuralgia (PHN) may correlate with damage to the central nervous system (CNS). According to Watson *et al.*, pain mechanisms may differ among patients.[2]

The therapy of acute herpes zoster (AHZ) has been controversial for many years, and as yet an ideal treatment to prevent postherpetic neuralgia has been not found. [3★★★,4★★★,5,6★★★,7★★★,8★★★,9★★★,10★,11★★★,12★★★]

Pain relief should be obtained by using techniques which are common for acute pain management. The efficacy of the treatment in the acute phase of herpes zoster should prevent transformation of acute pain into a chronic pain syndrome – postherpetic neuralgia.[13,14]

PATHOPHYSIOLOGY

Herpes zoster is an acute viral infection of a DNA type affecting the ganglion of the posterior spinal root or the ganglion of the cranial nerves. The infection may not remain in the posterior horn but can spread into the anterior horn, producing paresis. It can also spread into the bulbar region or into the brain, producing a generalized fatal encephalitis. From the ganglion, the virus spreads along the nerve fiber to the skin, where one can observe the herpes affecting certain dermatomes. The peripheral nerve of the affected ganglion is also the site of the demyelinization, degeneration, fibrosis, and cellular infiltration.[2,15] In the months following acute herpes zoster infection, areas of regeneration and degeneration

in the involved peripheral nerves can be observed. The virus destroys the afferent fibers. The damage in herpes zoster is caused by acute inflammation, which produces injury mostly in the large fast-conducting fibers. The small fibers regenerate faster than larger fibers, and many of the latter become slow conducting when they regenerate. The majority of the nerve fibers left have a diameter of about 5 μm instead of 13 μm. When the large fibers are lacking, a burning pain of long duration mediated via the small fibers results.[16]

Primary infection with the varicella-zoster virus (VZV) results in chickenpox – a common childhood condition. In 1948, the herpes zoster virus (HZV) was classified morphologically as a varicella-zoster virus (VZV) by Rake *et al.* using an electron microscope.[17] This observation was confirmed by complement fixation tests and described by Taylor-Robinson and Downie in 1959.[18] Gold reported in 1966 on the differences in the immune and antibody responses between the clinical course of VZV and that of HZV.[19] Patients with VZV infection produce immunoglobulin M (IgM) complement-fixing antibody. This type of antibody is produced by the first exposure to an infecting agent. Patients with HZV produce IgG antibody, the type of antibody which is produced as a secondary response. Also, serum from patients recovering from HZV infection has a higher antibody titer than serum from patients with VZV infections. Gold suggested that HZV produces a secondary antigenic stimulus.[19] The varicella-zoster virus remains in the body after clinical recovery, lying dormant in the dorsal root ganglion. After reactivation, the virus migrates along one or two sensory nerves. Reactivation of the latent virus leads to intense inflammation of the sensory nerve and to the eruption of the rash in the skin distribution of the affected nerves.[20]

EPIDEMIOLOGY

Acute herpes zoster is quite a common neurological disease of elderly or immunosuppressed patients. It can be associated with general illness or physical trauma, but often no cause can be found.[1,21] The incidence is 3–4 cases per year per 1,000 individuals, but it increases very dramatically with advancing age (Table 33.1).

The high incidence with increasing age has been attributed to the general waning of the immune system with age and to decline in cellular immunity against the varicella-zoster virus. There are no significant differences concerning ethnic or racial incidence. Both sexes are equally afflicted. Patients with immune systems that are compromised by disease or drug therapy are more sensitive to the herpes zoster virus infection. The incidence rate increases with the severity of the disease and the aggressiveness of chemotherapy or radiation, and has been noted in 30–50% of patients.[22]

In 10% of herpes zoster patients, the affected individuals have identifiable risk factors such as:

- advancing age;
- cancer;
- stress;
- transplantation;
- surgery;
- radiotherapy;
- preceding illness;
- chemotherapy;
- immunosuppression;
- high-dose corticosteroids;
- human immunodeficiency virus (HIV) infection;
- others.

Herpes zoster can be the first presenting illness of HIV infection and has been shown to be a prognostic indicator toward the development of acquired immunodeficiency syndrome (AIDS).[23]

In cancer patients, the most affected are those with:

- Hodgkin's disease;
- non-Hodgkin's lymphoma;
- multiple myeloma;
- chronic lymphatic leukemia.

An increase of primary varicella-zoster infection is also noticed in patients receiving high-dose corticosteroid therapy in such conditions as nephritic syndrome and rheumatic fever.

The number of deaths owing to varicella virus in immunosuppressed patients is not known yet. However, there was a report from Preblud and D'Angelo in 1979 describing approximately 100 cases of deaths each year in the USA associated with VZV infection.[24]

CLINICAL MANIFESTATION

The first clinical symptom of acute herpes zoster infection is pain with paresthesiae and dysesthesiae in the affected dermatome followed a few days later by a vesicular eruption.[25,26] The reactivation of varicella-zoster virus causes intense inflammation, often with hemorrhagic necrosis of nerve cells and partial destruction of the ganglion. The virus spreads along the sensory nerve to the skin and produces the characteristic herpes zoster rash. The skin lesion is mostly unilateral and limited to the area of skin innervated by the affected sensory ganglion. The pain syndrome increases sharply as the vesicular rash progresses, and decreases slowly with the healing of the lesions. Severe pain in the acute stage is more characteristic in older patients and might be of such severity that control of the pain is difficult to achieve even with regular doses of narcotics. In most patients, the duration of the skin eruption is until the separation of the last crust, which is about 10–14 days, but in patients over 50 years of age the skin lesions can be present for a few weeks. In some patients, irreversible skin damage and sensory loss occurs.

In AHZ, the frequently affected dermatomes are in the thoracic region and the facial region, mostly in the first division – ophthalmic branch – of the trigeminal nerve. Generalized lesions may occur several days after the onset of herpes zoster, especially in immunosuppressed individuals, and can lead to cutaneous or visceral dissemination with death as a result.

Some other neurological complications (1%) can occur, such as:

- infection of the central nervous system (encephalomyelitis);
- meningitis;
- transverse myelitis;
- necrotizing myelopathy;
- Guillain–Barré syndrome;
- motor complication with temporary paralysis (facial palsy);
- ophthalmic complications (50–70%).

Ocular complications may occur in any structure in the eye or orbit:[27]

- corneal hypesthesia or anesthesia (50%);
- corneal ulceration (neurotrophic keratitis) (41–60%).

Table 33.1 *Increasing incidence of acute herpes zoster with age*

Age of affected individuals (years)	Number of cases per year per 1,000
10–19	1.4
40–49	2.9
60–69	6.8
80–84	10.1

- epidural hematoma;
- epidural abscess;
- neurological deficit owing to a spinal nerve or to spinal cord lesion;
- epidurally broken needle;
- local anesthetic toxicity;
- headache;
- others.

Nerve root and nerve branch blocks

To perform paravertebral blocks, local anesthetics with or without other drugs (steroids, analgesics) should be injected near the foramen intervertebralis, where nerves leave the vertebral column prior to their division into somatic and autonomic parts. Nerve branch blocks such as facet blocks are performed with a small amount of local anesthetic to the rami posterior as a diagnostic procedure. Commonly, 0.5–1 ml of 2% lidocaine (lignocaine) will be used for this procedure. Spread of local anesthetics to other parts of the nerve root can cause many complications such as:

- hypotension owing to sympathetic block;
- temporary motor dysfunction;
- other neurologic disturbances;
- pneumothorax when performing intercostal nerve blocks.

Accuracy of the nerve blocks, especially nerve root blocks, nerve branch blocks, and sympathetic blocks, can be achieved by using:

- a C-arm with image intensifier;
- radiological medium contrast;
- if necessary, nerve stimulation with an insulated needle and an appropriate current (2 Hz) to stimulate a motor response or to stimulate a sensory response (50 or 100 Hz).

The use of radiological medium contrast for the visualization of the nerve and the position of the needle and its control by using the image intensifier and also the nerve stimulation is recommended by many authors.[10*]

As mentioned above, nerve root and nerve branch blocks performed with local anesthetics with or without steroids or analgesics can be useful in the treatment of acute herpes zoster.

Sympathetic blocks

Except for intradural sympathetic blocks such as epidural or subarachnoidal blocks, sympathetic interruption can be achieved through blocking the sympathetic chain, peripheral nerve blocks, or pharmacologically using different drugs such as α-receptor blockers, norepinephrine activity blockers, and β-receptor blockers.[85]

Good therapeutic results can be achieved by blocking the sympathetic chain with local anesthetics, neurolytic agents, or with radiofrequency thermolesion.[67***,70,86*,87*]

Sympathetic blocks can be used as diagnostic and therapeutic tools. The efficacy of a local anesthetic agent should always be determined before performing sympathetic block with neurolytic agents (phenol 6% or alcohol 96%). A complication often observed is that of neuritis of the somatic nerves.

In patients not achieving prolonged pain relief with local anesthetic sympathetic block, surgical or neurolytic sympathectomy usually provides this. Poor results can occur when technical difficulties result in an incomplete sympathectomy, and the possibility of complications is always present following both surgical and chemical sympathectomy.[88] Recently, for permanent denervation of the sympathetic chain, a radiofrequency thermolesion technique has been used.[87*]

As mentioned above, sympathetic blocks are very popular in the treatment of AHZ.[66**,67***,68–72] The most frequently used blocks are stellate ganglion and lumbar sympathetic block.[69,77**]

Stellate ganglion block (cervicothoracic sympathetic block)

The stellate ganglion has two parts:

- inferior cervical ganglion;
- first thoracic ganglion.

These two parts form the single structure lying in front of the seventh cervical transverse process and on the first rib. The stellate ganglion is part of the sympathetic trunk, which lies in the cervical region behind the carotic sheath on the fascia covering the muscle close to the processus transversus of the cervical vertebrae. The pleura is in front and below. A single-shot technique is usually performed with 10 ml of 0.25% bupivacaine. A stellate ganglion block is an easy procedure, however some complications can occur:

- intravascular injection;
- brachial block;
- laryngeal recurrent nerve block;
- pneumothorax;
- temporary Horner block;
- epidural or subarachnoidal injection.

Stellate ganglion block has good efficacy in acute and chronic pain in herpes zoster ophthalmicus.[77**,86*]

Thoracic sympathetic block

This procedure is commonly performed as a permanent block via neurolytic radiofrequency thermolesion or surgical sympathectomy. Because of frequent complications such as intrathecal injection and pneumothorax, thoracic sympathetic block is not regularly used in the management of pain. However, with all precautions concerning the safety and use of contrast medium and image-intensifier techniques, thoracic sympathetic block can also be useful in the treatment of pain in AHZ.[72,86]*

Lumbar sympathetic block

The lumbar sympathetic chain lies on the anterolateral surface of the lumbar vertebrae. Anterior to the left side lies the aorta, and on the right side the vena cava inferior, which is covered by the retroperitoneal fascia. This fascial compartment is limited by the vertebral column, psoas sheath, and retroperitoneal fascia. Local anesthetics used for sympathetic blocks can easily spread in this compartment and have a wide effect. There are different techniques of lumbar sympathetic blocks.[69–72]

The following complications can occur:

- subarachnoidal injection;
- genitofemoral neuralgia;
- somatic nerve damage;
- perforation of a disk;
- puncture of major vessel;
- puncture of renal pelvis;
- others.

To avoid the above-mentioned complications, a diagnostic sympathetic block has to be performed and an image-intensifying technique must be used.

Cranial nerves blocks and cranial ganglionic blocks

The most common nerve blocks and ganglion blocks of the head used in the treatment of AHZ are:

- trigeminal nerve blocks – Gasserian ganglion block;
- trigeminal nerve branches block;
- ophthalmic nerve block;
- maxillary nerve block;
- mandibular nerve block.

Trigeminal nerve block – Gasserian ganglion block

The Gasserian ganglion lies at the apex of the petrous bone at the junction of the middle and posterior cranial fossa. A Gasserian ganglion block is easy to perform using Hartel's anterior approach technique, which was described in 1914. This technique of trigeminal block should be performed under slight anesthesia using radiological contrast medium and image-intensifier control. For trigeminal block, local anesthetics, neurolytic agents, and steroids can be used. Very good results of these methods have been reported in the treatment of pain in herpes zoster.[5]

The following complications of Gasserian ganglion block may occur:

- injection of local anesthetics or neurolytic agents into the cerebrospinal fluid (CSF);

- unconsciousness;
- temporary paralysis of the ipsilateral cranial nerve system;
- hematoma;
- encephalitis;
- others.

Patients with AHZ undergoing Gasserian ganglion block should be hospitalized and observed for 24 h.

Trigeminal nerve branches

Ophthalmic nerve block
Ophthalmic nerve block is very easy to perform. The ophthalmic nerve branch of the trigeminal nerve involves the supraorbital and supratrochlear branches. The injection of small doses (2–4 ml) of local anesthetic can offer acceptable analgesia.

Maxillary nerve block
This nerve is usually blocked by the lateral approach. Using local anesthetics, profound analgesia can be obtained in the upper jaw and in the teeth on the ipsilateral side of face.

Some complications such as hematoma or temporary blindness owing to the spread of local anesthetic to the optic nerve can occur.

Mandibular nerve block
Using local anesthetics for the mandibular nerve block, analgesia occurs in the skin of the lower jaw except in some small areas of the auricle. Possible complications are hematoma, temporary anesthesia of the muscles of mastication, which causes some incoordination or ipsilateral movements of the jaw, and others.

Trigeminal nerve branches blocks can be useful as an additional treatment to antiviral therapy in the management of acute herpes zoster pain, especially in cases where VZV infection is present only in one division of the trigeminal nerve.

Intrapleural blocks

The effectiveness of pleural analgesia for the treatment of acute herpes zoster in the thoracic region has been reported by some authors.[89,90]

The mechanism of action of this procedure is based on blocking different nerves, such as:

- intercostal nerves;
- sympathetic nerves;
- parietal pleural nerve endings;
- possibly phrenic nerve and phrenic nerve endings.

Other peripheral blocks and local infiltration

Generally, nerve blocks of different types produce analgesia in the tissue which is supplied by the nerve. Local infiltration of local anesthetics with or without steroid is very popular and been reported to be effective in the treatment of AHZ.[41*,42*,65,74*,81*]

Laser

In the last few years, the use of the laser has gained popularity. The word "laser" means light amplification by stimulated emission of radiation. The development of the laser technique dates from 1967.[91]

According to the type of the active medium, the wavelength, and the heating effect of the laser light, there are different kinds of the laser.

In practice, those most commonly used are:

- power lasers – for surgical use;
- medium-power lasers (midlaser);
- low-power lasers (soft laser).

Soft lasers carry out their activity in the upper layers of the derma. Laser penetration can activate and normalize the basic regulatory function of the connective tissue. The intensity of the laser beam is reduced by the tissue, but the mechanism of action is not yet completely understood.[92] Clinically, an anti-inflammatory, antiedemic, analgesic effect and an increase in cell proliferation could be shown.

Effective treatment of inflammatory diseases including AHZ has been reported in some clinical publications.[93,94**] Recently, in a preliminary report, very good efficacy of a low-power helium–neon laser was shown in patients with AHZ. After 10 days' therapy, a significant reduction of allodynia, constant deep burning, and aching pain was achieved.[94**]

As low-power laser seems to be a simple, effective, and harmless therapy, it can be recommended as an adjunctive therapy in AHZ.

Transcutaneous electric nerve stimulation

Transcutaneous electrical nerve stimulation (TENS) is a noninvasive pain-relieving method that is almost free of side-effects and that involves the application of pulsed square wave electrical current through surface electrodes to the skin. TENS stimulates the large myelinated nerve fibers, which causes the presynaptic inhibition of conduction in thin nociceptive afferents (according to the gate control theory[95]), and which also causes an increase in endorphin levels in the CSF.[96]

TENS equipment allows adjustment of frequency and amplitude. The three most often applied stimulation patterns are:

- conventional with high frequency (40–150 Hz) and low intensity 10–30 mA;
- pulsed with low frequency (bursts of 100 Hz at 1–2 Hz) and low intensity (10–30 mA);
- acupuncture-like with low frequency and high intensity (15–50 mA).

The ideal frequency and amplitude parameters have not yet been established. The amplitude is usually adjusted by the patient until a comfortable tingling sensation is felt. The stimulator may be used almost continuously, or intermittently. In order to obtain the maximum benefit from this form of therapy, it is important to use a variety of frequencies, electrode placement methods, and also to change the duration and frequency of treatment. Often, small differences in these parameters will produce large alterations in the clinical effect.

The most common problem encountered is that of skin irritation at the electrode site due to an allergic reaction to the electrodes. In addition, the prolonged use of an electrode at high output intensity may also cause skin irritation, but periodic changing of the electrode position can solve this problem. There are some reports describing the effectiveness of TENS in the treatment of chronic pain, and especially in patients with postherpetic neuralgia.[97,98] In AHZ, the use of TENS is not the preferred technique because of difficulty with the placement of electrodes on painful affected dermatomes. However, a recently published preliminary study[99**] in immunocompetent patients with AHZ showed better efficacy of percutaneous electrical nerve stimulation (PENS) than antiviral therapy with famciclovir with respect to pain relief, healing of the skin lesions, improvement in physical activity, and sleep quality. Moreover, PENS was also more effective than famciclovir in preventing PHN-related pain symptoms 3 and 6 months after resolution of the cutaneous lesions.

Other stimulation techniques

Other stimulation techniques such as deep brain stimulation and spinal cord stimulation have no value in AHZ.

Acupuncture

Acupuncture, which has been used for more than 3,000 years as a pain-relieving method, has become very popular in the last 20 years in the Western hemisphere. There are only a few reports, most of them uncontrolled, suggesting that acupuncture begun in the acute phase of herpes zoster, i.e. within 72 h of the appearance of the skin eruption, could produce a substantial reduction in the incidence and severity of PHN if combined with antiviral medication.[100–102]

Miscellaneous therapy

Other reported therapeutic modalities include:

- immune globulin prophylaxis in compromised patients;[103**]

- ultrasonic therapy;[104]
- iontophoresis;[105]
- levodopa.[106]**

CONCLUSIONS AND CLINICAL SUGGESTIONS

Despite wide and various treatment modalities in the management of AZH, an ideal treatment for AZH and prevention of PHN has not yet been found. A number of drugs and methods which have been reported and discussed in this chapter are effective and useful in clinical practice, but they do not have documented evidence of their preventive role in the development of PHN.

It is very important to recognize that herpes zoster is triggered by immune status, age, physical or mental stress, malignancy, and infections or diseases. The choice of the therapy should depend on the immune status and age of the patient.

Patients should be categorize in four groups:

- immunocompetent young;
- immunocompetent old;
- immunocompromised young;
- immunocompromised old.

Immunocompetent young patients

In this group, patients are less than 50 years old, possess normal immunologic responsiveness, and other serious illnesses are excluded. The goal of the treatment is to relieve their pain and prevent inflammatory damage of the nerves and tissues. The most accepted treatment in this group is the use of antiviral therapy, which diminishes or stops the viral replication and spread of the infection to the peripheral nerves. Anti-inflammatory agents are useful in decreasing tissue damage. Also, steroids can be administered locally, systemically, or epidurally. If necessary, pain relief should be administered according to the WHO analgesic ladder. Sympathetic blocks may be also performed.

Immunocompetent old patients

In this older group of patients, no defined disease should be found. However, a higher incidence of the spread of the infection can be expected. The main goal of the therapy in this group is prevention of PHN. Antiviral therapy combined with anti-inflammatory therapy and antidepressants may be efficient and effective in preventing PHN. Eaglstein et al. reported that corticosteroids prevented the development of PHN in this group of patients.[38]* Some other authors have recommended the use of epidural blocks[39]* with corticosteroids, with or without antiviral therapy. Also, sympathetic nerve block can be useful in the treatment of pain and prevention of PHN.[67]***,[70] If necessary, pharmacotherapy with a combination of non-narcotic and narcotic analgesics with antidepressants or anticonvulsants should be applied.

Immunosuppressed young patients

The goal of therapy in young patients who are immuno-deficient is to reduce or to diminish the spread of virus within and outside the primary ganglion nerve dermatome segment. Therefore, antiviral therapy is the first choice of treatment. Additional pain relief should be achieved by techniques which are used for acute pain treatment, including pharmacotherapy and invasive therapy modalities.

Immunosuppressed old patients

The risk of viral dissemination is more often present in this group. Also, there is a high incidence of postherpetic neuralgia. Antiviral therapy is necessary, and prevention of postherpetic neuralgia should be the goal. However, corticosteroids must be used with caution. These patients are more susceptible to viral spread and attendant CNS and visceral complications. Data suggest that steroids do not prevent postherpetic pain in this group. Pain relief by nerve blocks is recommended.

Special attention should be given to the treatment of AHZ in the trigeminal region in all groups of patients as, according to Loeser,[3]*** postherpetic neuralgia is more frequently observed in this region. However, methylprednisolone injection into the Gasserian ganglion in the very early stage of acute herpes zoster can significantly reduce the incidence of PHN.[5] Taking into consideration that in AHZ and PHN there is a close relationship between the duration of neuralgia and therapeutic efficacy, early aggressive treatment of acute pain is necessary. According to Watson,[13,14] antiviral therapy should be administered within 72 h and analgesics including opioids (if necessary), nerve blocks, and early antidepressants[49]**,[50]* should be used.

REFERENCES

◆ 1. Dworkin RH, Portenoy RK. Pain and its persistence in herpes zoster. Pain 1996; 65: 241–51.

2. Watson CPN, Deck JH, Morshead C, et al. Postherpetic neuralgia: further post-mortem studies of cases with and without pain. Pain 1991; 44: 105–17.

● 3. Loeser JD. Herpes zoster and postherpetic neuralgia. Pain 1986; 25: 149–164.

● 4. Portenoy RK, Duma C, Foley KM. Acute herpetic and postherpetic neuralgia: clinical review and current management. Ann Neurol 1986; 20: 651–64.

5. Pernak J, Erdmann W, Bryant JD. Acute herpes zoster of the trigeminal nerve and its treatment. *J Pain Ther* 1993; **3**: 101–7

● 6. Higa K. Acute herpetic pain and postherpetic neuralgia. *Eur J Pain* 1993; **14**: 79–90.

◆ 7. Stankus SJ, Dlugopolski M, Packer D, Management of herpes zoster (shingles) and posthepertic neuralgia. *Am Fam Phys* 2000; **61**: 2437–44.

● 8. Raj PP. Management of pain due to herpes zoster and postherpetic neuralgia. In: Parris WCV ed. *Cancer Pain Management: Principles and Practice*. Boston, MA: Butterworth-Heinemann, 1997: 335–55.

◆ 9. Heald PW. Current treatment practice of herpes zoster. *Expert Opin Pharmacother* 2001; **2**: 1283–7.

10. Johnson RW. Current and future management of herpes zoster. *Antiviral Chem Chemother Suppl* 1997; **8**: 19–29.

● 11. Alper BS, Lewis PR. Does treatment of acute herpes zoster prevent or shorten postherpetic neuralgia? A systematic review of the literature. *J Fam Pract* 2000; **49**: 255–64.

● 12. Fouchard N. Which optimal management for patients with herpes zoster? A review of randomized, controlled trials on acute herpes zoster and postherpetic neuralgia therapy. *Med Mal Infect* 1998; **28**: 738–45.

13. Watson CPN, Watt VR, Chipman M, *et al*. The prognosis with postherpetic neuralgia. *Pain* 1991; **46**: 195–9.

◆ 14. Watson CPN, Gershon AA. Postherpetic neuralgia: the importance of preventing this intractable end-stage disorder. *J Infect Dis* 1998; **178** (Suppl. 1): S91–4.

15. Zacks SI, Langfitt TW, Elliott FA. Herpetic neuritis: a light and electron microscopic study. *Neurology* 1964; **14**: 744–50.

16. Noordebos W. Physiological correlates of clinical pain syndromes. In: Soulairac A, Cahn J, Charpentier J eds. *Pain*. New York, NY: NY Academic, 1968: 465–75.

17. Rake G, Blank H, Corriell LL, *et al*. Relationship of varicella and herpes zoster. Electron microscopic studies. *J Bacteriol* 1948; **56**: 293.

18. Taylor-Robinson D, Downie AW. Chickenpox and herpes zoster. I. Complement-fixation studies. *Br J Exp Pathol* 1959; **40**: 398.

19. Gold E. Serologic and virus isolation studies of patients with varicella or herpes zoster infection. *New Engl J Med* 1966; **274**: 181–5.

20. Hope-Simpson RE. The nature of herpes zoster: a long-term study and a new hypothesis. *Proc R Soc Med* 1965; **58**: 9–20.

21. Glynn C, Crockford G, Gavaghan D, *et al*. Epidemiology of shingles. *J R Soc Med* 1990; **83**: 617–19.

22. Choo PW, Galil K, Donahue JG, *et al*. Risk factors for postherpetic neuralgia. *Arch Intern Med* 1997; **157**: 1217–24.

23. Melbye M, Boedert J, Brossman RJ, *et al*. Risk of AIDS after herpes zoster. *Lancet* 1987; **728**: 730.

24. Preblud SR, D'Angelo LJ. Chickenpox in United States 1972–1977. *J Infect Dis* 1979; **140**: 257–60.

25. Sklar SH, Wigand JS. Herpes zoster. *Br J Dermatol* 1981; **104**: 351–2.

26. Lycka BSA. Dermatologic aspects of herpes zoster. In: Watson CPN ed. *Herpes Zoster and Postherpetic Neuralgia*, vol. 5. Amsterdam: Elsevier, 1993: 59–72.

27. Liesegang TJ. Diagnosis and therapy of herpes zoster ophthalmicus. *Ophthalmology* 1991; **98**: 1216–19.

● 28. Lancaster T, Silagy C, Gray S. Primary care management of acute herpes zoster: systematic review of evidence from randomized controlled trials. *Br J Gen Pract* 1995; **45**: 39–45.

◆ 29. Herne K, Cirelli R, Lee P, Tyring SK. Antiviral therapy of acute herpes zoster in older patients. *Drugs Aging* 1996; **8**: 97–112.

30. Tyring SK. Efficacy of famciclovir in the treatment of herpes zoster. *Semin Dermatol* 1996; **15** (Suppl. 2): 27–31.

● 31. Jackson JL, Gibbons R, Meyer G, Inouye L. The effect of treating herpes zoster with oral acyclovir in preventing postherpetic neuralgia: a meta-analysis. *Arch Intern Med* 1997; **157**: 909–12.

● 32. Wood MJ, Kay R, Dworkin RH, *et al*. Oral acyclovir therapy accelerates pain resolution in patients with herpes zoster: a meta-analysis of placebo-controlled trials. *Clin Infect Dis* 1996; **22**: 341–7.

33. Beutner KR, Friedman DJ, Forszpaniak C, *et al*. Valaciclovir compared with acyclovir for improved therapy for herpes zoster in immunocompetent adults. *Antimicrob Agents Chemother* 1995; **39**: 1546–53.

◆ 34. Wood MJ, Shulda S, Fiddian AP, Crooks RJ. Treatment of acute herpes zoster: effect of early (<48 h) versus late (48–72 h) therapy with acyclovir and valaciclovir on prolonged pain. *J Infect Dis* 1998; **178** (Suppl.): S 81–4.

35. Gnann Jr JW, Crumpacker CS, Lalezari JP, *et al*. Sorivudine versus acyclovir for treatment of dermatomal herpes zoster in human immunodeficiency virus-infected patients: results from a randomized, controlled clinical trial. *Antimicrob Agents Chemother* 1998; **42**: 1139–45.

36. Perry CM, Wagstaff AJ. Famciclovir. A review of its pharmacological properties and therapeutic efficacy in herpes virus infection. *Drugs* 1995; **50**: 396–415.

37. Dworkin RH, Boon RJ, Griffin DRG, Phung D. Postherpetic neuralgia: impact of famciclovir, age, rash severity, and acute pain in herpes zoster patients. *J Infect Dis* 1998; **178** (Suppl.): S 76–80.

38. Eaglstein WH, Katz R, Brown JA. The effects of early corticosteroids therapy on the skin eruption and pain of herpes zoster. *JAMA* 1970; **211**: 1681–3.

39. Moesker A, Boersma FP. The effect of extradural administration of corticosteroids as pain treatment of acute herpes zoster and to prevent postherpetic neuralgia. In: Erdmann W, Oyama T, Pernak J eds. *The Pain Clinic*, vol. 1. Utrecht: VNU Science Press, 1985: 273–9.

40. Pernak J. Treatment of acute herpes zoster for the prevention of postherpetic neuralgia. *Pain* 1990; **Suppl.**: S60.

41. Epstein E. Treatment of zoster and postzoster neuralgia by the intralesional injection of triamcinolone. A computer analysis of 199 cases. *Int J Dermatol* 1976; **15:** 762–9.

42. Chiarello SE. Tumescent infiltration of corticosteroids, lidocaine, and epinephrine into dermatomes of acute herpetic pain or postherpetic neuralgia. *Arch Dermatol* 1998; **134:** 279–81.

43. Pasqualucci A, Pasqualucci V, Galla F, *et al*. Prevention of postherpetic neuralgia: acyclovir and prednisolone versus epidural local anesthetic and methylprednisolone. *Acta Anaesthesiol Scand* 2000; **44:** 910–18.

● 44. Gill KS, Wood MJ. The value of steroids in the treatment of herpes zoster. *Expert Opin Invest Drugs* 1994; **3:** 791–7.

45. Wood MJ, Johnson RW, McKendrick MW, *et al*. A randomized trail of acyclovir for 7 days or 21 days with and without prednisolone for treatment of acute herpes zoster. *New Engl J Med* 1994; **330:** 896–900.

46. Kishore-Kumar R, Max MB, Schafer SC, *et al*. Desipramine relieves postherpetic neuralgia. *Clin Pharmacol Ther* 1990; **47:** 305–12.

47. Watson CPN, Vernich L, Chipman M, Reed K. Nortriptyline versus amitriptyline in postherpetic neuralgia: a randomized trial. *Neurology* 1998; **51:** 1166–71.

48. Watson CPN, Chipman M, Reed K, *et al*. Amitryptyline versus maprotiline in postherpetic neuralgia: a randomised, double-blind crossover trial. *Pain* 1992; **48:** 29–36.

● 49. Bowsher D. The effects of pre-emptive treatment of postherpetic neuralgia with amitriptyline: a randomized, double-blind, placebo-controlled trial. *J Pain Symptom Manage* 1997; **13:** 327–31.

50. Bowsher D. Acute herpes zoster and postherpetic neuralgia: effects of acyclovir and outcome of treatment with amitriptyline. *Br J Gen Pract* 1992; **42:** 244–6.

51. Avery AJ, Reeves J. Acute herpes zoster, postherpetic neuralgia, acyclovir and aminotriptyline. *Br J Gen Pract* 1992; **42:** 493–4.

52. Segal AZ, Rordorf G. Gabapentin as a novel treatment for postherpetic neuralgia. *Neurology* 1996; **46:** 1175–6.

53. Rowbotham M, Harden N, Stacey B, *et al*. Gabapentin for the treatment of postherpetic neuralgia: a randomized controlled trial. *JAMA* 1998; **280:** 1837–42.

54. Filadora VA, Sist TC, Lema MJ. Acute herpetic neuralgia and postherpetic neuralgia in the head and neck: response to gabapentin in five cases. *Reg Anesth Pain Med* 1999; **24:** 170–4.

55. Weis O, Sriwatanakul K, Weintraub M. Treatment of postherpetic neuralgia and acute herpetic pain with amitriptyline and perphenazine. *South Afr Med J* 1982; **62:** 274–5.

◆ 56. Sunshine A, Olsen Z. Nonnarcotic analgesic. In: Wall PD, Melzack R eds. *Textbook of Pain*. Edinburgh: Churchill Livingstone, 1994: 923–43.

57. Bareggi SR, Pirola R, De Benedittis G. Skin and plasma levels of acetylsalicylic acid: a comparison between topical aspirin/diethyl ether mixture and oral aspirin in acute herpes zoster and postherpetic neuralgia. *Eur J Clin Pharmacol* 1998; **54:** 231–5.

58. Vickers MD, O'Flaherty D, Szekely SM, *et al*. Tramadol: pain relief by an opioid without depression of respiration. *Anaesthesia* 1992; **47:** 291–6.

● 59. Portenoy RK. Chronic opioid therapy in nonmalignant pain. *J Pain Symptom Manage* 1990; **5** (Suppl.1): S46–62.

60. Zenz M, Strumpf M, Tryba M. Long-term oral opioid therapy in patients with nonmalignant pain. *J Pain Symptom Manage* 1992; **7:** 69–77.

61. Riopelle JM, Lopez-Anaya A, Cork RC, *et al*. Treatment of the cutaneous pain of acute herpes zoster with 9% lidocaine (base) in petrolatum paraffin ointment. *J Am Acad Dermatol* 1994; **30:** 757–67.

62. Rowbotham MC, Davies L, Fields HL. Topical lidocaine gel relieves postherpetic neuralgia. *Ann Neurol* 1995; **37:** 246–53.

63. De Benedittis G, Besana F, Lorenzetti A. A new topical treatment for acute herpetic neuralgia and postherpetic neuralgia: the aspirin/diethyl ether mixture: an open-label study plus a double-blind controlled clinical trial. *Pain* 1992; **48:** 383–90.

64. De Benedittis G, Lorenzetti A. Topical aspirin/diethyl ether mixture versus indomethacin and diclofenac/diethyl ether mixtures for acute herpetic neuralgia and postherpetic neuralgia. *Pain* 1996; **65:** 45–51.

65. Rosenak S. Procain injection treatment of herpes zoster. *Lancet* 1938; **5:** 1056–8.

66. Tenicela R, Lovasik D, Eaglstein W. Treatment of herpes zoster with sympathetic blocks. *Clin J Pain* 1985; **1:** 63–7.

● 67. Ali NMK. Does sympathetic ganglionic block prevent postherpetic neuralgia? Literature review. *Reg Anesth* 1995; **20:** 227–33.

68. Colding A. The effect of regional sympathetic blocks in the treatment of herpes zoster: a survey of 300 cases. *Acta Anaesthesiol Scand* 1969; **13:** 133–41.

69. Colding A. Treatment of pain: organisation of a pain clinic: treatment of acute herpes zoster. *Proc R Soc Med* 1973; **66:** 541–3.

70. Winnie AP, Hartwell PW. Relationship between time of treatment of acute herpes zoster with sympathetic blockade and prevention of postherpetic neuralgia: clinical support for a new theory of the mechanism by which sympathetic blockade provides therapeutic benefit. *Reg Anesth* 1993; **18:** 277–82.

71. Koh WS, Park SM, Kim BS, Shin DY. The effect of sympathetic blocks in the prevention of postherpetic neuralgia. *Korean J Dermatol* 1997; **35:** 620–6.

72. Whizar-Lugo VM, Carrada-Perez S, Martinez-Andrade-MA, *et al*. Sympathetic nerve blocks with 0.25% ropivacaine in acute herpes zoster pain. *Rev Mex Anesthesiol* 1998; **21:** 151–8.

● 73. Wu CL, Marsh A, Dworkin RH. The role of sympathetic

nerve blocks in herpes zoster and postherpetic neuralgia. *Pain* 2000; **87:** 121–9.

74. Dan K. Nerve block therapy and postherpetic neuralgia. *Crit Rev Phys Rehabil Med* 1995; **7:** 93–112.

75. Hadzic A, Vloka JD, Saff GN, *et al.* The "three-in-one block" for treatment of pain in a patient with acute herpes zoster infection. *Reg Anesth* 1997; **22:** 575–8.

76. Rutgers MJ, Dirksen R. The prevention of postherpetic neuralgia: a retrospective view of patients treated in the acute phase of herpes zoster. *Br J Clin Pract* 1988; **42:** 412–14.

77. Lipton JR, Harding SP, Wells JCD. The effect of early stellate ganglion block on postherpetic neuralgia in herpes zoster ophthalmicus. *Pain Clin* 1986/1987; **1:** 247–52.

78. Bauman J. Prevention of postherpetic neuralgia. *Anesthesiology* 1987; **67:** 441–2.

79. Manabe H, Dan K, Higa K. Continuous epidural infusion of local anaesthetics and shorter duration of acute zoster-associated pain. *Clin J Pain* 1995; **11:** 220–8.

80. Hwang SM, Kang YC, Lee YB, *et al.* The effects of epidural blockade on the acute pain in herpes zoster. *Arch Dermatol* 1999; **135:** 1359–64.

81. Pasqualucci V, Del Sindaco F, Cirulli P. The rationale for the use of peridural local anesthetics in the therapy of herpes zoster. *Minerva Anesthesiol* 1991; **57:** 433–6.

82. Sung SY, Hong-Yong K, Han-Uk K, Chull-Wan I. Comparative evaluation of the treatment of herpes zoster with and without sympathetic block. *Korean J Dermatol* 1998; **36:** 1–6.

83. Boas RA. Sympathetic nerve blocks: In search of a role. *Reg Anesth Pain Med* 1998; **23:** 292–305.

84. Yanagida H, Suwa K, Corssen G. No prophylactic effect of early sympathetic blockade on postherpetic neuralgia. *Anesthesiology* 1987; **66:** 73–6.

85. Visitsunthorn U, Prete P. Reflex sympathetic dystrophy of the lower extremity. A complication of herpes zoster with dramatic response to propranolol. *West J Med* 1981; **135:** 62–6.

86. Higa K, Hori K, Harasawa I, *et al.* High thoracic epidural block relieves acute herpetic pain involving the trigeminal and cervical regions: comparison with effects of stellate ganglion block. *Reg Anesth* 1998; **23:** 25–9.

87. Pernak J. Percutaneous radiofrequency thermal lumbar sympathectomy. *Pain Clinic* 1995; **8:** 99–106.

88. Swerdlow M. *Relief of Intractable Pain*, vol. 1, 2nd edn. Amsterdam: Elsevier, 1978: 169–71.

89. Johnson LR, Rocco AG, Ferrente FM. Continuous sub-

pleural-paravertebral block in acute thoracic herpes zoster. *Anesth Analg* 1988; **67:** 1105–8.

90. Reiestad F, Kvalheim L, McIlvaine WB. Pleural analgesia for the treatment of acute severe herpes zoster. *Reg Anesth* 1989; **14:** 244–6.

91. Goldman JA. *Biomedical Aspects of the Laser.* Berlin: Springer Verlag, 1967.

92. Palmieri B. Mid-laser action mechanism: facts and hypothesis. *Med Laser Rep* 1985; **2:** 3–5.

93. Landthaler M, Haina D, Waidelich W. Behandlung von Zoster, postzosterischen Schmerzen und Herpes simplex recidivans in loco mit Laser-Licht. *Fortschr Med* 1983; **101:** 1039–41.

94. Stoklas S, Galehr E, Lerche A, *et al.* Effect of repeated irradiation with low power helium–neon laser on acute herpetic pain. *Anesth Analg* 1998; **86** (Suppl. 2): S317.

95. Melzack R, Wall PD. Pain mechanisms: a new theory. *Science* 1965; **150:** 971–8.

96. Salar G, Job I, Mingrino S. *et al.* Effect of transcutaneous electrotherapy on CSF: β-endorphin content in patients without pain problems. *Pain* 1981; **10:** 169–72.

97. Nathan PW, Wall PD. Treatment of postherpetic neuralgia by prolonged electric stimulation. *Br Med J* 1974; **3:** 645–7.

98. Taverner D. Alleviation of postherpetic neuralgia. *Lancet* 1960; **2:** 671–3.

99. Ahmed HE, Craig WF, White PF, *et al.* Percutaneous electrical nerve stimulation: an alternative to antiviral drugs for acute herpes zoster. *Anesth Analg* 1998; **87:** 911–14.

100. Coghlan CJ. Herpes zoster treated by acupuncture. *Cent Afr J Med* 1992; **38:** 466–7.

101. Li H. 34 cases of herpes zoster treated by moxibustion at dazhui (du 14). *J Tradit Chin Med* 1992; **12:** 71.

102. Boaler J. Acupuncture in the management of herpes zoster. *Acupunct Med* 1996; **14:** 80–2.

103. Stevens DA, Merigan TC. Zoster immune globulin prophylaxis of disseminated zoster in compromised hosts. A randomised trial. *Arch Intern Med* 1980; **140:** 52–4.

104. Jones RJ, Silman GM. Trial of ultrasonic therapy for acute herpes zoster. *Practitioner* 1987; **231:** 1336–40.

105. Kodama K, Sakaguchi Y, Morioka T, *et al.* Iontophoresis using a local anesthetic for the treatment of pediatric acute herpetic pain. *J Anesth* 1998; **12:** 95–9.

106. Kernbaum S, Hauchecorne J. Administration of levodopa for relief of herpes zoster pain. *JAMA* 1981; **246:** 132–4.

treatment of HZ with antivirals and analgesics to reduce the extent of the nerve damage that likely correlates with intractable pain.

Live, attenuated varicella vaccine elicits protective immunity against varicella-zoster virus (VZV) in children and adults,[66-69] although mild breakthrough cases of varicella may occur. It has been suggested that waning VZV-specific cell-mediated immunity in the elderly can be stimulated by varicella vaccine in order to prevent the occurrence and severity of HZ and hence PHN.

Early treatment of varicella with the antiviral agent acyclovir may prevent or attenuate the occurrence of HZ.[69] Initially, studies of acyclovir were not impressive, but more recent trials that have paid more attention to persistent pain suggest a protective effect of this drug when used in high doses orally (800 mg five times daily). Newer antivirals such as famciclovir[70,71] and valaciclovir[72] may prove more effective than acyclovir in preventing PHN.

A number of controlled studies of small numbers of patients with HZ treated with corticosteroids have claimed a reduction in PHN. Two controlled trials have purported to prove such an effect.[73,74] These trials have been criticized, and more recent controlled trials have shown no effect.[75,76]

Uncontrolled trials of sympathetic blocks for HZ have claimed relief of the acute pain of HZ and a reduction in the subsequent development of PHN,[52,53,77,78] although one study showed no effect.[79] None of these trials was controlled, and with the marked natural tendency for improvement of pain with time, it is easy to confuse such an effect with a treatment effect.[80]

One placebo-controlled trial supports the preventative effect of amantadine hydrochloride against PHN when used in a dose of 100 mg twice daily at the onset of HZ.[81,82] Other unreplicated trials claim a prophylactic effect with levodopa[83] and adenosine monophosphate.[84] Good control with the acute pain of HZ with opioids, if necessary, may also be important in reducing PHN.

PROGNOSIS

A study of PHN with regard to prognosis[85] indicates that, even with long-duration PHN, about one-half of patients recover slowly over months to years, with most having no therapy. The bad news is that the other half continue to suffer despite therapy, sometimes even until death.

CONCLUSIONS

Although none of the putative preventive approaches to PHN can be regarded as conclusively established to be effective at significantly preventing this disorder, pend-

ing final proof, it is reasonable to treat patients early and aggressively to relieve the pain of HZ and to try to prevent PHN if the therapy is safe and well tolerated. It is important to recognize that the population at highest risk for PHN is the age group 60 years or over who may have a risk of 50% or more developing this complication. Valaciclovir or famciclovir appear to be safe and to modestly reduce the occurrence of PHN. Although no controlled trial has ever been carried out of nerve blocks to treat HZ pain or prevent PHN, they are reasonable and safe in experienced hands, and may be repeated if effective as symptoms dictate. The use of nonsteroidal anti-inflammatory drugs, such as acetaminophen (paracetamol) and opioids, are justified to relieve the severe pain that accompanies the acute illness on an as-needed basis. The initiation of low-dose amitriptyline may be considered at this stage.[86]

For established PHN (neuropathic pain persisting for more than 1 month after HZ), the most repeatedly effective agents in clinical trials appear to be antidepressants, and controlled trials support this approach. These data indicate that pain may be reduced from moderate or severe to mild in about two-thirds of patients. It is reasonable to commence with amitriptyline or nortriptyline in a dose of 10 mg at night in those over 65 years and with 25 mg in those aged 65 years or younger. The dose is increased by similar increments in a single dose at night every 7–10 days until relief is obtained or side-effects supervene. If these fail, one can try desipramine or maprotiline in similar doses. Two controlled trials support the use of the anticonvulsant gabapentin in PHN with a low occurrence of side-effects.[34,35]** Doses up to 3,600 mg/day may be required. Occasionally, patients failing these may benefit from a serotonergic drug such as trasodone, clomipramine, or fluoxetine, but no controlled trial has been done and these do not appear to be useful for the majority of the patients. It is also possible that the addition of a neuroleptic such as fluphenazine 1 mg up to three times daily may give added benefit in some. A trial-and-error approach in refractory patients may also include the anticonvulsants carbamazepine, phenytoin, clonazepam, or valproate. For resistant cases, opioids may be safely prescribed on an as-needed or round-the-clock basis. Long-acting oral forms of oxycodone, morphine, and hydromorphone and the fentanyl skin patch may be of advantage. There is evidence that topical capsaicin has a weak to moderate effect and may be an adjunctive treatment if carefully used. Recent evidence supports the use of a lidocaine skin patch. An RCT[87] has suggested that intrathecal methylprednisolone given in 4-weekly injections relieved more than 90% of patients with PHN of at least 1 year's duration. This dramatic effect needs to be duplicated. Unfortunately, in many parts of the world, methylprednisolone is not approved for intrathecal use because the preservative may be neurotoxic and a preservative-free preparation is not available.

REFERENCES

1. Kurzke JR. Neuroepidemiology. *Ann Neurol* 1984; **16:** 265–77.

◆ 2. Head H, Campbell AW. The pathology of herpes zoster, and its bearing on sensory localisation. *Brain* 1900; **23:** 353–529.

◆ 3. Watson CP, Deck JH, Morshead C, *et al.* Postherpetic neuralgia: further postmortem studies of cases with and without pain. *Pain* 1988; **34:** 129–38.

4. Noordenbos W. Problems pertaining to the transmission of nerve impulses which give rise to pain. In: *Pain,* vol. 10. Amsterdam: Elsevier, 1959: 68–80.

5. Baron R, Haendler G, Schulte H, Afferent large fibre polyneuropathy predicts the development of postherpetic neuralgia. *Pain* 1997; **73:** 231–8.

6. Oaklander AL, Romans K, Horasek S, *et al.* Unilateral postherpetic neuralgia with bilateral sensory damage. *Ann Neurol* 1998; **44:** 789–95.

7. Watson CPN, Midha R, Devor M, *et al.* Trigeminal postherpetic neuralgia: clinically unilateral, pathologically bilateral. In: Devor M, Rowbotham M, Wiesenfeld-Hallin Z eds. *Proceedings of the World Congress on Pain.* Vienna: Elsevier, 2000: 733–9.

8. Wall PD, Gutnick M. Ongoing activity in peripheral nerves. *Exp Neurol* 1974; **43:** 580–93.

● 9. Rowbotham M, Petersen KL, Fields HL. Is postherpetic neuralgia one disorder? *Pain Forum* 1998; **7:** 231–7.

◆ 10. Hope-Simpson RE. The nature of herpes zoster: a long-term study and a new hypothesis. *Proc R Soc Med* 1965; **58:** 9–20.

11. Ragozzino MW, Melton LJ, Kurland LT, *et al.* Population-based study of herpes zoster and its sequelae. *Medicine* 1982; **61:** 310–16.

12. Burgoon Jr CF, Burgoon JS, Baldridge GD. The natural history of herpes zoster. *JAMA* 1957; **164:** 265.

13. De Moragas JM, Kierland RR, The outcome of patients with herpes zoster. *Arch Dermatol* 1957; **75:** 193–6.

14. Watson CPN, Chipman M, Reed K, *et al.* Postherpetic neuralgia: 208 cases. *Pain* 1988; **34:** 289–98.

● 15. Feinmann C. Pain relief by antidepressants: possible modes of action. *Pain* 1985; **23:** 1–8.

● 16. Getto CJ, Sorkness CA, Howell T. Antidepressants and chronic non-malignant pain: a review. *J Pain Symptom Manage* 1987; **2:** 8–18.

● 17. Goodkin K, Gullion CM. Antidepressants for the relief of chronic pain: do they work. *Ann Behav Med* 1989; **11:** 75–80.

18. Woodforde JM, Dwyer B, McEwen BW, *et al.* The treatment of postherpetic neuralgia. *Med J Aust* 1965; **2:** 869–72.

19. Taub A. Relief of postherpetic neuralgia with psychotropic drugs. *J Neurosurg* 1973, **39:** 235–9.

20. Taub A, Collins WF. Observations on the treatment of denervation dysesthesia with psychotropic drugs. *Adv Neurol* 1974; **4:** 309–15.

◆ 21. Watson CPN, Evans RJ, Reed K, *et al.* Amitriptyline versus placebo in postherpetic neuralgia. *Neurology* 1982; **32:** 671–3.

◆ 22. Max MB, Schafer SC, Culnane M, *et al.* Amitriptyline but not lorazepam relieves postherpetic neuralgia. *Neurology* 1988; **38:** 1427–32.

23. Watson CPN, Evans RJ. A comparative trial of amitriptyline and zimelidine in postherpetic neuralgia. *Pain* 1985; **23:** 3887–994.

24. Kishore-Kumar R, Schafer SC, Lawlor BA, *et al.* Single doses of the serotonin agonists buspirone and m-chlorophenylpiperazine do not relieve neuropathic pain. *Pain* 1989; **37:** 223–7.

◆ 25. Kishore-Kumar R, Max MB, Schafer SC, *et al.* Desipramine relieves postherpetic neuralgia. *Clin Pharmacol* 1990; **47:** 305–12.

◆ 26. Watson CPN, Chipman M, Reed K, *et al.* Amitriptyline versus maprotiline in postherpetic neuralgia. *Pain* 1992; **18:** 29–36.

27. Watson CPN, Vernish L, Chipman M, Reed K. nortriptyline versus amitriptyline in postherpetic neuralgia: a randomised trial. *Neurology* 1998; **51:** 1166–71.

28. Faber GA, Burks JW. Chlorprothixene therapy for herpes zoster neuralgia. *South Med J* 1974; **67:** 808–12.

29. Nathan PW. Chlorprothixene Taractan in postherpetic neuralgia and other severe chronic pains. *Pain* 1978; **5:** 367–71.

30. Killian JM, Fromm GH. Carbamazepine in the treatment of neuralgia. *Arch Neurol* 1968; **19:** 219–36.

31. Hatangdi VS, Boad RA, Richards EG. Postherpetic neuralgia: management with antiepileptic and tricyclic drugs. In: Bonica JJ, Albe-Fessard D eds. *Advances in Pain Research and Therapy*, vol. 1. New York, NY: Raven Press, 1976: 583–7.

32. Gerson GR, Jones RB, Luscombe DK. Studies on the concomitant use of carbamazepine and clomipramine for the relief of postherpetic neuralgia. *Postgrad Med J* 1977; **54:** 104–9.

33. Raftery H. The management of postherpetic pain using sodium valproate and amitriptyline. *Irish Med J* 1979; **79:** 399–401.

34. Rice ASC, Maton S, and the Postherpetic Neuralgia Study Group. Gabapentin in postherpetic neuralgia: a randomised, double-blind, controlled study. *Pain* 2001; **94:** 214–25.

◆ 35. Rowbotham M, Harden N, Stacey B, *et al.* Gabapentin for the treatment of postherpetic neuralgia: a randomised controlled trial. *JAMA* 1998; **280:** 1837–42.

36. Taub A. Opioid analgesic in the treatment of chronic intractable pain of non-neoplastic origin. In: Kitahata LM, Collins D eds. *Narcotic Analgesics in Anesthesiology.* Baltimore, MD: Williams & Wilkins, 1982: 199–208.

37. Tennant FS, Uelmen GI. Narcotic maintenance for chronic pain: medical and legal guidelines. *J Postgrad Med* 1983; **71:** 81–94.

38. Tennant FS, Robinson D, Sagherian DL, Seecof R.

Table 35.3 *Pharmacotherapy for neuropathic pain associated with spasticity*

Drug	Dose range	Potential adverse effects
Tricyclic antidepressants**		
Amitryptyline	10–200 mg/q.h.s.	Dry mouth, urinary retention, sedation
Nortriptyline	10–100 mg/q.h.s.	Dry mouth, urinary retention, sedation
Anticonvulsants**		
Phenytoin	100–300 mg/day	Sedation, gum hypertrophy, hepatotoxicity
Carbamazepine	100–1,000 mg/day	Blood dyscrasia, sedation, confusion
Oxcarbazepine	150–200 mg/day	Blood dyscrasia, sedation, confusion
Gabapentin	100–3,600 mg/day	Sedation, nausea, ataxia, myoclonus
Valproate	250–1,500 mg/day	Nausea, tremor, weight gain, hepatotoxicity
Topiramate	15–400 mg/day	Weight loss, kidney stones, sedation, ataxia
Zonisamide	50–400 mg/day	Weight loss, kidney stones, sedation, ataxia

q.h.s., every hour until sufficient.

Table 35.4 *Spasticity assessments*

Adult patients	Pediatric patients
Tone intensity scales (e.g. Ashworth)	Tests of motor development and functional performance
Tone/spasm frequency scores	Comprehensive diagnostic developmental assessments
Global scales of motor impairment (e.g. Fugl–Meyer evaluation)	Motor assessments
Upper extremity dexterity and strength testing (e.g. Purdue pegboard test)	Assessments designed for children with disabilities
ADL/hygiene scales (e.g. Barthel)	
Clinical gait scores	
Pain scales (e.g. visual analog scales)	
Goniometry	
Electrophysiologic/biomechanical measures	
Global scales of disability (e.g. functional independence measure)	
Patient/caregiver assessment/report of adjustment and disability ("quality of life" measures, e.g. Sickness Impact Profile)	

ADL, activities of daily living.

TREATMENT OPTIONS FOR PAINFUL SPASTICITY

Interventions have been separated by category below. This compartmentalization rarely occurs in clinical practice as most patients with pain from spasticity require several interventions in combination. Treatments are scored with asterisks to denote the level of evidence supporting clinical efficacy in published literature.

Physiotherapy and nonpharmacological strategies*

The role of physical and occupational therapy (PT/OT) cannot be overemphasized for:

- prevention of contractures;
- strengthening of weak muscles;
- training in selective motor activation;
- use of safety techniques;
- reduction of noxious stimuli (e.g. pressure sores).

A wide range of interventions may be beneficial in reducing spastic muscle overactivity, including stretching, biofeedback, massage, and splinting. A multidisciplinary team with PT and OT input is crucial for success.

Oral medications**

Standard antispasticity medications are listed in Table 35.5.[9,10] Several medications may confer added benefit via modulations of central neurotransmitter systems. One example is tizanadine, an α_2-adrenergic agonist that may have analgesic as well as antispastic properties.[11–13] Some patients require chronic pain medication outside the realm of spasticity management. Such agents include antiepileptic compounds (e.g. carbamazepine, gabapen-

Table 35.5 *Uses, doses, and adverse effects of oral pharmacologic therapy for spasticity management*

Drug	Common use(s)	Daily adult dose (mg/day)	Maximum pediatric dose	Adverse effects
Baclofen**	MS, SCI, possibly stroke	60–120	30–60 mg	Decreased ambulation speed, muscle weakness, sedation, difficulty in seizure control
Tizanidine**	MS, SCI, stroke	2–36	NR	Sedation, dry mouth, rare hepatotoxicity
Dantrolene sodium**	MS, SCI, stroke	100–400	3 mg/kg	Decreased ambulation speed, muscle weakness, hepatotoxicity
Clonidine*	Possibly SCI	0.1–0.4	NR	Depression, hypotension
Cyproheptadine*	Possibly MS and SCI	12–108	0.5 mg/kg	Muscle weakness, sedation, dry mouth
Benzodiazepine				
Diazepam**	MS, SCI, possibly stroke	5–60	0.8 mg/kg	Sedation, decreased ambulation speed, cognitive effects
Clorazepate*	MS, stroke	5–10	NR	Minor sedation
Ketazolam*	SCI, TBI, CP	30–60	NR	Sedation
Clonazepam*	Possibly MS	0.5–3	NR	Sedation

CP, cerebral palsy; MS, multiple sclerosis; NR, not reported; SCI, spinal cord injury; TBI, traumatic brain injury.

tin), antidepressants, and opioids (e.g. fentanyl patch). In general, opioids are not a viable long-term strategy as they may interfere with bowel management and have unwanted psychotropic effects.

Surgery*

Several surgical interventions may assist in the reduction of painful spasticity, including ablation of the dorsal root entry zone in SCI patients, tendon transfer, neurectomy, shunting of hydrocephalus or syringomyelia, and even thalamic stimulator implantation (Table 35.6).[14-19]

Intrathecal medications**

Delivery of medication more directly to the spinal cord via the intrathecal space is effective in pain management. Several drugs of different pharmacologic classes have been infused by catheter with or without programmable pump devices. Most common is baclofen, followed by morphine, clonidine, and fentanyl. Intrathecal baclofen pump implantation (Table 35.7) has proven valuable when pain is due to widespread or generalized hypertonia and spasms.[20-23] Long-term results are satisfactory if a team approach is used and careful patient selection and follow-up are employed.[24]

Chemodenervation

If a patient has painful spasticity and it has been determined that the pain results from focal muscle overactivity, then a reduction in focal muscle overactivity may result in reduced pain. If pain is generated by a mechanism unrelated to muscle contraction, chemodenervation of muscle is unlikely to be of benefit, and treatment should be directed toward other pain generators.

Phenol and alcohol neurolysis**

Focal muscle overactivity may be reduced by neurolysis of the motor nerve to the target muscle. This may be carried out by specifically locating the motor nerve (e.g. the musculocutaneous nerve to the biceps brachii) and precisely placing 0.25–2.0 ml of phenol 5–6% solution (Table 35.8).[25] Alternatively, a larger volume of phenol solution may be infused into the belly of the target muscle. This results in neurolysis of multiple individual motor nerve endings. The former technique is known as *motor nerve block* and the latter as *motor point block*. Motor nerve blocks are most commonly restricted to relatively pure motor nerves such as the obturator nerve (for thigh adductor spasticity) and the musculocutaneous nerve (for elbow flexor spasticity). Unfortunately, phenol blocks of mixed sensorimotor nerves have a higher risk of iatrogenic neuropathic pain. Motor point blocks have a greater risk of local tissue trauma or necrosis, phlebitis, and pain owing to the volume of phenol required. Although phenol is relatively inexpensive, the technical expertise necessary on the part of the clinician has limited this form of chemodenervation.

Botulinum toxin injections**

Chemodenervation may be produced with localized infusion of a potent neurotoxin. When minute quantities are injected into a target muscle, botulinum toxin (BTX) produces a dose-dependent controlled amount of muscle relaxation or weakness. The toxin acts by blocking the release of acetylcholine from the neuromuscular junction. The pharmacology of BTX is described elsewhere.[26] Three serotypes of BTX have been used clinically, including types A, B, and F. Their pharmacology, duration of effect, and potency differ; therefore, the reader is cautioned to be clear as to which agent is used when reviewing the literature.

Published trials and reports for spasticity include two different formulations of type A botulinum toxin:

Table 35.6 *Surgical techniques tested in the treatment of spasticity*

Procedure	Target	Results
Stereotactic encephalotomy*	Globus pallidus Ventrolateral thalamic nuclei Cerebellum	Variable to poor
Cerebellar stimulation*	Cerebellum	Poor
Longitudinal myelotomy*	Conus medullaris	Variable
Cervical posterior rhizotomy*	C1–C3	Slight improvements Significant potential for complications
Selective posterior rhizotomy**	Selected roots of L2–S2	Variable, encouraging
Neurectomy*	Involved nerves	Variable, high recurrence, possibility of permanent painful dysesthesiae
Tendon lengthening, release or transfer*	Contracted or spastic muscle	Variable but generally effective

Reproduced with permission from Chambers HG. The surgical treatmnt of spasticity. *Muscle Nerve* 1997; **6** (Suppl.): 5121–8.

Table 35.7 *Guidelines for intrathecal baclofen infusion***

Useful for generalized spasticity, especially leg adduction, extension, and hip flexion

Conduct test dose to predict response (delayed response possible)

Use programmable infusion rates and doses

Initial continuous infusion 25 μg/day

Titrate up to 400–500 μg/day or until satisfactory reduction in spasticity

Common side-effects: drowsiness, dizziness, nausea, hypotension, headache, and weakness

Requires ITB team and patient commitment

ITB, intrathecal baclofen.

Botox (Allergan, Inc.) and Dysport (available in Europe only; Ipsen, Inc.). Both are effective, but the dose equivalency is approximately 300–500 units of Dysport to 100 units of Botox (Table 35.8). Clinical trials evaluating the type B toxin [Myobloc (USA), NeuroBloc (Europe); Elan Pharmaceuticals] have been conducted,[27,28] and the product has obtained Food and Drug Administration (FDA) approval for the treatment of cervical dystonia. In these studies, the type B toxin was found to significantly decrease the pain from cervical dystonia. Clinical trials are currently under way with type B toxin for spasticity as well as myofascial pain and conditions involving involuntary muscle contractions. A treatment algorithm to determine when to use of botulinum toxin for painful spasticity is provided in Fig. 35.1.

BTX has been used for a variety of clinical disorders, including hemifacial spasm, blepharospasm, cervical dystonia (torticollis), limb dystonia, spasticity, and sphincter dyssynergia. In the early 1980s, it became clear that pain reduction was quite common in patients receiving BTX for cervical muscle contraction. Review of the spasticity literature reveals that pain reduction may be an important result of such treatment.[29] Painful clonus, painful cocontraction of agonist and antagonist muscles, joint position abnormalities, and focal nerve compression by muscle may be reduced in select patients. Perioperative pain may be reduced by BTX injection. Ballieau and colleagues have reported reduced analgesic need, lessening of pain, and shorter length of hospital stay in children with cerebral palsy undergoing adductor tendon lengthening surgery.[30]

It has been suggested that BTX may have some effect on pain via mechanisms other than simple muscle cholinergic blockade. The empiric observation that migraine was reduced in some patients receiving frontalis injections has led to controlled clinical trials that were under way at the time of writing. Preliminary results suggest that there may be a prophylactic benefit; however, the mechanism of action is unclear.[31] Further research is needed prior to indiscriminate use of BTX for management of pain (see Chapter P22).

CLINICAL OUTCOMES

Intervention for painful spasticity should be assessed for:

- technical effect;
- functional effect;
- clinical outcome.

For example, chemodenervation at the muscle (technical effect) may result in reduced spasm or clonus (functional effect) that may translate into improved independence in activities of daily living (clinical outcome). Clearly, treatment success depends upon appropriate patient selection, goal determination, and technical skill. Treatment failure may result from deficiency at any level: inappropriate patient selection, goal determination, or technical problems. The most common failure of chemodenervation is mismatch of treatment and patient goal. Technical failure

Table 35.8 *Characteristics of chemodenervation techniques for spasticity*

Parameter	Botulinum toxin**	Phenol motor nerve block*	Phenol motor point block*
Extent of chemodenervation	Controlled, dose dependent Best for small- and medium-sized muscles	"All or none" Limited to muscle supplied by "pure" motor nerves	Variable Requires infusion of large dose of phenol
Technical skill	Simple to inject	Technically difficult	Moderately difficult
Dosage range	Type A toxin, Botox ≤400 U Type A toxin, Dysport ≤1,200–2,000 U Type B toxin, Myobloc 5,000–15,000 U	0.25–2 ml of 5–6% phenol	<1 g (10 ml of 5% phenol)
Risk of side-effects	Low risk, except weakness	High risk, including chronic dysesthesiae and pain and injection	Similar to motor nerve block + tissue necrosis
Cost	High	Low	Low

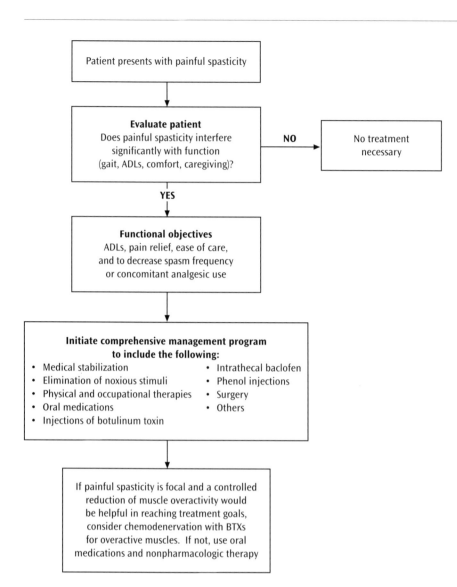

Figure 35.1 *Algorithm for use of botulinum toxin in the treatment of painful spasticity. BTX, botulinum toxin; ADL, activities of daily living.*

may be due to incorrect selection or localization of target muscle or insufficient dose of botulinum toxin. An assessment of response and a detailed algorithm for use of botulinum toxin in spasticity have been published.[32]

FUTURE RESEARCH

Improved management of painful spasticity will ultimately depend on strategies aimed at reducing the extent of neurologic injury. Acute injury management and neuroprotective therapies may save vulnerable tissue and perhaps block the cascade of neurotoxic events initiated by trauma and disease. In the near future, a clearer understanding of the pathophysiology of pain will allow refinement of pharmacological and surgical interventions. Today, chemodenervation with botulinum toxin is an integral part of our armamentarium against painful spasticity. More precise BTX injection techniques, improved criteria for patient selection, and a combination of chemodenervation with other treatment modalities hold promise for the treatment of painful spasticity.

REFERENCES

1. Maynard FM, Karnas RS, Waring WP. Epidemiology of spasticity following traumatic spinal cord injuries. *Arch Phys Med Rehab* 1990; **71:** 566–9.
2. Mayer NH. Clinicophysiologic concepts of spasticity and motor dysfunction in adults with an upper motorneuron lesion. *Muscle Nerve* 1997; **6** (Suppl.): S1–13.
3. Little JW, Micklesen P, Umlauf R, Britell C. Lower extremity manifestations of spasticity in chronic spinal cord injury. *Am J Phys Med Rehab* 1989; **68:** 32–6.
4. Yarkony G. Spinal cord injury. In: Lazar R ed. *Principles of Neurologic Rehabilitation.* New York, NY: McGraw-Hill, 1998: 121–42.
5. Costa JL, Wetzel FT. Chronic pain. In: Lazar R ed. *Principles of Neurologic Rehabilitation.* New York, NY: McGraw-Hill, 1998: 209–24.
6. Gaviria M, Frumaga K. Clinical aspects and treatment of neuropsychiatric disturbances in patients with chronic neurologic disorders. In: Lazar R ed. *Principles of Neurologic Rehabilitation.* New York, NY: McGraw-Hill, 1998: 553–64.

● 7. Pierson SH. Outcome measures in spasticity management. *Muscle Nerve* 1997; **6** (Suppl.): S36–60.

8. Wade DT. Measurement and assessment: what and why? In: Wade DT ed. *Measurement in Neurological Rehabilitation*. Oxford: Oxford University Press, 1992: 15–26.

● 9. Kita M, Goodkin DE. Drugs used to treat spasticity. *Drugs* 2000; **59**: 487–95.

● 10. Taricco M, Adone R, Pagliacci C, Telaro E. Pharmacological interventions for spasticity following spinal cord injury. *Cochrane Database Syst Rev* 2000; **2**: CD001131.

◆ 11. Groves L, Shellenberger MK, Davis CS. Tizanidine treatment of spasticity: a meta-analysis of controlled, double-blind, comparative studies with baclofen and diazepam. *Adv Ther* 1998; **15**: 241–51.

12. Hirata K, Koyama N, Minami T. The effects of clonidine and tizanidine on responses of nociceptive neurons in nucleus ventralis posterolateralis of the cat thalamus. *Anesth Analg* 1995; **81**: 259–64.

13. Medical Letter. Tizanidine for spasticity. *Med Lett* 1997; **39**: 62.

14. Boop FA. Evolution of the neurosurgical management of spasticity. *J Child Neurol* 2001; **16**: 54–7.

15. Jeanmonod D, Sindou M. Somatosensory function following dorsal root entry zone lesions in patients with neurogenic pain or spasticity. *J Neurosurg* 1991; **74**: 916–32.

16. Midha M, Schmitt JK. Epidural spinal cord stimulation for the control of spasticity in spinal cord injury patients lacks long-term efficacy and is not cost-effective. *Spinal Cord* 1998; **36**: 190–2.

17. Sindou MP, Mertens P. Neurosurgery for spasticity. *Stereotact Funct Neurosurg* 2000; **74**: 217–21.

18. Sindou M. Microsurgical DREZ-otomy for the treatment of spasticity and pain in the lower limbs. *Neurosurgery* 1989; **24**: 655–70.

● 19. Smyth MD, Peacock WJ. The surgical treatment of spasticity. *Muscle Nerve* 2000; **23**: 153–63.

20. Becker R, Alberti O, Bauer BL. Continuous intrathecal baclofen infusion in severe spasticity after traumatic or hypoxic brain injury. *J Neurol* 1997; **244**: 160–6.

◆ 21. Meythaler JM, Guin-Renfroe S, Brunner RC, Hadley MN. Intrathecal baclofen for spastic hypertonia from stroke. *Stroke* 2001; **32**: 2099–109.

22. Middleton JW, Siddall PJ, Walker S, *et al*. Intrathecal clonidine and baclofen in the management of spasticity and neuropathic pain following spinal cord injury: a case study. *Arch Phys Med Rehabil* 1996; **77**: 824–6.

23. Stempien L, Tsai T. Intrathecal baclofen pump use for spasticity: a clinical survey. *Am J Phys Med Rehabil* 2000; **79**: 536–41.

24. Middel B, Kuipers-Upmeijer H, Bouma J, *et al*. Effect of intrathecal baclofen delivered by an implanted programmable pump on health-related quality of life in patients with severe spasticity. *J Neurol Neurosurg Psychiatry* 1997; **63**: 204–9.

25. Gracies JM, Elovic E, McGuire J, Simpson DM. Traditional pharmacological treatments for spasticity. Part 1. Local treatments. *Muscle Nerve* 1997; **6** (Suppl.): S61–91.

● 26. Coffield JA, Considine RV, Simpson LL. The site and mechanism of action of botulinum neurotoxin. In: Jankovic J, Hallet M eds. *Therapy With Botulinum Toxin*. New York, NY: Marcel Dekker, 1994: 3–14.

◆ 27. Brashear A, Lew MF, Dykstra DD, *et al*. Safety and efficacy of Neurobloc (botulinum toxin type B) in type-A responsive cervical dystonia. *Neurology* 1999; **53**: 1439–46.

◆ 28. Brin MF, Lew MF, Adler CH, *et al*. Safety and efficacy of NeuroBloc (botulinum toxin type B) in type-A resistant cervical dystonia. *Neurology* 1999; **53**: 1431–8.

● 29. O'Brien CF. Overview of clinical trials and published reports of botulinum toxin for spasticity. *Eur J Neurol* 1997; **4** (Suppl. 2): S11–13.

◆ 30. Barwood S, Baillieu C, Boyd R, *et al*. Analgesic effects of botulinum toxin A: a randomized, placebo-controlled clinical trial. *Dev Med Child Neurol* 2000; **42**: 116–21.

31. Mathew NT, Saper JR, Silberstein SD, *et al*. A multicenter, double-blind, placebo-controlled trial of two doses of botulinum toxin type A (Botox) in the prophylactic treatment of migraine. *Neurology* 1998; **52** (Suppl. 2): A256.

● 32. Brin M, Spasticity Study Group. Dosing, administration, and a treatment algorithm for use of botulinum type A for adult-onset spasticity. *Muscle Nerve* 1997; **6** (Suppl.): S208–20.

Headache

RIGMOR JENSEN AND PEER TFELT-HANSEN

Headache is one of the most frequent pain disorders and is known by almost everyone. Despite its widespread prevalence, the pathophysiology behind primary headache disorders is widely unknown and treatment strategies are still unspecific, although acute migraine therapy has improved considerably in the last decade.

Until 1988, there was no internationally accepted classification of headache disorders – scientific results varied considerably and were practically incomparable owing to imprecise classification. With the introduction of the International Headache Classification in 1988[1] various headache disorders were classified as primary or secondary headaches on the basis of their clinical symptoms and by means of a hierarchical and operational diagnostic system. This system is now used and accepted worldwide and has improved headache research considerably.

Migraine and tension-type headache are the most prevalent primary headaches; operational diagnostic criteria were introduced for these types of headache in 1988.[1] Migraine was formerly divided into either a common or a classical migraine, but is now classified as migraine either with or without aura. Tension-type headache is the term designated by The International Headache Society (IHS) to describe what previously was called tension headache, muscle contraction headache, psychomyogenic headache, stress headache, etc.[1] The characteristics of tension-type headache have been described extensively,[2–4] but diagnostic criteria and subtyping (i.e. episodic vs. chronic) were also introduced in the IHS classification.[1] Distinguishing episodic from chronic tension-type headache and tension-type headache from migraine has practical implications in the management strategies. Chronic tension-type headache is often associated with more severe pain, with more accompanying symptoms, is often combined with medication overuse, and is less influenced by daily hassles and stress. Studies from specialized clinics led to the conclusions that chronic tension-type headache evolves from migraine, along a continuum of the same disease with evolving manifestations. Population studies, however, paint a different picture.[5–8] These studies show that tension-type headache and migraine differ in gender ratio, age distribution, and clinical presentation. Therefore, it could be argued that the "continuum theory" is an artifact of referral bias.[9,10] It is most likely that migraine and tension-type headache are two different entities, although they may coexist in the same predisposed individual. Furthermore, as tension-type headache is more frequent and severe in migraineurs than in nonmigraineurs, migraine may be a precipitant to tension-type headache and not part of a continuum.[10–12] It can be extremely difficult to distinguish between various headache disorders in the severely affected patients attending highly specialized headache clinics, and a headache diary and a long-term follow-up are therefore mandatory.[13]

EPIDEMIOLOGY

Migraine has a quite uniform worldwide prevalence, with a life time prevalence of 16% and a 1-year prevalence of 10%.[6,7,14,15] In contrast to prevalence studies, there is a general lack of population-based data on the incidence of migraine, but retrospectively recorded data indicate that the annual incidence per 1,000 person–years is around 2 in males and 6 in females.[15] The male–female ratio in migraine in general varies from 1:2 to 1:3, with a more pronounced female preponderance in migraine without aura than in migraine with aura.[15]

The prevalence of migraine increases with age until peak prevalence is reached during the fourth decade of life and thereafter declines; again, this is more pronounced in females than in males.[6,15] The most common age of onset is during the second or third decade of life.[6,15] The previous theory of a higher prevalence of migraine in well-educated persons from higher social levels could not be confirmed in properly designed population studies, and is probably a reflection of an artifact of referral bias.

In its milder and infrequent forms, tension-type headache is a nuisance, not a disease; however, in its frequent forms, it becomes distressing and socially disturbing like other primary headaches such as migraine or cluster headache. The prevalence of episodic tension-type headache varies considerably among population-based studies, and ranges from 38.3% in one recent American study[8] to 74% in a Danish cross-sectional study.[6] In contrast, the prevalence of chronic tension-type headache is quite uniform – 2–3% in most studies.[6-8]

The male–female ratio of tension-type headache is 4:5, indicating that, unlike migraine, females are only slightly more affected.[6-8] The mean duration of tension-type headache has been reported to be 10.3 years in a German population study[7] and 19.9 years in a clinical study,[16] illustrating the considerable referral bias and the life time consistency of this disorder. The median frequency of the episodic form varies from 2.2 to 6 days per month,[5,7] whereas the vast majority of patients with chronic tension-type headache suffer from an almost daily constant headache. In contrast to migraine, there is no consistent decline in prevalence with increasing age.[6]

CLINICAL FEATURES

The clinical variability of migraine between patients is fairly low, and the migraine attack is very similar within the same subject independent of whether there is an attack once a year or once a week, i.e. an all-or-nothing phenomenon that runs its course once started. In contrast, tension-type headache is usually more graded, varying from a mild short-lasting episode on one day to a long-lasting moderate to severe pain on another.[10] It is still unknown what mechanism can explain such a periodicity in otherwise healthy subjects.

PAIN CHARACTER, SEVERITY, AND LOCATION

The typical migraine attack is often characterized by a severe, pulsating, unilateral pain which is intensely aggravated by physical activity,[1,17] although various clinical manifestations have been described. The prominent associated symptoms as photophobia, phonophobia, nausea, and sometimes also vomiting are often just as incapacitating as the pain itself.

In tension-type headache, the patient usually describes their pain as a "dull," "nonpulsating" headache. Terms

such as a sensation of "tightness," "pressure," or "soreness" are often used. Some patients refer to a "band" or a "cap" compressing their head, whereas others mention a big "weight" over their head and/or their shoulders.[2-4,17,18] The pain of tension-type headache is typically bilateral: 90% of subjects in one population-based study reported bilateral pain.[17] Nevertheless, pain does not always occur in the same location. Strictly unilateral pain accounts for pain in 4–12.5% of patients.[4,5,17-19] In patients complaining of pain of this type, an associated localized abnormality such as trigger points, oromandibular dysfunction, or intracranial disorder should be suspected.

PATHOPHYSIOLOGY

Migraine

The following pathophysiological mechanisms have been suggested to be responsible for migraine: genetic, neurogenic, vascular, inflammatory, or combinations of these. These mechanisms may be peripherally or centrally located or there may be interactions between the periphery and the brain that are altered during the attack.

In the genetic field, very exciting data have been published.[20] In the very rare condition familial hemiplegic migraine, mutations in the P/Q calcium channel complex have been described, but it is not known whether these mutations play a role in the much more frequent migraine with or without aura. A genetic mechanism is undoubtedly involved as Russell has found an increased familial risk in first-degree relatives to migraineurs, although this varies from 1.9 in migraine without aura to 3.8 in migraine with aura and to 14 in cluster headache.[21] These data indicate that the mode of inheritance is multifactorial, and that the primary headache disorders have somewhat different pathophysiological mechanisms.

Can the precipitating factors provide any important clues to reveal the pathophysiology? The most frequently reported precipitating factors are stress, mental tension, hormones, certain foods, wine and spirits, and smoking.[11,12] However, these factors are quite nonspecific, can only be identified in some patients, and vary considerably between and within patients. Precipitating factors are therefore only of limited use, although the frequent reports of mental and biochemical stressors along with accompanying symptoms such as nausea, photophobia, and phonophobia indicate central mechanisms.

For decades, the migraine aura has been linked to a cortical hyperexcitability, but neurophysiological evidence for this likely mechanism has actually been scarce and results are conflicting. More advanced methods, such as transcranial magnetic stimulation, have demonstrated consistently and significantly lowered thresholds and have recorded visual symptoms as phosphenes in all migraine patients, in contrast to only 27.3% of the controls,[22] in favor of an increased excitability.

The previous theory of cortically spreading depression, which has mainly been demonstrated in animal models, is also very likely to play a role in the migraine aura.[23] Whether this cortical and neuronal hyperexcitability exists in migraine both with and without aura, and whether it is the causative mechanism for the entire attack or just a triggering factor, is not yet known. More recent very exciting data using a functional magnetic resonance imaging (MRI) technique demonstrated a subcortical activation spreading from the red nucleus to the cortical occipital structures in migraine patients both with and without aura.[24]

With regard to the peripheral factors, the cranial vessels have been extensively studied. Patients never doubt that their pain is a vascular pain because of the throbbing, pulsating quality and the transient comfort of compressing the temporal artery on the painful site. Simple dilatation of the large intracranial arteries plays a role in the pain process, as dilation of various segments of the middle cerebral artery can produce referred pain in the relevant areas but the pain is transient and not a migraine. Ictally, a strictly unilateral dilation of the temporal artery on the painful site has been demonstrated,[25] and there is also indirect evidence of dilatation of the middle cerebral artery on the migraine site by means of transcranial Doppler measurements in some but not in all studies.[26] Infusion of the nitric oxide (NO) donor nitroglycerine (NTG) also gives rise to a dilation of the cephalic arteries, and a delayed headache indistinguishable from genuine migraine attack is elicited in most migraine patients after 5–6 h.[27,28] However, the NO molecule acts on multiple systems, including the cortical and the brainstem neurons, and the vascular effect may therefore represent another epiphenomenon. Nevertheless, the NTG model is a very useful human model for the study of various aspects of the entire migraine episode.[27-29] The highly prominent vasoconstrictor effect of specific and effective acute migraine drugs, such as the triptans, ergotamine, and dihydroergotamine (DHE), also supports a prominent vascular mechanism.

Neurogenic inflammation and the activation of the trigeminal ganglion and the trigeminal nucleus have been intensively studied in animal models[30,31] and are also highly involved in migraine attacks, leading to migraine being described as a trigeminovascular disease. Whether the activation of the trigeminal system is primary or secondary to the migraine pain is as yet unknown, but these models have also been very useful in the study of pain-producing mechanisms and for screening possible therapeutic agents.

In conclusion, migraine is a highly transient, complex disorder in otherwise healthy individuals, and the most likely mechanism that can unify the numerous existing hypotheses is a neuronal depolarization. This depolarization is probably due to a genetically inherited membrane channel dysfunction in the neurons, in the form of either increased excitability or a lack of inhibitory transmitters. If a certain number and combination of probably very individual external triggers are present, a migraine attack can be initiated. Except for the attacks, there are no clinical signs of any underlying neuronal dysfunction, as trigger factors are required to start the process. Similarly, the trigger factors alone cannot initiate the migraine attack because a genetic disposition is required, thus both conditions should be fulfilled. The activation of the trigeminal and vascular systems is most likely to be secondary to the basic migraine process, although it is highly involved in the elicited central–peripheral–central migraine cascade. At present, acute pharmacological intervention in these systems is quite effective as it minimizes and interferes with this cascade reaction, but it has no preventive effect on the next attack, indicating that other basic neuronal or transmitter systems are involved. Future studies using more advanced neurophysiological and neuroimaging techniques will hopefully, along with genetic studies, shed more light on the basic mechanisms of migraine.

Tension-type headache

The etiology of tension-type headache is also far from elucidated. Tension-type headaches generally occur with emotional conflict and psychosocial stress, but the cause–effect relationship is not clear. Stress and mental tension are thus the most frequently reported precipitating factors, occurring with a frequency in tension-type headache similar to that in migraine.[11,12] Widely normal personality profiles are found in subjects with episodic tension-type headache, whereas studies of subjects with the chronic form often reveal a higher frequency of depression and anxiety.[32,33] In a controlled study, Holroyd et al. reported that depression, anxiety, and somatization were highly abnormal during ongoing pain, and were normalized when patients were retested outside the pain period.[34] In general, psychological abnormalities in tension-type headache may therefore be viewed as secondary or comorbid to the pain disorder, although they are closely related in most subjects.

Increased tenderness in pericranial muscles is the most consistent abnormal physical finding in patients with tension-type headache; it increases with increasing frequency and intensity of the headache.[35] Subjects with the episodic form have increased tenderness compared with migraineurs and healthy controls, but are less tender than subjects with chronic tension-type headache.[35-37] The texture of pericranial, shoulder, and chewing muscles is often altered in tension-type headache, with generalized increased consistence.[38] Such findings have previously only been detected by manual palpation, but a newly invented and validated instrument – a hardness meter – has confirmed this observation.[39,40] The pathophysiological background and significance of these findings are not yet clarified. Pain sensitivity assessed by a pressure algometer is widely used in research, but plays no role in routine practice. Concerning pain thresholds recorded by pressure algometry, most studies report normal pain thresholds in episodic tension-type headache but decreased values in patients with the chronic form.[35,36,41] A recent study demonstrated for the first time that chronic tension-type headache has a physiological basis and is caused at least partly by qualitative changes in the central processing of sensory information.[42]

On this basis, it can be concluded that the underlying pain mechanisms in tension-type headache must be highly dynamic as they represent a wide variety of frequency and intensity not only between subjects but also within the individual subject over time. The initiating stimulus may be a condition of mental stress, nonphysiological motor stress, a local irritative process, or a combination of these. Secondary to the peripheral stimuli, the supraspinal pain perception structures may become activated, and owing to central modulation of the incoming stimuli a self-limiting process will be the result in most subjects. As most cases of chronic tension-type headache evolve from the episodic form, it is postulated that prolonged peripheral input sensitizes the central nervous system,[43] and a disturbance in the complex interaction between peripheral and central mechanisms is therefore of major importance for the conversion of episodic into chronic tension-type headache.[43,44]

DIAGNOSIS

A diagnosis of primary headaches as migraine or tension type requires exclusion of other organic disorders. The absence of specific and distinguishing features of tension-type headache may explain why physicians, and subsequently patients, question the diagnosis whereas the migraine symptoms are more characteristic. Consequently, paraclinical investigations to exclude other organic disease are more frequently performed in tension-type headache (and probably should be) than in other headaches such as migraine. If an intracranial lesion is suspected on the basis of a clinical history and/or examination, a computed tomography (CT) or MRI scan should be performed. At present, there are no reliable paraclinical tests that are useful in the differential diagnosis. Therefore, a careful history and examination as well as a prospective follow-up using diagnostic headache diaries[13] are of utmost importance to reach the diagnosis.

An early migraine attack should be treated quite differently from an episode of tension-type headache, and a separation between these disorders is therefore important. The intensity of pain, the aggravation by physical activity, and the pronounced accompanying symptoms are some of the main features of migraine, although recall bias often influences the history. It has to be kept in mind that tension-type headache and migraine often coexist in the same patient, and an exact diagnosis can only seldom be applied at the initial consultation.

There is usually little difficulty in distinguishing symptomatic headache due to sinus or eye disease from tension-type headache or migraine. Chronic sinusitis cannot be accepted as a cause of headache on the basis of a simple radiological thickening of sinus mucosa. At least intermittent radiological or clinical signs of ongoing sinus disease have to be present. Similarly, radiological evidence of cervical spondylosis is rarely a satisfactory explanation for a headache since it can be found with equal prevalence in age-matched nonheadache subjects and in other headache patients.[45,46] The relation between oromandibular dysfunction and headache also remains controversial as a similar prevalence of oromandibular dysfunction in subjects from the general population suffering from tension-type headache or migraine or devoid of headache suggests that a causal relationship with primary headaches must be rare.[47]

Changes in intracranial pressure are well-known causes of headache. Although spontaneous or symptomatic intracranial hypotension is most often distinguishable from other headache types by its clear-cut accentuation in the erect position ("orthostatic headache"), the syndrome of idiopathic intracranial hypertension, also known as pseudotumor cerebri or benign intracranial hypertension, may mimic chronic tension-type headache. It is vital to remember that idiopathic intracranial hypertension may occur without papilledema, and patients with obesity and pulsatile tinnitus may suggest this diagnosis.[48]

Although brain tumors represent only a very small minority among the causes of headache, they obviously are a major concern to patients and clinicians. Headache occurs at presentation in approximately 36–50% of patients with brain tumors and develops in the course of the disease in 60%. Headaches are a more common symptom of brain tumor in children. Headaches awakening the patient from sleep or that are present on awakening, associated with vomiting, are frequent characteristics of brain tumors, but may also occur in some migraineurs.

In clinical practice, the most frequent cause for chronic daily headache is chronic analgesic and/or ergotamine or triptan abuse, to which patients may evolve after having presented initially with migraine or episodic/chronic tension-type headache.[49] Although the mechanism of drug-induced headache is not clear, it is a very widespread phenomenon complicating the primary headache disorders. The prevalence of drug-induced headache is 3% in the general population, and up to 50% in headache clinic populations.[49,50] Recognizing this condition is of crucial importance because it has been demonstrated that a short time interval between the onset of drug abuse and first withdrawal is the most important predictor for a favorable long-term outcome.[50] In contrast, gender, family history, type of headache, and number of tablets do not influence the outcome.

TREATMENT

First, it is important to establish an accurate diagnosis in which the individual headache episode is identified and separated from a secondary headache, most frequently drug-induced headache. The treatment of primary headache disorders consist primarily of prevention by avoidance of any possible trigger factors, of treatment of the acute attack, and of pharmacological prophylactic treatment. One of the most important elements in treating headache patients in general is, however, to take their complaints seriously, show empathy, and examine them thoroughly as most have been met with medical ignorance and lack of interest for years.

The acute episode

Migraine

Migraine attacks can be treated with nonspecific drugs such as analgesics and nonsteroidal anti-inflammatory drugs (NSAIDs), which have an effect on headaches generally, or with specific antimigraine drugs such as ergot alkaloids, ergotamine and dihydroergotamine, and triptans (5-HT$_{1B/1D}$ receptor agonists), which only are effective in migraine.[51***] Worldwide, most migraine attacks are treated with nonspecific drugs. The absorption of orally administered drugs is delayed during migraine attacks.[51***] If nonspecific drugs are used, we therefore recommend that they are combined with a prokinetic antiemetic drug such as metoclopramide in order to normalize the absorption. In several randomized clinical trials (RCTs), nonspecific drugs, often combined with metoclopramide, were compared with sumatriptan, see Table 36.1. Oral ergotamine has a very low bioavailability (<1%) and, as expected, was inferior to oral triptans in two RCTs (Table 36.2). In contrast, rectal ergotamine was superior to rectal sumatriptan (Table 36.2), but because it also acts on dopamine and 5-hydroxytryptamine (5-HT$_2$) receptors it causes more side-effects than the triptans. The benefit–tolerability ratio for effective doses of ergotamine is thus less than that for triptans. Ergotamine was recently only recommended in patients who already use it, are responding satisfactorily to the drug, with no contraindications to its use and with no signs of dose escalation.[52***] Long-lasting migraine attacks (>48h) may be usefully treated with ergotamine as headache recurrence (primary successful treatment within 2h with subsequent increase to moderate or severe headache within 24h) is probably less likely with ergotamine.[52***] If ergotamine is used, the rectal route, provided it is acceptable to the patient, can be recommended.[52***]

Triptans

The triptans are a completely new class of compounds which act as agonists on the 5-HT$_{1B/1D}$ receptor. The first of this family, sumatriptan, was undoubtedly a significant advance in migraine therapy.[53**,54***,55***] After oral administration of sumatriptan, the bioavailability is rather low (~14%).[56***,57**] The oral bioavailability of the second-generation 5-HT$_{1B/1D}$ receptor agonists, especially naratriptan (~70%) and almotriptan (~80%), is much improved.[58***,59***] The action of the latter can be partly attributed to the more lipophilic nature of these drugs.[56***,57,58,59***]

The mechanisms of actions of triptans in migraine are mainly constriction of dilated cranial extracerebral blood vessels,[60] reduction of neuropeptide release and plasma protein extravasation across dural vessels,[61] and inhibition of impulse transmission centrally within the trigeminovascular system.[62,63] However, the possible contribution of the neuronal effect of triptans mediated via the 5-HT$_{1D}$ receptor has been put in doubt because PNU142633, a selective 5-HT$_{1D}$ receptor agonist, has not proved effective in the acute treatment of migraine.[64]

Efficacy of triptans in randomized clinical trials

The relative efficacy of the different triptans has only been investigated in 15 comparative RCTs.[58***,59***] In addition to direct comparative trials, one can get some information about the efficacy of different drugs by calculating the mean therapeutic gain (response rate of active drug minus response rate of placebo) based on several RCTs carried out with the same methodology, as shown in Table 36.1. When judging the mean therapeutic gain with 95% confidence intervals (CI) in Table 36.1, only definite differences, i.e. no overlapping CI, should be taken into account. Oral sumatriptan 50–100mg is usually regarded as the standard drug for comparisons, and as shown in Table 36.1 6mg subcutaneous sumatriptan (51%) and 80mg eletriptan orally (42%) have higher therapeutic gains than oral sumatriptan, whereas 2.5mg of naratriptan (22%) and 2.5mg of frovatriptan (16%) have lower therapeutic gains. Direct comparative RCTs gave essentially the same results: 80mg eletriptan was superior to 50mg and 100mg sumatriptan, whereas 2.5mg naratriptan was inferior to 100mg sumatriptan and 10mg rizatriptan.[58***,59***] Zolmitriptan (2.5mg and 5mg), rizatriptan (5mg and 10mg), and almotriptan (12.5mg) were found to be similar to sumatriptan (50mg and 100mg), whereas 40mg eletriptan was found to be better than 50mg sumatriptan in one RCT but the same as sumatriptan in another RCT.[58***,59***,65***] Rizatriptan, probably because of its faster absorption than sumatriptan, resulted in headache relief in 20% more patients within 2h than sumatriptan.[58***,59***,66***]

Table 36.1 *Mean therapeutic gain[a] for different triptans and forms of administration based on published papers and abstracts[58,59]*

Drug	Dose	Mean therapeutic gain (%)[b]	95% Confidence interval
Sumatriptan	Subcutaneous 6 mg	51	48–51
Sumatriptan	Oral 100 mg	32	29–34
Sumatriptan	Oral 50 mg	29	25–34
Sumatriptan	Oral 25 mg	24	18–29
Sumatriptan	Nasal 20 mg	30	25–34
Sumatriptan	Rectal 25 mg	31	25–37
Zolmitriptan	Oral 2.5 mg	32	26–38
Naratriptan	Oral 2.5 mg	22	18–26
Rizatriptan	Oral 10 mg	37	34–40
Rizatriptan	Oral 5 mg	28	23–34
Rizatriptan	Wafer[c] 10 mg	37	29–45
Eletriptan	Oral 80 mg	42	37–47
Eletriptan	Oral 40 mg	37	32–42
Almotriptan	Oral 12.5 mg	26	20–32
Frovatriptan	Oral 2.5 mg	16	8–25

a. Percentage headache relief after active drug minus percentage headache relief after placebo.
b. Based on headache relief (a decrease from severe or moderate headache to none or mild after 2 h; for subcutaneous sumatriptan, after 1 h).
c. A rapidly dissolving wafer.

Table 36.2 *Randomized clinical trials comparing triptans with nontriptans[58,59]*

Drug	Dose	Headache relief (%)[a]	Difference (%)	95% Confidence interval
Sumatriptan	Oral 100 mg	66	*+18*	*+9 to +27*
Ergotamine + caffeine	Oral 2 mg + 200 mg	48		
Sumatriptan	Oral 100 mg	56	*+11*	*–1 to +23*
Aspirin + metoclopramide	Oral 900 mg + 10 mg	45		
Sumatriptan	Oral 100 mg	53	–4	–17 to +8
L-ASA[b] + metoclopramide	Oral 1,620 mg + 10 mg	57		
Sumatriptan	Oral 100 mg	79	+2	–17 to +20
Tolfenamic acid[c]	Oral 200 mg + 200 mg	77		
Sumatriptan	Subcutaneous 6 mg	80	*+30*	*+19 to +41*
Dihydroergotamine	Nasal 1 mg + 1 mg	50		
Sumatriptan	Subcutaneous 6 mg	85 (83[d])	*+12*	*+3 to +21*
Dihydroergotamine	Subcutaneous 1 mg + 1 mg	73 (86[d])	(–3[d])	(–11 to +5[d])
Sumatriptan	Nasal 20 mg	63	*+12*	*+4 to +20*
Dihydroergotamine	1 mg + 1 mg	51		
Sumatriptan	Subcutaneous 6 mg	91	*+17*	*+8 to +27*
L-ASA[b]	Intravenous 1,800 mg	74		
Sumatriptan	Rectal 25 mg	63	*–10*	*–18 to –2*
Ergotamine + caffeine	Rectal 2 mg + 200 mg	73		
Eletriptan	80 mg	68	*+35*	*+26 to +44*
Ergotamine + caffeine	2 mg + 200 mg	33		
Eletriptan	40 mg	54	*+21*	*+11 to +30*
Ergotamine + caffeine	2 mg + 200 mg	33		

Significant differences are shown in bold italics.
a. A decrease from severe or moderate headache to none or mild after 2 h.
b. Lysine acetylsalicylate.
c. Rapid release formulation.
d. After 4 h.

How do the triptans compare with other drugs for acute migraine treatment? As shown in Table 36.2, sumatriptan (100 mg) and eletriptan (40 mg and 80 mg) were superior to oral ergotamine plus caffeine (2 mg + 200 mg). Oral sumatriptan (100 mg) was not more effective than aspirin plus metoclopramide for the first-treated attack (but superior for the second and third attacks), and was similar to lysine acetylsalicylate plus metoclopramide [1,620 mg (~900 mg aspirin) + 10 mg] and to a rapid release formulation of tolfenamic acid (200 mg + 200 mg). Subcutaneous sumatriptan (6 mg) was superior to nasal dihydroergotamine (1 mg + 1 mg), to subcutaneous dihydroergotamine (1 mg + 1 mg), after 2 h but not after 4 h, and to intravenous lysine acetylsalicylate [1,800 mg (~ 1,000 mg aspirin)]. In contrast, rectal sumatriptan (25 mg) was inferior to rectal ergotamine plus caffeine (2 mg + 200 mg) but caused less adverse events (8% versus 27%). In all five RCTs where a triptan and an ergot alkaloid were compared, there were fewer recurrences after the ergot alkaloid than after the triptan.[58]***

In one RCT, not shown in Table 36.2 because its design differed from the RCTs that are shown, diclofenac–potassium (50 mg and 100 mg) was equivalent to 100 mg sumatriptan.[58]*** There is clearly a need for more comparative trials with second-generation triptans and current nontriptan drugs to definitively establish the place of triptans in migraine therapy.[58]***

Therapeutic use of triptans

The triptans used clinically at the time of writing are sumatriptan, zolmitriptan, naratriptan, eletriptan, almotriptan, and rizatriptan. Soon, frovatriptan will probably be introduced, but the recommended dose is as yet unknown. The first and easy point is *when not to use triptans,* and the contraindications to triptans are shown in Table 36.3.

The recommended doses of sumatriptan, zolmitriptan, naratriptan, and rizatriptan are shown in Table 36.3. There is no doubt that subcutaneous sumatriptan (6 mg), as shown in Table 36.1, has the highest therapeutic gain (50%) among currently available forms of a triptan. Oral (50 and 100 mg), intranasal (20 mg), and rectal sumatriptan (25 mg) have the same therapeutic gain (30–35%) as oral zolmitriptan (2.5 mg) and rizatriptan (10 mg), see Table 36.1. In contrast, the recommended 2.5-mg dose of naratriptan has a lower therapeutic gain of approximately 20%. It should be noted, however, that this is a low dose of naratriptan, deliberately chosen to have no more side-effects than placebo. In doses of 7.5 and 10 mg, naratriptan is equivalent to 100 mg sumatriptan.[58]***,[59]***

Daily intakes of triptans that, apart from in patients with chronic cluster headache, must be considered an abuse or inappropriate use of the drug have been reported and are most often observed in patients who have previously abused drugs such as ergotamine or analgesics. A study using prescription data suggests that sumatriptan abuse is a real problem, with 1% of sumatriptan users taking 60 doses of sumatriptan or more within 30 days.[67]*** In these patients, sumatriptan is often used for drug-induced headache.[68] Migraine patients should not be allowed to use triptans daily, with an upper limit of 10 doses of a triptan per month being adhered to. In previous drug abusers, it has been recommended that the use of triptans should be limited to one dose per week.[58]***

Finally, with several triptans on the market, one has the opportunity to try several of these in the treatment of the migraine patient. It is our clinical experience that, if one triptan is not effective, one can often have success with another triptan or another mode of administration.

Treatment of tension-type headache

Owing to the lack of pathophysiological knowledge of tension-type headache, there is no selective or specific therapy. Pharmacological treatment of the acute episode includes simple analgesics, NSAIDs, and muscle relaxants. The efficacy of these drugs in treating tension-type headache has only rarely been systematically tested using modern-day methodology.[69]***

The effect of solid aspirin compared with effervescent aspirin was investigated in a placebo-controlled study which demonstrated that aspirin was significantly better than placebo but that there was no significant difference between solid and effervescent aspirin.[70]** In another placebo-controlled study, it was noted that acetaminophen (paracetamol) and aspirin were more effective than placebo, but did not differ from each other.[71]** However, as the gastric side-effect profile is much better with acetaminophen than with aspirin, acetaminophen may be recommended as the first drug of choice for these mild or moderate headache episodes. Although simple over-the-counter (OTC) drugs are the most commonly used drugs for headache, excessive and frequent use, often combined with caffeine and/or sedatives, should clearly be avoided because of the high risk of drug-induced headache. Therefore, thorough information and an upper daily/weekly limit of such drug consumption are essential to these patients.

The value of NSAIDs in treating tension-type headache is scarcely substantiated in RCTs. Some comparative studies indicate that various doses of ibuprofen are significantly more effective than placebo, and that they are at least as effective, but not superior to, aspirin or acetaminophen.[72]**,[73]** When different doses of ketoprofen, ibuprofen, and naproxen sodium were compared with each other, no significant difference between the NSAIDs was demonstrated.[74]**,[75]** Finally, the use of muscle relaxants is only on an empirical basis and cannot be recommended.

Nonpharmacological treatment

Physical therapy, including treatment modalities such as hot and cold packs, ultrasound and electrical stimulation, improvement of posture, relaxation, and exercise programs, have all been used. However, the majority of these treatments have not been properly evaluated, and most of the reported studies are not controlled. In one open-label study, the beneficial long-term effect of physical therapy was excellent,[76]* whereas a controlled study reported only a minor effect on headache frequency after 8 weeks of standardized treatment.[77]** A recent controlled study concluded that there was no significant effect of spinal manipulation on patients with episodic tension-type headache.[78]**

Table 36.3 *Therapeutic use of marketed triptans (as of 1 March 2000) in currently recommended doses (see text for details)*

Contraindications to triptans	Ischemic heart disease, variant angina, cerebral and peripheral vascular disease, and uncontrolled hypertension. Pregnancy. Use of ergot alkaloids within 24 h. Current use or use of MAO-inhibitors within the last 2 weeks. Hypersensitivity to the triptan. Hemiplegic and basilar migraine
Cautious use	Patients on SSRIs can be treated with triptans but should be warned about the symptoms of serotonin syndrome
Recommended doses of triptans	**Maximum daily dosage**
	6 mg subcutaneous sumatriptan — 12 mg
	50–100 mg oral sumatriptan — 300 mg
	(25-mg tablets available in the USA)
	20 mg intranasal sumatriptan — 40 mg
	25 mg sumatriptan as suppositories — 50 mg
	2.5–5 mg oral zolmitriptan — 10 mg
	2.5 mg oral naratriptan — 5 mg
	10 mg oral rizatriptan[a] — 20 mg
	10 mg oral rizatriptan wafer[a] — 20 mg
Clinical efficacy in the treatment of migraine attacks	Subcutaneous sumatriptan (6 mg) > oral sumatriptan (50–100 mg) = intranasal sumatriptan (20 mg) = rectal sumatriptan (25 mg) = oral zolmitriptan (2.5–5 mg) = oral rizatriptan (10 mg) > oral sumatriptan (25 mg), oral naratriptan (2.5 mg)
Speed of onset of effect compared with placebo	Subcutaneous sumatriptan (10 min) > intranasal sumatriptan (15 min) > oral sumatriptan = oral rizatriptan (30 min) > rectal sumatriptan (30–60 min) > oral zolmitriptan and oral naratriptan (60 min). It should be noted, however, that these "early responses," apart from subcutaneous sumatriptan, are often of relatively small magnitude
Speed of onset of effect compared directly among two triptans or two administration forms of a triptan	Oral rizatriptan > oral sumatriptan. Intranasal sumatriptan (>) oral sumatriptan.
Adverse events with triptans	So-called "triptan" symptoms: tingling, numbness, warm/hot sensation, pressure or tightness in different part of the body, including chest and neck. Rarely regular chest pain. Dizziness and sedation
Choice of form of administration	Tablets generally most convenient. If severe nausea/vomiting is present, the patient could alternatively use an injection, nasal spray, or a suppository
Additional dose if the first dose of a triptan is not effective	There is no evidence that a second dose of a triptan increases the efficacy. Instead, if the chosen dose of a triptan is ineffective, patients should try another dose or different forms of administration or another triptan
Recurrence or secondary treatment failure	Most triptans have the same recurrence rate of 20–40%. Naratriptan has in some trials a lower recurrence rate than sumatriptan and could be tried in recurrence-prone patients
Use of a second dose for the treatment of a recurrence when the first dose of a triptan is primarily effective	A second dose of a triptan will probably be effective, but, with multiple recurrence for days, alternative drugs should probably be tried
Abuse or inappropriate use of triptans	Triptans should not be used on a daily basis (except in the treatment of chronic cluster headache). Set an upper limit of 10 doses per month. Use triptans with extreme caution in previous drug abusers
Breast feeding	Sumatriptan can be used if milk is expressed and discarded for 8 h after the dose. Not recommended with the other triptans
Possible drug interactions	Except the interaction between rizatriptan and propranolol, there are no drug interactions of triptans and currently used prophylactic drugs for migraine and some SSRIs (see text)

MAO, monoamine oxidase; SSRIs, selective serotonin reuptake inhibitors.
a. 5 mg rizatriptan in patients on propranolol.

Baclofen has been evaluated in double-blind trials, which have not been randomized. It is effective in some patients and, provided the drug is not withdrawn rapidly, it has fewer side-effects than carbamazepine.[89]** It is a useful drug to use in newly diagnosed patients whose pain severity is still relatively low and in those who find it difficult to tolerate carbamazepine. It can be used in combination with carbamazepine. Fromm *et al.*[90]** also compared racemic baclofen with L-baclofen in a double-blind crossover trial with 15 patients and found that L-baclofen was effective in 9 out of 15 patients, whereas only one patient found the racemic form more effective. Mild side-effects were reported in five patients.

Topical proparcaine (local anesthetic) was used in a placebo-controlled trial in patients with ophthalmic trigeminal neuralgia, but was not found to be effective.[91]*

All other drugs, including clonazepam, gabapentin, oxcarbazepine, phenytoin, and valproic acid, have only been reported in open studies and all claim to be effective; however, in many reports the outcome measures are very poorly defined and long-term follow-up is missing. Gabapentin has been shown to be effective in the treatment of other neuropathic pains, and a randomized controlled trial in patients with trigeminal neuralgia is now needed.

The reader is referred to three review articles on medical management of trigeminal neuralgia for details of rarer drugs that have been tried.[92-94] The efficacy and tolerability of these drugs as well as recommended dosages are in shown in Table 37.16, but it must be remembered that the methodology of many of these studies is very poor. Based on these data some guidelines on management are put forward in Fig. 37.1.

Surgical

All these treatments are kept up to date in *Clinical Evidence*.[84] Treatment can be aimed at three levels: peripheral nerve branches, Gasserian ganglion, and posterior fossa, as shown in Table 37.17. Of all the treatments, only microvascular decompression causes no destruction of the trigeminal nerve and attempts to correct the presumed causative factor. With the increasing number of case reports showing good long-term pain control and decreased mortality and morbidity, it would appear that this is the treatment of choice, but the objective evidence is lacking, although data are now emerging. Not all patients, however, are suitable for this procedure because of either advanced age or complex medical problems. Less invasive treatments at the level of either the Gasserian ganglion or the peripheral nerve ending then need to be considered. Gamma knife radiosurgery is the latest technique to be used, and some long-term and objective data are now available.[95]

Randomized controlled trials at the peripheral level have showed that injections of streptomycin are no better than lidocaine (lignocaine).[96,97] No randomized controlled trials have been performed on any other surgical treatment. Despite the large quantity of literature, most of the data are retrospective and of poor quality, and attempts have been made to analyze them in several textbooks.[98-100] General descriptions of the techniques used and the advantages and disadvantages of the major procedures, based on an extensive review of the literature, are summarized in Table 37.17. More detailed surgical data can be found in textbooks such as Rovit *et al.*[99]

The following details should be included in articles on the surgical management of trigeminal neuralgia:

- The diagnostic criteria used, including types of cases included, e.g. multiple sclerosis, tumors.
- The inclusion/exclusion criteria for the study.
- Description of the population, i.e. age at onset of disease or surgery, length of disease, location of pain, details of previous surgery.
- Daily drug dosage prior to surgery, preoperative measure of pain, preoperative investigations, including sensory testing.
- Description of surgical technique, operative findings, peroperative complications, and technical failures.
- Length of follow-up, mean/median time of follow-up, and accounting of all patients.
- Definitions of what constitutes a recurrence, a good outcome measure, and a complication.
- Statement on data collection: who, how, what, when.
- Recurrence rates analyzed, ensuring that life table analysis, i.e. Kaplan–Meier, and analysis by intention to treat, i.e. patients lost to follow-up or dead, are used.
- Mortality reported, report absence/presence of standard complications.

Articles lacking a substantial proportion of these details should be excluded from any analysis. Quality of life measures and patient satisfaction surveys would enhance the data.

There is only one paper that attempts to measure pre- and postoperative pain, to assess patient satisfaction, and to follow up patients longitudinally in a prospective trial.[101] This has shown that selection of patients prior to radiofrequency thermocoagulation does affect outcome and that complications change over time. At present, it is not possible to give evidenced-based information to patients on the rates of complications and the time to their resolution as longitudinal data have not been reported. There are no quality-of-life data and the economic evaluations are only just being considered.

Patients themselves are unsure of which treatment to choose, as shown during a survey carried out at the Trigeminal Neuralgia Association Support Group meetings.[102]* This is partly the result of lack of information, and it remains the responsibility of neurosurgeons and other health care professionals to give patients as much detailed information as possible and to be able to offer

Table 37.16 *Drugs used in the management of trigeminal neuralgia*

Drug	Other names	Type of evidence (no. treated in each report)	Daily dosage range	Short-term outcome reported in each study (reference)
Baclofen	Lioresal	Controlled trials (10, 14); case reports (50, 16)	50–80 mg	7/10 (89); 10/14 (126); 37/50 (89); 9/16 excellent or good (127)
Capsaicin	Zostrix	Case reports (12, 5)	3 g for 21–28 days	6/12 complete; 4/12 partial; 4/10 relapses (128); 1/5 partial; 4/5 nil or little (129)
Carbamazepine	Tegretol	Randomized controlled trials (315)	300–1,200 mg	NNT 2.6 (2.2–3.3) (83)
Clonazepam	Rivotril, Klonopin	Case reports (19, 25)	2–8 mg	13/19 excellent or good (130); 63% complete/partial (131)
Gabapentin	Neurontin	Case reports (2, 7)	1,200–3,600 mg	2/2 (132); 6/7 (133)
Lamotrigine	Lamactal	RCT (13); case reports (20, 4)	200–400 mg	NNT 7 (88); 16/20 excellent; 4/20 partial (134); 4/4 excellent (135)
Oxcarbazepine	Trileptal	Case reports (13, 6, 21)	300–1,200 mg	13/13 excellent or good (136); 6/6 excellent (137); 16/21 excellent or good (138); 15/15 excellent (103)
Pimozide	Orap	RCT (48)	4–12 mg	18/48 improved (87)
Proparcaine	Proxy-metacaine	RCT (47); case reports (60, 15)	Two drops of 0.5% solution	0/47 (91); 24/60 good; 17/60 nil; 9/60 lost (139); 13/15 (140)
Phenytoin	Epanutin	Case report (4, 20)	200–300 mg	4/4 excellent (141); 8/20 excellent; 6/20 partial (142)
Tizanidine		RCT (5); controlled trial (11)	6–18 mg	1/5 excellent (85); 8/10 (143)
Tocainide	Tonocard	RCT (12)	60 mg/kg	Results same for carbamazepine as tocainide, 12/12 (86)
Valproic acid	Epilim, Depakote	Controlled trial (10); case reports (4)	600–2,000 mg	9/20 excellent/good (144) 75% excellent, 25% partial (145)

RCT, randomized controlled trial; NNT, number needed to treat; NS, not stated – case reports, poor data, no clear outcome measures, making comparisons impossible so the results have not been totaled.

a range of treatments and not just one form (www.tna-uk.org.uk, www.tna-support.org). Because of the rarity of the disease, patients often feel very isolated and say that dentists and primary care physicians lack knowledge about this condition. With this in mind, a support group was set up in 1991 in the USA, and it now has over 8,000 members. Canada, Finland, Australia, and the UK have also set up support groups. Patients now have access to an excellent web page on trigeminal neuralgia as well as an email chat group. The usefulness of this group has been shown not only by its rapidly increasing membership but also in the poems and pictures some patients have presented as a way of sharing their sufferings.

Prognosis

There are no reports in the English language on the natural history of the disease, but most experts are agreed that the disease is progressive.[76] It is suggested that with time the condition becomes more intractable and bears similarities to other neuropathic pains. It becomes more difficult to treat not only medically but also surgically. In a cohort study of 15 patients followed over 16 years, 12 out of 15 eventually required surgery as oxcarbazepine

did not control their symptons. Two patients died while on oxcarbazepine.[103] There are currently no markers that could be used to predict progression for individual patients.

OPHTHALMIC POSTHERPETIC NEURALGIA

Postherpetic neuralgia has been covered in detail (see Chapter Ch34). Up to 20% of herpes zoster cases will present with symptoms in the ophthalmic region, and of these up to 50% will have ocular problems. The short- and long-term problems can be not only pain but also the loss of sight. Treatment is mainly aimed at reducing ocular problems rather than at reducing the postherpetic neuralgia, but there is, as yet, no conclusive evidence that it does so.[104]

OTHER CAUSES OF FACIAL PAIN

The IASP definitions[12] of some rare causes of facial pain are listed below; others are listed in Table 37.18.

Table 37.16 *Continued from facing page*

Side-effects/withdrawals (no. of side-effects in reports)	Comments	References
Ataxia, lethargy, fatigue, nausea, vomiting (1/10, 2/14, 6/50, 1/16)	Slow dose escalation as withdrawal symptoms occur	89**, 126*,127*
Burning sensation (NS)	Rub on the skin, temporary relief in majority, avoid contact with the eye	128*, 129*
Ataxia, dizziness, diplopia, lethargy NNT 3.4 (2.5–5.2) for side-effects, NNT 24 (13–110) for withdrawal	Reduced white cell count, hyponatremia higher doses, folate deficiency in prolonged use	83***
Lethargy, fatigue, dizziness, personality change (4/19, 22/25)	Thrombocytopenia can occur	130*, 131*
Ataxia, dizziness, drowsiness, nausea, headache (0, 0)	Patients in the larger series all had multiple sclerosis	132*, 133*
Dizziness, drowsiness, constipation, ataxia, diplopia, irritability (7/13, 1/20, 0/4)	Rapid dose escalation increases incidence of rashes	88**, 134*, 135*
Ataxia, dizziness, diplopia, lethargy which may be related to hyponatremia (1/13, 2/6, 10/21)	Side-effects less severe than with carbamazepine, hyponatremia is dose dependent	103*, 136*– 138*
Extrapyramidal, e.g. tremor, rigidity (40/48)	Side-effects too severe to recommend routine use	87**
Toxic keratopathy in long-term use (ns, 0/15)	Short-lasting even if given repeatedly	91**, 139*, 140*
Ataxia, lethargy, nausea, headache, behavioral changes (1/4, NS)	Folate deficiency in prolonged use, gingival hypertrophy, could be used intravenously for immediate effect	141*, 142*
Dizziness (NS, 3/11)	Effect is short-lasting	85**, 143*
Nausea, paresthesiae, rash (3/12)	Risk of aplastic anemia precludes its routine use	86**
Irritability, restlessness, tremor, confusion, nausea (1/20, NS)	Rash; prolonged use alopecia, weight gain, increase efficacy with baclofen.	144*, 145*

Geniculate neuralgia

Severe lancinating pains felt deeply in the external auditory canal subsequent to an attack of acute herpes zoster.

Tolosa–Hunt syndrome

Episodes of unilateral pain in the ocular and periocular area combined with ipsilateral paresis of oculomotor nerves (ophthalmoplegia) and of the first branch of the Vth cranial nerve. The episodes are most often circumscribed in time, but may be repetitive.

Short-lasting unilateral neuralgiform pain with conjunctival injection and tearing (SUNCT)

This condition is defined as repetitive paroxysms of unilateral short-lasting pain of, usually, 15–120 s duration, mainly in the ocular and periocular area, of a neuralgiform nature and moderate to severe intensity, usually appearing only during daytime, and accompanied by ipsilateral marked conjunctival injection, lacrimation, a low to moderate degree of rhinorrhea, and (subclinical) forehead sweating. SUNCT is not responsive to indomethacin or carbamazepine, and has, so far, mostly been observed in males.

Raeder syndrome

Horner-type syndrome of the IIIrd cranial nerve type combined with aching steady pain in the ocular and periocular area, with or without parasellar cranial nerve involvement; the Vth nerve is most often involved, but also the IInd, IIIrd, IVth, and VIth cranial nerves may be affected, all on one side. The cases with and without parasellar cranial nerve involvement have been placed in two groups: I and II respectively. Sweating is reduced on the symptomatic side in IIIrd nerve disorders, including Raeder syndrome, but apparently only in the medial part of the forehead (corresponding to the sympathetic fibers that follow the internal carotid and ultimately perhaps the supraorbital arteries).

Table 37.17 *Surgical treatments in current use for trigeminal neuralgia*

Type	Procedure	Mortality	Morbidity	Recurrence rate (average)	Advantages	Disadvantages
Peripheral therapies: these are performed in most cases using local anesthesia, trigger area carefully defined, in some cases direct exposure of the nerve involved (intra- or extraorally)						
Cryotherapy, neurectomy, alcohol injections	Alcohol or streptomycin injected; neurectomy includes obliteration of the canal; cryotherapy is applied three times (during one surgical treatment) at temperatures ranging from −60°C to −120°C	Nil	Low and local, mainly mild sensory loss which may be permanent; if intraoral incisions are made then patients will have discomfort for up to 2 weeks similar to that after extraction of wisdom teeth	10–24 months. Pain may recur but in a different branch, which then may need treatment	Any age and level of medical fitness; relatively easy to perform, some immediately; most do not require GA; most are reversible and repeatable; minor side-effects and no mortality	Only of value if single trigger point; often adjuvant therapy needs to be used; short-term relief only, months; cannot keep repeating procedure; sensory loss can be permanent; small number anesthesia dolorosa or dysesthesiae; pain migrates
Gasserian ganglion: short-acting general anesthesia or heavy sedation; a cannula is inserted through the skin into the foramen ovale; the position of the cannula is checked by radiograph before a procedure is carried out						
Radiofrequency thermo-coagulation	Gasserian ganglion is subjected to temperature from 60°C to 80°C	Low (two reported)	Within the trigeminal nerve; related to sensory loss; anesthesia dolorosa; eye sensation reduced or lost; masseteric dysfunction; temporary hearing loss	3–5 years	Few patients are not regarded medically fit; easy to perform; can vary extent of lesion; immediate effect; relatively low recurrence rate; repeatable; few complications outside the trigeminal nerve	Need to wake patient during procedure, making it difficult; expensive equipment; radiographic facility required intraoperatively; destructive procedure and so can induce neuropathic pain; sensory loss is inevitable and a problem in 60% of patients; anesthesia dolorosa is difficult to manage; eye complications as well as others in the trigeminal area

Table 39.3 *Differential diagnosis for chronic low back pain*

Extraspinal
Abdomen
    Peritoneal cavity: neoplasm
    Retroperitoneal space: aortic aneurysm, neoplasm
Pelvis
    Gynecological disorders
Orthopedic
    Hip arthritis
Vascular
    Insufficiency
    Aneurysm
Neurological
    Neuropathy (diabetic, zoster)

Intraspinal
Infection
    Abscess
    Diskitis
Neoplasm
Arachnoiditis
Ruptured intervertebral disk

naires are available to assess disability, and have the advantage of applying a score so that changes with treatment can be evaluated. The Oswestry Disability Index asks questions on physical, social, and personal activity.[21] Although it has been updated on at least two occasions, it remains popular and is easy and quick to complete. Other questionnaires target specific areas such as depression.[22] More formal assessments of disability may be made, usually for the purposes of disability benefit.

Psychosocial risk factors (yellow flags)

The concept of red flags indicating serious pathology has been extended to the idea of yellow flags indicating psychosocial barriers to recovery.[23] Risk factors for chronicity are included in Table 39.4. The *New Zealand Acute Back Pain Guide* also includes a guide to assessing psychosocial risk factors for the *development* of chronic disability following *acute* back pain.[24] The guide identifies the following factors that consistently predict poor outcomes:

- presence of a belief that back pain is harmful or potentially severely disabling;
- fear-avoidance behavior and reduced activity levels;
- tendency to low mood and withdrawal from social interaction;
- an expectation of passive treatment(s) rather than a belief that active participation will help.

There is evidence to suggest that fear of pain is a better predictor of disability than negative affect or general negative beliefs.[25]

Abnormal illness behavior

Psychosocial distress may be expressed as inappropriate behavior. This may be confirmed through either a self-reported questionnaire or identification of nonorganic signs on examination. The Illness Behaviour Questionnaire[26] is not restricted to chronic low back pain and may identify hypochondriasis, somatic fixation, and disturbances of affect. A group of nonorganic physical signs were described by Waddell *et al.* in patients with chronic low back pain.[27] These include inappropriate tenderness, weakness, sensory disturbance, and overreaction. The presence of multiple nonorganic signs suggest that psychosocial factors are important and should be addressed, however they do not mean that there is no physical cause for pain nor do they mean that patients are deliberately faking pain for secondary gain.

Key point

- There are no diagnostic features that identify the source of low back pain for most patients.
- The presence of red flags suggests serious spinal pathology.
- The presence of yellow flags suggests an increased likelihood of developing chronic disability.

RADIOLOGICAL INVESTIGATION

Plain radiographs

Plain radiographs (usually anteroposterior and lateral views of the complete lumbosacral spine and lateral view of the lower two disks) are primarily helpful in identifying structural problems in the bones, including vertebral fractures and dislocations and bony destruction secondary to tumor or infection. A normal radiograph does not rule out serious spinal pathology, nor does it demonstrate soft tissue problems such as disk prolapse or abnormalities involving the nerve roots.[17] Guidelines regarding the use of lumbar spine radiography are based on limited to moderate evidence and mainly relate to back pain of between 4 and 6 weeks' duration. These guidelines essentially state that there is no indication for routine radiographs in acute low back pain in the absence of clinical red flags.[20,23,28] The Clinical Standards Advisory Group states that "X-rays may be performed in simple backache if symptoms and disability are not improving after six weeks."[29] However, a recent health technology assessment evaluated the role of radiography in primary care patients with low back pain of at least 6 weeks' duration.[30] This randomized but unblinded trial comparing lumbar spine radiographs plus usual care with usual care alone concluded that lumbar spine radiography was not associated with improved functioning, severity of pain, or overall health status and was associated with an increase in general practitioner (GP) workload. There were no cases of serious pathology identified in any of the 421 patients. The overall conclusion from this study was that lumbar spine radiography should not be recommended for low back pain in the absence of red flags for serious spinal pathology, even if the pain has persisted for at least 6 weeks.

Bone scans

A bone scan may be helpful as a second-line screening test for serious spinal pathology and does not have a place in the diagnostic evaluation of back pain in the absence of red flags.

Cross-sectional imaging (magnetic resonance imaging and computed tomography)

The Scottish Back Trial Group randomized 145 patients with simple low back pain into an "imaging" [magnetic resonance imaging (MRI) or computed tomography (CT)] or "no imaging" group. They found no differences between the groups with respect to diagnosis or treatment plans and concluded that there is a need for evidence-based guidelines for imaging in low back pain (LBP) treatment.[31] Controversy still prevails about the relationship between disk degeneration and low back pain. In 164 symptomatic men, MRI of the lumbar spine found low back pain to be associated with signs of disk degeneration, and nerve root pain with posterior disk bulges.[32] However, radiological evidence of disk and bony abnormalities are also present in the normal population and are only weakly associated with back pain.[33] Indeed, radiological evidence of prolapsed intervertebral disks occurs in over 25% of asymptomatic subjects.[34] If the result of an investigation is not going to change management, why do the test?

EVIDENCE-BASED EVALUATION OF MANAGEMENT

Well-established guidelines exist for the management of acute low back pain.[20***,23***,29***] Successful treatment of acute back pain will hopefully lead to a reduction in the number of people developing chronic low back pain, although convincing evidence is lacking. However, for the 2–10% of the population who presently have chronic low back pain, and for those who fail "acute back pain pathways," there needs to be a management strategy aimed at reducing both pain and disability. Of the many studies on the management of chronic back pain, many are

methodologically flawed. There has been little good evidence on therapeutic efficacy. In 1987, the Quebec Task Force on Spinal Disorders published management guidelines for activity-related spinal disorders on the basis of the strength of the evidence.[35***] They considered the randomized controlled trials (RCTs) to be the strongest proof of effectiveness and, as poor quality is associated with bias, also considered the methodologic quality of the studies. They found that no single therapeutic intervention was demonstrated to be effective in the treatment of chronic low back pain! Things appear to have moved forward – a more recent systematic review found evidence for effectiveness of some conservative interventions for chronic low back pain, although the problem with poor methodological quality persists.[36***] Methodological issues are being addressed and the overall quality of research is improving.

For this chapter, where possible, the information has been obtained from meta-analyses, systematic reviews, and RCTs. The supporting evidence for efficacy is graded in Table 39.5, thereby providing an evidence-based evaluation of the following treatments:

- pharmacology;
- physical therapies;
- surgery;
- injection therapies;
- neuromodulation;
- complementary therapies;
- psychological therapies.

Pharmacology

Analgesics

In two systematic reviews, there was little strong evidence regarding drug therapy for chronic low back pain.[36***,37***] No RCTs evaluating acetaminophen (paracetamol) alone were found. In a high-quality

Table 39.4 *Risk factors for chronicity (including yellow flags)*

Previous history of low back pain
Total work loss (owing to low back pain) in past 12 months
Radiating leg pain
Reduced straight-leg raising
Signs of nerve root involvement
Reduced trunk muscle strength and endurance
Poor physical fitness
Self-rated health poor
Heavy smoking
Psychological distress and depressive symptoms
Disproportionate illness behavior
Low job satisfaction
Personal problems – alcohol, marital, financial
Adversarial medicolegal proceedings

Table 39.5 *Evidence-based evaluation of treatments*

Treatment	Effective	Strength of evidence	Comment
Pharmacology			
Analgesics			
Acetaminophen	N/K	No evidence	Low likelihood of harm
NSAIDs	Moderately	***	
Opioids	Yes	**	Low likelihood of abuse
Adjuvant therapy			
Antidepressants	For nerve pain	***	
Anticonvulsants	For nerve pain	***	
Physical therapies			
Spinal manipulation	Yes	***	
Traction	No	**	
Exercise	Yes	***	
Functional restoration	Yes	**	
Back school	Possibly	***	Half the studies – effective
Surgery			
Decompression/fusion	No	***	Poor-quality studies in systematic review
Diskectomy	Yes	***	Unknown whether superior to conservative management
Injection therapies			
Epidurals	Possibly	***	Two systematic reviews: different conclusions
Facet injections	Possibly	**	Conflicting evidence
Nerve root injections	Yes	**	One study only
Botulinum A toxin	Yes	**	One study only
Neuromodulation			
TENS	Possibly	***	Poor-quality studies, probably short-term benefit
SCS		N/K	No RCTs
Complementary therapies			
Acupuncture	No	***	Poor-quality studies in systematic review
Massage	Moderately	***	Increasing evidence
Relaxation	N/K	No evidence	
Psychological	Yes	***	Inpatient and outpatient interventions effective

N/K, not known; NSAID, nonsteroidal anti-inflammatory drug; TENS, transcutaneous electrical nerve stimulation; SCS, spinal cord stimulation; RCT, randomized controlled trial.
Acetaminophen (paracetamol).

RCT, acetaminophen was found to be as effective as the nonsteroidal anti-inflammatory drug (NSAID) diflunisal.[38]*** A systematic review found moderate evidence that NSAIDs are effective for chronic low back pain, and there is strong evidence that the various types of NSAIDs are equally effective.[39]*** A double-blind, crossover RCT found that a combination of acetaminophen 1,000 mg/codeine 60 mg 4-hourly was as effective as tramadol 100 mg 4-hourly in patients with refractory chronic back pain, with 80% of patients obtaining good or satisfactory short-term pain relief.[40]** An RCT comparing tramadol with placebo demonstrated that for those patients tolerating tramadol it was more effective than placebo for the treatment of chronic low back pain.[41]** In the open-label, run-in phase prior to randomization, 20% of patients were unable to tolerate tramadol. Oxycodone and morphine compared with naproxen were found to have a positive effect on mood and pain, but did not affect activity level in an open RCT lasting 16 weeks.[42]** No adverse events occurred and there was no significant risk of abuse. Twenty-eight of 33 patients found strong opioids to be effective and had sustained improvements in pain and function at 32 months in an open (nonrandomized) trial for patients with severe refractory back pain.[43]* There was no evidence of addictive behavior or organ toxicity in any patient.

Adjuvant medication

Tricyclic antidepressants were found to be effective in neuropathic pain (not specifically low back pain) in a systematic review of RCTs.[44]*** In a double-blind, placebo-controlled RCT, nortriptyline reduced pain intensity scores for low back and nerve root pain in nondepressed men.[45]** However, health-related quality of life, mood, and physician ratings of overall outcome did not differ significantly between treatments, and four patients withdrew because of adverse effects. Schreiber et al. randomized 40 nondepressed patients suffering from low back pain and whiplash-associated neck pain to receive either fluoxetine 20 mg daily or amitriptyline 50–75 mg daily and found them to be equally effective in providing pain relief.[46]** There were no published RCTs evaluating anticonvulsants in low back pain. However, anticonvulsants were found to be effective in neuropathic pain (not specifically low back pain) in a systematic review of RCTs.[47]*** Although the two systematic reviews were not evaluating chronic low back pain specifically, one could extrapolate that antidepressants and anticonvulsants might be effective for nerve root pain. Trials are needed to establish the relative efficacy and harm associated with different antidepressants and anticonvulsants. A double-blind N-of-1 study found that intramuscular (i.m.) ketamine 0–40 mg added to i.m. morphine eight times per day reduced chronic low back pain due to osteoporosis.[48]* This caused only mild side-effects and the patient experienced substantial benefit.

Bisphosphonates

Bisphosphanates, while not analgesic, reduce the risk of risk of vertebral fractures in osteoporosis.[49]*

Other

A double-blind RCT found parenteral vitamin B_{12} more effective than placebo in alleviating low back pain in patients with no signs of nutritional deficiency.[50]** Two different doses of willow bark extract (low dose, 120 mg; high dose, 240 mg) were found to be more analgesic than placebo in patients with chronic low back pain in a double-blind RCT.[51]**

Key points

- Simple analgesics such as acetaminophen (paracetamol) and NSAIDs should be tried.
- Weak opioids should be added for moderate pain and strong opioids should be tried for severe pain.
- Strong opioids, when used for pain relief, are not generally associated with addictive behavior.
- Adjuvant analgesics such as tricyclic antidepressants and/or anticonvulsants should be tried for neuropathic pain.

Physical

Spinal manipulation

There is evidence from two systematic reviews that manipulation is more effective than placebo treatment, usual care by the general practitioner, bed-rest, analgesics, and massage.[36]***,[52]***

Traction

An RCT published in the Lancet in 1995[53]** and in Spine in 1997[54]** found that for patients with back pain of at least 6 weeks' duration, traction was no better than sham traction in terms of the patient's global perceived effect, severity of main complaints, functional status, and pain.

Exercise

A Cochrane review found strong evidence that exercise therapy was more effective than usual GP care and equally effective as conventional physiotherapy.[55]*** A systematic review found three trials reporting positive results with different types of exercises and two trials reporting better results with intensive exercising than with low-grade exercising.[56]*** It was concluded that graded exercise programs and different types of exercising should be evaluated in patients with chronic back pain. A subsequent RCT found that exercise (physiotherapy-run exercise classes combined with a relaxation and education session) was more clinically effective and cost-effective at 1 year than traditional GP management regardless of patient preference.[57]** Those in the exercise group had less disability and pain, nearly 50% fewer days off work, and used fewer health care resources. In another trial, patients were randomized into three groups to receive modern active physiotherapy, muscle conditioning using training devices, or low impact aerobics. Significant reductions in pain and disability occurred in all groups to a similar degree, and these differences were maintained at 1 year. This has important financial implications, as the costs associated with physiotherapy and use of devices were three to four times greater than those for aerobics. Aerobics therefore has the potential to relieve some of the financial burden associated with chronic low back pain.[58]**,[59]** An RCT found that sedentary postmenopausal women with back problems may benefit from regular long-term therapeutic exercise in terms of subjective back complaints and slowed loss of bone mass.[60]**

Functional restoration

Functional restoration programs are intensive multidisciplinary programs that last several weeks. Patients randomized to a functional restoration program had less pain and disability, remained more physically active, used fewer analgesics, and visited health care professionals less often than patients randomized either to a nontreated control group or to less intensive but different training programs.[61]** These differences were sustained at 1 year.

Back schools

There is moderate evidence that back schools have better short-term effects than other treatments for low back pain and that intensive back school programs in occupational settings are more effective than placebo or waiting list controls.[36**,62***] In an earlier systematic review, seven studies found positive results and seven found negative results for back schools when compared with a reference treatment.[63***]

Key points

- Exercise therapy should be recommended for the treatment of chronic low back pain. Low-impact aerobics is cheap and effective.
- Some evidence exists to support the use of manipulation, back schools, and functional restoration programs, but these are more expensive than exercise.
- There is no evidence to support the use of traction.

Surgery

Decompression/fusion

A Cochrane review evaluating all forms of surgical treatment for degenerative conditions affecting the lumbar spine revealed only 14 RCTs and the quality of these was poor.[64***] These trials dealt primarily with short-term technical outcomes rather than patient-centered outcomes such as pain, disability, and capacity for work. There were no trials comparing any form of surgery with natural history, placebo, or any form of conservative treatment. Instrumented fusion was found to give a higher fusion rate than noninstrumented fusion but did not improve clinical outcomes and may be associated with higher complication rates. Despite the fact that surgical investigations and interventions account for up to 30% of health care costs for spinal disorders,[29] surgical treatment of degenerative lumbar spondylosis is still not substantiated by good scientific evidence.[64***] The fastest growing indication for surgery in those over 65 years of age is spinal stenosis. A meta-analysis of published case series suggests that 64% of patients obtained good to excellent results from surgery, however major deficits in study design and reporting preclude firm conclusions.[65***]

Diskectomy/chemonucleolysis

Epidemiological and clinical studies show that most lumbar disk prolapses resolve naturally with the passage of time and conservative management.[1***] A Cochrane review found 27 RCTs evaluating surgical interventions for the treatment of lumbar disk prolapse.[1***] Although there were methodological weaknesses in many, there were some good-quality trials. There was strong evidence that chemonucleolysis produces better clinical outcomes than placebo, and one trial showed this benefit was maintained at 10 years.[1***] Surgical diskectomy was in turn superior to chemonucleolysis and was associated with fewer requirements for a second intervention.

There is some evidence that the complication rate of chemonucleolysis is lower than that of surgical diskectomy, however the final result of chemonucleolysis followed by surgery is poorer than that of primary diskectomy. There were no differences in clinical outcomes between microdiskectomy and standard diskectomy. A 10-year retrospective follow-up of microdiskectomy found successful outcomes, defined as complete relief of or occasional back/leg pain in 91% of cases at 6 months and 83% at 10 years.[66*] There was moderate evidence suggesting that percutaneous diskectomy produced poorer clinical outcomes than standard diskectomy or chemonucleolysis.[1***] There were no published RCTs evaluating laser diskectomy.

Intradiskal electrothermy

Intradiskal electrothermy (IDET) is a novel method for managing diskogenic low back pain using controlled thermal energy via an intradiskal delivery device.[67*] Targeted thermal energy can shrink collagen fibrils, cauterize granulation tissue, and coagulate nerve tissue. IDET can raise the annulus temperature to achieve these effects. A prospective nonrandomized clinical trial evaluated this technique in patients who met the criteria for lumbar fusion and found a significant improvement in pain and functional outcome at 7 months.[67*] However, a more recent RCT evaluated this technique in 28 patients with at least 1 year of chronic diskogenic back pain and concluded that it is not effective in reducing pain or disability.[68**] This study was a prospective double-blind RCT in which patients were randomized to receive percutaneous intradiskal radiofrequency (RF) thermocoagulation or the same procedure without the RF current.

Artificial disk replacement

Artificial disk replacement is a relatively novel addition to the classical surgical procedures of diskectomy and fusion. The advantage of this technique is the restoration of the natural biomechanics of the segment after disk excision, thus relieving pain and preventing further degeneration at adjacent segments. Two-year results of 50 prospectively studied patients found that 70% had satisfactory pain relief, the best results occurring in patients with an isolated diskopathy, without previous spinal operations or other spinal pathology.[69**] However, 13% had permanent side-effects or complications related to the procedure. The authors conclude that, for patients with isolated symptomatic diskopathies resistant to conservative treatment, disk prosthesis is worth considering as an alternative to conventional surgery. There are no published RCTs evaluating this technique.

Gene transfer therapy

Gene therapy may have potential applications in the treatment of spinal disorders, particularly those associated with disk degeneration and spinal fusion.[70]* Work to date has been in the laboratory and there are no human studies available.

Key points

- There is no evidence about the clinical effectiveness of any form of surgical decompression or fusion for degenerative lumbar spondylosis compared with natural history, placebo, or conservative treatment. Surgery should not be undertaken in the absence of neurological signs.
- Most lumbar disk prolapses resolve spontaneously with time or conservative treatment.
- Diskectomy in carefully selected patients provides faster relief from the acute attack than conservative management. It is not clear who should be treated conservatively and who should undergo diskectomy.
- Chemonucleolysis is less effective than diskectomy for lumbar disk prolapse but more effective than placebo.
- Intradiskal electrothermy and artificial disk replacement are two novel techniques requiring further evaluation.

Injection techniques

A Cochrane review found a lack of evidence on the effectiveness of injection therapy for subacute and chronic benign low back pain of more than 1 month's duration.[71]*** This review distinguished between three injection sites: epidural, facet joint, or local injections and included 21 RCTs, many of which had poor methodological quality.

Epidural injections

The Cochrane review by Nelemans *et al.* found that no conclusion could be drawn regarding the effect of epidural steroid injection (ESI) therapy.[71]*** There have been two systematic reviews of ESIs for low back pain and sciatica and they drew somewhat conflicting conclusions despite a substantial overlap in the included RCTs. Koes *et al.* systematically reviewed 12 RCTs evaluating ESIs for patients with low back pain and sciatica. Half of the studies found ESIs to be better and half found them to be no better or worse than the reference treatment.[72]*** This finding was independent of the methodological scores of the trials. Watts and Silagy undertook a meta-analysis of 11 placebo-controlled trials (nine of which were reviewed by Koes) on the efficacy of epidural corticosteroids in the treatment of sciatica.[73]*** In their quantitative findings of pooled data, they found that ESIs were effective at 6 and 12 months in the management of lumbosacral nerve root pain of variable duration (1–63 months). There were no RCTs evaluating the relatively new technique of ESIs via epiduroscopy. For further information on ESI, please see Chapter P33.

Facet injections

The Cochrane review by Nelemans *et al.* also found only one well-designed RCT evaluating facet joint injections. This study compared injections of corticosteroid into the facet joints with isotonic saline.[74]** There were no differences in pain or disability between the groups at 1 or 6 months. An RCT comparing facet joint and facet nerve injections with local anesthetic and steroid in patients with refractory chronic low back pain found no difference between the groups.[75]** A systematic review of radiofrequency procedures for the treatment of spinal pain found moderate evidence that RF lumbar facet denervation is more effective for chronic low back pain than placebo.[76]*** One double-blind RCT found that radiofrequency lumbar facet denervation to be effective for patients with chronic low back pain of more than 1 year's duration.[77]** In this study, patients were required to have had a positive response to diagnostic neural blockade prior to randomization. This study demonstrates the potential importance of patient selection prior to evaluating treatment. However, another study found that radiofrequency facet joint denervation was found to be no better than sham therapy for relieving pain or disability in an RCT of patients with chronic back pain also having had a good response after intra-articular facet injections under fluoroscopy.[78]**

Nerve root injections

A double-blind RCT found that selective nerve root injection of bupivacaine plus corticosteroid was significantly more effective than bupivacaine alone in obviating the need for decompression in patients with radicular pain who were otherwise considered to be operative candidates.[79]** There were no outcome measures of pain or disability in this study.

Botulinum toxin

A double-blind RCT of 31 patients found that paravertebral administration of botulinum toxin was more effective at relieving pain and improving function at 3 and 8 weeks than placebo in patients with chronic low back pain.[80]**

Other

The Cochrane review by Nelemans *et al.* found that overall there was insufficient evidence for the effectiveness of local injection therapy (e.g. trigger points, ligaments).[71]** No RCTs evaluating lumbar plexus (psoas compartment) block or autonomic block for the treatment of low back pain were found.

Key points

- Evidence on the effectiveness of epidural steroid injections and facet joint injections is lacking; there is a need for large RCTs with good methodology.
- Evidence on radiofrequency lumbar facet denervation is conflicting; there is a need for large RCTs with good methodology.
- Nerve root injections appear to be helpful in preventing surgery for patients with radicular pain (one RCT only).
- Botulinum toxin A injections appear to be helpful in chronic low back pain, at least in the short term.

Neuromodulation

Transcutaneous electrical nerve stimulation

Transcutaneous electrical nerve stimulation (TENS), originally based on the gate-control theory of pain, is widely used for the treatment of chronic low back pain. There is a Cochrane review that examined the available evidence from randomized placebo-controlled trials on TENS for the treatment of chronic back pain. Of 68 identified studies, only six were suitable for inclusion owing to poor methodology. TENS reduced pain and improved function in the short term, but studies evaluating longer term follow-up at 3 and 6 months showed a near return to baseline conditions.[81]*** There is little evidence that TENS causes harmful side-effects apart from mild skin reactions and occasional temporary worsening of the perception of pain. TENS is more effective than placebo for reducing pain and improving function in the short term, has low capacity to cause harm, is inexpensive, and therefore may have a role to play as part of an overall treatment program.

Percutaneous electrical nerve stimulation

Percutaneous electrical nerve stimulation (PENS) is a novel nonpharmacologic pain therapy which uses acupuncture-like needle probes positioned in the soft tissues and/or muscles to stimulate peripheral sensory nerves at dermatomal levels corresponding to local pathology.[82]** PENS was found to be more effective than sham PENS, TENS, and exercise in decreasing pain scores, reducing daily analgesic medication, and improving physical activity, quality of sleep, and sense of well-being in a randomized crossover study of 60 patients with chronic back pain.[82]**

Spinal cord stimulation

There are no meta-analyses, systematic reviews, or completed RCTs evaluating spinal cord stimulation (SCS) in back pain. Initial results on 27 patients have been reported from an RCT comparing SCS and reopera-

tion for failed back surgery syndrome.[83]** In this trial, patients selected for reoperation by standard criteria were randomly assigned to either SCS or reoperation, the primary outcome measure being the frequency of crossover to the alternative procedure if the results from the first were unsatisfactory. Although a significant advantage for SCS over reoperation at the 6-month crossover point was found, the completed study has not yet been reported. A systematic literature synthesis of 39 case series found that approximately 50–60% of patients with failed back surgery syndrome report at least 50% pain relief with SCS at long-term follow-up.[84]** There was, however, no evidence upon which to draw conclusions about the efficacy of SCS relative to placebo or other treatments or about the effects of spinal cord stimulation on functional disability, medication use, or work status. A prospective multicenter study of SCS for relief of back and extremity pain similarly found that 55% of patients obtained pain relief and improved quality of life. Neither of these reports included studies that were randomized, and therefore may be overestimating treatment effect by as much as 40%.[47]***

Key points

- TENS should be tried as part of an overall treatment program, but does not provide long-term relief.
- PENS, a novel therapy, was beneficial in one RCT and therefore worth trying if available. Its use requires further evaluation.
- There is a lack of evidence regarding the efficacy and safety of spinal cord stimulation in chronic back pain with or without leg pain.

Complementary medicine

Acupuncture

A recent National Institutes of Health (NIH) consensus panel concluded that, although there is clear scientific evidence that acupuncture is effective for chemotherapy and pregnancy induced nausea and vomiting and postoperative dental pain, there is insufficient evidence to support the use of acupuncture in chronic pain. The results of a systematic review,[85]*** also contained in a Cochrane review,[86]*** confirm that there is no scientific evidence that acupuncture is an effective treatment for low back pain. However, most of the 11 studies reviewed were of very poor methodological quality, and therefore there is a need for quality RCTs. A meta-analysis found that acupuncture was superior to various control interventions, although there was insufficient evidence to state whether it was superior to placebo.[87]*** An RCT in elderly patients with low back pain lasting more than 6 months found that acupuncture and TENS had demonstrable benefits on visual analog scale (VAS) scores and analgesic consumption.[88]*** There was, however, no placebo group, so it is possible that these were placebo effects.

Massage

A systematic review found only four RCTs evaluating the role of massage therapy in back pain, and all had major methodological flaws.[89]*** One of the trials found that massage was superior to no treatment, two implied that it was as effective as spinal manipulation and TENS, and one study found that it was less effective than manipulation. A more recent RCT comparing traditional Chinese medical acupuncture, therapeutic massage, and self-care education for chronic low back pain found that therapeutic massage was more effective at 10 weeks than self-care and acupuncture for pain and disability.[90]** Longer term follow-up at 1 year found that massage was still more effective than acupuncture, but not self-care, and also that patients in the massage group consumed less medication and had the lowest costs of subsequent care. In another study, 24 patients with back pain for at least 6 months were randomized to receive two 30-min massage or relaxation therapy sessions per week for 5 weeks.[91]** Patients receiving massage therapy reported less pain, depression, and anxiety and their sleep had improved at the end of the study. There was no long-term follow-up reported from this study. Patients with back pain of between 1 week and 8 months' duration randomized to a comprehensive massage therapy group (massage, exercise, and posture education) reported less pain and disability after a 4-week treatment period than patients randomized to receive massage, remedial exercise, and posture or placebo (sham laser) alone.[92]**

Relaxation

A systematic review found little evidence to support the effectiveness of relaxation in the relief of chronic pain generally.[93]*** There were no RCTs evaluating relaxation specifically in the treatment of back pain.

Spa therapy

Spa therapy was found to be beneficial in terms of pain intensity, disability, and analgesic consumption in an RCT comparing spa therapy and routine drug therapy with routine drug therapy alone in patients with low back pain. Significant differences were present at 6 months.[94]** Perhaps funding for the surgical treatment of back pain should be diverted to fund programs of spa therapy in France!

Key points

- Massage seems to have some potential as a treatment in persistent back pain but further investigation is required.
- There is inadequate evidence regarding acupuncture, relaxation, and spa therapy for the treatment of back pain.
- Large valid studies of complementary therapies are needed.

Psychological

Chronic back pain leads to functional and psychological disability that in turn can lead to an increased perception of pain, thus a vicious cycle may be established. Therefore, in addition to treating nociceptive components of pain, therapeutic modalities also need to address the contributing psychosocial factors. Behavioral therapy, cognitive therapy, and psychophysiological therapy are the three commonly used psychological approaches to pain management. These techniques may be used individually or in combination, in either inpatient or outpatient settings.

Behavioral therapy

Behavioral approaches are based on the operant conditioning principles of Skinner and applied to pain management by Fordyce.[95] Behavioral therapy includes the positive reinforcement of healthy behaviors (e.g. encouraging activity) and the negative reinforcement of, or withdrawal of attention toward, pain behaviors. Family and health professionals can all adopt this approach of reinforcing healthy behavior and ignoring pain behavior; the ultimate aim is to increase the frequency of "well" behavior and to extinguish "pain" behavior.

Cognitive therapy

Behavioral therapy alone tends to ignore the thought processes involved in the interpretation of pain. Cognitive therapy aims to change or restructure the thought processes surrounding a patient's pain and disability, e.g. conveying to a patient that pain is not necessarily a sign of on-going damage or that pain associated with exercise may be a sign of muscles strengthening, thereby leading to improved fitness. Cognitive–behavioral therapy is a combination of both the behavioral and cognitive approaches.

Psychophysiological therapy/respondent therapy

This approach aims to modify the physiological system directly, e.g. by decreasing muscle tension using hypnotherapy, biofeedback, or relaxation techniques.

A meta-analysis of RCTs evaluating psychological approaches to pain management found them to be an effective treatment for patients with chronic low back pain, but that it is unknown which interventions are most beneficial for which patients. Only six of the 25 trials were of high quality.[96]*** A review of behavioral interventions for back pain in primary care found that cognitive and behavioral treatments were superior to no treatment on measures of pain and disability, although the meta-analysis did not find these therapies different from other active treatments on specific outcome measures.[97]*** Six of the trials included in the van Tulder review were also included in the Turner review. An RCT compared inpatient and outpatient cognitive pain management programs for mixed chronic pain patients.[98]** Patients were randomly allocated to an inpatient program, outpatient program, or a waiting list control. Inpatients and outpatients made significant improvements in physical performance, psychological function, and reduced medication use. Inpatients made greater gains and maintained them better at 1 year while using less health care than outpatients. There were no improvements in the waiting list group.

There is increasing evidence, therefore, that individual and group psychological interventions are effective in the management of back pain. Large RCTs are required to evaluate which patients benefit most from which type of psychological intervention.

Key points

- Psychological interventions are helpful in treating patients with chronic back pain.
- Inpatient and outpatient pain management programs are effective for chronic pain patients.
- It is not known which interventions are most beneficial for which patients.

REFERENCES

● 1. Gibson JNA, Grant IC, Waddell G. *Surgery for Lumbar Disc Prolapse (Cochrane Review)*. The Cochrane Library. Oxford: Update Software, 2000: Issue 2.

2. Raspe H. Back pain. In: Silman AJ, Hochberg MC eds. *Epidemiology of the Rheumatic Diseases*. Oxford: Oxford University Press, 1993.

3. Bogduk N. The sources of low back pain. In: Jayson MIV ed. *The Lumbar Spine and Back Pain*. Edinburgh Churchill Livingstone, 1992.

4. Kaplan M, Dreyfuss P, Halbrood B, Bogduk N. The ability of lumbar medial branch blocks to anesthetize the zygapophyseal joint. A physiologic challenge. *Spine* 1998; **23:** 1847–52.

◆ 5. Schwarzer AC, Wang SC, Bogduk N, *et al.* Prevalence and clinical features of lumbar zygapophyseal joint pain – a study in an Australian population with chronic low back pain. *Ann Rheum Dis* 1995; **54:** 100–6.

6. Schwarzer AC, Aprill CN, Derby R, *et al.* The prevalence and clinical features of internal disc disruption in patients with chronic low back pain. *Spine* 1995; **20:** 1878–83.

● 7. Bogduk N. Precision diagnosis of spinal pain. In: Camp-

bell JN ed. *Pain 1996 – an Updated Review*. Seattle, WA: IASP, 1996: 313–23.

8. Dreyfuss P, Michaelsen M, Pauza K, *et al.* The value of medical history and physical examination in diagnosing sacroiliac join pain. *Spine* 1996; **21:** 2594–602.

9. Morinaga T, Takahashi K, Yamagata M, *et al.* Sensory innervation to the anterior portion of lumbar intervertebral disc. *Spine* 1996; **21:** 1848–51.

10. Nakamura SI, Takahashi K, Takahashi Y, *et al.* The afferent pathways of discogenic low back pain. Evaluation of L2 spinal nerve infiltration. *J Bone Joint Surg Br* 1996; **78:** 606–12.

11. Omarker K, Myers RM. Pathogenesis of sciatic pain: role of herniated nucleus pulposus and deformation of spinal nerve root and dorsal root ganglion. *Pain* 1998; **78:** 99–105.

12. Nachemson A. Lumbar mechanics as revealed by lumbar intradiscal pressure measurements. In: Jayson MIV ed. *The Lumbar Spine and Back Pain*. Edinburgh: Churchill Livingstone, 1992.

◆ 13. Bogduk N. The innervation of the lumbar spine. *Spine* 1983; **8:** 286–93.

14. Andersson GBJ. Epidemiological features of low back pain. *Lancet* 1999; **354:** 581–5.

15. Papageorgiou AC, Croft PR, Ferry S, *et al.* Estimating the prevalence of low back pain in the general population. *Spine* 1995; **20:** 1889–94.

16. Papageorgiou AC, Croft PR, Thomas E, *et al.* Influence of previous pain experience on the episode incidence of low back pain. Evidence from the South Manchester back pain survey. *Pain* 1996; **66:** 181–5.

◆ 17. Waddell G. *The Back Pain Revolution*. Edinburgh: Churchill Livingstone, 1998.

18. Flor H, Birbaumer N. Comprehensive assessment and treatment of chronic back-pain patients without physical disabilities. In: Bond MR, Charlton JE, Woolf CJ eds. *Proceeding of the VIth World Congress on Pain*. Amsterdam: Elsevier Science Publishers, 1991.

19. Fields HL. *Core Curriculum for Professional Education in Pain*. Seattle, WA: IASP Press, 1995.

◆ 20. Bigos S, Bowyer O, Braen G, *et al.* Acute low-back pain problems in adults. Clinical Practice Guidelines No. 14. In: *Agency for Health Care Policy and Research Publication No. 95–0642*. Rockville, MD: AHCPR, 1994.

21. Fairbank JCT, Couper J, Davis JB, O'Brien JP. The Oswestry Low Back Pain Disability questionnaire. *Physiotherapy* 1980; **66:** 271–3.

22. Zung WWK. A self rated depression scale. *Arch Gen Psychiatry* 1965; **32:** 63–70.

◆ 23. Waddell G, Feder G, McIntosh A, *et al. Low Back Pain Evidence Review*. London: Royal College of General Practitioners, 1999.

◆ 24. Accident Rehabilitation and Compensation Insurance Corporation of New Zealand and the National Health Committee. *New Zealand Acute Back Pain Guide*. Wellington, NZ: Accident Rehabilitation and Compensation Insurance Corporation of New Zealand and the National Health Committee, 1997.

25. Crombez G, Vlayen JWS, Heuts PHTG, Lysens R. Pain-related fear is more disabling than pain itself: evidence on the role of pain-related fear in chronic back pain disability. *Pain* 1999; **80:** 329–39.

26. Pilowski I, Spence N. *Manual for the Illness Behaviour Questionnaire*, 3rd edn. Adelaide: University of Adelaide, 1994.

27. Waddell G, McCulloch JA, Kummel E, Venner RM. Nonorganic signs in low back pain. *Spine* 1980; **5:** 117–25.

28. The Royal College of Radiologists. *Making the Best Use of a Department of Clinical Radiology: Guidelines for Doctors*, 4th edn. London: The Royal College of Radiologists, 1998.

◆ 29. Clinical Standards Advisory Group. *Back Pain: Report of a CSAG Committee on Back Pain*. London: HMSO, 1994.

30. Kendrick D, Fielding K, Bentley E, *et al.* The role of radiography in primary care patients with low back pain of at least 6 weeks duration: a randomised (unblinded) controlled trial. *Health Technol Assess* 2001; **5:** 30.

31. Gillan MG, Gilbert FJ, Andrew JE, *et al.* Influence of imaging on clinical decision making in the treatment of lower back pain. *Radiology* 2001; **220:** 393–9.

32. Luoma K, Riihimaki H, Luukkonen R, *et al.* Low back pain in relation to lumbar disc degeneration. *Spine* 2000; **25:** 487–92.

◆ 33. Deyo RA. Magnetic resonance imaging of the lumbar spine. Terrific test or tar baby? *N Engl J Med* 1994; **331:** 115–16.

34. Gorman WF, Hodak JA. Herniated intervertebral disc without pain. *J Okla State Med Assoc* 1997; **90** (5): 185–90.

35. Spitzer WO, LeBlanc FE, Dupuis M. Scientific approach to the assessment and management of activity-related spinal disorders. *Spine* 1987; **7** (Suppl.): 1–59.

● 36. van Tulder MW, Koes BW, Bouter LM. Conservative treatment of acute and chronic nonspecific low back pain: a systematic review of randomized controlled trials of the most common interventions. *Spine* 1997; **22:** 2128–56.

37. Deyo RA. Drug therapy for back pain: which drugs help which patients? *Spine* 1996; **21:** 2840–50.

38. Hickey RFJ. Chronic low back pain: a comparison of diflunisal with paracetamol. *N Z Med J* 1982; **95:** 312–14.

● 39. van Tulder MW, Scholten RJPM, Koes BW, Deyo RA. Nonsteroidal anti-inflammatory drugs for low back pain (Cochrane Review). The Cochrane Library. Oxford: Update Software, 2002: Issue 2.

40. Muller FO, Odendaal CL, Muller FR, *et al.* Comparison of the efficacy and tolerability of a paracetamol/codeine fixed-dose combination with tramadol in patients with refractory chronic back pain. *Arzneimittelforschung* 1998; **48:** 675–9.

41. Schnitzer TJ, Gray WL, Paster RZ, Kamin M. Efficacy of tramadol in treatment of chronic low back pain. *J Rheumatol* 2000; **27:** 772–8.

◆ 42. Jamison RN, Raymond SA, Slawsby EA, *et al.* Opioid therapy for chronic noncancer back pain: a randomized prospective study. *Spine* 1998; **23:** 2591–60.

43. Schofferman J. Long-term opioid analgesic therapy for severe refractory lumbar spine pain. *Clin J Pain* 1999; **15:** 136–40.

● 44. McQuay HJ, Tramer M, Nye BA, *et al.* A systematic review of antidepressants in neuropathic pain. *Pain* 1996; **68:** 217–27.

45. Atkinson JH, Slater MA, Williams RA, *et al.* A placebo-controlled randomized clinical trial of nortriptyline for chronic low back pain. *Pain* 1998; **76:** 287–96.

46. Schreiber S, Vinokur S, Shavelstozon V, *et al.* A randomized trial of fluoxetine versus amitriptyline in musculo-skeletal pain. *Isr J Psychiatry Relat Sci* 2001; **38:** 88–94.

47. McQuay HJ, Moore RA. *An Evidence-based Resource for Pain Relief*. Oxford: Oxford University Press, 1998.

48. Cherry DA, Plummer JL, Gourlay GK, *et al.* Ketamine as an adjunct to morphine in the treatment of pain. *Pain* 1995; **62:** 119–21.

49. Liberman UA, Weiss SR, Broll J, *et al.* Effect of oral alendronate on bone mineral density and the incidence of fractures in postmenopausal osteoporosis. *N Engl J Med* 1995; **333:** 1437–43.

50. Mauro GL, Martorana U, Cataldo P, *et al.* Vitamin B12 in low back pain: a randomised, double-blind, placebo-controlled study. *Eur Rev Med Pharmacol Sci* 2000; **4:** 53–8.

51. Chrubasik S, Eisenberg E, Balan E, *et al.* Treatment of low back pain exacerbations with willow bark extract: a randomized double-blind study. *Am J Med* 2000; **109:** 9–14.

● 52. Koes BW, Assendelft MD, van der Heijden GJMG, Bouter LM. Spinal manipulation for back pain: an updated systematic review of randomised clinical trials. *Spine* 1996; **21:** 2860–73.

53. Beurskens AJ, de Vet HC, Koke AJ, Lindeman E, *et al.* Efficacy of traction for non-specific low back pain: a randomised clinical trial. *Lancet* 1995; **346:** 1596–600.

54. Beurskens AJ, de Vet HC, Koke AJ, *et al.* Efficacy of traction for nonspecific low back pain. 12-week and 6-month results of a randomised clinical trial. *Spine* 1997; **22:** 2756–62.

● 55. van Tulder MW, Malmivaara A, Esmail R, Koes BW eds. *Exercise Therapy for Low Back Pain (Cochrane Review)*. Oxford: Update Software, 2000.

56. Faas A. Exercises: which ones are worth trying, for which patients, and when? *Spine* 1996; **21:** 2874–8.

◆ 57. Moffett JK, Torgerson D, Bell-Syer S, *et al.* Randomised controlled trial of exercise for low back pain: clinical outcomes, costs, and preferences. *Br Med J* 1999; **319:** 279–83.

◆ 58. Mannion Af, Muntener M, Taimela S, Dvorak J. Comparison of three active therapies for chronic low back

other disorders, including osteoarthritis of the same hip, lumbar spondylosis, and rheumatoid arthritis.[122] Since no findings are pathognomonic of trochanteric bursitis, the diagnosis is generally based on the clinical picture, which includes pain along the lateral side of the upper thigh that is aggravated by activity or lying on the affected side. Physical examination reveals tenderness over the greater trochanter. Less frequent soft-tissue disorders in this area include iliopsoas bursitis, iliogluteal bursitis ("weaver's bottom"), and adductor tendinitis, which tends to occur as a sporting injury, particularly in gymnasts and horseback riders.[123]

Chronic knee pain is common at all ages: osteoarthritis is the major determinant in the elderly, whereas anterior knee pain syndrome (chondromalacia patella) is more important in adolescents and children. There are also a large number of soft-tissue structures within the knee giving rise to symptoms including ligamentous injuries, meniscal tears, bursitis, popliteal cysts, iliotibial band syndrome, and synovial plicae.[124] Prepatellar bursitis is among the commonest of these and is usually related to repetitive trauma. Diagnosis is usually obvious, with a fluctuant swelling over the front of the patella. Anserine bursitis is also common, although in practice the term tends to be used loosely to describe any pain over the medial aspect of the upper tibia in the region of the bursa and so may include lesions of the medial ligament or pes anserus insertion.[125]

Soft-tissue disorders of the ankle include Achilles tendinitis, which is generally associated with repetitive trauma due to excessive use of the calf muscles during sporting activities. There may be an associated Achilles bursitis, which can also arise spontaneously or in association with a systemic arthropathy such as rheumatoid arthritis. One of the most common causes of pain around the heel is plantar fasciitis, which generally also results from repetitive microtrauma with risk factors being obesity, athletics, and poor footwear.[111] The disorder may coexist with subcalcaneal bursitis.

Treatment

Treatment options are similar to those discussed in the section on upper limb soft-tissue disorders, except that there are even fewer controlled trials demonstrating efficacy of particular therapeutic modalities. For the most part, primary care management consists of rest, simple analgesia, and NSAIDs. Physical therapy may be used in both acute and chronic disorders, but evidence for efficacy remains scant. Uncontrolled studies have shown infiltration of local anesthetics and steroids to be helpful in confirming the diagnosis and in bringing relief to a number of these disorders, but definitive studies are awaited.

REFERENCES

1. Liang MH, Esdaile JM. Impact and cost-effectiveness of rheumatologic care. In: Kippel JH, Dieppe PA eds. *Rheumatology*, 2nd edn, vol. 1. London: CV Mosby, 1998: 2.1–2.4.

2. Bradley EM, Tennant A. Impact of disablement due to rheumatic disorders in a British population: estimates of severity and prevalence from the Calderdale rheumatic disablement survey. *Ann Rheum Dis* 1993; **52:** 6–13.

3. Dieppe P, Sergent J. History. In: Kippel JH, Dieppe PA eds. *Rheumatology*, 2nd edn, vol. 1. London: CV Mosby, 1998.

4. Helliwell PS. The semeiology of arthritis: discriminating between patients on the basis of their symptoms. *Ann Rheum Dis* 1995; **54:** 924–6.

5. Doherty M, Dacre J, Dieppe P, Snaith M. The "GALS" locomotor screen. *Ann Rheum Dis* 1992; **51:** 1165–9.

◆ 6. Arnett FC, Edworthy SM, Bloch DA, *et al.* The American Rheumatism Association 1987 revised criteria for the classification of rheumatoid arthritis. Arthritis Rheum 1988; **31:** 315–24.

◆ 7. Lawrence RC, Helmick CG, Arnett FC, *et al.* Estimates of the prevalence of arthritis and selected musculoskeletal disorders in the United States. *Arthritis Rheum* 1998; **41:** 778–81.

8. Symmons DP, Barrett EM, Bankhead CR, *et al.* The United Kingdom: results from the Norfolk Arthritis Register. *Br J Rheumatol* 1994; **33:** 735–9.

9. Winchester R, Dwyer E, Rose S. The genetic basis of rheumatoid arthritis; the shared epitope hypothesis. *Rheum Dis Clin North Am* 1992; **18:** 761–83.

10. Fleming A, Crown JM, Corbett M. Early rheumatoid disease. I. Onset. II. Patterns of joint involvement. *Ann Rheum Dis* 1976; **35:** 357–63.

11. Schumacher HR. Palindromic onset of rheumatoid arthritis: clinical, synovial fluid and biopsy studies. *Arthritis Rheum* 1982; **25:** 361–9.

12. Matteson EL, Cohen MD, Conn DL. Rheumatoid arthritis: clinical features and systemic involvement. In: Klippel JH, Dieppe PA eds. *Rheumatology*, 2nd edn. London: Mosby, 1998: 5.4.1–5.4.8.

13. Resnick D. Rheumatoid arthritis. In: Resnick D ed. *Bone and Joint Imaging*, 2nd edn. Philadelphia, PA: WB Saunders, 1996: 195–209.

14. Weissberg DL, Resnick D, Taylor A, *et al.* Rheumatoid arthritis and its variants: analysis of scintiphotographic, radiographic and clinical examinations. *Am J Radiol* 1978; **131:** 665–73.

◆ 15. Donnelly S, Scott DL, Emery P. Management of early inflammatory arthritis. *Baillère's Clin Rheumatol* 1992; **6:** 251–60.

16. Silverstein FE, Faich G, Goldstein JL, *et al.* Gastrointestinal toxicity with celecoxib vs nonsteroidal anti-

inflammatory drugs for osteoarthritis and rheumatoid arthritis: the CLASS study. A randomized controlled trial. Celecoxib Long-term Arthritis Safety Study. *JAMA* 2000; **284:** 1247–55.

17. Bombardier C, Laine L, Reicin A, *et al.* Comparison of upper gastrointestinal toxicity of rofecoxib and naproxen in patients with rheumatoid arthritis. VIGOR Study Group. *N Engl J Med* 2000; **343:** 1520–8.

18. Moreland LW, St Clair EW. The use of analgesics in the management of pain in rheumatic diseases. *Rheum Dis Clin North Am* 1999; **25:** 153–91.

19. Ash G, Dickens CM, Creed FH, *et al.* The effects of dothiopin on subjects with rheumatoid arthritis and depression. *Rheumatology* 1999; **38:** 959–67.

20. The British Society for Rheumatology. *Guidelines for Monitoring Second Line Drugs in Rheumatoid Arthritis.* London: BSR Publications, 1993.

◆ 21. American College of Rheumatology ad hoc Committee on Clinical Guidelines. Guidelines for the management of rheumatoid arthritis. *Arthritis Rheum* 2002; **46:** 328–46.

22. Van Der Heide A, Jacobs JWG, Bijlsma JWJ, *et al.* The effectiveness of early treatment with "second line" anti-rheumatic drugs: a randomised controlled trial. *Ann Intern Med* 1996; **124:** 600–7.

23. Egsmose C, Lund B, Borg G, *et al.* Patients with rheumatoid arthritis benefit from early second line therapy: 5 year follow-up of a prospective double-blind placebo controlled study. *J Rheumatol* 1995; **22:** 2208–13.

24. Saurez-Almazor ME, Belseck E, Shea B, *et al.* Rheumatoid arthritis (RA): anti-malarials vs. placebo. In: Tugwell P, Brooks P, Wells G, *et al.* eds. *Musculoskeletal Module of The Cochrane Database of Systematic Reviews*, issue 3. Oxford: Update Software, The Cochrane Library, 1998.

25. Felson DT, Anderson JJ, Meenan RF. The comparative efficacy and toxicity of second-line drugs in rheumatoid arthritis: results of two meta-analyses. *Arthritis Rheum* 1990; **33:** 1449–61.

26. Easterbrook M. The ocular safety of hydroxychloroquine. *Semin Arthritis Rheum* 1993; **23:** 62–7.

27. Saurez-Almazor ME. Rheumatoid arthritis. *Clin Evid* 1999; **1:** 225–37.

● 28. Felson DT, Anderson JJ, Meenan RF. Use of short-term efficacy/toxicity trade-offs to select second-line drugs in rheumatoid arthritis: a meta-analysis of published clinical trials. *Arthritis Rheum* 1992; **35:** 1117–25.

29. Clark P, Tugwell P, Bennet K, *et al.* Meta-analysis of injectable gold in rheumatoid arthritis. In: Tugwell P, Brooks P, Wells G, *et al.* eds. *Musculoskeletal Module of The Cochrane Database of Systematic Reviews*, issue 3. Oxford: Update Software, The Cochrane Library, 1998.

30. Rau R. Does parenteral gold retard radiological progression in rheumatoid arthritis? *J Rheumatol* 1996; **55:** 307–18.

● 31. Saurez-Almazor ME, Soskolne CL, Saunders LD, Russell AS. Use of second line drugs in the treatment of rheumatoid arthritis in Edmonton, Alberta: patterns of prescription and long-term effectiveness. *J Rheumatol* 1995; **22:** 836–43.

32. Suarez-Almazor ME, Belseck E, Shea B, *et al.* Rheumatoid arthritis (RA): penicillamine vs. placebo in RA. In: Tugwell P, Brooks P, Wells G, *et al.* eds. *Musculoskeletal Module of The Cochrane Database of Systematic Reviews*, issue 1. Oxford: Update Software, The Cochrane Library, 1999.

33. Suarez-Almazor ME, Belseck E, Shea B, *et al.* Rheumatoid arthritis (RA): methotrexate vs. placebo. In: Tugwell P, Brooks P, Wells G, *et al.* eds. *Musculoskeletal Module of The Cochrane Database of Systematic Reviews*, issue 3. Oxford: Update Software, The Cochrane Library, 1998.

34. Pincus T, Marcum SB, Callahan LF. Long-term drug therapy for rheumatoid arthritis in seven rheumatology private practices. II. Second line drugs and prednisone. *J Rheumatol* 1992; **19:** 1885–94.

◆ 35. Wolfe F, Hawley DJ, Cathey MA. Termination of slow acting anti-rheumatoid therapy in rheumatoid arthritis: a 14 year prospective evaluation of 1017 starts. *J Rheumatol* 1990; **17:** 994–1002.

36 Gotzsche PC, Podenphant J, Olesen M, Halbert P. Meta-analysis of second-line anti-rheumatic drugs: sample size bias and uncertain benefit. *J Clin Epidemiol* 1992; **45:** 587–94.

37. Alarcon GS, Lopez-Mendez A, Walter J, *et al.* Radiographic evidence of disease progression in methotrexate treated and non-methotrexate disease modifying anti-rheumatic drug treated rheumatoid arthritis patients: a meta-analysis. *J Rheumatol* 1992; **19:** 1868–73.

38. Suarez-Almazor ME, Belseck E, Shea B, *et al.* Rheumatoid arthritis (RA): azathioprine vs. placebo in RA. In: Tugwell P, Brooks P, Wells G, *et al.* eds. *Musculoskeletal Module of The Cochrane Database of Systematic Reviews*, issue 1. Oxford: Update Software, The Cochrane Library, 1999.

39. Suarez-Almazor ME, Belseck E, Shea B, *et al.* Rheumatoid arthritis (RA): cyclophosphamide vs. placebo in RA. In: Tugwell P, Brooks P, Wells G, *et al.* eds. *Musculoskeletal Module of The Cochrane Database of Systematic Reviews*, issue 1. Oxford: Update Software, The Cochrane Library, 1999.

40. Jawad ASM, Scott DGI. Second-line agents in the treatment of systemic vasculitis. In: Dixon JS, Furst DE eds. *Second-line Agents in the Treatment of Rheumatic Diseases.* New York, NY: Marcel Dekker, 1992: 503–53.

41. Wells G, Haguenauer D, Shea B, *et al.* Rheumatoid arthritis (RA): cyclosporine vs. placebo. In: Tugwell P, Brooks P, Wells G, *et al.* eds. *Musculoskeletal Module of The Cochrane Database of Systematic Reviews*, issue 3. Oxford: Update Software, The Cochrane Library, 1998.

42. Smolen JS, Kalden JR, Scott DL, *et al.* Efficacy and safety of leflunomide compared with placebo and sulphasalazine in active rheumatoid arthritis: a double-

blind, randomised, multicentre trial. *Lancet* 1999; **353:** 259–66.

◆ 43. Elliott MJ, Maini RW, Feldmann M, *et al*. Randomised, double-blind comparison of chimeric monoclonal antibody to tumour necrosis factor alpha (cA$_2$) vs. placebo in rheumatoid arthritis. *Lancet* 1994; **344:** 1105–10.

44. Lipsky PE, van der Heijde DM, St Clair EW, *et al*. Infliximab and methotrexate in the treatment of rheumatoid arthritis. Anti-Tumor Necrosis Factor Trial in Rheumatoid Arthritis with Concomitant Therapy Study Group. *N Engl J Med* 2000; **343:** 1594–602.

◆ 45. Moreland LW, Baumgartner SW, Schiff MH, *et al*. Treatment of rheumatoid arthritis with a recombinant human tumour necrosis factor receptor (p75)–Fc fusion protein. *N Engl J Med* 1997; **337:** 141–7.

46. Moreland LW, Schiff MH, Baumgartner SW, *et al*. Phase III trial of DMARD failing rheumatoid arthritis patients with TNF receptor P75 Fc fusion protein (TNFR: Fc, ENBREL). *J Invest Med* 1998; **46:** 228A.

47. Weinblatt ME, Kremer JM, Bankhurst AD, *et al*. A trial of etanercept, a recombinant tumour necrosis factor receptor: Fc fusion protein, in patients with rheumatoid arthritis receiving methotrexate. *N Engl J Med* 1999; **340:** 253–9.

48. Bathon JM, Martin RW, Fleischmann RM, *et al*. A comparison of etanercept and methotrexate in patients with early rheumatoid arthritis. *N Engl J Med* 2000; **343:** 1586–93.

● 49. Gotzsche PC, Johanson HK. Meta-analysis of short term low dose prednisolone vs. placebo and non-steroidal anti inflammatory drugs in rheumatoid arthritis. *Br Med J* 1998; **316:** 811–18.

50. Criswell LA, Saag, KG, Sems K, *et al*. Rheumatoid arthritis (RA): moderate-term low dose corticosteroids. In: Tugwell P, Brooks P, Wells G, *et al*. eds. *Musculoskeletal Module of The Cochrane Database of Systematic Reviews*, issue 1. Oxford: Update Software, The Cochrane Library, 1999.

◆ 51. Kirwan JR. Arthritis and Rheumatism Council low dose glucocorticoid study group: the effect of glucocorticoids on joint destruction in rheumatoid arthritis. *N Engl J Med* 1995; **333:** 142–6.

52. Alexander GJM, Hortas C, Bacon PA. Bed rest, activity and the inflammation of rheumatoid arthritis. *Br J Rheumatol* 1983; **22:** 134–40.

53. Million R, Kellgren JH, Poole P, Jayson MIV. Long-term study of management of rheumatoid arthritis. *Lancet* 1984; **i:** 812–16.

54. Gautt SJ, Spyker JM. Beneficial effect of immobilization of joints in rheumatoid and related arthritides: a splint study using sequential analysis. *Arthritis Rheum* 1969; **12:** 34–44.

● 55. Ytterberg SR, Mahowald KL, Krug HE. Exercise for arthritis. *Ballière's Clin Rheumatol* 1994; **8:** 161–89.

56. Machover S, Sapecky AJ. Effect of isometric exercise on the quadriceps muscle in patient with rheumatoid arthritis. *Arch Phys Med Rehabil* 1996; **47:** 737–41.

57. Panush RS, Webster EM. Food allergies and other adverse reactions to foods. *Med Clin North Am* 1985; **69:** 533–46.

58. Conn DL, Arnold WJ, Hollister JR. Alternative treatments and rheumatic diseases. *Bull Rheum Dis* 1999; **48** (7): 1–4.

59. Simkin PA. Zinc, again (editorial). *J Rheumatol* 1997; **24:** 626–8.

● 60. Scott DL, Long AF. An overview of studies of disease outcome. In: Long AF, Scott DL eds. *Measuring Outcomes in Rheumatoid Arthritis*. London: Royal College of Physicians, 1996: 35–44.

61. Masi AT. Articular patterns in the early course of rheumatoid arthritis. *Am J Med* 1983; **75** (6A): 16–26.

◆ 62. Rasker JJ, Cosh JA. The natural history of rheumatoid arthritis: a fifteen year follow-up study. *Clin Rheumatol* 1984; **3:** 11–20.

63. Yelin E, Henke C, Epstein W. The work dynamics of the person with rheumatoid arthritis. *Arthritis Rheum* 1987; **30:** 507–12.

◆ 64. Mutru O, Laakso M, Isomäki H, Koota K. Ten year mortality and causes of death in patients with rheumatoid arthritis. *Br Med J* 1987; **30:** 507–12.

65. Keuttner K, Goldberg VM eds. *Osteoarthritic Disorders*. American Academy of Orthopedic Surgeons, 1995: 21–5.

66. Dieppe P, Chard J. Osteoarthritis. *Clin Evid* 1999; **1:** 219–24.

67. Spector T, MacGregor AJ. Epidemiology of rheumatic diseases. In: Snaith ML ed. *ABC of Rheumatology*, 2nd edn. London: BMJ, 1999: 82–6.

68. Silman AJ, Hochberg MC. *Epidemiology of the Rheumatic Disease*. Oxford: Oxford University Press, 1993.

69. Pinals RS. Mechanism of joint destruction, pain and disability in osteoarthritis. *Drugs* 1996; **52** (Suppl. 3): 14–20.

70. Doherty M, Dieppe P. Clinical aspects of calcium pyrophosphate crystal deposition. *Rheum Dis Clin North Am* 1988; **14:** 395–414.

71. Dieppe PA, Doherty M, MacFarlane DG, *et al*. Apatite-associated destructive arthritis. *Br J Rheumatol* 1984; **3:** 84–91.

72. Campion J, Watt J. Imaging and laboratory investigations. In: Klippel JH, Dieppe PA eds. *Rheumatology*. London: Mosby Year Book Europe, 1994: 7.5.1–5.14.

73. Freemont AJ, Denton J, Chuk A, *et al*. Diagnostic value of synovial fluid microscopy: a reassessment and rationalisation. *Ann Rheum Dis* 1991; **50:** 101–7.

74. McCrae F, Should J, Dieppe P, *et al*. Scintigraphic assessment of osteoarthritis of the knee joint. *Ann Rheum Dis* 1992; **51:** 938–42.

75. Pendleton A, Arden N, Dougados M, *et al*. EULAR recommendations for the management of knee osteoarthritis: report of a task force of the Standing Committee for International Clinical Studies Including Therapeutic Trials (ESCISIT). *Ann Rheum Dis* 2000; **59:** 936–44.

76. American College of Rheumatology. Subcommittee on

osteoarthritis guidelines: recommendations for the medical management of osteoarthritis of the hip and knee. *Arthritis Rheum* 2000; **43:** 1905–15.

◆ 77. Moore RA, Tramer MR, Carroll D, *et al.* Review: topical nonsteroidal anti-inflammatory drugs are effective and safe for pain. *Br Med J* 1998; **316:** 333–8.

78. Zhang WY, Po ALW. The effectiveness of topically applied capsaicin: a meta-analysis. *Eur J Clin Pharmacol* 1994; **46:** 517–22.

79. Deal CL, Schnitzer TJ, Lipstein JR, *et al.* Treatment of arthritis with topically applied capsaicin; a double-blind trial. *Clin Ther* 1991; **13:** 383–95.

80. Anonymous. What can be done about osteoarthritis? *Drugs Ther Bull* 1996; **34:** 33–5.

81. Anonymous. Articular and periarticular corticosteroid injections. *Drugs Ther Bull* 1995; **33:** 67–70.

82. Anonymous. Hyaluronan or hylans for knee osteoarthritis? *Drugs Ther Bull* 1999; **37:** 71–2.

◆ 83. Huskisson EC, Berry H, Gishen P, *et al.* Effects of anti-inflammatory drugs on the progression of osteoarthritis of the knee. *J Rheumatol* 1995; **22:** 1941–6.

84. Eccles M, Freemantle N, Mason J, for the North of England Non-steroidal Anti-Inflammatory Drug Guidelines Development Group. North of England evidence based guideline development project: summary guidelines for non-steroidal anti-inflammatory drugs versus basic analgesia in treating the pain of degenerative arthritis. *Br Med J* 1998; **317:** 526–30.

85. Chard J, Dieppe P. Glucosamine for osteoarthritis: magic hype or confusion. *Br Med J* 2001; **322:** 1439–40.

86. Reginster JY, Deroisy R, Rovati LC, *et al.* Long-term effects of glucosamine sulphate on osteoarthritis progression: a randomised, placebo-controlled clinical trial. *Lancet* 2001; **357:** 251–6.

87. McAlindon TE, LaValley MP, Felson DT. Efficacy of glucosamine and chondroitin for treatment of osteoarthritis. *JAMA* 2000; **284:** 1241.

● 88. Wollheim FA. Current pharmacological treatment of osteoarthritis. *Drugs* 1996; **52** (Suppl. 3): 27–38.

89. Superio-Cabulslay E, Ward MM, Lorig KR. Patient education interventions in osteoarthritis and rheumatoid arthritis: a meta analytic comparison with nonsteroidal anti-inflammatory drug therapy. *Arthritis Care Res* 1996; **9:** 292–301.

90. Gallo F. The effects of social support networks on the health of the elderly. *Soc Work Health Care* 1982; **8:** 65–74.

91. Keefe FJ, Caldwell DS, Baucom D, *et al.* Spouse-assisted coping skills training in the management of osteoarthritic knee pain. *Arthritis Care Res* 1996; **9:** 279–91.

92. Rene J, Weinberger M, Mazzuca SA, *et al.* Reduction of joint pain in patients with knee osteoarthritis who have received monthly telephone calls from lay personnel and whose medical treatment regimes have remained stable. *Arthritis Rheum* 1992; **35:** 511–15.

93. Ettinger Jr WH, Burns R, Messier SP, *et al.* A randomized

trial comparing aerobic exercise and resistance exercise with a health education program in older adults with knee osteoarthritis. *JAMA* 1997; **277:** 64–6.

94. Cushnaghan J, McCarthy C, Dieppe P. Taping the patella medially: a new treatment for osteoarthritis of the knee joint. *Br Med J* 1994; **308:** 753–5.

95. Perrot S, Menkes CJ. Nonpharmacological approaches to pain in osteoarthritis: available options. *Drugs* 1996; **52** (Suppl. 3): 21–6.

◆ 96. Felson DT, Zhang Y, Anthony JM, *et al.* Weight loss reduces the risk for symptomatic osteoarthritis in women. The Framingham study. *Ann Intern Med* 1992; **116:** 772–9.

97. Taylor P, Hallett M, Flaherty L. Treatment of osteoarthritis of the knee with transcutaneous electrical nerve stimulation. *Pain* 1981; **11:** 233–40.

98. Lewis B, Lewis D, Cumming G. The comparative analgesic efficacy of transcutaneous electrical nerve stimulation and a non-steroidal anti-inflammatory drug for painful osteoarthritis. *Br J Rheumatol* 1994; **33:** 455–60.

99. Ernst E. Acupuncture as a symptomatic treatment of osteoarthritis. *Scand J Rheumatol* 1997; **26:** 444–7

100. Sasaki T, Yasuda K. Clinical evaluation of the treatment of osteoarthritic knees using a newly designed wedge insole. *Clin Orthop* 1987; **221:** 181–7.

101. Maratz V, Muncie Jr HL, Walsh MH. Occupational therapy in the multi-disciplinary assessment and management of osteoarthritis. *Clin Ther* 1986; **9:** 24–9.

102. Anonymous. What can be done about osteoarthritis? *Drugs Ther Bull* 1996; **34:** 33–5.

103. Ike RW, Arnold WJ, Rothschild EW. Tidal irrigation versus conservative medical management in patients with osteoarthritis of the knee: a prospective randomised study. *J Rheumatol* 1992; **19:** 772–9.

104. Anonymous. Hip and knee joint replacements. *Drugs Ther Bull* 1992; **30:** 57–60.

◆105. Palmer K, Coggon D, Cooper C, Doherty M. Work related upper limb disorders: getting down to specifics. *Ann Rheum Dis* 1998; **57:** 1–2.

◆106. Allander E. Prevalence, incidence and remission rates of some common rheumatic diseases or syndromes. *Scand J Rheumatol* 1974; **3:** 145–53.

107. Croft P, Pope D, Silman A The clinical course of shoulder pain: prospective cohort study in primary care. *Br Med J* 1996; **313:** 601–2.

●108. van der Heijden GJMG. Shoulder disorders: a state of the art review. *Ballière's Clin Rheumatol* 1999; **13:** 287–309.

109. Cyriax J. *Textbook of Orthopaedic Medicine.* London: Ballière Tindall, 1981.

110. Bamji AN, Erhart CC, Price TR, Williams PL. The painful shoulder: can consultants agree? *Br J Rheumatol* 1996; **35:** 1172–4.

◆111. Winters JC, Groenier HK, Sobel JS, *et al.* Classification of shoulder complaints in general practice by means of cluster analysis. *Arch Phys Med Rehabil* 1997; **78:** 1369–74.

112. van der Windt DAWM, van der Heijden GJMG, Scholten RJPM, *et al*. The efficacy of non-steroidal anti-inflammatory drugs for shoulder complaints: a systemic review. *J Clin Epidemiol* 1995; **48:** 691–704.

113. van der Heijden GJMG, van der Windt DAWM, Kleijnen J, *et al*. Steroid injections for shoulder disorders: a systematic review of randomised clinical trials. *Br J Gen Pract* 1996; **46:** 309–16.

114. van der Heijden GJMG, van der Windt DAWM, De Winter AF. Physiotherapy for patients with soft-tissue shoulder disorders: a systematic review of randomised clinical trials. *Br Med J* 1997; **315:** 25–30.

115. Takala J, Sievers K, Klaukka T. Rheumatic symptoms in the middle aged population in south-western Finland. *Scand J Rheumatol* 1982; **47:** 15–29.

●116. Linaker CH, Walker-Bone K, Palmer K, Cooper C. Frequency and impact of regional musculoskeletal disorders. *Ballière's Clin Rheumatol* 1999; **13:** 197–215.

117. Hamilton PG. The prevalence of humeral epicondylitis: a survey in general practice. *J R Coll Gen Pract* 1986; **36:** 464–5.

●118. Helliwell PS. The elbow, forearm, wrist and hand. *Ballière's Clin Rheumatol* 1999; **13:** 311–28.

119. Stock SR. Workplace ergonomic factors and the development of musculoskeletal disorders of the neck and upper limbs: a meta-analysis. *Am J Ind Med* 1991; **19:** 87–107.

●120. Fedorczyk J. The role of physical agents in modulating pain. *J Hand Ther* 1997; **10:** 110–21.

121. Chard MD, Hazelman BL. Tennis elbow: physical methods of treatment. In: Schlapback P, Gerber NJ eds. *Physiotherapy: Controlled Trials and Facts*. Basel: Karger, 1991: 99–107.

122. Shapira D, Nahir M, Scharf Y. Trochanteric bursitis: a common clinical problem. *Arch Phys Med Rehabil* 1986; **67:** 470–8.

123. Mazieres B, Carette S. The hip. In: Kippel JH, Dieppe PA eds. *Rheumatology*, 2nd edn, vol. 1. London: CV Mosby, 1998.

●124. McAlindon TE. The knee. *Ballière's Clin Rheumatol* 1999; **13:** 329–44.

125. Graham GP, Fairclough JA. The knee. In: Kippel JH, Dieppe PA eds. *Rheumatology*, 2nd edn, vol. 1. London: CV Mosby, 1998.

Chronic chest pain

ALF COLLINS

This chapter concentrates on pain anterior to the midaxillary line and/or pain referred from structures within the precordium. Primary dorsal chronic chest pains are likely to be referred from the spine and are not discussed. Malignant disease must always be considered as a cause of chest pain, but again will not be further discussed.

EPIDEMIOLOGY

There are no epidemiological studies on chronic chest pain *per se*. However, a US study of all types of chronic pain in a large health maintenance organization showed that chest pain had occurred for more than a whole day in the previous 6 months in 12% of the population under investigation.[1]

The majority of patients with chest pain who are referred for specialist opinion will present to a cardiac clinic. The cause of the pain in more than 50% of such patients is noncardiac.[2] In a recent survey of over 600 referrals to a "one stop" chest pain clinic, only 27% had a cardiac cause for their symptoms.[3]

Patients reassured that they do not have heart disease have a poor outcome in terms of distress, disability, and continuing concern that they have a cardiac disorder.[4] Few are given an explanation for, or management of, the underlying minor medical disorders that might be causing their pain, and only a minority are directly referred for psychological intervention.[5]

ETIOLOGY

Chronic chest pain can arise from the following structures:

- Visceral
  - heart, pericardium, great vessels;
  - pleura;
  - esophagus;
  - upper gastrointestinal tract.
- Primary somatic
  - muscle, sternal and costal joints, periosteum.
- Referred somatic
  - cervical spine;
  - thoracic spine and nerve roots.

ASSESSMENT AND MANAGEMENT OF THE PATIENT WITH CHRONIC CHEST PAIN

Most patients with chronic chest pain are managed by primary care physicians or by cardiologists. Few cardiologists work in multidisciplinary pain management teams, yet the majority of patients with chronic chest pain have complex somatopsychic disorders. Many of these patients present a considerable diagnostic and management challenge to their care givers.

The following management guideline is recommended in the care of these patients:

Identify specific pain syndromes and treat accordingly.
Many syndromes have a somatopsychic basis, and the patient's fears, beliefs, and expectations must be assessed and managed while a diagnosis is being sought. Many patients believe that their pain is due to their heart, even after a cardiac source for the pain has been discounted.[4,6,7]

Patients often present with more than one chest pain syndrome.
Patients with a combination of ischemic heart disease and noncardiac chest pain are particularly

difficult to manage.[8] Ischemic heart disease and gastroesophageal reflux disorder often coexist.[9]

Assess and manage any underlying psychological predisposition to chronic chest pain.

Approximately 25% of patients with ischemic heart disease have demonstrable psychological comorbidity (Table 41.1). The figure rises to over 60% for patients with noncardiac chest pain.[4] Patients who display overt psychological disorders, or who fail to respond to simple interventions, may need true multidisciplinary management or referral for cognitive–behavioral therapy.[10,11]**

Use a patient-centered approach to management.[12]

Offer a full explanation of the diagnosis and potential management strategies at all stages.[5] Encourage the patient to become involved in the decision-making process. Promotion of self-efficacy will improve outcomes from all interventions.[13]***

PAIN SYNDROMES

The following pain syndromes will be described:

- cardiac-related chest pain;
- gastroesophageal reflux disease;
- musculoskeletal chest pain;
- radicular neuropathic pain;
- postcardiothoracic surgery syndromes;
- psychological disorders associated with, or presenting as, pain.

Chronic pleural pain and mastalgia rarely present to chronic pain clinics and will not be discussed.

Chronic cardiac-related chest pain

The following pain syndromes will be described:

- angina pectoris;
- refractory angina pectoris;
- syndrome X.

Pericardial and aortic causes of chronic pain are rare and will not be discussed.

Angina pectoris

The word angina is derived from the Greek "αγχειν" (*anchein*, to choke) and was first used in a lecture to the

Table 41.1 *Psychological risk factors and chronic chest pain*

Pain beliefs and fears
Anxiety
Depression
Somatoform disorders

Royal College of Physicians of London by Heberden in 1668. The manuscript of the lecture – *Some Account of a Disorder of the Breast* – was published in 1772, and the author gives an accurate description of the clinical presentation of angina, despite not knowing that the pain came from the heart.

The etymology of the word is of interest, being derived from the same Greek root as "anxiety" and "anguish."

Hippocrates (in *Coacis*, 400 BC) and Pliny the Elder (in *Natural History*, AD 70) both provide us with accounts of chronic chest pain associated with sudden death.

There continued to be descriptions of angina through history (namely Harvey 1649, Desportes 1811), but it was not until 1912 that Herrick described the pain of myocardial infarction.[14]

Angina pectoris is a clinical diagnosis characterized by chest discomfort due to myocardial ischemia. Myocardial ischemia is commonly associated with coronary artery disease (CAD), but may be due to a decrease in myocardial oxygen supply or an increase in oxygen demand without evident CAD.

Clinical considerations

Character of angina pectoris Typical visceral pain, poorly localized, and often described as pressure, tightness, or heaviness. Patients may describe their symptoms with nonverbal gestures, e.g. laying the hands on the chest or clutching the throat.[15]

Localization In the anterior chest in 96% of cases; in 34%, this is the only site. In 33% of cases, pain refers to the left arm and in 23% to the right arm. In 30% of cases, pain refers to the jaw.[16] The character and site of pain varies little in individual patients, and the distribution of the angina is only loosely correlated with the region of ischemic myocardium.[17]

Accompanying symptoms Breathlessness and diaphoresis accompany the pain, along with apprehension, fear, and anxiety. Apprehension may be overwhelming (*angor animi*).

Severity In daily life, up to 70% of episodes of myocardial ischemia are asymptomatic.[18,19] There is no clear relationship between the degree of ischemia and the level of reported pain.[20]

Duration Often short-lived and relieved by rest.

Provoking and relieving factors Classically, unaccustomed exercise brings about angina, but anxiety and extreme emotion have been noted to provoke angina since the time of Heberden. Between 25% and 50% of episodes of angina in daily life are triggered by emotional, as opposed to physical, factors.[19,21]

Psychological aspects of angina pectoris Patients with angina have a lower quality of life than those with other chronic diseases such as arthritis, back pain, and stroke. This is despite angina sufferers having less pain than patients with other chronic disorders.[22]

Forty percent of patients who do not return to work

after an uncomplicated myocardial infarct have a fear of imminent death. Twenty-five percent of these patients have distorted health beliefs, fearing that every attack of angina damages the heart.[23] In fact, the reverse appears to be the case.[24,25]

Numerous studies have shown positive correlations between anxiety, depression, and neuroticism and the frequency and severity of angina, independent of the extent of the coronary disease.[26]

The affective domain of the experience of angina promotes a further increase in myocardial oxygen demand and a decrease in oxygen supply as a result of coronary vasoconstriction. This positive feedback loop causes further ischemia and pain, the so-called "cardiocardiac reflex" (Fig. 41.1).[27]

The operative intervention of internal mammary (IMA) ligation, which was popular in the 1950s, improved angina in a majority of patients. Subsequent randomized trials performed by Cobb[28] and by Dimond[29]** showed no benefit of IMA ligation over sham intervention. Any new intervention in ischemic heart disease must undergo intense scrutiny because of the complexity of the interaction between psyche and soma in the genesis of angina.

Assessment and management of the patient with angina pectoris

The management of uncomplicated angina lies within the domains of cardiology and cardiac surgery. The ischemia-based model of management prevails, and international clinical management guidelines exist.[30,31]**

Interventional techniques such as coronary artery surgery (CABG) and angioplasty improve quality of life,[8] but CABG only offers prognostic benefit (Table 41.2) if there is left mainstem disease, three-vessel disease with ventricular dysfunction, or two-vessel disease with proximal left mainstem stenosis and ventricular dysfunction.[32]**

A number of studies have shown significant improvement in angina using a cognitive–behavioral pain management program approach.[33,34]** Although these results are impressive, pain management approaches are not as yet accepted into mainstream cardiology.

Table 41.2 *Prognostic benefit from CABG*

Left mainstem disease
Three-vessel disease with left ventricular dysfunction
Two-vessel disease with proximal LAD stenosis and left
  ventricular dysfunction

LAD, left anterior descending artery.

Refractory angina pectoris

Refractory angina pectoris is angina associated with coronary artery disease that cannot be controlled by lifestyle adjustment, optimal medical therapy, angioplasty, or coronary bypass surgery.[35]

A national survey of patients referred for coronary angiography because of stable angina pectoris was performed by the Swedish Council of Technology Assessment in Health Care in 1994/1995. Of the patients referred, 9.6% were rejected for revascularization despite severe symptoms.[36]

No other reliable data on the prevalence of refractory angina exist at the time of writing.

Assessment and management of the patient with chronic refractory angina

One approach has been developed by a multidisciplinary working party of the European Society of Cardiology.[35] A similar approach is being implemented in the UK.[37]

It is recommended that the patient be managed by a multidisciplinary team, with assessment by an interventional cardiologist and cardiac surgeon, and by pain management specialists, psychiatrists, psychologists, and rehabilitation specialists as necessary.

Evaluate diagnosis Demonstrable myocardial ischemia temporally related to symptoms is a prerequisite. Methods used will depend on local expertise and availability.

Exclude noncardiac causes Anemia, hypertension, costochondritis, internal mammary artery syndrome (IMAS; see below) and gastroesophageal reflux disorder should be considered (see below). A trial of proton pump inhibitors should be offered (see below).

The cardiocardiac reflex

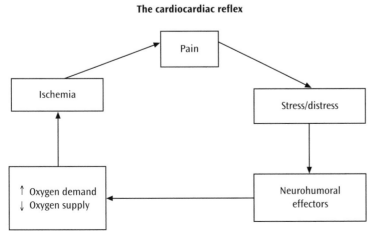

Figure 41.1 *The cardiocardiac reflex.*

Optimize anti-ischemic medication Optimization of antianginal medication in patients referred for transmyocardial laser revascularization considerably reduced symptoms in 44% of patients with "refractory" angina.[38]

Assess and address psychological distress Significantly distressed patients may need individual psychological management.

Assess and address pain-related beliefs and anxieties Twenty-five percent of patients believe that every attack of angina irreparably damages the heart. Many patients believe that moderate exercise is potentially harmful.[34]

Institute a rehabilitation program Rehabilitation programs emphasize risk factor reduction, exercise, and psychosocial support.[39] Cognitive–behavioral pain management programs emphasize a symptom-based approach to management. Choice will depend on local expertise and availability.

Consider other management strategies as outlined below Historically, management strategies have as their rationale an ischemia-based model of etiology.

Primary pain management has been rejected because of the fear that pain reduction might conceal a useful warning signal.

The concept of angina as a useful signal has recently been challenged.[24] Seventy percent of ischemic episodes in daily life are not perceived by the patient,[18,19] and there is no evidence of a direct relationship between the degree of ischemia and the level of pain.[20]

Additionally, there is strong evidence that short periods of ischemia both promote new vessel growth and protect the myocardium from further ischemic insult. This so-called "ischemic preconditioning" is related to adenosine release.[24,25]

Treatments for refractory angina

The following treatments, outlined in Table 41.3, will be considered. No data comparing any of these treatments exist at the time of writing.

- Transcutaneous electrical nerve stimulation (TENS).
  - Safety established: does not provoke dysrhythmia.[40]
  - Clinical effectiveness established: 40–70% of patients report significant symptom reduction compared with prestimulation.[41,42*]
  - Mode of action complex and unknown: pain and ischemia are reduced in tandem.[43] There is no good evidence for a primary anti-ischemic effect.[44]
  - Conventionally, electrodes are placed over the precordium in order to stimulate the area of pain: there are no randomized trials that test this hypothesis.
  - Conventionally, high-frequency stimulation is used (70–100 Hz): there are no trials of low-frequency TENS in angina pectoris.

- Conventionally, patients stimulate for 1 h, three times daily as prophylaxis, plus on-demand stimulation should angina occur: the evidence for this so-called "hangover effect" of TENS is based on nonrandomized trials,[44] and may represent ischemic preconditioning.
- A significant proportion of patients develop skin irritation because of high stimulation intensity during attacks of angina (M. J. DeJongste, personal communication).
- Caution should be exercised when the patient has an indwelling pacemaker or defibrillator (M. Chester, personal communication).[45]

- Spinal cord stimulation (SCS).
  - Safety established: there is no increase in overall mortality compared with matched, unimplanted groups.[46] Patients with indwelling spinal cord stimulators show no tendency to dysrhythmia,[47,48] ventricular dysfunction,[49] or sudden death[46] with the stimulator switched on compared with it switched off. Patients appear to feel the pain of myocardial infarction with the stimulator switched on.[50,51]
  - Clinical effectiveness established: 70–85% of patients report significant decreases in angina frequency[44,46,52*,53**] and improvement in quality of life[54,55*] compared with preimplant. Clinical effectiveness is sustained over long-term follow-up.[50] Mannheimer's group randomized patients with severe refractory angina to either high-risk coronary artery surgery or SCS. Symptom reduction was similar in both groups, with a much higher mortality rate in the CABG group.[56,57**]
  - Mode of action complex and unknown: SCS is anti-ischemic either primarily[58] or secondary to pain reduction,[57,59] thus causing a "winding down" of the cardiocardiac reflex. Although a reduction in oxygen demand has been inferred,[60] this is not always the case.[61] A redistribution of blood supply from epicardial to endocardial has been demonstrated by one group using positron emission tomography (PET),[62] but has not been found by others.[63]

Table 41.3 *Treatments for refractory angina*

Transcutaneous electrical nerve stimulation
Spinal cord stimulation
Thoracic epidural anesthesia
Endoscopic thoracic sympathectomy
Stellate ganglion blockade
Intermittent urokinase
Enhanced external counterpulsation
Myocardial revascularization by laser
Gene therapy and angiogenesis

– Conventionally, the area of pain is stimulated.[64] There are no randomized trials to test this hypothesis.

– Conventionally, high-frequency stimulation is used.[65] There are no randomized trials to tell us what is the "best frequency."

– Conventionally, stimulation three or four times daily helps to prevent angina. Stimulation is also used just before anticipated angina, and to treat established angina.[65] Trials attesting to the "hangover effect" of SCS in preventing angina were not randomized, and the hangover may represent ischemic preconditioning.[44]

– Caution should be exercised when the patient has an indwelling pacemaker[66] or defibrillator (M. Chester, personal communication) and when the patient is subjected to magnetic resonance imaging.[67]

• Thoracic epidural anesthesia.
  – The majority of studies are in acute myocardial ischemia. There is good symptom relief and reduction of ischemic indices in unstable angina.[68,69*] There is much less experience in chronic stable angina, and the reported complication rate is high.[70]

• Endoscopic thoracic sympathectomy.
  – Limited data are available: clinical effectiveness appears good, but operative morbidity is high.[71,72*]

• Left stellate ganglion injection.
  – Limited data available: clinical effectiveness of local anesthetic injection appears good and long lasting,[73*] although the rationale is obscure at present.

• Intermittent urokinase therapy.
  – Limited data available: clinical effectiveness appears good in small studies, although frequent admissions are needed and the cost is high.[74]

• Enhanced external counterpulsation (EECP).
  – EECP is based upon augmentation of coronary flow in diastole, using a computer-controlled system of externally applied pneumatic cuffs.[75] Patients initially require frequent treatments, but there are long-term improvements in ischemia and angina, particularly for patients who do not have three-vessel disease.[76*] An international registry exists, and results appear promising, with very low morbidity.[77]

• Myocardial revascularization by laser.
  – The rationale is based on the creation of channels between the ventricular cavity and the myocardium, either from epicardium to ventricle (TMLR) or from the ventricle to the myocardium (PMLR).
  – Transmyocardial laser revascularization (TMLR) is the most widely used to date. Six multicenter randomized controlled trials (RCTs) show early symptom improvement in the majority of survivors of the intervention.[78–82,83**] Myocardial perfusion was assessed in five of the six trials. No improvement in perfusion was found in four, and in the fifth trial the magnitude of symptom improvement was out of proportion to the improvement in perfusion. The duration of the angina-free period is usually less than 1 year. The mortality rate of the procedure is 5–20%.[84] The mechanism of action is now uncertain, and involves angiogenesis, cardiac denervation, and placebo effect.[83]
  – Percutaneous laser revascularization has a much lower mortality than TMLR. Initial results are promising, with early improvement in symptoms and low morbidity. The role of the placebo effect has not yet been determined.[85**]

• Gene therapy and angiogenesis.
  – Direct myocardial injection of DNA encoding for vascular endothelium growth factor (VEGF). Preliminary clinical data are encouraging.[86]

The plethora of treatment strategies for refractory angina reflects uncertainty about etiological factors underlying the disorder. The UK consensus-based treatment algorithm attempts to rectify this by providing a step-wise approach to management.[37]

Syndrome X

Clinical considerations

Syndrome X is typical angina associated with ischemia-like changes on the stress electrocardiogram (EKG) in the presence of normal coronary arteries. It is more common in women and is associated with a normal life expectancy.[87]

Syndrome X is a spectrum of clinical entities. Research has focused on the role of endothelial dysfunction in the etiology of the disorder, but only a minority of patients with syndrome X have demonstrable myocardial ischemia using the objective measure of continuous coronary sinus pH monitoring.[88]

The role of visceral hyperalgesia in the pathogenesis of syndrome X is becoming established.[89] Although patients with chest pain and normal coronary arteries have a tendency to psychological comorbidity (see below), the psychological characteristics of the subgroup of patients with typical syndrome X have not been systematically studied.[90]

Assessment and management of the patient with syndrome X (Table 41.4)

One approach has been suggested by Kaski and Valenzuela Garcia.[91**] Patients with exercise-induced chest pain or high resting heart rates as assessed by ambulatory EKG may benefit from β-blockade.[92**] A proportion of those others with evidence of ischemia will benefit from calcium channel blockers.[93**] Adenosine antagonists may

Table 41.4 *Management of syndrome X*

β-Blockers
Calcium channel blockers
Adenosine antagonists
Estrogen therapy
Tricyclic antidepressants
Transcutaneous electrical nerve stimulation
Spinal cord stimulation
Psychological intervention

be beneficial in patients with a positive response to dipyridamole stress testing.[94]**

The majority of patients with syndrome X do not have evidence of ischemia. The therapeutic options for these patients are estrogen therapy,[95]** tricyclic antidepressants,[96]** TENS,[91] spinal cord stimulation,[97,98]* or psychological intervention.[11,99]**

Chronic noncardiac chest pain

There are numerous studies on the assessment, management, and prognosis of patients with noncardiac chest pain. What many long-term follow-up studies fail to do, however, is to identify that these patients are a heterogeneous group. The following diagnoses should be considered when a patient presents with noncardiac chest pain as assessed by history, examination, and stress EKG.

Gastroesophageal reflux disorder

Between 36% and 50% of patients referred to a cardiologist with chest pain have an esophageal disorder as the primary cause for their pain.[4,100]

The evidence for esophageal motility disorders as a cause of chest pain is poor.[101,102] Noncardiac chest pain associated with esophageal motility disorders does not respond to motility-modifying drugs.[103]** Additionally, studies of prolonged ambulatory motility monitoring show that chest pain is rarely accompanied by disturbances of motility.[104]

Visceral hypersensitivity or hypervigilance is an increasingly recognized cause of chest pain,[105] but the most common disorder resulting in esophageal pain is gastroesophageal reflux disorder (GERD) (Table 41.5).[106]

Assessment and management of the patient with esophageal chest pain
The history is classically of intermittent retrosternal burning pain, often with radiation across the precordium. The predictive value of the history is, however, poor.[107,108]

Table 41.5 *Esophageal pain*

Gastroesophageal reflux disorder
Visceral hypersensitivity

Esophageal pain can refer into the jaw and arms, can be related to exercise, and can be relieved by both nitrates and calcium channel blockers (Table 41.6).[9,109]

GERD is more common in patients with coronary heart disease than in the general population.[9] A study of two groups of patients – one with chest pain and normal coronary angiograms and the other with chest pain and abnormal angiograms – subjected both groups to 24-h pH monitoring (see below). No significant difference was found in episodes of reflux-associated chest pain between the two groups. The authors suggest that esophageal pain is perhaps underdiagnosed.[110]

In patients without an evident cardiac cause for their pain, esophageal pain should be suspected. The most sensitive test to correlate chest pain and reflux is 24-h pH monitoring.[106,111] But endoscopy is most frequently used, as it is simple and straightforward; the detection of esophagitis at endoscopy should not necessarily infer causality but should prompt a trial of acid suppression.

Omeprazole in a dose of 60 mg daily for 1 week, crossing over to placebo for a further week, has a diagnostic sensitivity of 78% and specificity of 86% in patients with chest pain of uncertain origin (Table 41.7).[112]

Esophageal acid perfusion, intravenous edrophonium, and balloon distension tests are used to more accurately define diagnosis in specialist gastroenterology practice (J. de Caestecker, personal communication).

Management is by reassurance and explanation that there is no underlying cardiac cause for their pain. Many patients do not accept that the source of their pain is esophageal.[6]

Proton pump inhibitors have been shown to reduce the pain related to GERD.[113] Other management strategies are within the domain of the gastroenterologist (Table 41.8).

Musculoskeletal chest pain syndromes

Up to 70% of patients referred to a chest pain clinic have normal coronary angiograms.[3] Of these patients, 40–70% have a primary musculoskeletal source for their pain, with myofascial pains being three times more common than joint pains (Table 41.9).[114,115]

Assessment and management of patients with musculoskeletal chest pain

- The diagnosis is in all cases clinical, and should be based on positive evidence. Musculoskeletal chest pain should not be a diagnosis made by exclusion.
- Provide reassurance and a full explanation of the diagnosis.
- Assess and manage psychological risk factors.
- Provide specific treatment of the organic disorder.

Bone pains

Chronic pain can occur after sternal fracture[116] or after cardiac surgery (see below). A history of significant

Table 41.6 *Comparison of classical angina and esophageal pain*

Pain description	Angina	Esophageal pain
Time-course	Often short	Often prolonged
Site and radiation	Precordium, jaw, arms	Retrosternal, precordium, jaw, arms
Character	Pressure, tight, band-like	Burning, pressure
	Associated with fear	Less pronounced fear
Provoking factors	Exercise, stress, food, cold; rare at night	Food, posture, rarely exercise related; often at night
Relieving factors	Rest, trinitrates	Trinitrates, antacids

trauma is nearly always present, but fractures may occur spontaneously in the elderly.[117]

Anecdotally, simple analgesics and TENS have been used to manage persistent pain after sternal injury.[116]

Joint pains

Pain syndromes in sternal and costal joints are in general idiopathic, but can occur after trauma or surgery, particularly cardiac surgery where the sternum is split.

These syndromes can also occur as part of a systemic disorder, and on occasion can be mimicked by tumor or infection in the joint space.

Adolescents who present with chest pain have been shown to have tender costal cartilages in 14–79% of cases.[118-120]

Table 41.7 *Diagnosis of esophageal chest pain*

No evidence of cardiac, musculoskeletal, or primary psychological disorder
Trial of PPI
Upper gastrointestinal tract endoscopy
24-h pH monitoring

PPI, proton pump inhibitor.

Table 41.8 *Management of esophageal chest pain*

Reassurance
Proton pump inhibitor
Specialist referral

Table 41.9 *Musculoskeletal chronic chest pains*

Bone pain
  Sternal fracture
Joint pain
  Manubriosternal pain
  Costochondral pain
  Tietze syndrome
  Twelfth rib syndrome
Myofascial pain
  Intercostal myofascial syndrome
  Pectoralis major myofascial syndrome
  Pectoralis minor myofascial syndrome
Referred pain
  Cervical spine referred pain
Radicular pain
  Intercostal neuralgia

Anecdote suggests that management of these pains should be by simple analgesics or anti-inflammatories, TENS,[120] or acupuncture.[121] Local infiltration with steroid has been reported to be beneficial.[122]

Manubriosternal pain

- Rare.
- Usually occurs as part of a systematic syndrome, such as psoriatic arthropathy or ankylosing spondylitis.[123]
- Monoarthritis of the joint has been described.[124]
- Disease-modifying therapy may be helpful if a systematic disorder is present.

Costochondral pain

- Present in 10% of those patients attending cardiac clinics who have normal coronary angiograms.[114]
- Pain and tenderness in a number of costal cartilages, often without evidence of swelling.[115]
- Unilateral or bilateral.
- Candida costochondritis has been described in intravenous drug abusers.[125]
- Common in adolescents who present with chest pain.[118-120]
- Usually self-limiting.[120]

Tietze syndrome (chondropathia tuberosa, costosternal chondrodynia)

- Pain, swelling, and tenderness in the sternoclavicular joint or in the upper costochondral or sternochondral joints.
- Usually unilateral, usually only one or two joints affected.
- Usually idiopathic, but can occur postoperatively (e.g. CABG, major breast surgery[126]).
- Has been described in children.[127]
- Usually self-limiting.[127]

Twelfth rib syndrome[128]

- Pain in twelfth rib plus its costal cartilage.
- Pain reproduced by manipulation of the rib.
- Usually unilateral.
- Anecdote suggests symptomatic treatment.

Myofascial pains

Pain in the chest can be secondary to myofascial disorder in intercostal muscles, pectoralis major, or pectoralis minor. Assessment and management of these pains will be considered in the chapter devoted to myofascial pain (see Chapter Ch44).

Referred pain

Chest pain referred from the cervical spine will usually be provoked by neck movement. Assessment and management will be considered in the chapter devoted to neck pain (see Chapter Ch38).

Radicular pain

Intercostal neuralgia has the typical features of neuropathic pain. Postherpetic neuralgia will be considered in a separate chapter (see Chapter Ch34).

Slipping rib syndrome[129,130]

- Radicular pain in approximately T8–T10 distribution, leading to chest or abdominal pain.
- The syndrome has been described in adults and children.
- The pathology is slipping of costal cartilage onto the adjacent intercostal nerve.
- Management is symptomatic, although surgical intervention has been described.

Postcardiothoracic surgery chronic pain syndromes

Chronic chest pain is common after coronary artery bypass surgery[131] (Table 41.10).

- Patients may present with a number of pain syndromes.
- Many patients demonstrate psychological comorbidity (see below).
- Pain may be caused by, or incidental to, the surgery.

Assessment and management of post cardiac surgery pain (Table 41.11)

- Assess and address fears and beliefs. Many patients fear that ongoing pain is cardiac in origin.
- Assess for refractory angina or gastroesophageal reflux disorder and treat accordingly.
- Treat other specific syndromes as below.

Left internal mammary artery pain syndrome
- Stripping of the left internal mammary artery (LIMA) is associated with damage to the anterior

Table 41.10 *Post cardiac surgery chronic pain syndromes*

Refractory angina
Chronic scar pain
Anterior chest wall musculoskeletal pain
Left internal mammary artery syndrome

intercostal nerves in T1–6 territory in over 70% of patients after CABG.
- Persistent neuropathic pain over left anterior chest wall occurs in 15% of patients after cardiac surgery.[132]
- Anecdotal evidence suggests that this should be treated as neuropathic pain.

PSYCHOLOGICAL ASPECTS OF CHRONIC CHEST PAIN

All aspects of the care of people suffering from chronic chest pain should follow a patient-centered approach (see above). There should be an emphasis on sharing of information between physician and patient, and the patient should be encouraged to participate in the decision-making process at all stages.

- Patients with cardiac chest pain may suffer from anxiety, depression, fear avoidance behavior, and distorted pain beliefs (see above).[34]
- Over 60% of patients with chest pain and no evident organic pathology have demonstrable psychological morbidity, commonly anxiety, depression, or somatoform pain disorder.[133]
- Sixty percent of patients with noncardiac chest pain display a tendency to hyperventilation.[133]
- Patients with noncardiac chest pain often find it difficult to accept that their pain is not caused by their heart.[4,6,7]
- Patients with noncardiac chest pain are a heterogeneous group. The psychological characteristics of patients with specific chest pain syndromes have not been systematically studied.

Screening for psychological morbidity

- All patients who present with chronic chest pain should be screened for psychological morbidity. The screening process should include the use of validated questionnaires and a semistructured interview (Table 41.12).[133]
- Patients who present with evident psychological morbidity should be referred for management by a psychologist or psychiatrist.
- It is suggested that the screening process addresses pain-related beliefs and fears, anxiety, and depression.
- Distorted pain beliefs and fears should be addressed and managed. An adequate explanation of the triggers and causes of the pain experience is often all that is needed.
- Anxiety which is not specifically associated with abnormal pain beliefs is best treated by referral to a psychologist or psychiatrist (Table 41.13).
- Evident depression is best treated by referral to a psychologist or psychiatrist (Table 41.14).

Table 41.11 *Assessment and management of post cardiac surgery pain*

Problem	Assessment	Management
Stitch or sternal wire pain	Point tenderness	Surgical removal of stitch or wire
Sternum or drain scar pain	Pain ± hyperalgesia in and around scar	Management of neuropathic pain
Musculoskeletal pains	Point tenderness and pain on stressing joint	Acupuncture, dry needle, steroid injection
LIMA syndrome	Neuropathic pain in left anterior precordium	Management of neuropathic pain

LIMA, left internal mammary artery.

Table 41.12 *Assessment of chest pain beliefs and fears*

What do you understand is causing your pain?
Do you ever worry that the pain might be caused by a problem with your heart?
Does the pain stop you doing things you enjoy?

Table 41.13 *Assessment of anxiety*

Previous history of irritable bowel syndrome, migraine, or fibromyalgia
Hospital anxiety and depression questionnaire
Do you feel you are an anxious person?
Have you ever had a panic attack?
Do you ever hyperventilate?
What goes through your mind when you have chest pain?
What other symptoms do you experience when you get chest pain?

Table 41.14 *Assessment of depression*

Hospital anxiety and depression questionnaire
Do you suffer from low energy or mood?
Do you suffer from feelings of hopelessness?
Do you feel slowed up?
Do you wake early in the morning?

Table 41.15 *Suggested guideline for the management of chronic chest pain*

Assess and manage angina according to national protocol
Treat evident musculoskeletal pain with simple analgesia or injection therapy if appropriate
Trial of PPI if angina excluded and no evident musculoskeletal cause
Address fears and beliefs
Assess anxiety and depression and refer to psychologist if necessary
Follow-up: persistent symptoms? – consider individual psychological management or cognitive–behavioral therapy

PPI, proton pump inhibitor.

GUIDELINE FOR THE MANAGEMENT OF CHRONIC CHEST PAIN

All patients should have an adequate explanation of their condition and its potential management and should have their fears and beliefs addressed. A patient-centered model should be adopted (Table 41.15).[133]

REFERENCES

1. Von Korff M, Dworkin DF, Le Resche LL, Kruger A. An epidemiologic comparison of pain complaints. *Pain* 1988; **32:** 173–83.
2. Mayou R, Bryant B, Forfar C, *et al.* Non-cardiac chest pain and benign palpitations in the cardiac clinic. *Br Heart J* 1994; **72:** 548–53.
3. Jain D, Fluck D, Sayer JW, *et al.* Ability of a one-stop chest pain clinic to identify patients with high cardiac risk in a district general hospital. *J R Coll Phys Lond* 1997; **31:** 401–4.
4. Chambers J, Bass C. Chest pain with normal coronary anatomy: a review of natural history and possible etiologic factors. *Prog Cardiovasc Dis* 1990; **33:** 161–84.
5. Mayou R, Bass C, Hart G, *et al.* Can clinical assessment of chest pain be made more therapeutic? *Q J Med* 2000; **93:** 850–11.
6. Rose S, Achkar E, Easly KA. Follow up of patients with noncardiac chest pain: value of esophageal testing. *Dig Dis Sci* 1994; **39:** 2063–8.
7. Dart AM, Alban Davies HA, Griffith T, *et al.* Does it help to underdiagnose angina? *Eur Heart J* 1983; **4:** 461–2.
8. Mayou R, Bryant B. Quality of life after coronary artery surgery. *Q J Med* 1987; **239:** 239–48.
9. Mehta A, de Caestecker JS, Camm AJ, Northfield TC. Gastro-oesophageal reflux in patients with coronary artery disease: how common is it, and does it matter? *Eur J Gastroenterol Hepatol* 1996; **8:** 973–8.
◆ 10. Mayou R, Bryant B, Sanders D, *et al.* A controlled trial of cognitive behavioural therapy for non-cardiac chest pain. *Psychol Med* 1997; **27:** 1021–32.
11. Potts SG, Lewin R, Fox K, Johnstone E. Group psychological treatment for chest pain and normal coronary arteries. *Q J Med* 1999; **92:** 81–6.
12. Stewart M. Towards a global definition of patient-cen-

tred care. *Br Med J* 2001; **322:** 468–72.

● 13. Crow R, Gage H, Hampson S, *et al*. The role of expectancies in placebo effect and their role in the delivery of healthcare. *Health Technol Assess* 1998; **3:** 3.

14. Herrick JB. Clinical features of sudden obstruction of the coronary arteries. *JAMA* 1912; **59:** 2015–18.

15. Martin WB. Patients use of gestures in the diagnosis of coronary insufficiency disease. *Minn Med* 1957; **40:** 691–4.

16. Sampson JJ, Cheitlin MD. Pathophysiology and differential diagnosis of cardiac pain. *Prog Cardiovasc Dis* 1971; **13:** 507–22.

● 17. Crea F, Gaspardone A. New look to an old symptom; angina pectoris. *Circulation* 1997; **96:** 3766–73.

18. Epstein S, Quyyumi A, Bonow R. Current concepts in myocardial ischemia: silent or symptomatic. *N Engl J Med* 1988; **318:** 1038–43.

19. Deanfield J, Maseri A, Selwyn A, *et al*. Myocardial ischemia during daily life in patients with stable angina: its relation to symptoms and heart rate changes. *Lancet* 1983; **2:** 753–8.

20. Klein J, Chao S, Berman D, Rozanski A. Is "silent" myocardial ischemia really as severe as symptomatic ischemia? The analytical effect of patient selection biases. *Circulation* 1994; **89:** 1958–66.

21. Freedman SB, Wong CK. Triggers of daily life ischaemia. *Heart* 1998; **80:** 489–92.

22. Lyons RA, Lo SV, Littlepage BNC. Comparative health status of patients with 11 common illnesses in Wales. *J Epidemiol Community Health* 119; **48:** 388–90.

23. Wynn A. Unwarranted emotional distress in men with ischaemic heart disease. *Med J Aust* 1967; **2:** 847–51.

◆ 24. Yellon DM, Baxter GF, Marber MS. Angina reassessed: pain or protector? *Lancet* 1996; **347:** 1159–62.

25. Dana A, Yellon DM. Ischaemic preconditioning: a clinical perspective. *Hosp Med* 1998; **59:** 216–20.

26. Lewin RJ, Ingleton R, Newens AJ, *et al*. Adherence to cardiac rehabilitation guidelines: a survey of cardiac rehabilitation programmes in the United Kingdom. *Br Med J* 1998; **316:** 1354–5.

◆ 27. Collins P, Fox K. Pathophysiology of angina. *Lancet* 1990; **335:** 94–6.

28. Cobb LA. Evaluation of internal mammary artery ligation by a double-blind technique. *N Engl J Med* 1959; **260:** 1115–18.

29. Dimond KG, Kirtel CF, Crockett JE. Comparison of internal mammary ligation and sham operation for angina pectoris. *Am J Cardiol* 1960; **5:** 483–6.

● 30. ACC/AHA/ACP-ASIM. Guidelines for the management of patients with chronic stable angina: executive summary and recommendations. A Report of the American College of Cardiology/American Heart Association Task Force on Practice Guidelines. *Circulation* 1999; **99:** 2829–48.

● 31. Task Force of the European Society of Cardiology. Management of stable angina pectoris. Recommendations of the Task Force of the European Society of Cardiology. *Eur Heart J* 1997; **18:** 394–413.

● 32. Eagle KA, Guyton RA, Davidoff R, *et al*. ACC/AHA guidelines for CABG surgery. *JACC* 1999; **34:** 1262–1347.

33. Lewin B, Cay EL, Todd I. The angina management programme: a rehabilitation treatment. *Br J Cardiol* 1995; **1:** 221–6.

◆ 34. Lewin RJ. Improving quality of life in patients with angina. *Heart* 1999; **82:** 654–5.

● 35. Mannheimer C, Camici P, Chester M, *et al*. The problem of refractory angina. *Eur Heart J* 2002; **23** (5): 355–7.

36. Brorsson B, Persson H, Landelius P, Werko L. *Smärtor i bröstet: operation, ballongvidgning, medicinsk behandling*. Stockholm: Statens beredning för utvärdering av medicinsk, 1998: report 140.

37. www.angina.org.uk.

38. Nagele H, Kalmar P, Labeck M, *et al*. Transmyokardiale Laserrevaskularisation-Behandlungsoption bei der koronaren Herzerkrankung. *Z Kardiol* 1997; **86:** 171–8.

39. Lewin RJ, Thompson DR, Taylor RS. Cardiac rehabilitation. *Eur Heart J* 2000; **21:** 860–1.

40. Mannheimer C, Carlsson CA, Ericson K, *et al*. Transcutaneous electrical nerve stimulation in severe angina pectoris. *Eur Heart J* 1982; **3:** 297–302.

41. Mannheimer C, Carlsson CA, Vedin A, Wilhelmsson C. Transcutaneous electrical nerve stimulation in angina pectoris. *Pain* 1986; **26:** 291–300.

42. Mannheimer C, Carlsson CA, Emanuelsson H, *et al*. The effects of transcutaneous electrical nerve stimulation in patients with severe angina pectoris. *Circulation* 1985; **71:** 308–16.

43. Emanuelsson H, Manheimer C, Waagstein F, Wilhelmsson C. Catecholamine metabolism during pacing induced angina pectoris and the effect of transcutaneous electrical nerve stimulation. *Am Heart J* 1987; **114:** 1360–6.

◆ 44. Murray S, Collins PD, James MA. Neurostimulation treatment for angina pectoris. *Heart* 2000; **83:** 217–20.

45. Chen D, Philip M, Philip PA, Monga TN. Cardiac pacemaker inhibition by transcutaneous electrical nerve stimulation. *Arch Phys Med Rehabil* 1990; **71:** 27–30.

◆ 46. Ten Vaarwerk IA, Jessurun GA, DeJongste MJ, *et al*. Clinical outcome of patients treated with spinal cord stimulation for therapeutically refractory angina pectoris. *Heart* 1999; **82:** 82–8.

47. DeJongste MJ, Haaksma J, Hautvast RW, *et al*. Effects of spinal cord stimulation on myocardial ischemia during daily life in patients with severe coronary artery disease. A prospective ambulatory electrocardiographic study. *Br Heart J* 1994; **71:** 413–18.

48. Hautvast RW, Brouwer J, DeJongste MJ, Lie KI. Effect of spinal cord stimulation on heart rate variability and myocardial ischemia in patients with chronic intrac-

table angina pectoris. A prospective ambulatory electrocardiographic study. *Clin Cardiol* 1998; **21:** 33–8.

49. Kujacic V, Eliasson T, Mannheimer C, *et al*. Assessment of the influence of spinal cord stimulation on left ventricular function in patients with severe angina pectoris: an echocardiographic study. *Eur Heart J* 1993; **14:** 1238–44.

50. Sanderson JE, Ibrahim B, Waterhouse D, Palmer RB. Spinal electrical stimulation for intractable angina-long-term clinical outcome and safety. *Eur Heart J* 1994; **15:** 810–14.

51. Andersen C, Hole P, Oxhoj H. Does pain relief with spinal cord stimulation for angina conceal myocardial infarction? *Br Heart J* 1994; **71:** 419–21.

52. Sanderson JE, Brooksby P, Waterhouse D, *et al*. Epidural spinal electrical stimulation for severe angina: a study of its effects on symptoms, exercise tolerance and degree of ischaemia. *Eur Heart J* 1992; **13:** 628–33.

53. Hautvast RW, DeJongste MJ, Staal MJ, *et al*. Spinal cord stimulation in chronic intractable angina pectoris: a randomised controlled efficacy study. *Am Heart J* 1998; **136:** 1114–20.

◆ 54. Eliasson T, Augustinsson LE, Mannheimer C. Spinal cord stimulation in severe angina pectoris- presentation of current studies, indications and clinical experience. *Pain* 1996; **65:** 169–79.

◆ 55. Jessurun G, DeJongste MJ, Blanksma PK. Current views on neurostimulation in the treatment of cardiac ischemic syndromes. *Pain* 1996; **66:** 109–16.

56. Mannheimer C, Eliasson T, Augustinsson LE, *et al*. Electrical stimulation versus coronary artery bypass surgery in severe angina pectoris: the ESBY study. *Circulation* 1998; **97:** 1157–63.

57. Norrsell H, Pilhall M, Eliasson T, Mannheimer C. Effects of spinal cord stimulation and coronary artery bypass grafting on myocardial ischaemia and heart rate variability: further results from the ESBY study. *Cardiology* 2000; **94:** 12–18.

58. Manheimer C, Eliasson T, Andersson B, *et al*. Effects of spinal cord stimulation in angina pectoris induced by pacing and possible mechanisms of action. *Br Med J* 1993; **307:** 477–80.

59. Chandler MJ, Brennan TJ, Garrison DW, *et al*. A mechanism of cardiac pain suppression by spinal cord stimulation: implications for patients with angina pectoris. *Eur Heart J* 1993; **14:** 95–106.

60. Norrsell H, Eliasson T, Mannheimer C, *et al*. Effect of pacing induced myocardial stress and spinal cord stimulation on whole body and norepinephrine spillover. *Eur Heart J* 1997; **18:** 1890–6.

61. Oosterga M, ten Vaarwerk IA, DeJongste MJ, Staal MJ. Spinal cord stimulation in refractory angina pectoris-clinical results and mechanisms. *Z Kardiol* 1997; **86:** 107–13.

62. Hautvast RW, Blanksma PK, DeJongste MJ, *et al*. Effect

of spinal cord stimulation on myocardial blood flow assessed by positron emission tomography in patients with refractory angina pectoris. *Am J Cardiol* 1996; **77:** 462–7.

63. De Landsheere C, Mannheimer C, Habets A, *et al*. Effect of spinal cord stimulation on regional myocardial perfusion assessed by positron emission tomography. *Am J Cardiol* 1992; **69:** 1143–9.

64. Murphy DF, Giles KE. Dorsal column stimulation for pain relief from intractable angina pectoris. *Pain* 1987; **28:** 365–8.

65. Mannheimer C, Augustinsson LE, Carlsson CA, *et al*. Epidural spinal electrical stimulation in severe angina pectoris. *Br Heart J* 1988; **59:** 56–61.

66. Iyer R, Gnanadurai V, Forsey P. Management of cardiac pacemakers in patients with a spinal cord stimulator implant. *Pain* 1998; **74:** 333–5.

67. Liem LA, van Dongen VC. Magnetic resonance imaging and spinal cord stimulation systems. *Pain* 1997; **70:** 95–7.

68. Blomberg S, Emanuelsson H, Herlitz J, *et al*. Thoracic epidural anesthesia in patients with unstable angina pectoris. *Anesth Analg* 1989; **69:** 559–62.

69. Olausson K, Magnusdottir H, Lurje L, *et al*. Anti-ischemic and anti-anginal effects of thoracic epidural anesthesia versus those of conventional medical therapy in the treatment of severe refractory unstable angina pectoris. *Circulation* 1997; **96:** 2178–82.

70. Gramling-Bebb P, Miller M, Reeves S, *et al*. Treatment of medically and surgically refractory angina pectoris with high thoracic epidural analgesia: initial clinical experience. *Am Heart J* 1997; **133:** 648–55.

71. Wetterwik C, Claes G, Drott C, *et al*. Endoscopic thoracic sympathectomy for severe angina. *Lancet* 1995; **345:** 97–8.

72. Tygesen H, Claes G, Drott C, *et al*. Effect of endoscopic transthoracic sympathectomy on heart rate variability in severe angina pectoris. *Am J Cardiol* 1997; **79:** 1447–52.

73. Chester M, Hammond C, Leach A. Long term benefits of stellate ganglion block in severe chronic refractory angina. *Pain* 2000; **87:** 103–5.

74. Peters AJ, Schoebel FC, Jax TW, *et al*. Long term urokinase therapy and isovolaemic hemodilution. A clinical and hemodynamic comparison in patients with refractory angina pectoris. *Int J Angiol* 1999; **8:** 44–9.

● 75. Soran O, Crawford LE, Schneider VM, Feldman AM. Enhanced external counterpulsation in the management of patients with cardiovascular disease. *Clin Cardiol* 1999; **22:** 173–8.

76. Michaels AD, Kennard ED, Kelsey SE, *et al*. Does higher diastolic augmentation predict clinical benefit from enhanced external counterpulsation?: Data from International EECP Patient Registry (IEPR). *Clin Cardiol* 2001; **24:** 453–8.

77. Barsness G, Feldman AM, Holmes Jr DR, *et al*. The International EECP Patient Registry (IEPR): design, methods, baseline characteristics and acute results. *Clin Cardiol* 2001; **24**: 435–42.

78. Aaberge L, Nordstrand K, Dragsund M, *et al*. Transmyocardial revascularization with CO2 laser in patients with refractory angina pectoris. Clinical results from the Norwegian randomised trial. *J Am Coll Cardiol* 2000; **35**: 1170–7.

79. Allen KB, Dowling RD, Fudge TL, *et al*. Comparison of transmyocardial revascularization with medical therapy in patients with refractory angina. *N Engl J Med* 1999; **341**: 1029–36.

80. Burkhoff D, Schmidt S, Schulman S, *et al*. Transmyocardial laser revascularisation compared with continued medical therapy for treatment of refractory angina pectoris: a prospective randomised trial. *Lancet* 1999; **354**: 885–90.

81. Frazier OH, March RJ, Horvath KA. Transmyocardial revascularization with a carbon dioxide laser in patients with end-stage coronary disease. *N Engl J Med* 1999; **341**: 1021–8.

82. March R. Transmyocardial laser revascularisation with the CO2 laser: one year results of a randomised controlled study. *Semin Thorac Cardiovasc Surg* 1999; **11**: 12–18.

83. Schofield PM, Sharples LD, Caine N, *et al*. Transmyocardial laser revascularisation in patients with refractory angina: a randomised controlled trial. *Lancet* 1999; **353**: 519–24.

84. Lange RA, Hillis LD. Transmyocardial laser revascularization. *N Engl J Med* 1999; **341**: 1075–6.

85. Oesterle SN, Sanborn TA, Ali N, *et al*. Percutaneous transmyocardial laser revascularisation for severe angina: the PACIFIC trial. Potential class improvement from intramyocardial channels. *Lancet* 2000; **356**: 1705–10.

86. Losordo D, Vale P, Isner J. Gene therapy for myocardial angiogenesis. *Am Heart J* 1999; **138**: 132–41.

87. Kemp HG, Vokonas PS, Cohn PF, Gorlin R. The anginal syndrome associated with normal coronary arteriograms. Report of a six year experience. *Am J Med* 1973; **54**: 735–42.

88. Rosano G, Kaski J, Arie S, *et al*. Failure to demonstrate myocardial ischaemia in patients with angina and normal coronary arteries. Evaluation by continuous coronary sinus pH monitoring and lactate metabolism. *Eur Heart J* 1996; **17**: 1175–80.

89. Chauhan A, Mullins PA, Thuraisinghjam SI, *et al*. Abnormal pain perception in syndrome X. *J Am Coll Cardiol* 1994; **24**: 329–35.

● 90. Potts S, Bass C. Chest pain with normal coronary arteries: psychological aspects. In: Kaski JC ed. *Angina Pectoris with Normal Coronary Arteries: Syndrome X*, 2nd edn. Boston, MA: Kluwer, 1999.

● 91. Kaski JC, Valenzuela Garcia LF. Therapeutic options for the management of patients with cardiac syndrome X. *Eur Heart J* 2001; **22**: 283–93.

92. Fragasso G, Chierchia SL, Pizzetti G, *et al*. Impaired left ventricular filling dynamics in patients with angina and angiographically normal coronary arteries: effect of β adrenergic blockade. *Heart* 1997; **77**: 32–9.

93. Cannon R, Watson RM, Rosing DR, Epstein SE. Efficacy of calcium channel blocker therapy for angina pectoris resulting from small-vessel coronary artery disease and abnormal vasodilator reserve. *Am J Cardiol* 1985; **56**: 242–6.

94. Yoshio H, Shimizu M, Kita Y, *et al*. Effects of short term aminophylline administration on cardiac functional reserve in patients with syndrome X. *JACC* 1995; **25**: 1547–51.

95. Albertsson PA, Emanuelsson H, Milson I. Beneficial effect of treatment with transdermal estradiol-17β on exercise induced angina and ST segment depression in syndrome X. *Int J Cardiol* 1996; **54**: 13–20.

96. Cannon RO, Quyyumi AA, Mincemoyer R, *et al*. Imipramine in patients with chest pain despite normal coronary arteriograms. *N Engl J Med* 1994; **330**: 1411–17.

97. Eliasson T, Albertsson P, Hardhammar P, *et al*. Spinal cord stimulation in angina pectoris with normal coronary angiograms. *Coronary Artery Dis* 1993; **4**: 819–27.

98. Lanza GA, Sestito A, Sandric S, *et al*. Spinal cord stimulation in patients with refractory anginal pain and normal coronary arteries. *Ital Heart J* 2001; **2**: 25–30.

99. Van Peski-Oosterbaan AS, Spinhoven P, Van Rood Y, *et al*. Cognitive behavioural therapy for non-cardiac chest pain: a randomised trial. *Am J Med* 1999; **106**: 424–9.

100. Voskuil JH, Cramer J, Breumelhof R, *et al*. Prevalence of esophageal disorders in patients with chest pain newly referred to a cardiologist. *Chest* 1996; **109**: 1210–14.

101. Goyal RK. Changing focus on unexplained esophageal chest pain. *Ann Intern Med* 1996; **124**: 1008–11.

102. Kahrilas PJ. Nutcracker esophagus; an idea whose time has gone? *Am J Gastroenterol* 1993; **88**: 167–9.

103. Richter JE, Dalton CB, Bradley LA, Castell DO. Oral nifedipine in the treatment of non-cardiac chest pain in patients with nutcracker esophagus. *Gastroenterology* 1987; **93**: 21–8.

104. Frobert O, Funch-Jensen P, Bagger JP. Diagnostic value of esophageal studies in patients with angina-like chest pain and normal coronary arteriograms. *Ann Intern Med* 1996; **124**: 959–69.

105. Rao SSC, Gregersen H, Hayek B, *et al*. Unexplained chest pain: the hypersensitive, hyperreactive and poorly compliant esophagus. *Ann Intern Med* 1996; **124**: 950–8.

106. de Caestecker JS, Blackwell JN, Brown J, Heading RC. The oesophagus as a cause of recurrent chest pain; which patients should be investigated and which tests used? *Lancet* 1985; **ii**: 1143–6.

107. Alban Davies H, Jones DB, Rhodes J, Newcombe RG. Angina-like esophageal pain: differentiation from

cardiac pain by history. *J Clin Gastroenterol* 1985; **7**: 477–81.

108. Wu EB, Chambers JB. Chest pain: is the history useful? *Int J Clin Pract* 2000; **54**: 74.

109. Mehta A, de Caestecker JS, Northfield TC. Effect of nifedipine and atenolol on gastro-oesophageal reflux. *Eur J Gastroenterol Hepatol* 1993; **5**: 627–9.

110. Cooke RA, Anggiansah A, Chamber JB, Owen WJ. A prospective study of oesophageal function in patients with normal coronary angiograms and controls with angina. *Gut* 1998; **42**: 323–9.

111. Ghillebert G, Janssens J, Vantrappen G, *et al*. Ambulatory 24 hour intraesophageal pH and pressure recordings v provocation tests in the diagnosis of chest pain of esophageal origin. *Gut* 1990; **31**: 738–44.

112. Fass R, Fennerty B, Ofmann JJ, *et al*. The clinical and economic value of a short course of omeprazole in patients with non-cardiac chest pain. *Gastroenterology* 1998; **115**: 42–9.

113. NICE Technology Appraisal. *Guidance on the Use of Proton Pump Inhibitors in the Treatment of Dyspepsia*. NHS National Institute for Clinical Excellence, 2001.

114. Mukerji B, Mukerji V, Alpert MA, Selukar R. The prevalence of rheumatologic disorders in patients with chest pain and angiographically normal coronary arteries. *Angiology* 1995; **46**: 425–30.

115. Wise CM, Semble EL, Dalton CB. Musculoskeletal chest wall syndromes in patients with non-cardiac chest pain: a study of 100 patients. *Ann Phys Med Rehabil* 1992; **73**: 147–9.

116. de Oliveira M, Hassan TB, Sebewufu R, *et al*. Long term morbidity in patients suffering a sternal fracture following discharge from the A and E department. *Injury* 1998; **29**: 609–12.

117. Schapira D, Nachtigal A, Scharf Y. Spontaneous fracture of the sternum simulating myocardial infarction. *Clin Rheumatol* 1995; **14**: 478–80.

118. Pantell RH, Goodman Jr BW. Adolescent chest pain: a prospective study. *Pediatrics* 1983; **71**: 881–7.

119. Driscoll DJ, Glicklich LB, Gallen WJ. Chest pain in children: a prospective study. *Pediatrics* 1976; **57**: 648–51.

120. Brown RT. Costochondritis in adolescents. *J Adolesc Health Care* 1981; **1**: 198–201.

121. Li B. 106 cases of non-suppurative costal chondritis treated by acupuncture at xuanzhong point. *J Tradit Chin Med* 1998; **18**: 195–6.

122. Kamel M, Kotob H. Ultrasonographic assessment of local steroid injection in Tietze's syndrome. *Br J Rheumatol* 1997; **36**: 547–50.

123. Fournie B, Boutes A, Dromer C, *et al*. Prospective study of anterior chest wall involvement in ankylosing spondylitis and psoriatic arthritis. *Rev Rheum Engl* 1997; **64**: 22–5.

124. Jurik AG, Graudal H. Monoarthritis of the manubriosternal joint. A follow-up study. *Rheumatol Int* 1987; **7**: 235–41.

125. Gimferrer JM, Callejas MA, Sanchez-Lloret J, *et al*. Candida albicans costochondritis in heroin addicts. *Ann Thor Surg* 1986; **41**: 89–90.

126. Kozlov MI. Chondroperichondritis of costal cartilages as a complication of surgical approaches to the thorax without direct injury of the cartilage. *Vestn Khir Im I Grek* 1998; **157**: 48–50.

127. Mukamel M, Kornreich L, Horev G, *et al*. Tietze's syndrome in children and infants. *J Pediatr* 1997; **131**: 774–5.

◆128. Cranfield KA, Buist RJ, Nandi PR, Baranowski AP. The twelfth rib syndrome. *J Pain Symptom Manage* 1997; **13**: 172–5.

129. Mooney DP, Shorter NL. Slipping rib syndrome in childhood. *J Pediatr Surg* 1997; **32**: 1081–2.

130. Lem-Hee N, Abdulla AJ. Slipping rib syndrome: an overlooked cause of chest and abdominal pain. *Int J Clin Pract* 1997; **51**: 252–3.

131. Eisenberg E, Pultorak Y, Pud D, *et al*. Prevalence and characteristics of post coronary artery bypass pain (PCP). *Pain* 2001; **92** (1–2): 11–17.

132. Mailis A, Umana M, Feindel CM. Anterior intercostal nerve damage after coronary artery bypass graft surgery with use of internal thoracic artery graft. *Ann Thorac Surg* 2000; **69**: 1455–8.

◆133. Chambers J, Bass C, Mayou R. Non-cardiac chest pain: assessment and management. *Heart* 1999; **82**: 656–7.

42

Chronic abdominal, groin, and perineal pain of visceral origin

TIMOTHY J NESS

Chronic pain localized to the abdomen, groin, and/or perineum can have multiple etiologies ranging from focal sites of inflammation to idiopathic systemic diseases (Table 42.1). These pains fall within the practice of virtually every medical specialty and are some of the most common presenting symptoms for the primary care physician. Pain experienced in the abdomen, groin, and/or perineum may arise from pathology of the nervous system innervating those structures or may originate in the viscera, vascular structures, or musculoskeletal–articular structures. Psychological disturbance frequently manifests as complaints of abdominal discomfort, as evidenced by common usage of the term *hypochondria* as "imagined illness" when the term anatomically refers to the mid-upper abdomen. Other chapters address gynecologic (pelvic) pain, chest (thoracic visceral) pain, neurologic pain, psychogenic pain, spine-related pain, and pain syndromes occurring as complications of surgery (e.g. a neuroma following hernia repair); all of which can be causes of abdominal, groin, and perineal pain. As a consequence, this chapter will focus on pains arising from nongynecologic abdominal and pelvic viscera. Following a brief review of the phenomenon of visceral pain, a general discussion relating to the evaluation of abdominal pain will be given. The disease states of chronic pancreatitis, irritable bowel syndrome, and interstitial cystitis will then be discussed in depth as "archetype" chronic disease states, since these entities are illustrative of general phenomena present in patients presenting with chronic or recurrent abdominal, groin, and/or perineal symptomatology and therefore serve as examples of diagnostic workups and therapeutic modalities. Numerous other painful disorders with abdominal, groin, or perineal symptomatol-

ogy will then briefly be discussed as "correlates" of the archetypal disorders. Various useful reviews have also addressed disorders discussed in this chapter and general statements will be referenced to those reviews.[1-10] Prior to the discussion of "chronic" disorders, a discussion of pancreatic cancer will be presented because it serves as a contrast to most of the other conditions which are considered to be nonlife-threatening and associated with significant psychopathology such as anxiety, depression, and substance abuse.

VISCERAL PAIN

Pains arising from the surface of the body are well localized and evoke localized motor responses such as flexion reflexes. In contrast, visceral pains are characterized by the following:

1 poor localization;
2 strong emotional responses;
3 immobility coupled with tonic increases in muscle tone;
4 vigorous, nonspecific, autonomic responses.

Stimuli that produce tissue damage or predict potential tissue damage (e.g. cutting, burning, pinching) universally produce reports of pain when applied to the skin but unreliably evoke reports of pain when applied to visceral structures. Stimuli which can produce pain from visceral structures such as distension of the gallbladder are also stimuli which occur naturally and daily (albeit at lower intensities) but which generally fail to evoke any sensations at all. Humans use tissue damage-related

Table 42.1 *Sources of chronic abdominal, groin, and perineal pain*

I   Infectious–inflammatory pain states
   A Esophagitis (XIX-4; XIX-5)
   B Gastritis and duodenitis (XXI-14)
   C Chronic gastric ulcer (XXI-4)
   D Chronic duodenal ulcer (XXI-5)
   E Radiation enterocolitis (XXI-16)
   F Crohn's disease (XXI-9)
   G Ulcerative colitis and other colitis/ulcer (XXI-17)
   H Diverticular disease of the colon (XXI-12)
   I Chronic pancreatitis (XXI-19)
   J Ulceration of anus and rectum (XXV-5)
   K Gallbladder disease (XXI-2)
   L Pain from urinary tract – kidney stones (XXIV-10)
   M Subphrenic abscess (XIX-1)
   N Tuberculous peritonitis (NC)

II Functional pain states
   A Postgastric surgery syndrome, dumping (XXI-18)
   B Postcholecystectomy syndrome (XXI-3)
   C Dyspepsia and other dysfunctional disorders in stomach (XXI-15)
   D Irritable bowel syndrome (XXI-11)
   E Chronic constipation – fecal impaction (XXI-10)
   F Proctalgia fugax (XXV-4)
   G "Adhesions" (NC)

III Musculoskeletal origin
   A Thoracic, lumbar, and sacral spinal disease (X, XXVI, XXVII)
   B Slipping rib syndrome (XVII-10)
   C Abdominal muscle wall (I-18, I-34)

IV Other pain states
   A Herniated abdominal organs (XIX-2)
   B Aneurysm of the aorta (XVII-7)
   C Chronic mesenteric ischemia (XXI-8)
   D Hepatic capsule distension secondary to cardiac failure (XXI-1)
   E Injury of external genitalia (XXV-6)
   F Pain due to hemorrhoids (XXV-3)
   G Hydronephrosis – urinary bladder distension (XXIV-10)
   H Interstitial cystitis (NC)

V   Abdominal pain of chest-related origin
   A Cardiac (XVII-4,5)
   B Pericarditis (XVII-6)
   C Diaphragm (XVII-8; XIX-2)
   D Esophageal (XIX-3,4,5)

VI Generalized disease origin
   A Familial Mediterranean fever (XXII-1)
   B Intermittent acute porphyria (XXII-3)
   C Variegate porphyria (XXII-5)
   D Hereditary coproporphyria (XXII-4)
   E Systemic rheumatologic (I-8; I-27)
   F Fibromyalgia (I-9)
   G Lead poisoning (NC)
   H Adrenal insufficiency (NC)

VII Due to cancer
   A Esophagus (XVII-9)
   B Stomach (XXI-6)
   C Colon (XXI-13)
   D Rectum (XXIX-5)
   E Pancreas (XXI-7)
   F Liver or biliary system (XXI-21)
   G Kidney (XXI-22)
   H Urinary bladder (XXIV-12)
   I Prostate (XXV-7)
   J Testicular (NC)
   K Spinal involvement (X-3, XXVI-3, XXIX)
   L Other metastatic, including carcinomatosis (NC)

VIII Gynecological pain
   A Mittelschmerz (XXIV-1)
   B Secondary dysmenorrhea (XXIV-2)
   C Primary dysmenorrhea (XXIV-3)
   D Endometriosis (XXIV-4)
   E Posterior parametritis (XXIV-5)
   F Tuberculous salpingitis (XXIV-6)
   G Retroversion of the uterus (XXIV-7)
   H Ovarian pain (XXIV-8)
   I Injury of female external genitalia (XXV-6)
   J Vaginismus or dyspareunia (XXIV-11)
   K Chronic pelvic pain without obvious pathology (XXIV-9)

IX Neurologic origin
   A Acute herpes zoster (XX-1)
   B Postherpetic neuralgia (XX-2)
   C Peripheral neuropathy (I-1)
   D Central pain (I-6)
   E Segmental or intercostal neuralgia (XX-3)
   F Twelfth rib syndrome (XX-4)
   G Abdominal cutaneous nerve entrapment syndrome (XX-5)
   H Abdominal migraine (XXII-2)
   I Postsurgical neuroma (NC)
   J Painful scar (I-26)
   K Neuralgias of iliohypogastric, ilioinguinal, genitofemoral nerves (XXV-1)
   L Guillain–Barré syndrome (I-36)

X   Pain of psychological origin (XXIII-2; XXIII-3; XXIII-4; XXV-2)

XI Pain of uncertain origin (NC)

Roman numerals in parentheses indicate classification per Merskey and Bogduk.[126] NC, indicates not classified.

descriptors (e.g. rending) when describing their visceral pain because a *perception* of tissue damage is present even if no tissue damage is occurring. The peripheral nervous system pathways of abdominal visceral sensation have been defined in humans and are summarized in Fig. 42.1.

Central nervous system pathways related to visceral sensation are not as well defined and include nontraditional pain pathways such as the dorsal columns.[11] Chronic visceral pains likely have both peripheral and central components.

Stimuli which have been employed in experimental studies of visceral nociception include electrical stimuli, chemical stimuli, ischemia, and mechanical stimuli. Electrical stimulation produces reports of pain in humans and has been used to evoke cerebral potentials in order to assess visceral sensory pathways. Chemical stimuli have been applied topically, intravascularly, or via "physiological" pathways (e.g. systemic cyclophosphamide-induced cystitis) in order to define the endogenous substances responsible for an altered sensitivity to mechanical or environmental stimuli (e.g. acidity of urine) which may occur spontaneously or secondary to inflammation. Ischemia of visceral structures has been produced by the occlusion of visceral vasculature. Experimentally and clinically, the effects of such occlusion are dependent upon collateral blood flow and metabolic activity of the selected organ. The most commonly utilized experimental visceral stimuli are mechanical stimuli such as the probing and stretch of visceral structures or the distension of hollow organs using fluids or foreign bodies. Mechanical stimuli may mimic what is observed in certain pathological pain states (e.g. bowel obstruction) and the *pattern* of mechanical stimulation has been proposed as the source of pain in functional bowel disorders.

Inflammation of visceral structures has proven to be a potent modifier of behavioral, neuronal, autonomic, and motor responses to visceral stimulation in experimental models.[12] The clinical correlate to this is that the presence of inflammation in visceral structures frequently, but not universally, leads to reports of pain. Cystitis, esophagitis, gastritis, duodenitis, ileitis, colitis, and proctitis all have as a hallmark evidence of mucosal inflammatory changes. However, ulcerative colitis, which is associated with profound inflammatory changes of the mucosal lining, may present with *non*painful, bloody stools. Hence, visceral pathology and symptomatology are not reliably linked.

GENERAL EVALUATION OF ABDOMINAL PAIN

Abdominal pain is a common presenting symptom for the clinician. Primary evaluation includes an interview to assess the acute versus chronic nature of the complaints, exacerbating and ameliorating factors, and definition of coexisting disease. Chronic use of medications which alter bowel motility is meaningful. The clinical history alone may allow for a functionally accurate diagnosis in up to 80% of patients.[13] Palpation of the abdomen can identify abdominal wall rigidity, suggesting a peritoneal process, distended bowel, or underlying masses suggestive of neoplastic, infectious, or obstructive processes; and localizable tenderness, which may suggest involvement of a particular organ system. Auscultation of bowel sounds may suggest the presence or absence of gastroin-

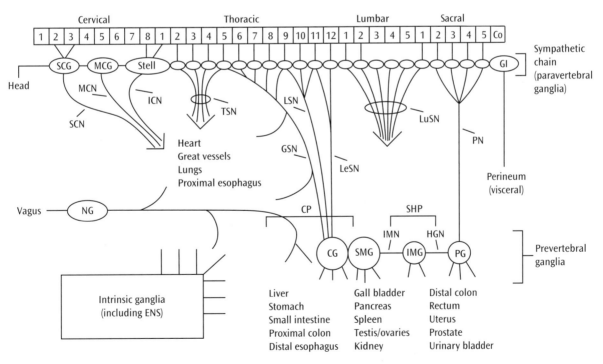

Figure 42.1 *Schematic diagram of the nervous supply of the viscera in humans. SCN, MCN, and ICN, superior, middle, and inferior cardiac nerves; TSN, GSN, LSN, LeSN, and LuSN, thoracic, greater, lesser, least, and lumbar splanchnic nerves; PN, pelvic nerve; IMN, intermesenteric nerve; HGN, hypogastric nerve; SCG and MCG, superior and middle cervical ganglia; Stell, stellate ganglion; CG, celiac ganglion; SMG and IMG, superior and inferior mesenteric ganglia; PG, pelvic ganglion; GI, ganglion impar; CP and SHP, celiac and superior hypogastric plexuses; NG, nodose ganglion; ENS, enteric nervous system. (Adapted from Ness and Gebhart.[128])*

testinal motility and give evidence for obstruction. Rectal and pelvic examinations may give additional information related to local pathology. Neurologic examination may demonstrate evidence of neuropathy or localized radiculopathy. Basic laboratory examinations include testing for fecal blood, urinalysis, blood cell count with white cell differential, serum amylase/lipase levels, electrolytes, and liver function tests. Radiographic evaluations, other tests, endoscopic evaluations, ultrasonography, paracentesis, or advanced imaging studies would be dependent upon the persistence or progression of complaints.

ARCHETYPE DISORDERS

Pancreatic cancer

Most tumors of the pancreas arise from exocrine tissue, primarily ductular epithelium, with only rare cases of endocrine pancreatic tumors. In experimental animals, pancreatic cancer can be induced by several compounds (e.g. nitrosoureas), but no specific agent has been conclusively linked to its development. There is indirect evidence that tobacco use increases the incidence of pancreatic carcinoma and links have been made with hepatobiliary disease, diabetes mellitus, fatty foods, and alcohol ingestion, but conclusive evidence is still lacking. Chronic pancreatitis is considered by some to be a premalignant condition for pancreatic cancer,[14] but this has only been definitively demonstrated for patients with hereditary pancreatitis.[15] Pancreatic cancer occurs more frequently in males (2:1), in blacks, and in peoples of developed countries. The mean age at diagnosis is 55. It is the second most common cancer of the gastrointestinal tract and ranks fifth among cancers as a cause of death.

The classic presentation of pancreatic cancer located at the head of the pancreas (70% of these tumors) is the triad of abdominal pain, weight loss, and jaundice due to obstruction of the biliary system. Epigastric tenderness and a palpable gallbladder or abdominal mass may be present, but in general there are no definitive findings on physical examination. Cancer in the body or tail of the pancreas may be associated with venous obstruction, portal hypertension, and/or bleeding. The abdominal pain is described as persistent and typically located in the middle of the upper abdomen and may have radiation through to the back. It can be dull and achy, gnawing, or have a cramping, colicky sensation. Pain is moderate to severe in 20–30% of patients at the time of presentation and is severe in > 80% with advanced disease.[16] Weight loss may be profound and malabsorption is frequently noted. Owing to its location and the typically asymptomatic nature of this cancer, tumors are often quite advanced and deemed unresectable at the time of presentation. Nonspecific and vague complaints normally attributed to anxiety or depression are often the earliest features in

up to 50% of patients.[17,18] Caraceni and Portenoy[16] have delineated several pancreatic cancer pain syndromes based on clinical characteristics and the pathology identified with appropriate imaging modalities (Table 42.2). Abdominal computed tomography or ultrasonography followed by surgical or endoscopic biopsy are the most frequent diagnostic modalities. Findings from endoscopic retrograde cholangiopancreatography, arteriography, and/or pancreatic function tests may warrant progression to surgical treatment (curative resection versus palliative treatment) prior to definitive biopsy results. The prognosis of advanced disease is poor.

Once a patient has received a definitive diagnosis of pancreatic cancer, they may enter into palliative treatments in which the cancer may be treated surgically, with chemotherapy, or with radiation therapy.[19] The indications for these treatments are beyond the scope of this chapter, but are dependent upon precise localization and tumor differentiation. Ample use of opioids, anti-inflammatories, and adjuvant agents constitute medical therapies and are extensively employed even to extremely high doses. Neuraxial opioids are considered appropriate. Psychological therapies and pastoral counseling become vitally important and the pharmacological treatment of anxiety and depression are considered to be standard care. Therapeutic options for pancreatic cancer pain are listed in Table 42.3.

Table 42.2 *Pancreatic cancer pain syndromes[a]*

I   Pain due to direct tumor involvement
A Visceral pain
1 Infiltration of pancreas
2 Infiltration of duodenum/stomach
3 Liver metastases: capsule distension, diaphragmatic irritation
4 Biliary tree distension–obstruction
5 Bowel obstruction
6 Ischemic pain due to mesenteric vessel involvement
B Somatic pain
1 Retroperitoneal involvement (direct, nodal)
2 Parietal peritoneum and abdominal wall involvement
3 Abdominal distension due to ascites
4 Bone metastases
C Neuropathic pain
1 Radiculopathy from retroperitoneal spread
2 Radiculopathy from metastases
3 Lumbosacral plexopathy
4 Epidural spinal cord compression
II Pain due to cancer therapies
A Postoperative pain syndromes
B Biliary prosthesis complications
C Postchemotherapy pain syndromes
D Postradiation pain syndromes

a. Adapted from Caraceni and Portenoy.[16]

Table 42.3 *Treatments for pancreatic cancer-related pain*

I Analgesics and side-effect management[a]
   A Opioids***
   B Anti-inflammatories***
   C Antiemetics***
   D Adjuvants[b]
      1 Antidepressants**
      2 Stimulants (methylphenidate)**
      3 Anticonvulsants**
      4 Antiarrhythmics**
II Curative surgery[c]
III Palliative treatments (surgery, radiotherapy, chemotherapy)***
IV Neurolysis (neurolytic celiac plexus block)***
V Biliary stenting procedures (for obstruction)*
VI Psychological interventions[†]

a. Assessed for cancer pain with pancreatic cancer patients as component.
b. As indicated by side-effects or nature of pain (e.g. neuropathic).
c. Disease often unresectable at time of diagnosis – "curative" implies abolition of pain apart from that which is surgery related.

Evidence-based scoring: [†]series reports; *limited controlled studies; **well-designed, randomized, controlled studies; ***systematic review, consensus statement, or meta-analysis.

A key modality of palliative treatment for patients with pancreatic cancer and other upper abdominal cancers is the neurolytic celiac plexus block (NCPB). It has been described as the single most effective neurolytic block,[20] and large series[21] have demonstrated it to be safe and with few complications. Several percutaneous techniques of NCPB have been described,[22–24] including those which are guided by fluoroscopy or computed tomography. The classic technique consists of the injection of a neurolytic agent (typically alcohol or phenol) into the retroperitoneal periaortic region of the upper abdomen/lower thorax. The nerve supply to the upper abdominal viscera traverses this region, and so this technique results in deafferentation of sensory input from the region and also affects bowel motility and systemic blood pressure because of efferent effects. Eisenbert et al.[25]*** performed a meta-analysis of available studies related to NCPBs and concluded that the block was effective in most patients independent of the period of follow-up. Commonly cited success rates range from 80% to 90% with success measured as a reduction of opioid requirement.[18,26] When used alone, the NCPB abolishes the pain of pancreatic cancer in 10–24% of patients.[27] Quality of life measures show a progressive deterioration in patients with pancreatic cancer, but in a randomized prospective study Kawamata et al.[28] demonstrated that patients who received an NCPB as part of their pain management had less deterioration than those treated exclusively with systemic medications. Other neurolytic procedures such as chemical and/or surgical splanchnicectomy have also been demonstrated to be similarly effective with success rates of 63–81%, but have had less use historically.[26] Ischia et al.[27] evaluated three different techniques for percutaneous neurolysis (transaortic plexus block versus classic retrocrural versus bilateral splanchnicectomy) in a prospective randomized study of 61 patients and found no differences in the efficacy or morbidity of the various techniques. There is a case report of the effectiveness of bilateral vagotomy.[29]

The treatment of pain due to pancreatic cancer forms one end of the spectrum of pain management options. Aggressive surgical, medical, and other interventional treatments such as neuraxial opioids and neurolysis are not only considered acceptable but are also ethically mandated in many cases. Presenting symptoms of pancreatic cancer may be protean in nature and similar to other abdominal pain disorders with a high incidence of anxiety and depression.

Chronic pancreatitis

Symptomatic pancreatitis can be associated with pancreatic cell death and/or with ductal fibrosis and calcification. Acute pancreatitis, such as that induced by passage of a gallstone, is thought to be pathogenetically and morphologically different from chronic pancreatitis[30] and generally resolves without permanent structural abnormalities. Chronic pancreatitis *is* associated with permanent abnormalities, but may present with an acute necrotic episode. Excessive alcohol consumption is the primary etiology in 70–80% of the cases of chronic pancreatitis in developed nations, although the precise mechanism of action of alcohol has not been determined. First described in 1788 by Cawley in his description of "a free living young man" who developed severe pancreatic disease, it has been described as a "drunkard's pancreas" since 1878. Only 5–10% of heavy drinkers develop symptomatic chronic pancreatitis and so there are likely genetic, infectious, and/or nutritional factors that also contribute to its development. The other 20–30% of cases of chronic pancreatitis are predominantly idiopathic in origin, although other etiologies include a pancreas divisum, genetic causes (hereditary type), previous trauma, previous obstructive episodes, hyperparathyroidism, hyperlipidemia, and α-antitrypsin deficiency. In certain third world nations, a tropical variety of chronic pancreatitis is common and has been associated with specific dietary patterns.

Various theories have been put forward related to the precise pathophysiology of chronic pancreatitis. Experimentally, chronic pancreatitis may be induced in animals by the administration of toxins, but similar links have not been conclusively identified in humans. Alterations in the protein components of pancreatic fluids have been noted that may result in the formation of "sludge" or intraductal "plugs" that become calcified into "stones," which produce inflammatory and fibrotic reactions. Braganza[31] proposed that oxidative stress underlies chronic pancreatitis with periodic bursts of free radical formation leading to chronic injury. Genetic factors have been clearly identified in hereditary pancreatitis and in association with such diseases as cystic fibrosis, but no specific marker has been identified in association with other etiologies. Intraductal hypertension is a common sequel of stone formation/fibrosis and has been proposed as a source of the continuous pain that may develop in chronic pancreatitis. However, relief of ductal obstruction and hypertension does not invariably result in pain relief. Similarly, pancreatic intraparenchymal pressure, a correlate to myofascial compartment syndromes with associated ischemia and neural compression, has also been proposed as the source of pain. As stated before, for most cases of chronic pancreatitis, a common finding is a high level of chronic alcohol ingestion. The average latent period is 18 years and a comorbidity is cirrhosis of the liver (to complement "cirrhosis" of the pancreas). Cigarette smoking is associated with increased incidence of chronic pancreatitis and diets with too much or too little fat and/or protein have been implicated.

Histopathologically, chronic pancreatitis is identified by the presence of intraductal calcification (stones), acinar cell loss, fibrosis, and inflammation. Proliferation of unmyelinated nerve fibers and mononuclear cell infiltrates around nerve sheaths has been noted,[32] and elevated levels of the neuropeptides substance P and calcitonin gene-related peptide (CGRP) have been identified.[33] Identifiable pathology does not firmly correlate with reports of pain.[34]

The primary presenting complaint is pain. Classically, it is deep, boring, and epigastric with frequent radiation through to the back. It may be episodic in nature but may advance until it is continuous and may be precipitated by eating. Sitting upright or leaning forward may decrease the pain. It is often coupled with nausea and vomiting, which may lead to dehydration, malnutrition, and an inability to take oral analgesics. Steatorrhea due to pancreatic insufficiency may result with advanced disease, as may glucose intolerance and eventual diabetes mellitus with associated clinical history. Subjects with alcoholic chronic pancreatitis are generally thin individuals (often emaciated) and may have stigmata associated with extensive alcohol use and associated liver failure. An inflammatory mass may be palpable, but typically abdominal guarding precludes adequate deep palpation. There are no definitive findings on physical examination.

Diffuse intraductal calcium deposition is pathognomonic of chronic pancreatitis and this may be demonstrated by plain abdominal radiographs in 30% of cases. Ultrasonographic evaluation is 60–70% sensitive for intraductal abnormalities and computed tomography is 90% sensitive. Endoscopic retrograde cholangiopancreatography (ERCP) is the "gold standard" for chronic pancreatitis based on ductal abnormalities, which are graded by severity. Newer, noninvasive imaging studies include magnetic resonance cholangiopancreatography. Elevated serum amylase and lipase levels indicate a pancreatic exocrine cell-damaging process. Pancreatic function tests have found less utility with improved sensitivity of other diagnostic modalities.

A system of stratification or subgroupings of patients by morphological or functional criteria has never been agreed upon.[30] Differential diagnoses must include pancreatic cancer but also include peptic ulcer disease, irritable bowel syndrome, gallstones, and endometriosis. An initial first step in the management of pain in patients with chronic pancreatitis is the exclusion of complications that can be the cause of the pain such as pseudocysts or compression of adjacent visceral structures.[35]

The literature related to the treatment of pain in chronic pancreatitis consists of numerous retrospective collections of patients subjected to treatments determined by interest in applying a certain method.[30] Few studies of chronic pancreatitis pain have employed placebo-controlled methodologies. Those studies that have employed these methodologies generally demonstrated limited effects of the studied treatment. Procedural studies have generally not had controls performed. The symptomatology of chronic pancreatitis is episodic in nature, with frequent exacerbations and spontaneous resolution. Hence, any "open" study that is initiated during an exacerbation (when the patient presents to the study physician for treatment) is likely to be deemed effective in some patients owing to the natural course of the disease. Therapeutic options for chronic pancreatitis are listed in Table 42.4 and a suggested treatment pathway given in Fig. 42.2.

For alcoholic chronic pancreatitis, the initial treatment is abstinence from alcohol. If the patient continues to drink, their 5-year mortality rate approaches 50%; if they do not drink, it takes 25 years to achieve a mortality rate of 50%. Psychological therapies directed toward developing alternative coping mechanisms and abstaining from alcohol are considered vitally necessary, but outcomes related to substance abuse treatment are mixed and not

Table 42.4 *Treatment options for chronic pancreatitis pain*

I	Abstinence from alcohol*
II	Opioids*
III	Anti-inflammatories†
IV	Antioxidants and micronutrients**
V	Endoscopic management (stents, sphincterotomy, stone removal)
VI	Oral pancreatic enzyme treatment*
VII	Neurolysis*
VIII	Intraceliac steroid injections*
IX	Surgical diversion or resection*
X	Pseudocystic drainage (percutaneous, endoscopic, surgical)*

Evidence-based scoring: †series reports; *limited controlled studies; **well-designed, randomized, controlled studies.

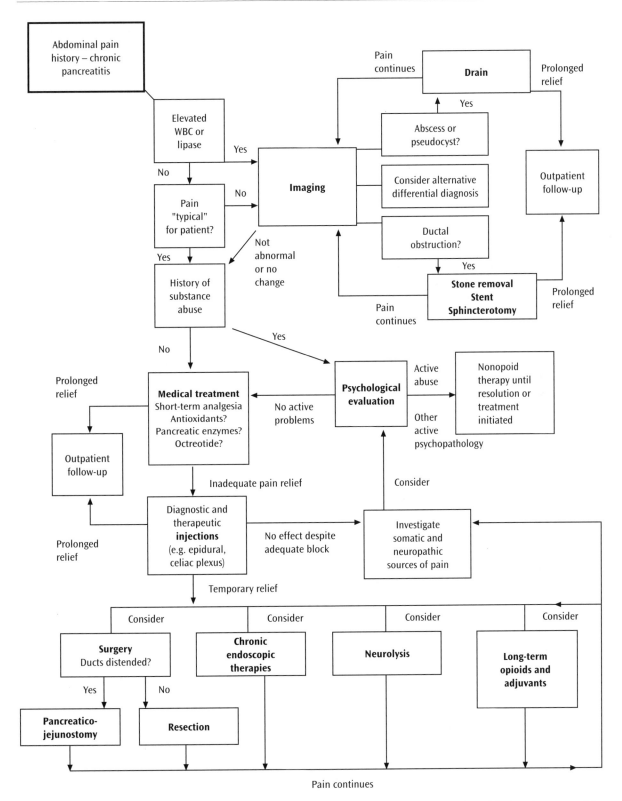

Figure 42.2 *Proposed flow diagram for the evaluation and treatment of the patient presenting with chronic pancreatitis-related pain. WBC, white blood cell count.*

limited to this specific population. It has been commonly reported that total abstinence from alcohol achieves pain relief in up to 50% of patients, particularly those with mild to moderate disease,[35–38] but even this tenet of care has been questioned.[39]

The endoscopic placement of stents, sphincterotomy, dilation, and/or stone removal are well-established alternatives to surgery in the treatment of biliary tract diseases, and similar techniques for the relief of chronic pancreatic pain have been developed.[40] However, prolonged stenting of pancreatic ducts as a therapy is still viewed as in the realm of clinical research.[30] Extracorporeal shock-wave lithotripsy has been coupled with endoscopic procedures to remove stones from the main pancreatic duct with reported pain reduction in some patients.[41]

Opioids are the primary analgesic therapy of advanced chronic pancreatitis, although some have suggested use of adjuvants such as antidepressants. There is the unfortunate but common experience of clinicians that patients who have alcoholic pancreatitis may exchange their alcohol addiction for an opioid addiction. Patients with substance abuse histories develop painful diseases and ethically require treatment, but clinicians still experience significant angst in association with their patients' symptomatic treatment. Both corticosteroids and nonsteroidal anti-inflammatory drugs would seem logical choices in the treatment of a chronic inflammatory process. However, case reports[42,43] of pancreatitis induced by these agents has temporized their use.

Based on the oxidative stress hypothesis, placebo-controlled medical trials of antioxidants and micronutrients such as vitamins C and E, β-carotene, S-adenosylmethionine, and selenium have produced favorable results.[44,45] Braganza[31] has made the statement that antioxidant therapy has made surgery for pancreatic pain "obsolete" at his institution (University of Manchester Royal Infirmary, Manchester, UK). This provocative statement will require testing at other institutions. It is notable that a trial of allopurinol,[46] which reduced oxidative stress through an inhibition of xanthine oxidase, was not effective at reducing the symptomatology of chronic pancreatitis.

Oral pancreatic enzyme treatments have been utilized as inhibitors of pancreatic enzyme secretion with a resultant decrease in intraductal pressure. This negative feedback strategy has been effective at reducing pain in some studies,[47,48] but four of six randomized, prospective, placebo-controlled, double-blind studies failed to observe any effect of this treatment.[30] In one study,[49] pain improved in a majority of patients whether or not they were receiving the pancreatic enzymes of placebo. Negative feedback inhibition of pancreatic secretion can also be provided by somatostatin or its analog octreotide, but two randomized, prospective, double-blind, placebo-controlled studies failed to see any statistically significant improvement in pain and so octreotide cannot be recommended for general use.[30,35]

Celiac plexus blocks with local anesthetics have been used for diagnostic purposes,[50] as part of protocols for the determination of eligibility for surgical treatment,[51] and as primary therapies when coupled with steroids.[50,52] It is notable that series reporting the efficacy of intraceliac plexus steroids did not compare their treatment with systemic steroids, although significant central nervous system effects of the steroids (i.e. acute mania) have been reported.[53] Neurolytic celiac plexus blocks (NCPBs) have been performed using alcohol or phenol. NCPB for the treatment of nonmalignant pancreatic pain has both proponents[54] and opponents.[55] Fugere and Lewis[56] reviewed 20 series in which NCPBs were utilized for chronic pancreatitis and concluded that there were deficiencies in every report, stating that most of the studies were not prospective, randomized, or controlled. They also noted that results of NCPB on chronic pancreatitis pain were not as good as those for cancer-related pain. Enthusiasm for NCPB for chronic pancreatitis has also been tempered by the apparent limited duration of effect requiring retreatment (e.g. 2–6 months),[55] secondary side-effects such as chronic diarrhea,[57] and the occurrence of uncommon but catastrophic neurological sequelae.[58–60] Other forms of injection therapy have also been employed, including bilateral splanchnic nerve blocks, intrapleural anesthetics, and epidural infusions in open trials and anecdotal reports.

Surgical treatment is often viewed as the definitive treatment of chronic pancreatitis despite the absence of prospective randomized studies. Relief of ductal hypertension/obstruction by surgical means via pancreaticojejunostomy is reported as effective in relieving pain for at least 5 years in 70–93% of appropriately selected patients who had dilated pancreatic ducts as demonstrated by ERCP and in 40% of patients with nondilated ducts. Morbidity/mortality associated with the surgical procedure is stated as 0–5%. Partial or total resection of the pancreas leads to pain relief for at least 5 years in 54–95% of patients, with 0–5% morbidity/mortality.[30,35] Following total resection, the loss of the endocrine function of the pancreas leads to diabetes mellitus with its own associated morbidity and mortality.

Pancreatic pseudocysts are nonepithelialized sacs of pancreatic fluids and/or blood and necrotic debris with apparently inadequate drainage. They enlarge, are frequently painful, and risk rupture of their contents into the peritoneal cavity. Treatments have been predominantly procedural with open or percutaneous drainage, followed by marsupialization (connection of the cyst to nearby gastrointestinal structure) if recurrent. Following surgical drainage of pseudocysts, it has been reported that 96% of patients report short-term relief of pain and 53% remain pain free for many years.[61] Lehman et al.[60] reviewed six series in which pseudocysts were treated endoscopically and stated that results were excellent in appropriate candidates, with 81–94% of attempted cases reported as successful. No prospective, randomized studies related to pseudocyst drainage have been reported.

Visceral neurolysis via surgical splanchnicectomy or celiac ganglionectomy has been reported. The best results have been reported by Mallet-Guy[62] in a series of 215 patients treated with a combination of surgery and/or neurolysis. Ninety-eight patients had biliary diversions, biliary–enteric bypasses, or external drainage performed in addition to neurolysis; the other 117 patients had only exploratory surgery and neurolysis. Results were not stratified between groups. Five years after their surgery, 5% of the patients had died, 8% had recurrence of their pain, 13% were lost to follow-up, and 74% were characterized as free from pain and relapsing effects (90% of living/available patients). Thoracoscopic splanchnic nerve resections have been reported.[63] Surgical neurolysis as a treatment for pain due to chronic pancreatitis has not been subjected to a randomized, controlled trial.

It has been proposed that the pain of chronic pancreatitis will eventually "burn out" and subside as the disease process progresses to total organ failure.[64] Whereas this may occur in some patients, it occurs at a variable rate and may not occur at all.[65] Hence, delay of treatment in the hopes of disease resolution is neither realistic nor ethical.

Interstitial cystitis

At present, there is no agreed etiology or pathophysiology for interstitial cystitis (IC). The only defining pathology is the presence of mucosal ulcers or "glomerulations" (small submucosal petechial hemorrhages) viewed cystoscopically after hydrodistension (sustained distension of the bladder). The presence of Hunner's (mucosal) ulcers, so named after the first clinician to describe them, separates IC patients into those with ulcerative and those with nonulcerative types. Glomerulations are not unique to IC, but occur in other forms of cystitis (e.g. radiation cystitis). Theories related to the development of IC have centered around four primary hypotheses:

1 that a disruption of the normal urothelial barrier has occurred and bladder sensory nerves are being activated by urinary constituents;
2 that a systemic autoimmune disease is presenting as a local manifestation;
3 that abnormal mast cell activity occurs within the bladder;
4 that alterations in peripheral and/or central nervous system structures have led to a neuropathic type of pain.

The frequent association of IC with other chronic diseases and pain syndromes such as inflammatory bowel disease, systemic lupus erythematosus, irritable bowel syndrome, "sensitive" skin, fibromyalgia, and allergies[66] speaks to the fact that there may be multiple different pathophysiologies grouped together under one diagnosis. Recent studies have demonstrated some histopathological differences in bladder biopsies from patients with IC compared with normal controls, with increased expression of substance P-containing nerve fibers and substance P receptor-encoding mRNA,[67,68] increased nerve growth factor content,[69] and altered mast cell activity.[70] The meaning of these findings is still to be determined.

Prevalence of IC is estimated to be 2 in 10,000.[71] It has a female–male ratio of 10:1, although some are proposing that, in males, IC may be misdiagnosed as prostatodynia (see below).[72] Patients with IC are 10–12 times more likely to report childhood bladder problems than the general population. Although a history of urinary tract infection is twice as common in IC patients as in non-IC patients, most report infrequent urinary trace infections (< 1/year) prior to the onset of their IC symptoms. Urgency, frequency, nocturia, and associated pain are the primary symptoms of IC. Pain may be localized to the lower abdomen, pelvis, groin, and/or perineum. The onset of the disease is normally abrupt with rapid progression of symptomatology, often following an "event" such as a prolonged episode of severe urgency while searching for a lavatory. Anxiety and depression are frequent comorbidities. Suprapubic tenderness to palpation may accompany a diagnosis of IC. As a diagnosis of exclusion, other physical findings and examinations should be negative for identifiable pathology, with the exception of abnormal cystometry and cystoscopy.

A reasonable approach for evaluation and treatment has been proposed by Pontari et al.,[73] which includes urine cultures, pelvic and rectal examinations, cystometry, and cystoscopy. Criteria for IC have been suggested by a consensus panel (Table 42.5). Parsons et al.[74] proposed the use of intravesical potassium solutions as a provocative diagnostic test for IC with a sensitivity of 75%, but at present this serves only as a research tool.

The ultimate goal of therapy is to neutralize the factor(s) responsible for a disease process. In the absence of any known causative factors, the treatments for IC have been guided by prudence, and a given patient's therapy typically progresses from the least invasive treatments and proceeds to the more invasive.[73] A listing of treatments for IC is given in Table 42.6. Some studies of treatments have employed placebo-controlled methodologies, but most have been open trials and generally without controls. Up to 50% of patients diagnosed with IC have spontaneous remissions with durations of 1–80 months.[71] Any treatment of IC must factor these patients into the "success" rate of that treatment.

Avoidance of foods that exacerbate symptoms (e.g. acidic foods such as cranberry juice) have proven to have great value in individuals, but has not been tested in a controlled fashion in large populations. As part of the diagnostic process, hydrodistension is performed and this procedure often proves to be therapeutic with short-term reductions in frequency and pain in more than half of the patients. Patients with symptomatic improvement for 6 months or more are considered can-

Table 42.5 *Interstitial cystitis diagnostic criteria*[a]

I   Inclusion criteria (both required)
   1   Hunner's (mucosal) ulcer or glomerulations on cystoscopy
   2   Pain associated with the bladder or urinary urgency

II Exclusion criteria (any of the following):

Age < 18 years	Symptomatic urethral diverticulum
Radiation cystitis	Uterine/cervical cancer
Cyclophosphamide cystitis	Vaginal or urethral cancer
Tuberculous cystitis	Benign or malignant bladder
Bacterial cystitis or prostatitis in last 3 months	tumors
Active genital herpes	Bladder or lower ureteral calculi
Vaginitis	Duration < 9 months
Involuntary bladder contractions	Absence of nocturia
No urgency with bladder fill > 350 cm³	Frequency < 8 times per day
Absence of urgency with 100 cm³ air or 150 cm³ water	Symptoms relieved by antibiotics, urinary antiseptics,
(fill rate 30–100 cm³/min)	anticholinergics, or antispasmodics

a. Criteria proposed by NIDDK Workshop on Interstitial Cystitis.[127]

Table 42.6 *Interstitial cystitis treatment options*

I   Hydrodistension†
II   Dietary modification†
III   Intravesical treatments
   A   Dimethyl sulfoxide*
   B   Heparin†
   C   Corticosteroids†
   D   Bicarbonate†
   E   Clorpactin†
   F   Bacille Calmette–Guérin†
IV   Antidepressants†
V   Antihistamines†
VI   Cyclosporine†
VII   Opioids†
VIII   Nonsteroidal anti-inflammatories†
IX   Transcutaneous electrical nerve stimulation†
X   Pentosanpolysulfate*
XI   Epidural local anesthetics†
XII   Neurolysis*
XIII   Surgical resection/diversion†
XIV   Behavioral therapies†

Evidence-based scoring: †series reports; *limited controlled studies.

roids and/or bicarbonate has been proposed as effective therapy,[73] as has clorpactin (a derivative of hypochlorous acid in a buffered base),[80] with success rates ranging from 50% to > 90%. A controlled comparison of intravesical DMSO with intravesical saline by Perez-Marrero et al.[81] demonstrated improvements in symptomatology in 53% of the DMSO-treated group and in only 18% of the saline-treated group. DMSO produces a distinct taste and smell on the patient's breath, so blinded comparisons were not performed. Based on the hypothesis that IC is a local manifestation of a systemic autoimmune disease, immunosuppressant therapies such as systemic cyclosporine[82] and intravesical bacille Calmette–Guérin immunotherapy[83] have been utilized in open trials with near 100% success rates reported.

Long-term treatment with opioids is an option in patients with IC, but this treatment remains controversial for all nonmalignant processes. Transcutaneous electrical nerve stimulation has been used in open trials and demonstrated to produce good results or remission in 26–54% of patients.[84] Behavioral therapies and self-care strategies such as timed voiding have proven to have value in some individuals.[85,86] A report by Irwin et al.[87] of a series of 13 patients suggests that lumbar epidural local anesthetic blocks may have short-term efficacy in up to 75% of patients.

Neurolysis by percutaneous injection or surgical resection has been described. The most positive results are those of Gillespie,[88] who reported on 175 women diagnosed with IC treated with laser obliteration of the vesicoureteric plexus bilaterally. One hundred and twelve patients reported complete relief and 58 partial relief following the procedure. Two-year follow-up in 45 patients in the "complete relief" group demonstrated no recurrence of symptoms. Considered a last resort, surgery in the form of supravesical diversions or cystectomy has also received mixed reports of efficacy. For example, Peeker et al.[89] reported excellent results in patients with classic (ulcerative) IC and poor results in nonulcerative IC.

didates for repeat hydrodistension.[73] Open trials or tricyclic antidepressants have produced reported success rates of 64–90%,[75] and oral antihistamines have been reported to produce a reduction in symptoms.[76] The oral, renally excreted heparin-like agent pentosanpolysulfate (Elmiron) has been examined in several placebo-controlled, double-blind studies. One, by Holm-Bentzen et al.,[77] failed to see any beneficial effects of a 4-month treatment with the drug. However, two other studies observed an overall symptomatic improvement (> 25%) in 28–32% of patients treated with the drug compared with a similar improvement in only 13–16% of patients treated with placebo.[78,79] Intravesical installation of dimethyl sulfoxide (DMSO) and/or heparin and/or corticoste-

Webster *et al.*[90] reported that only two of their 14 patients treated surgically with urinary diversion and cystourethrectomy had symptom resolution, and Baskin and Tanagho[91] have reported on patients with continued bladder pain despite the absence of a bladder.

Irritable bowel syndrome

Irritable bowel syndrome (IBS) is a diagnosis of exclusion that is based on symptomatology and has been demonstrated to have associated abnormalities of motility and/or sensation in different subpopulations. A frequent companion of other disorders without identifiable histopathology such as fibromyalgia, noncardiac chest pain, functional dyspepsia, and mixed headaches, it has similarly been associated with significant neuroses and psychoses such as anxiety and depression. There exist many diverse hypotheses related to the etiology of IBS. These propose that the pain may be psychosocial in origin, that the pain my be due to motility dysfunction at one or multiple sites in the gut (with dietary modifiers), or that the pain is a manifestation of visceral hyperalgesia. This visceral hyperalgesia may be due to peripheral sensitizers (e.g. mast cells) or altered central nervous system processing. Like many diagnoses of exclusion, it is likely that multiple pathophysiologies are present in different subgroups and that all of these hypotheses may be correct for different subgroups.

IBS is a common diagnosis given to 40–70% of referrals to gastroenterologists. In general populations, up to 20% of women and 10% of men experience symptomatology consistent with IBS, but most people with these symptoms do not seek medical care. Of those who do seek care, 50–60% have significant symptomatology consistent with depression and/or an anxiety disorder. IBS typically presents in the third or fourth decades of life and has a female to male ratio of 2:1. It is present in many cultures, with similar prevalences noted in the UK, China, India, Japan, New Zealand, the USA, and South America.

At least three different clinical presentations are given the diagnosis of IBS, two of which have no pain or pain as a minor component (watery diarrhea group and alternating constipation–diarrhea group respectively). The third subgroup has abdominal pain as their primary symptom and altered bowel movements as a secondary or exacerbating complaint. In this group, pain is typically in the left lower quadrant or in the suprapubic region and may be precipitated by food ingestion and a need to defecate. Bloating, mucus in the stools, and flatulence are often prominent and anxiety may exacerbate symptoms. Although there is great variation between patients, the particular symptom complex for a given patient generally remains constant. Generalized abdominal tenderness to palpation is common. The classic physical finding is a tender, palpable mass (the sigmoid colon) in the left lower quadrant. As a diagnosis of exclusion, physical examination, imaging, and laboratory findings should be negative for neoplasm, inflammatory bowel disease, infection, diverticulosis, or other intra-abdominal process. Colonoscopy and/or barium enema radiography should not demonstrate focal lesions. Stool samples should not have occult blood or infectious agents present. It is generally agreed that the colons of patients with IBS are exceptionally reactive to physiological stimuli (e.g. eating), but the finding is not pathognomonic. There are no absolute criteria for the diagnosis of IBS except for a report of abdominal pain and altered bowel habit in the absence of identifiable pathology, but criteria have been proposed to facilitate a "positive" diagnosis (Table 42.7). Motility studies and sensation evocation with a distending balloon in the rectum or sigmoid colon may prove valuable in the stratification of patients to different groups, but at present still serve as research tools.

IBS has exacerbations and spontaneous resolution of pains and so "open" trials initiated when the patient presents with an exacerbation can easily demonstrate the effectiveness of virtually any therapy. Placebo rates of 40–70% have been quoted.[92] Unlike chronic pancreatitis or interstitial cystitis, procedural treatments have not been a major component of therapy because, by definition of the disease, there is no structural pathology to treat. Controlled studies have been performed, but are likely hampered by the multiple pathophysiologies that are all diagnosed as IBS. Without definitive, objective diagnostic criteria by which to stratify patients, it is likely that effective treatments will similarly be difficult to demonstrate. Owing to the typically stable nature of a patient's symptom complex, once significant pathology has been ruled out, additional or repeat investigation is probably not necessary unless the symptom complex was to change.[93,94]

As in any chronic disorder, an important (but not particularly testable) component to the management of IBS is a stable, trusting patient–physician relationship. Life-threatening pathology may be simply ruled out with-

Table 42.7 *Diagnostic criteria[a] for irritable bowel syndrome*

I	No identifiable neoplastic, infectious, or inflammatory etiology for symptoms
II	Three months of continuous or recurrent symptoms of abdominal pain which is
	A Relieved by defecation, *or*
	B Associated with a change in stool consistency, *or*
	C Associated with a change in stool frequency with two of the following:
	1 Altered stool frequency (> 3/day or < 3/week)
	2 Altered stool form
	3 Altered stool passage (straining, urgency, incomplete evacuation)
	4 Passage of mucus
	5 Abdominal bloating

a. Rome criteria.[92]

out an exhaustive investigation and the patient needs to be assured that their symptoms are believed. Therapeutic options for IBS are listed in Table 42.8. As part of a diagnostic/therapeutic trial, patients are generally advised to engage in dietary modifications such as avoiding milk products, avoiding excessive legume consumption (associated with gas production), increasing fiber and bran in those with constipation,[95] avoiding caffeine- or sorbitol-containing foods, and establishing a stable dietary pattern in the hope of establishing a stable evacuation routine. Anticholinergics/antidiarrheals have been extensively employed clinically and extensively studied. Reviews of the efficacy of these agents have concluded that their benefit is unproven.[95,96] Traditional advice has been to keep analgesic therapy to a minimum, with the use of opioids particularly discouraged.[95] Recently, a prospective, placebo-controlled, multicenter study demonstrated efficacy of the peripheral κ-opioid receptor selective agonist fedotozine in the treatment of IBS as well as other functional bowel disorders.[97,98] Tricyclic antidepressants have been demonstrated to have efficacy in controlled studies, but it is unclear whether it is due to their antidepressant, sedative, anticholinergic, or analgesic effects. Farthing[99] has proposed the use of serotonin-specific reuptake inhibitors (e.g. paroxetine) in patients with significant constipation-related symptoms because of a motility-promoting effect. Gastrokinetic agents, antidiarrheals, serotonin receptor antagonists, osmotic laxatives, naloxone, cholecystokinin antagonists, and peppermint oil have all been proposed as effective. Injection therapies have not been generally employed in the treatment of IBS, but a neurolytic celiac plexus block has been reported as useful in the treatment of idiopathic abdominal pain.[100]

Behavioral treatments such as hypnotism, cognitive therapy, and supportive psychotherapy have proven valuable, especially if pain is intermittent and there is identified psychiatric disease such as anxiety or depression.[101] Swedlund et al.,[102] in a prospective, randomized study of 99 patients with the diagnosis of IBS, demonstrated that those patients who received eight psychotherapy sessions (and antispasmodics and bulking agents) had less abdominal pain, better bowel movements, and less psychological distress at both 3 and 15 months following treatment than similar patients treated only with anti-spasmodics and bulking agents. Other studies have been less supportive of behavioral treatments.[103]

OTHER PAINFUL DISORDERS

General

The disorders of pancreatic cancer, chronic pancreatitis, irritable bowel syndrome, and interstitial cystitis have been presented as archetypal examples illustrative of most of the problems facing the clinician in the diagnosis and management of this type of pain. In the case of pancreatic cancer, we have a disorder that has definable histopathology, is accepted as pain producing by all caregivers, and elicits intensive and aggressive treatment. Palliative surgery, high-dose opioids, and therapeutic interventions such as neurolysis are considered standards of care. This contrasts with interstitial cystitis and irritable bowel syndrome – disorders for which reassurance and "watchful waiting" are considered appropriate care with aggressive treatments reserved for the patients who complain loudest and longest. For these disorders, opioids have been viewed as controversial at best and contraindicated in many patients. Chronic pancreatitis is somewhere intermediate to these other disorders in that definable pathology is present but it does not correlate with pain symptomatology. Chronic pancreatitis has the additional factor of having a high incidence in substance abusers. It also has a frequent association with life-threatening complications such as pancreatic necrosis, malnutrition, and pseudocyst formation, and so frequently may lead to hospitalization. Other sources of chronic abdominal visceral pain as well as urogenital and rectal pain syndromes producing groin and perineal symptomatology[104] all have correlates with these disorders, and their diagnostic workups and therapies are similar. A limited discussion of several of these painful disorders and their correlation to the above four archetype disorders is given below.

Other visceral cancers (Table 42.1, VII)

Cancer can arise in all visceral structures. Symptomatology related to these cancers is similar for all sites, with dull constant pain a common "early" symptom. Pain is generally localized to the chest or upper abdomen for upper gastrointestinal tract lesions and organs located in the upper abdomen. It is generally localized to lower abdomen/perineum for lower gastrointestinal tract lesions and pelvic organs. The key statement is "generally" because no symptomatology or location is pathognomonic for any specific disease site because of the frequent presence of metastatic extension prior to diagnosis. Visceral cancers are frequently asymptomatic

---

Table 42.8 *Treatment options for irritable bowel syndrome*

I   Dietary modification
   A   Food avoidance (caffeine, milk products, legumes)[†]
   B   Addition of fiber/bran/bulking agents*
II Behavioral therapies**
III Antidepressants**
IV Anticholinergics/antispasmodics*
V   κ-Opioid receptor agonists**

Evidence-based scoring: [†]series reports; *limited controlled studies; **well-designed, randomized, controlled studies.

until obstruction or invasion of other structures occurs. Anorexia, weight loss, fatigue, nausea, and virtually every other nonspecific symptom can be noted at presentation. Amenia, hematemesis, melena, hematuria, and palpable masses on physical examination may direct further investigation. Appropriate imaging and surgical exploration/biopsy are the definitive diagnostic modalities.

Even definitive evidence of complications such as endoscopic confirmation of radiation changes or nerve conduction studies consistent with neuropathy do not absolve the clinician of the need for ongoing care. What constitutes appropriate care is somewhat fuzzy as the distinction between palliative care for pain due to metastatic cancer and that for chronic "benign" pain in a patient with a history of cancer is unclear and lapses into the realm of opinion.

Inflammatory bowel disease (Table 42.1, I-F,G)

Ulcerative colitis (UC) and Crohn's disease (CD) are two recurrent gastrointestinal inflammatory disorders with many similarities in symptomatology and histopathology, but significant differences in extent of the disease process, relapse incidence, and associated complications such as fistula formation. Common presenting symptoms include abdominal pain, fever, and altered bowel habits such as bloody diarrhea. Inflammatory bowel disease is more common in whites than blacks or Asians, and 3–6 times more common in Jews than non-Jews. UC is three to five times more common than CD, but recurrent exacerbations are much less frequent. In UC, the gastrointestinal component of the disease process is restricted to the colon, whereas in CD there is involvement in all portions of the gastrointestinal tract. Extracolonic features of inflammatory bowel disease include arthritis, skin changes, and evidence of liver disease. Half of the patients with CD and 20% of the patients with UC studied by Buskila et al.[105] had diagnostic criteria for fibromyalgia. The diagnosis of inflammatory bowel disease is based on biopsy, colonoscopic/endoscopic appearances, and/or surgical evaluation. Other causes of inflammatory changes such as radiation enteritis or local infection (e.g. Shigella, Salmonella, amebiasis, Clostridium difficile) must be ruled out. Local complications of inflammatory bowel disease include the formation of fistulas, abscesses, strictures, perforation, and toxic dilation, all of which are more common in CD than UC. With a prolonged clinical course, there is a potential for the development of carcinoma. There is a stated incidence of colon cancer of 0.5–1% per year for every year after the initial 10 years of active inflammatory bowel disease. Surgical treatment of inflammatory bowel disease is normally reserved for the treatment of complications, with 20–25% of UC patients requiring colectomy and 70% of patients with CD. Colectomy presumably resolves UC, but does not resolve all of the symptoms of CD since the disease process is pan-enteric.

Dietary alterations may have some acute effects during a "flare," but have not been demonstrated to alter overall disease progression. Neurolysis is typically avoided since symptoms may act as early indicators of life-threatening complications. Regional anesthetic techniques, although of possible short-term benefit during a flare, have the same risks as neurolysis in that they may mask disease complications. Surgery has remained an integral component in the management of inflammatory bowel disease. Pain treatment related to inflammatory bowel disease forms a limited-choice corollary to chronic pancreatitis (Table 42.4). Whereas UC is potentially "cured" by colectomy, CD continues for a life time. Surgical resection of portions of inflamed bowel, strictures, or abscesses/fistulas are not uncommon in CD, but the strategies associated with surgical treatment continue to evolve. Surgical interventions may result in temporary relief until another site is affected, but such resections may also result in a "short bowel" with associated nutritional compromise. Since reports of pain may be associated with life-threatening complications, these patients may have frequent hospitalizations. The use of opioids and other motility-altering drugs carries the perception of an increased risk of toxic dilation with an associated increase in morbidity and mortality. Similar to other diseases with unknown etiologies, genetic influences, immunologic abnormalities, and infectious agents have all been implicated and used as rationales for treatment. Primary treatment for exacerbations is typically bowel rest, anti-inflammatories (e.g. oral sulfasalazine, possibly corticosteroids), nutritional/fluid/electrolyte management, and treatment of complications. No universal consensus appears to exist in relation to preventative treatment. Multiple therapies such as oral sulfasalazine, oral olsalazine, oral metronidazole, systemic corticosteroids, and mesalamine enemas/suppositories have been utilized not only as reactive treatments for exacerbations but also as prophylactic measures. Although results related to use of these agents are encouraging for UC, a multicenter study failed to observe any decrease in the recurrence of CD exacerbations even with sulfasalazine. Immunosuppressants such as azothioprine and cyclosporine have been used for a presumed immunologic etiology. Psychological treatments are justified by the presence of a life-long, recurrent disease process.

Chronic mesenteric ischemia: ischemic colitis

Inadequate blood supply to meet the energy demands of viscera can lead to reports of pain, such as that which occurs with cardiac angina. A similar phenomenon has been noted in the gastrointestinal system whereby severe abdominal pain may be precipitated by the ingestion of a meal.[106] Fear of eating with subsequent weight loss and poor nutritional status may further compromise patients already in ill health as a result of atherosclerotic disease in multiple sites. Poor peripheral pulses, abdominal bruits, and arteriographic evidence of stenosis or occlusion in the three main mesenteric arteries are all consistent with the diagnosis of *abdominal* angina. Similar to cardiac disease, abdominal angina may precede infarction, which has devastating life-threatening consequences. Arterial thrombosis, embolic events, venous occlusion, and low flow states due to poor cardiac output may all lead to the same disastrous results. Ischemic colitis represents approximately half of the cases of morbidity due to mesenteric vascular disease.[107] Although usually diagnosed by colonoscopy, 20% of patients with ischemic colitis develop evidence of peritonitis requiring surgical diagnosis and treatment. Initial presentation may be with persistent diarrhea, rectal bleeding, or weight loss. Surgical revascularization, thrombectomy, or angioplasty are definitive treatments for mesenteric vasculopathy, but as for all patients with widespread vascular disease comorbidity may dictate outcome as much as the specific procedure performed.

Diverticular disease

Diverticula can occur throughout the gastrointestinal tract, but prove to be most common in the colon where they exist as small sac-like herniations of mucosa through the muscular wall, typically at the site of penetrating blood vessels. Duodenal, jejunal, and ileal diverticula can occur with Meckel's diverticulum forming a special congenital abnormality present in 2% of the population. Meckel's diverticula are particularly notable since they may contain acid-producing gastric mucosa and lead to enteral ulcer formation. Colonic diverticula are generally pain free, but with the development of inflammation and/or obstruction of their mouth severe abdominal pain and infection may result. Peridiverticular abscesses, obstruction, colonic distension, bleeding, and altered bowel habit (diarrhea, constipation) are not uncommon. Painful diverticulosis classically presents as recurrent left lower quadrant colicky pain without evidence of inflammation. Like chronic pancreatitis, diverticular disease can produce pain which is episodic and which can have life-threatening consequences, if ignored. Bleeding diverticula are the most common sources of lower gastrointestinal tract bleeding,[108] and segmental colonic resection has the highest success rate at stopping bleeding. However, effects on pain are unclear. Reports of pain do not always correlate with observable pathology and symptoms can be nonspecific. A European surgical consensus panel was not able to definitively state when surgery was indicated for symptomatic reasons and called for randomized, controlled trials.[109]

Familial Mediterranean fever (Table 42.1, VI-A)

An autosomal recessive genetic disease linked to chromosome 16, familial Mediterranean fever begins at age 5–15 years.[110,111] Referred to as a trait of the sons of Shem (one of Noah's sons), owing to its increased incidence in Sephardic Jews, Armenians, Turks and Arabs, the known gene mutations have also been found in substantial numbers of people from other Mediterranean populations. Features that are classic include periodic febrile episodes without other cause, serous peritonitis, pleuritis, synovitis, and a rash that may resemble erysipelas. Abdominal pain of varying intensity occurs in 95% of the episodes, with chest pain and arthralgias in 75% of episodes. The frequency of the episodes may vary from twice per week to once per year, but most commonly occur at 2- to 4-week intervals with acute episodes typically lasting 1–3 days. Amyloidosis with associated kidney failure and arthralgia are the most severe associated sequelae. Leukocytosis and elevated sedimentation rate may be present on laboratory examination. Typical treatment is episodic with the use of systemic analgesics. In controlled studies, colchicine has been demonstrated to decrease the frequency of attacks and risks of amyloidosis.[112] Prophlylactic antibiotics, hormones, antipyretics, immunotherapy, psychotherapy, dietary alterations, chloroquine, and phenylbutazone have all been tried without success.

Porphyria (Table 42.1, VI-B,D)

Several related genetic disorders, all characterized by the increased formation of porphyrins of their precursors, are termed porphyria.[113,114] Three subgroups have been identified that all have similar symptomatology: intermittent acute porphyria (IAP), hereditary coproporphyria, and variegate porphyria. Of these, IAP is the most frequently encountered with attacks of colicky abdominal pain that are intermittent, that may be associated with environmental exposures, and that can last for days to months. Transmitted as an autosomal dominant disorder with incomplete penetration, family history may or may not be helpful in the diagnosis. Certain drugs such as barbiturates, benzodiazepines, alcohol, phenytoin, ketamine, etomidate, meprobamate, and corticosteroids have been particularly implicated as "triggers," although use of many of these agents without the precipitation of a crisis has been reported. Constipation, abdominal distension, and profuse vomiting are common. Neurological dysfunction may occur principally as a result of demyelination effects,[113] with emotional disturbance a nonspecific symptom. Urine and blood tests related to porphyria may only be diagnostic during crises. Genetic testing of asymptomatic members in IAP families may allow for avoidance of triggers. Treatment is avoiding known triggers, treating crises with intravenous fluids, hematin, and/

or increased carbohydrate intake, and treating pain and nausea with "safe" analgesics/antiemetics. Most opioids are alleged to be nontriggering, a notable exception is the mixed agonist–antagonist pentazocine. Chlorpromazine, promethazine, and droperidol have all been reported to be safe as antiemetics.

Orchialgia

Like abdominal pain, pain localized to the testes has a wide differential diagnosis. Local processes such as tumor, infection (e.g. epididymitis), varicocele/hydrocele/spermatocele, and testicular torsion are all potentially acute and chronic sources of pain. Previous surgeries such as inguinal hernia repair and vasectomy as well as noniatrogenic trauma can all lead to chronic inflammatory processes as well as altered sensation and associated chronic pain. Neuropathic etiologies ranging from diabetic neuropathy and entrapment neuropathies to spinal disk disease may all present with testicular pain. Scrotal pain should be differentiated from testicular pain since the nerve supplies differ and may represent differing sites of pathology along sacral versus thoracolumbar pathways. Owing to the "personal" nature of the site of pain, concerns related to psychological etiologies or sequelae of this chronic pain are maintained.

Treatment of chronic orchialgia forms a correlate to the disease entity of interstitial cystitis (Table 42.6) with numerous treatments proposed for a disease of unknown but presumably localized etiology. Traditional pain management has started with anti-inflammatories and/or antibiotics. Surgical procedures including epididymectomy, orchiectomy, or denervation procedures have been recommended, but long-term outcomes are unknown and retrospective series[115] have suggested limited benefit in "pain-prone" patients. Wesselmann et al.[104] have suggested that there may be benefit from low-dose antidepressants, anticonvulsants, membrane-stabilizing agents, opiates, and, in some patients, repeated lumbar sympathetic blocks, oral sympatholytics, and repeated infusions of phentolamine. Because of the wide differential diagnosis of testicular pain, no specific treatment will be universally effective.

Prostadynia

This disorder is defined as pain attributed to the prostate in the absence of identifiable pathology. Hallmark features consist of persistent complaints of urinary urgency, dysuria, poor urinary flow, and perineal discomfort without evidence of bacteria or white blood cells in prostatic fluids. It serves as a male-specific corollary to interstitial cystitis in that it has similar symptomatology, is a diagnosis of exclusion, and has a presumed site of pain

generation. Infectious, inflammatory, neurological, and referred gastroenterological etiologies of the pain need to be ruled out. Interestingly, Miller et al.[72] found cystoscopic findings of interstitial cystitis in 12 of 20 males referred to their clinic with the diagnosis of prostadynia. Wesselmann et al.[104] have suggested that interstitial cystitis, prostadynia (male), and vulvodynia (female) may all be variations of a generalized disorder of the epithelium of the urogenital sinus. To further quote Wesselmann et al.,[104] "No strikingly successful treatment options have been described and like interstitial cystitis, treatments may be empiric trials of medications employed in the treatment of chronic pain." Antibiotics are commonly employed despite the absence of evidence for a microbiological etiology. If urodynamic measures indicate abnormalities, use of α-adrenergic-blocking agents and/or transurethral balloon dilation of the prostate have been suggested as therapeutic. Transurethral microwave hyperthermia, pelvic floor relaxation techniques, and use of muscle-relaxing agents have also been suggested as therapeutic.

Postcholecystectomy syndrome

Gallbladder inflammation, gallstones, and associated pathology of the biliary tract are known sources of acute pain that is typically coupled with dyspepsia and, occasionally, jaundice when obstructive. However, even after surgical resection of the gallbladder, pain may continue, which is termed postcholecystectomy syndrome.[116-118] Typically in the right upper quadrant of the abdomen, its symptomatology is similar to that of cholecystitis in that it may be exacerbated by eating, may be associated with nausea, is described as continuous during the day, and is dull and frequently colicky. Appropriate workup will rule out definable pathology such as a retained bile duct stone or secondary pancreatitis. It is a correlate to chronic pancreatitis in that there may be abnormal pressures or motility within the biliary duct.

Endoscopic demonstration of elevated sphincter of Oddi pressures suggest sphincter dysfunction as the cause of the syndrome.[119] During endoscopic retrograde cholangiopancreatography, it may be possible to reproduce the pain by producing intraductal distention.[120] Endoscopic or surgical sphincterotomy or sphincteroplasty have been beneficial in series reports,[121,122] and calcium channel blockers or long-acting nitrates have been proposed as therapeutic when sphincterotomy is not possible.[119] Other treatment options are similar to chronic pancreatitis, with dietary alterations, surgical reexplorations, focal injections/neurolysis, and traditional analgesics all suggested as therapeutic options. In many cases, there is no objective identification of a site of pain generation so treatment is empiric. In many cases, the cholecystectomy was one aspect of this empiric treatment.

Proctalgia fugax

Episodic spasms of pain localized to the rectum/anus, occurring at irregular intervals and without identifiable cause, are termed proctalgia fugax.[123] Highly prevalent, occurring in 14–19% of healthy subjects, the episodes are brief (seconds to minutes) and infrequent (normally < 6/year). They may be precipitated by bowel movements, sexual activity, stress, and temperature changes and so may lead to avoidance behavior on the part of the patient. No etiology or method of treating/preventing proctalgia fugax has been universally accepted, although spasms of the sigmoid colon, levator ani, and/or pelvic floor musculature have been postulated as sources of the pain. Local anorectal pathology such as fissures or abscesses need to be ruled out as alternate sources of pain and spasm. Owing to the brief nature of most episodes, most reactive pharmacological treatments have usually proved inadequate, although clonidine, nitroglycerin, antispasmodics, and calcium channel blockers have all been reported as effective.[124] Heat or pressure applied to the perineum, food/drink consumption, dilation of the anal sphincter, assumption of a knee–chest position, and assumption of other postures have been anecdotally reported as beneficial. Inhaled salbutamol was demonstrated to shorten the duration of severe pain in a double-blind, placebo-controlled, crossover trial of 18 patients with the diagnosis of proctalgia fugax.[125]

Other

Abdominal pain may also result from nonabdominal sites. Abdominal migraine is a variant of the more typical migraine. Rather than headache and nausea, symptomatology may consist of abdominal pain and nausea. Treatment is similar to that of other migraines. Another source of abdominal pain may be cardiac failure, which produces congestion-related hepatomegaly and associated distension of the hepatic capsule. Similarly, low cardiac output may be associated with ischemia of the bowel. Chronic ulceration of the stomach or duodenum may also produce recurrent epigastric pain. Potentially life-threatening because of their potential for hemorrhage and perforation, they are generally viewed as acute events, diagnosed with endoscopy or contrast radiology and treated with antacids, mucosal coating agents, bowel rest, and drugs blocking gastric acid secretion/formation. Following abdominal or groin surgeries, nerve injury or entrapments can occur, resulting in neuralgias, neuroma formation, or referred pains (e.g. testicular pain following an inguinal hernia repair). Evaluation and treatment is similar to that of other neuropathic pains, which are discussed elsewhere.

SUMMARY

Chronic pain with abdominal, groin, or perineal localization is a common clinical entity with multiple etiologies, both known and unknown. Four archetypal disorders have been presented in depth, as well as multiple other disorders as correlates. Each of the sources of pain listed in Table 42.1 has its own unique aspects, but similarities in evaluation and treatment are apparent. All forms of cancer have their correlate in pancreatic cancer with defined pathology and a desire for aggressive palliative treatment. Infectious and inflammatory pain states are correlates to chronic pancreatitis in that they have definable pathology but variable symptomatology. They also have associated potentially life-threatening complications such as abscess formation, fistula formation, and hemorrhage. Functional and undefined pain conditions have their correlates in irritable bowel syndrome and interstitial cystitis with presumably defined *sites* of pain generation but minimal or absent definable pathology at those sites. All therapies are both disorder dependent and patient dependent. Outcome studies for many therapies are nonexistent, and so the challenge for the clinician treating pain is to define the most appropriate therapy for an individual patient. It is beyond the scope of this chapter to delineate every option every tried, but the general maxim of starting "simple" and advancing as needed is prudent for all of the disorders.

Key points

- Abdominal, groin and perineal pain can be of visceral, neuropathic, musculoskeletal or psychogenic origins.
- Visceral pain is poorly localized and evokes strong autonomic and emotional responses.
- There is a poor correlation between visceral pathology and reports of visceral pain.
- The principles of the management of visceral pain are similar to those of other painful conditions.

REFERENCES

1. Alter CL. Palliative and supportive care of patients with pancreatic cancer. *Semin Oncol* 1996; **23:** 229–40.
2. Caraceni A, Portenoy RK. Pain management in patients with pancreatic carcinoma. *Cancer* 1996; **78** (Suppl.): 639–53.
3. Farthing MJG. Irritable bowel, irritable body or irritable brain? *Br Med J* 1995; **310:** 171–5.
4. Hanno PM, Staskin DR, Krane RJ, Wein AJ eds. *Interstitial Cystitis*. New York, NY: Springer-Verlag, 1990.

● 5. Jansen JBMJ, Kuijpers JH, Zitman FJ, van Dongen R. Pain in chronic pancreatitis. *Scand J Gastroenterol* 1995; **30** (Suppl. 212): 117–25.

● 6. Maxwell P, Mendall MA, Kumar D. Irritable bowel syndrome. *Lancet* 1997; **350:** 1691–5.

● 7. Murray, JJ. Controversies in Crohn's disease. *Baillière's Clin Gastroenterol* 1998; **12:** 133–55.

● 8. Steer ML, Waxman I, Freedman S. Medical progress: chronic pancreatitis. *New Engl J Med* 1995; **332:** 1482–90.

● 9. Warshaw AL, Banks PA, Fernandez-Del Castillo C. AGA technical review: treatment of pain in chronic pancreatitis. *Gastroenterology* 1998; **115:** 765–76.

● 10. Wesselmann U, Burnett AL, Heinberg LJ. The urogenital and rectal pain syndromes. *Pain* 1997; **73:** 269–94.

◆ 11. Al-Chaer ED, Lawand NB, Westlund KN, Willis WD. Visceral nociceptive input into the ventral posterolateral nucleus of the thalamus: a new function for the dorsal column pathway. *J Neurophysiol* 1996; **76:** 2661–74.

12. Ness TJ. Models of visceral pain. *Inst Lab Animal Res J* 1999; **40:** 119–28.

13. Bynum TE. Abdominal pain. In: Stein JH ed. *Internal Medicine*, 2nd edn. Boston, MA: Little Brown and Co., 1987: 88–93.

14. Pitchumoni CS. Chronic pancreatitis: a historical and clinical sketch of the pancreas and pancreatitis. *Gastroenterologist* 1998; **6:** 24–33.

15. Andren-Sandberg A, Dervenis C, Lowenfels B. Etiologic links between chronic pancreatitis and pancreatic cancer. *Scand J Gastroenterol* 1997; **32:** 97–103.

16. Caraceni A, Portenoy RK. Pain management in patients with pancreatic carcinoma. *Cancer* 1996; **78** (Suppl.): 639–53.

17. Regan PT, Go VLW. Pancreatic diseases. In: Stein JH ed. *Internal Medicine*, 2nd edn. Boston, MA: Little Brown and Co., 1987: 261–71.

18. Alter CL. Palliative and supportive care of patients with pancreatic cancer. *Semin Oncol* 1996; **23:** 229–40.

19. Gastrointestinal Tumor Study Group. Radiation therapy combined with adriamyacin or 5-fluorouracil for the treatment of locally unresectable pancreatic carcinoma. *Cancer* 1985; **56:** 5623–8.

20. Thompson GE, Moore DC, Bridenbaugh LD, Artin RY. Abdominal pain and alcohol celiac plexus nerve block. *Anesth Analg* 1977; **56:** 1–5.

◆ 21. Brown DL, Bulley CK, Quiel EL. Neurolytic celiac plexus block for pancreatic cancer pain. *Anesth Analg* 1987; **66:** 869–73.

22. Kappis M. Sensibilitat und lokale anaesthesic im chirugischen gobect der bauchhohle mit besonder berucksichrigung der splanchnicusanethesia. *Beitr Klin Chir* 1919; **115:** 161–75.

23. Moore DC. *Regional Block: A Handbook for Use in the Clinical Practice of Medicine and Surgery*, 3rd edn. Springfield, IL: Charles C. Thomas, 1961.

24. Sharfman WH, Walsh TD. Review article: has the analgesic efficacy of neurolytic celiac plexus block been demonstrated in pancreatic cancer pain? *Pain* 1990; **41:** 267–71.

25. Eisenberg E, Carr DB, Chalmers TC. Neurolytic celiac plexus block for treatment of cancer pain: a meta-analysis. *Anesth Analg* 1995; **80:** 290–2.

26. Lebovits AH, Lefkowitz M. Pain management of pancreatic cardinoma: a review. *Pain* 1989; **36:** 1–11.

27. Ischia S, Ishia A, Polati E, Finco G. Three posterior percutaneous celiac plexus block techniques. A prospective, randomized study in 61 patients with pancreatic cancer pain. *Anesthesiology* 1992; **76:** 534–40.

◆ 28. Kawamata M, Ishitani K, Ishikawa K, *et al*. Comparison between celiac plexus block and morphine treatment on quality of life in patients with pancreatic cancer pain. *Pain* 1996; **64:** 597–602.

29. Merandino KA. Vagotomy for the relief of pain secondary to pancreatic carcinoma. *Am J Surg* 1964; **108:** 1–2.

30. Warshaw AL, Banks PA, Fernandez-Del Castillo C. AGA Technical Review: treatment of pain in chronic pancreatitis. *Gastroenterology* 1998; **115:** 765–76.

31. Braganza JM. The pathogenesis of chronic pancreatitis. *Q J Med* 1996; **89:** 243–50.

32. Bockman DE, Buchler M, Malfertheiner P, Beger HG. Analysis of nerves in chronic pancreatitis. *Gastroenterology* 1998; **94:** 1459–69.

33. Buchler M, Weihle E, Freiss H, *et al*. Changes in peptidergic innervation in chronic pancreatitis. *Pancreas* 1992; **7:** 183–92.

34. Walsh TN, Rode J, Theis BA, Russell RCG. Minimal change chronic pancreatitis. *Gut* 1992; **33:** 1566–71.

35. Malfertheiner P, Dominguez-Munoz JE, Buchler MW. Chronic pancreatitis: management of pain. *Digestion* 1994; **55** (Suppl. 1): 29–34.

36. Little JM. Alcohol abuse and chronic pancreatitis. *Surgery* 1987; **101:** 357–60.

37. Hayakawa T, Kondo T, Shibata T, *et al*. Chronic alcoholism and evolution of pain and prognosis in chronic pancreatitis. *Dig Dis Sci* 1989; **34:** 33–8.

38. Gullo L, Barbara L, Labo G. Effect of cessation of alcohol use on the course of pancreatic dysfunction in alcoholic pancreatitis. *Gastroenterology* 1988; **95:** 1063–8.

◆ 39. Lankisch PG, Seindensticker F, Lohr-Happe A, *et al*. The course of pain is the same in alcohol- and nonalcohol-induced chronic pancreatitis. *Pancreas* 1995; **10:** 338–41.

40. Lehman GA, Sherman S, Hawes RH. Endoscopic management of recurrent and chronic pancreatitis. *Scand J Gastroenterol* 1995; **30** (Suppl. 208): 81–9.

41. Sauerbruch T, Holl J, Sackmann M, Paumgartner G. Extracorporeal lithotripsy of pancreatic stones in

patients with chronic pancreatitis and pain: a prospective follow up study. *Gut* 1992; **33:** 969–72.

42. Castiella A, Lopez P, Bujanda L, Arenas JI. Possible association of acute pancreatitis with naproxen. *J Clin Gastroenterol* 1995; **21:** 258.

43. Felig DM, Topazian M. Corticosteroid-induced pancreatitis (letter). *Ann Intern Med* 1996; **124:** 1016.

44. Bilton D, Schofield D, Mei G, *et al.* Placebo-controlled trials of antioxidant therapy including S-adenosyl-methionine in patients with recurrent non-gallstone pancreatitis. *Drug Invest* 1994; **8:** 10–20.

45. Uden S, Bilton D, Nathan L, *et al.* Antioxidant therapy for recurrent pancreatitis: placebo-controlled trial. *Aliment Pharmacol Ther* 1990; **4:** 357–71.

46. Banks PA, Hughes M, Ferrante FM, *et al.* Does allopurinol reduce pain in chronic pancreatitis? *Int J Pancreatol* 1997; **22:** 171–6.

47. Isaksson G, Ihse I. Pain reduction by an oral pancreatic enzyme preparation in chronic pancreatitis. *Dig Dis Sci* 1983; **28:** 97–102.

48. Halgreen H, Pederson TN, Worning H. Symptomatic effect of pancreatic enzyme therapy in patients with chronic pancreatitis. *Scand J Gastroenterol* 1986; **21:** 104–8.

49. Mossner J. Is there a place for pancreatic enzymes in the treatment of pain in chronic pancreatitis? *Digestion* 1993; **54** (Suppl. 2): 35–9.

50. Hanowell ST, Kennedy SF, MacMamara TF, Lees DE. Celiac plexus block: diagnostic and therapeutic application in abdominal pain. *South Med. J* 1980; **73:** 1330–2.

51. Little JM. Chronic pancreatitis: results of a protocol of management. *Aust N Z J Surg* 1983; **53:** 403–9.

52. Busch EH, Atchison SR. Steroid celiac plexus block for chronic pancreatitis: results in 16 cases. *J Clin Anesth* 1989; **1:** 431–3.

53. Fishman SM, Catarau EM, Sachs G, *et al.* Corticosteroid-induced mania after single regional application at the celiac plexus. *Anesthesiology* 1996; **85:** 1194–6.

54. Bell SN, Cole R, Roberts-Thomson IC. Coeliac plexus block for control of pain in chronic pancreatitis. *Br Med J* 1980; **281:** 1604.

55. Leung JWC, Bowen-Wright M, Aveling W, *et al.* Coeliac plexus block for pain in pancreatic cancer and chronic pancreatitis. *Br J Surg* 1983; **70:** 730–2.

56. Fugere F, Lewis G. Coeliac plexus block for chronic pain syndromes. *Can J Anaesth* 1993; **40:** 954–63.

57. Chan VWS. Chronic diarrhoea: an uncommon side effect of celiac plexus block. *Anesth Analg* 1996; **82:** 205–7.

58. Takeda J, Namai H, Fukushima K. Anterior spinal artery syndrome after left celiac plexus block. *Anesth Analg* 1996; **83:** 178–9.

59. Cherry DA, Lamberty J. Paraplegia following coeliac plexus nerve block. *Anaesth Intensive Care* 1984; **12:** 59–61.

60. Galiazia EJ, Lahiri SK. Paraplegia following celiac plexus

block with phenol. *Br J Anaesth* 1974; **46:** 539–40.

61. Lohr-Happe A, Peiper M, Lankisch PG. Natural course of operated pseudocysts in chronic pancreatitis. *Gut* 1994; **35:** 1479–82.

62. Mallet-Guy PA. Late and very late results of resections of the nervous system in the treatment of chronic relapsing pancreatitis. *Am J Surg* 1983; **145:** 234–8.

63. Maher JW, Johlin FC, Pearson D. Thoracoscopic splanchnicectomy for chronic pancreatitis pain. *Surgery* 1996; **120:** 603–10.

64. Ammann RW, Akovbiantz A, Largiader F, Schueler G. Course and outcome of chronic pancreatitis. *Gastroenterology* 1984; **86:** 820–88.

65. Lankisch PG, Lohr-Happe A, Otto J, Creutzfeld W. Natural course in chronic pancreatitis: pain, exocrine and endocrine pancreatic insufficiency and prognosis of the disease. *Digestion* 1993; **54:** 148–55.

66. Alagiri M, Chottiner S, Ratner V, *et al.* Interstitial cystitis: unexplained associations with other chronic disease and pain syndromes. *Urology* 1997; **49** (Suppl. 5A): 52–7.

67. Pang X, Marchand J, Sant GR, *et al.* Increased number of substance P positive nerve fibres in interstitial cystitis. *Br J Urol* 1995; **75:** 744–50.

68. Marchand JE, Sant GR, Kream RM. Increased expression of substance P receptor-encoding mRNA in bladder biopsies from patient with interstitial cystitis. *Br J Urol* 1998; **81:** 224–8.

69. Lowe EM, Anand P, Terenghi G, *et al.* Increased nerve growth factor levels in the urinary bladder of women with idiopathic sensory urgency and interstitial cystitis. *Br J Urol* 1997; **79:** 572–7.

70. Theoharides TC, Sant GR, el-Mansoury M, *et al.* Activation of bladder mast cells in interstitial cystitis: a light and election microscopic study. *J Urol* 1995; **153:** 629–36.

71. Held PJ, Hanno PM, Wein AJ. Epidemiology of interstitial cystitis. In: Hanno PM ed. *Interstitial Cystitis.* London: Springer-Verlag, 1990: 29–48.

72. Miller JL, Rothman I, Bavendam TG, Berger RE. Prostadynia and interstitial cystitis: one and the same? *Urology* 1995; **45:** 587–90.

◆ 73. Pontari MA, Hanno PM, Wein AJ. Logical and systemic approach to the evaluation and management of patients suspected of having interstitial cystitis. *Urology* 1997; **49** (Suppl. 5A): 114–20.

74. Parsons CL, Greenberger M, Gaball L, *et al.* The role of urinary potassium in the pathogenesis and diagnosis of interstitial cystitis. *J Urol* 1998; **159:** 1862–7.

75. Hanro PM. Amitriptyline in the treatment of interstitial cystitis. *Urol Clin North Am* 1994; **21:** 121–30.

76. Theoharides TC. Hydroxyzine in the treatment of interstitial cystitis. *Urol Clin North Am* 1994; **21:** 113–20.

◆ 77. Holm-Bentzen M, Jacobsen F, Nerstromn B, *et al.* A prospective double-blind clinically controlled multicentre trial of sodium pentosanpolysulfate in the treatment of interstitial cystitis and related painful bladder disease.

J Urol 1987; **138:** 503–7.

78. Mulholand SG, Hanno P, Parsons CL, *et al*. Pentosan polysulfate sodium for therapy of interstitial cystitis. *Urology* 1990; **35:** 552–8.

79. Parsons CL, Benson G, Childs SJ, *et al*. A quantitatively controlled method to study prospectively interstitial cystitis and demonstrate the efficacy of pentosanpolysulfate. *J Urol* 1993; **150:** 845–8.

80. Messing EM, Stamey TA. Interstitial cystitis, early diagnosis, pathology and treatment. *Urology* 1978; **12:** 381–92.

81. Perez-Marrero R, Emerson LE, Feltis JT. A controlled study of dimethyl sulfoxide in interstitial cystitis. *J Urol* 1988; **140:** 36–9.

82. Forsell T, Ruutu M, Isoniemi H, *et al*. Cyclosporine in severe interstitial cystitis. *J Urol* 1996; **155:** 1591–3.

83. Zeidman EJ, Helfrick B, Pollard C, Thompson IM. Bacillus Calmette–Guerin immunotherapy for refractory interstitial cystitis. *Urology* 1994; **43:** 121–4.

84. Fall M, Lindstrom S. Transcutaneous electrical nerve stimulation in interstitial cystitis. *Urol Clin North Am* 1994; **21:** 131–9.

85. Whitmore KE. Self-care regimens for patients with interstitial cystitis. *Urol Clin North Am* 1994; **21:** 121–30.

86. Chaiken DC, Blaivas JG, Blaivis ST. Behavioural therapy for the treatment of refractory interstitial cystitis. *J Urol* 1993; **149:** 1445–8.

87. Irwin PP, Hammonds WD, Galloway NTM. Lumbar epidural blockade for management of pain in interstitial cystitis. *Br J Urol* 1993; **71:** 413–16.

88. Gillespie, L. Destruction of the vesicoureteric plexus for the treatment of hypersensitive bladder disorders. *Br J Urol* 1994; **74:** 40–3.

◆ 89. Peeker R, Aldenborg F, Fall M. The treatment of interstitial cystitis with supratrigonal cystectomy and ileocystoplasty: difference in outcome between classic and nonulcer disease. *J Urol* 1998; **159:** 1479–82.

90. Webster GD, MacDiarmid SA, Timmons SL. Impact of urinary diversion procedures in the treatment of interstitial cystitis and chronic bladder pain. *Neurourol Urodyn* 1992; **11:** 417.

91. Baskin LS, Tanagho EA. Pelvic pain without pelvic organs. *J Urol* 1992; **147:** 683–6.

92. Maxwell P, Mendall MA, Kumar D. Irritable bowel syndrome. *Lancet* 1997; **350:** 1691–5.

93. Ouyang A, Cohen S. Diarrhoea, constipation and the irritable bowel syndrome. In: Stein JH ed. *Internal Medicine*, 2nd edn. Boston, MA: Little Brown and Co., 1987: 120–8.

94. Longstreth GF. Irritable bowel syndrome. Diagnosis in the managed care era. *Dig Dis Sci* 1997; **42:** 1105–11.

95. Pattee PL, Thompson WG. Drug treatment of the irritable bowel syndrome. *Drugs* 1992; **44:** 200–6.

96. Klein KB. Controlled clinical trials in the irritable bowel syndrome: a critique. *Gastroenterology* 1988; **95:** 232–41.

97. Fraitag B, Homerin M, Hecketsweiler P. Double-blind dose-response multicentre comparison of fedotozine and placebo in treatment of nonulcer dyspepsia. *Dig Dis Sci* 1994; **39:** 1072–7.

98. Dapoigny M, Abitnbol JL, Fraitag B. Efficacy of peripheral kappa agonist fedotozine versus placebo in treatment of irritable bowel syndrome. A multicentre dose-response study. *Dig Dis Sci* 1995; **40:** 2244–9.

99. Farthing MJG. Irritable bowel, irritable body or irritable brain? *Br Med J* 1995; **310:** 171–5.

100. Hastings RH, McKay WR. Treatment of benign chronic abdominal pain with neurolytic celiac plexus block. *Anesthesiology* 1991; **75:** 156–8.

101. Guthrie E, Creed F, Dawson D, Tomenson B. A controlled trial of psychological treatment for the irritable bowel syndrome. *Gastroenterology* 1991; **100:** 450–7.

102. Swedlund J, Sjoden L, Ottosson JO, Doteval G. Controlled study of psychotherapy in irritable bowel syndrome. *Lancet* 1983; **2:** 589–91.

◆103. Talley NJ, Owen BK, Boyce P, Paterson K. Psychological treatments for irritable bowel syndrome: a critique of controlled treatment trials. *Am J Gastroenterol* 1996; **91:** 277–83.

104. Wesselmann U, Burnett AL, Heinberg LJ. The urogenital and rectal pain syndromes. *Pain* 1997; **73:** 269–94.

105. Buskila D, Odes LR, Neumann L, Odes HS. Fibromyalgia in inflammatory bowel disease. *J Rheumatol* 1999; **26:** 1167–71.

106. Montgomery RA, Venbrux AC, Bulkey GB. Mesenteric vascular insufficiency. *Curr Probl Surg.* 1997; **34:** 941–1025.

107. Cappell MS. Intestinal (mesenteric) vasculopathy. II. Ischemic colitis and chronic mesenteric ischemia. *Gastroenterol Clin North Am* 1998; **27:** 827–60.

108. Vernava III AM, Moore BA, Longo WE, Johnson FE. Lower gastrointestinal bleeding. *Dis Colon Rectum* 1997; **40:** 846–58.

109. Kohler L, Sauerland S, Neugebauer E. Diagnosis and treatment of diverticular disease: results of a consensus development conference. The Scientific Committee of the European Association for Endoscopic Surgery. *Surg Endosc* 1999; **13:** 430–6.

110. Samuels J, Aksentijevich I, Torosyan Y, *et al*. Familial Mediterranean fever at the millennium. Clinical spectrum, ancient mutations, and a survey of 100 American referrals to the National Institutes of Health. *Medicine* 1998; **77:** 268–97.

111. Ben-Chetrit E, Levy M. Familial Mediterranean fever. *Lancet* 1998; **351:** 659–64.

112. Livney A, Langevitz P, Zemer D, *et al*. The changing face of familial Mediterranean fever. *Semin Arthritis Rheum* 1996; **26:** 612–27.

113. Meyer UA, Schuumans MM, Lindberg RL. Acute porphyrias: pathogenesis of neurological manifestations. *Semin Liver Dis* 1998; **18:** 43–52.

114. Grandchamp B. Acute intermittent porphyria. *Semin Liver Dis* 1998; **18:** 17–24.

115. Costabile RA, Hahn M, McLeod DG. Chronic orchialgia

in the pain prone patient: the clinical perspective. *Am Urol Assoc* 1991; **146:** 1571–4.

116. Lasson A, Fork FT, Ekberg O. Decision-making in postcholecystectomy pain and biliary dyskinesia. *Dig Dis* 1989; **7:** 288–300.

117. Bates T, Ebbs SR, Harrison M, A'Hern RP. Influence of cholecystectomy on symptoms. *Br J Surg* 1991; **78:** 964–7.

118. Jorgensen T, Teglbjerg JS, Wille-Jorgensen P, *et al.* Persisting pain after cholecystectomy. A prospective investigation. *Scand J Gastroenterol* 1991; **26:** 124–8.

119. Burton FR. Postcholecystectomy syndrome. How to determine if the sphincter of Oddi is the cause. *Postgrad Med* 1992; **91:** 255–8.

120. Schmalz MJ, Geenen JE, Hogan WJ, *et al.* Pain on common bile duct injection during ERCP: does it indicate sphincter of Oddi dysfunction? *Gastrointest Endosc* 1990; **36:** 358–61.

121. Bozkurt T, Orth KH, Butsch B, Lux G. Long-term clinical outcome of post-cholecystectomy patients with biliary-type pain: results of manometry, non-invasive techniques and endoscopic sphincteroplasty. *Eur J Gastroenterol Hepatol* 1996; **8:** 245–9.

122. Wehrmann T, Wirmer K, Lembcke B, *et al.* Do patients with sphincter of Oddi dysfunction benefit from endoscopic sphincterotomy? A 5 year prospective trial. *Eur J Gastroenterol Hepatol* 1996; **8:** 251–6.

123. Vincent C. Anorectal pain and irritation: anal fissure, levator syndrome, proctalgia fugax and pruritus ani. *Primary Care Clin Office Pract* 1999; **26:** 53–68.

124. Swain R. Oral clonidine for proctalgia fugax. *Gut* 1987; **28:** 1039–40.

125. Eckardt VFR, Dodt O, Kanzler G, Bernhard G. Treatment of proctalgia fugax with salbutamol inhalations. *Am J Gastroenterol* 1996; **91:** 686–9.

126. Merskey H, Bogduk N eds. *Classification of Chronic Pain*, 2nd edn. Seattle, WA: IASP Press, 1994.

127. Wein AJ, Hanno PM, Gillenwater JY. Interstitial cystitis: an introduction to the problem. In: Hanno *et al.* eds. *Interstitial Cystitis*. New York, NY: Springer-Verlag, 1990: 3–16.

128. Ness TJ, Gebhart GF. Visceral pain: a review of experimental studies. *Pain* 1990; **41:** 167–234.

43

Chronic pelvic pain

ANDREA J RAPKIN AND TRICIA E MARKUSEN

Chronic pelvic pain (CPP) can be defined as pelvic pain that persists for more than 6 months. It may occur in individuals with no apparent physical abnormalities or, if disease is present, the pain is frequently more pronounced than the degree of pathology might suggest. Maladaptive behavior is often present, including the presence of dysfunctional relationships, dependent personality disorders, and/or mood disturbances. Although it cannot be accurately measured, the impact of CPP on society as a whole is clearly significant, e.g. more than $881.5 million is spent each year on outpatient visits associated with CPP in the USA alone.[1] Despite the attention CPP receives, its etiology remains obscure, test results are typically inconclusive, and traditional treatment is often unsuccessful.[1] Furthermore, CPP patients are commonly perceived negatively by the medical professional as they are often considered to be drug seeking and difficult to treat. The purpose of this chapter is to review the pelvic anatomy, differential diagnosis, and management of chronic pelvic pain.

EPIDEMIOLOGY

The exact incidence of chronic pelvic pain is unknown. In the USA, an estimated 12–15% of women report signs and symptoms suggestive of CPP, or have been diagnosed with the disease.[1,2] Approximately 10% of referrals to gynecologists and 44% of laparoscopies are performed to evaluate CPP.[3,4] Furthermore, the impact of CPP on society is not be measured only by the amount spent on the

diagnosis and treatment of disease but also by the opportunity cost it exacts. For example, Mathias and colleagues reported a 45% reduction in work productivity and a 15% increase in time lost from work in women with CPP.[1]

ETIOLOGY AND PATHOPHYSIOLOGY

Neuroanatomy

Visceral innervation

Proper evaluation and treatment of CPP requires an understanding of the abdominopelvic anatomy and its innervation. The reproductive organs are innervated primarily by the sympathetic (thoracolumbar) and parasympathetic (sacral) systems, with contributions from the somatic sensory nervous system.[5,6] The visceral afferent fibers travel the same route as their corresponding efferent sympathetic and parasympathetic fibers. Table 43.1 lists the pelvic structures and their innervation. The afferent innervation of the upper vagina, cervix, uterus, proximal fallopian tubes, upper bladder, terminal ileum, and distal large bowel travels with the thoracolumbar sympathetics through the inferior hypogastric plexus to the hypogastric nerve to the superior hypogastric plexus and on to the lower thoracic and lumber splanchnic nerves which enter the spinal cord at T10–L1. Other pathways of afferent innervation from the pelvis travel via the pelvic (parasympathetic) splanchnic nerves (nervi erigentes) to S2–4. The perineum, anus, and pelvic floor muscles are supplied by somatic branches of the pudendal nerve (S2–4). Urogenital sinus structures, including the lower vagina, lower bladder, and rectosigmoid, are innervated by both the thoracolumbar and sacral afferents.[5]

The outer fallopian tube, ovary, and upper ureter are innervated by sympathetic nerves traveling with the ovarian artery, and enter the sympathetic nerve chain at L4, ascend with the chain, and enter the spinal cord at T9 and T10. Of importance, one should appreciate:

1   The overlap of innervation among the reproductive, genitourinary, and gastrointestinal systems, via the sympathetic nerves to spinal segments T10–L1.
2   The lower abdominal wall, lower back, anterior vulva, urethra, and clitoris share a common innervation via L1 and L2 and are therefore the region of referred pain for the pelvic viscera.
3   The afferents from the ovary and outer fallopian tube bypass the inferior hypogastric nerve and superior hypogastric plexus, of which the latter is the site for presacral neurectomy.

Somatic versus visceral pain

The origin of pain in CPP may arise from a visceral disorder [which may then be referred to a specific dermatome(s)], or it may arise directly from the musculature or somatic nerves supplying the abdomen, pelvic floor, or perineum. The neurophysiology of pain transmission from the viscera (internal organs such as bowel, bladder, rectum, uterus, ovaries, and fallopian tubes) differs from that of somatic structures (cutaneous elements, fascia, muscles, parietal peritoneum, external genitalia, anus, and urethra). Visceral pain, in contrast to somatic pain, is usually deep, difficult to localize, and in an acute process is frequently associated with various autonomic reflexes such as restlessness, nausea, vomiting, and diaphoresis.[7] However, visceral pain can evoke a somatic component secondary to the viscerosomatic convergence of the visceral and somatic nerves at the level of the sec-

ond-order neurons in the dorsal horn. In the dorsal horn, these neurons receive input from somatic afferents or a combination of both somatic and visceral afferents. There is, therefore, a tremendous impact of somatic input at this level, which helps to explain the phenomenon of referred pain.

The type of pain receptor in the periphery further defines visceral and somatic responses to painful stimuli. Pain evoked at somatic nerves is received by nociceptors, whereas nonspecific wide dynamic range receptors are predominant in the viscera.[8,9] Visceral pain therefore likely evolves from enhanced pain sensitivity associated with repetitive or increasingly intense stimuli. For example, the repeated distention of the rat uterine horn or application of algesic agents has been shown to produce increased responsiveness of hypogastric afferent fibers.[10]

Knowledge of the innervation of the specific pelvic organs can provide further insight into the etiology of the primary disease. Acute and chronic gynecologic pain conditions are characterized by referred pain to the dermatomes associated with pelvic organ innervation, i.e. T10–L2 (anterior abdominal wall and anterior thighs) and dorsal rami of L1–L2 (lower back).[11–13] Referred pain is well localized, superficial in location, and appears to arise in the same spinal cord segment receiving the pain input.

Neuronal modulation

An important site of neuronal modulation of pain (and likely critical in the pathogenesis of chronic pelvic pain) is the dorsal horn, where neural cell bodies receive afferent input from somatic and visceral structures. Evidence from animal studies indicates that supraspinal factors can interact at the level of the dorsal horn to modulate the sensory perception of pain from the pelvic viscera.[14,15] Also, neuropeptides and neurotransmitters, including serotonin, substance P, and opiates, can further modulate pain perception.[16] Other factors that can influence pain presentation stem from variations in the

Table 43.1 *Pelvic structures and their innervation*

Organ	Spinal segment	Nerves
Outer two-thirds of fallopian tubes, upper ureter	T9–10	Thoracolumbar splanchnic nerves through mesenteric plexus
Ovaries	T9–10	Thoracolumbar splanchnic nerves traveling with ovarian vessels via renal and aortic plexus and celiac and mesenteric ganglia
Uterine fundus, proximal fallopian tubes, broad ligament, upper bladder, cecum, appendix, terminal large bowel	T11–12, L1	Thoracolumbar splanchnic nerves through uterine and hypogastric plexus
Lower abdominal wall	L1–2	Iliohypogastric, ilioinguinal
Perineum, vulva, lower vagina, anus, rectum	L1–L2, S2–S4	Pudendal, ilioinguinal, genitofemoral, posterior femoral cutaneous, anococcygeal
Upper vagina, cervix, lower uterine segment, posterior urethra, bladder trigone, uterosacral and cardinal ligaments, rectosigmoid, lower ureters	S2–S4	Sacral afferents traveling through the pelvic plexus

pelvic neural anatomy. Prior to entering the dorsal horn, the axons from the afferent nerves may extend upward or downward two or more spinal cord segments along the paravertebral ganglion, thus innervating a different dermatome. Further, intermingling of afferent nerve fibers from different visceral nerve plexuses (i.e. afferent fibers from the uterovaginal plexus and inferior hypogastric plexus may communicate with the ovarian plexus) can influence how pain presents. Crosstalk is another mechanism whereby pain presentation may be altered. With crosstalk, nociceptive stimuli (electrical potentials) from adjacent poorly myelinated or unmyelinated nerves (Aδ- and C-fibers) can incite messages in adjacent unmyelinated nerves originating from other viscera, thus evoking a pain response.[16] The role of the parasympathetic system in the transmission of painful stimuli is not fully known, however its main function is in the control and sensation of micturition, defecation, and reflex regulation of the reproductive organs.[5] The transmission of painful stimuli therefore relies on an intact sympathetic system with modulation of the pain by peripheral and central factors, including psychological factors.

Peripheral causes of chronic pelvic pain

The differential diagnosis of CPP encompasses many organ systems. It is therefore important to assess other pelvic anatomic structures in addition to the reproductive organs. Table 43.2 lists the differential diagnosis of the peripheral (noncentral) components of pelvic pain.

Gynecologic: noncyclic

Adhesions
Incidence The precise role of adhesions in the genesis of CPP is unclear. Several studies have investigated the incidence of adhesions in patients undergoing laparoscopy for CPP, with adhesions reported in 16–51% of cases.[17-21] The marked variation in incidence of adhesions noted in these studies may relate to the use of dissimilar control groups and/or a failure to recognize other causes of "occult" pelvic pain (abdominal wall or pelvic floor muscle pain, pelvic congestion, irritable bowel syndrome, and interstitial cystitis) prior to laparoscopy. Kresch and colleagues[19] retrospectively compared 100 women with chronic pelvic pain with 50 women undergoing laparoscopy for sterilization. Adhesions were present in 51% of CPP patients compared with 14% in the sterilization group. The adhesions in the CPP group more often involved bowel.[19] Keltz *et al.* in a combined retrospective/prospective study found colon-to-sidewall adhesions in a higher proportion of patients (93% versus 13%) with pelvic pain than the control group (sterilization).[22] Rapkin, however, reported adhesions in 26% of CPP patients and 39% of asymptomatic infertility patients, with no significant differences in the location or density of adhesions

between the two groups.[18] In summary, although women with CPP have a higher prevalence of adhesions than women undergoing sterilization, one cannot confidently conclude that these findings are causal, or even highly associated with CPP, as other populations (i.e. infertility patients) have been demonstrated to have higher adhesion rates.

Symptoms and signs Abdominal/pelvic pain in women with adhesions is generally noncyclical, and commonly associated with dyspareunia. A clinical presentation synonymous with partial or complete obstruction of the bowel may be seen. Uterine immobility and adnexal mass/tenderness may be noted during physical examination.[23]

Diagnosis Diagnosis is by exploratory laparoscopy or laparotomy. The new technique, known as "pain mapping" (office microlaparoscopy with local anesthesia/conscious sedation), may allow physicians to better locate the adhesions associated with pelvic pain. In an observational pain mapping study of 50 women under local anesthesia, manipulation of appendiceal and pelvic adhesions was observed to contribute significantly to pelvic pain.[24] However, correlation between lysis of adhesions or removal of these adhesions and long term pain outcome has yet to be established.

Treatment The mechanism by which adhesions contribute to chronic pain is thought to be secondary to the restriction of bowel mobility and distention.[25] Therefore, adhesiolysis should improve subjective pain symptoms; indeed, in several retrospective, noncontrolled studies, pain was improved in 50–90% of these patients.[25-29] However, some "adhesions" may be physiologic, such as the tethering of the ileum and ascending colon to the right sidewall and sigmoid colon to the left sidewall. Peters and colleagues performed the only randomized controlled study of adhesiolysis for the treatment of pelvic pain and found that surgery did not benefit those women with mild or moderate degrees of pelvic adhesions.[30] Forty-eight women with CPP and laparoscopically confirmed stage III or IV adhesions were randomized to undergo laparotomy or expectant management. Nine to 12 months postoperatively, pain response was evaluated. Adhesiolysis was of no more benefit than expectant management, except in those patients with severe, vascularized, and dense adhesions involving the serosa of the small bowel and, to a lesser extent, the colon. These patients tended to have symptoms and physical findings consistent with intermittent partial small bowel obstruction.[30] The patient's degree of psychosocial functioning may also influence the effectiveness of adhesiolysis. For example, Steege and Scott, in a small ($n = 30$), prospective, but nonrandomized, noncontrolled study found that after 8 months chronic pelvic pain patients with "CPP syndrome" had not benefited from surgery.[31] They defined women with

Table 43.2 *Peripheral causes of chronic pelvic pain*

Gynecologic	Infectious diarrhea
Noncyclic	Recurrent partial small bowel obstruction
Adhesions	Diverticulitis
Endometriosis	Hernia
Salpingo-oophoritis	Abdominal angina
Ovarian remnant syndrome	Recurrent appendiceal colic
Pelvic congestion syndrome (varicosities)	
Ovarian neoplasms	*Genitourinary*
Pelvic relaxation	Recurrent or relapsing systourethritis
Cyclic	Urethral syndrome
Primary dysmenorrhea	Interstitial cystitis
Secondary dysmenorrhea	Ureteral diverticula or polyps
Imperforate hymen or transverse vaginal septum	Carcinoma of the bladder
Cervical stenosis	Ureteral obstruction
Uterine anomalies (congenital malformation,	Pelvic kidney
bicornuate uterus, blind uterine horn)	
Intrauterine synechiae (Asherman syndrome)	*Neurologic*
Endometrial polyps	Nerve entrapment syndrome
Uterine leiomyoma	Neuroma
Adenomyosis	Trigger points
Pelvic congestion syndrome (varicosities)	
Endometriosis	*Musculoskeletal*
Atypical cyclic	Low back pain syndrome
Endometriosis	Myofascial syndrome
Adenomyosis	Fibromyalgia
Ovarian remnant syndrome	Pelvic floor muscle tension/spasm or trigger points
Chronic functional ovarian cyst formation	Hernia
Gastrointestinal	*Systemic*
Irritable bowel syndrome	Acute intermittent porphyria
Ulcerative colitis	Abdominal migraine
Granulomatous colitis (Crohn's disease)	Systemic lupus erythematosus
Carcinoma	Lymphoma
	Neurofibromatosis

CPP syndrome as those presenting with four or more of the following: (1) pain duration >6 months; (2) incomplete relief by previous treatments; (3) impaired physical functioning secondary to pain; (4) vegetative signs of depression; and (5) altered family roles.

Prevention Postoperative adhesions occur in 60–90% of patients following major pelvic surgery.[23,32] Animal and human studies have been used to evaluate various procedures designed to reduce adhesion formation. The benefits of corticosteroids, nonsteroidal anti-inflammatory drugs, irrigation, barrier methods [oxidized cellulose ("Interceed"), polytetrafluoroethylene (PTFE, known as "Gore-Tex")] and early second-look laparoscopy 1–2 weeks following surgery have been examined.[32,33] At this time, meticulous surgical technique is the only recommendation for prevention.

Endometriosis

Incidence The incidence of endometriosis varies with the population studied. In the general female population, prevalence is estimated at approximately 10%, and with infertile women it is 15–25%. Of those patients with CPP, endometriosis has been noted in 28–74% of women

undergoing diagnostic laparoscopy.[18–21,34] Overall, the exact prevalence of endometriosis is unknown, in part owing to the fact that diagnosis is typically only made during surgery. In the past decade, the incidence has increased, perhaps reflecting the increasing use of laparoscopy and greater awareness of various types of endometriotic lesions.[35] Endometriosis may present in any age group (from adolescents to postmenopausal women on hormonal therapy), however most diagnoses are made in women in their thirties or forties.[36,37]

Etiology In women with endometriosis, endometrial glands and stroma are located outside the uterine cavity, most commonly at the cul-de-sac, ovaries, and the pelvic visceral and parietal peritoneum. The favored theory, proposed by Sampson in the 1920s, is that endometriosis results from retrograde menses with implantation of endometrium on the peritoneum and nearby organs. Retrograde menses occur in 70–90% of women, however endometriosis does not necessarily result. It may be that reduced immune function contributes to the progression of endometriosis.[38] Proliferation occurs with each menstrual cycle, with resultant inflammation, scarring, fibrosis, and adhesion formation. Thus, the risk of endometriosis is thought to increase with abnormal menstrual activity, such as shorter menstrual cycle, menorrhagia, obstruction to outflow, and reduced parity.[37] The appropriate hormonal environment further permits proliferation. Further theories include celomic metaplasia of the peritoneum and hematogenous/lymphatic spread to extrapelvic sites.[38]

Symptoms and signs The most common symptoms of endometriosis are:

- Dysmenorrhea: pelvic pain may or may not be associated with menstruation, although most commonly it is most intense with menses and may start 7 days prior. Pain is sharp/pressure-like and located in the lower abdomen, back, and rectum.
- Deep dyspareunia.
- Infertility: although not necessarily associated with pelvic pain.
- Abnormal uterine bleeding: usually from a secretory endometrium.
- Nongynecologic symptoms: dyschezia or cyclic hematochezia with involvement of intestine/rectum. Urinary urgency, frequency, bladder pain, and hematuria with urinary tract involvement. Patients may occasionally develop bowel or ureteral obstruction.

Classic physical findings with endometriosis include uterosacral nodularity and focal tenderness on rectovaginal examination. This reflects the prevalence of posterior cul-de-sac disease. With severe disease, fibrosis can result in a fixed, retroverted uterus. Adnexal masses may be palpated, consistent with an endometrioma.[38]

Diagnosis A definitive diagnosis of endometriosis is made by laparoscopy or laparotomy.[39] On surveying the pelvis and abdomen, typical endometriotic lesions (from the early, active petechial lesions to the older and less active powder-burn, fibrotic lesions) may be visualized.[40] These findings may be present to help confirm the clinical diagnosis of endometriosis that is accurate approximately 50% of the time.[35] Histologic confirmation is approximately 60%.[41] Deep infiltrating lesions are most prevalent in the pouch of Douglas and the uterosacral ligaments and may cause pain by stimulating nerve endings.[41] Other diagnostic options include ultrasound, however this is limited to diagnosis of ovarian endometriomas, and an elevated CA-125 and erythrocyte sedimentation rate (ESR), however the specificity is low.

Treatment The chronic, recurring nature of endometriosis makes effective treatment difficult. However, there are several medical and surgical options available. Untreated, minimal to moderate endometriosis may progress in 30% of patients, regress in 30%, or remain static in 40%.[42] With medical treatment, the goal is to induce a pseudomenopause or pseudopregnancy state to reduce the hormonal/cyclic stimulation of endometriotic lesions.

Initial therapy often includes a short trial of cyclic or oral contraceptive pills. If unsuccessful, high-dose progestins, androgenic hormones (danazol), or gonadotropin-releasing hormone (GnRH) agonists are used to induce atrophy of implants.[38] Bergqvist and colleagues in a randomized double-blind controlled trial looked at 6-month GnRH-agonist therapy in 48 women with laparoscopically confirmed endometriosis. At follow-up, decreased pain was associated with GnRH-agonist treatment as well as a decrease in the size of the endometriotic lesions.[43] GnRH-agonist therapy may be initiated without laparoscopically confirmed endometriosis if it is clinically suspected. Hormonal add-back therapy (i.e. norethindrone acetate 2–5 mg daily with or without estrogen) has also been utilized to prevent the long-term hypoestrogenic side-effects (bone loss) of long-term (12 months) therapy, with continued relief of pelvic pain.[44] However, with long-term discontinuation of GnRH-agonist treatment, recurrence of symptoms may return in up to 36–75% of patients over a 5-year period, most commonly in patients with severe disease.[45]

Surgical intervention involves laparotomy or, commonly now, laparoscopy. At the time of the diagnostic laparoscopy, electrodissection, laser vaporization, or excision should be performed to remove lesions. Endometriomas should be removed with their capsule to prevent recurrence. In a prospective, randomized, double-blind study with 63 women, laparoscopic laser treatment was noted to benefit 90% of those women who initially responded at 1-year follow-up.[42] A more radical approach in women who have finished childbearing includes total abdominal hysterectomy with bilateral salpingo-oophorectomy, appendectomy, and removal of any residual gastrointestinal, genitourinary, or peritoneal disease. Additional benefit in pain reduction may be derived from adjunctive acupuncture or multidisciplinary pain management (Table 43.3).[46]

Outcome with respect to CPP The relationship of endometriosis to chronic pelvic pain is unclear as endometriosis is a common finding in reproductive-age women without pain, and other pathology (i.e. adhesions, pelvic floor muscle spasm, abdominal wall pain) may be simultaneously present.[39] Furthermore, the severity of disease does not significantly correlate with the degree of pain.[47,48] However, vaginal and uterosacral endometriosis was associated with complaints of deep dyspareunia.[48] In contrast, Stovall *et al.* found at a mean follow-up of 15 years in a population of 48 reproductive-age women that stage of disease was associated with persistence and intensity of chronic pelvic pain.[49] Furthermore, deeply infiltrating lesions, particularly of the uterosacral ligaments, was strongly associated with pain.[41] In summary, pain that is not cyclical and/or does not respond to adequate surgical and medical management of endometriosis should be reevaluated for another source of pain and/or other contributing factors.

Table 43.3 *Treatment approach when endometriosis suspected*

Trial of low-dose monophasic combination oral contraceptive pills (one pill/day for 3–6 months)

If no improvement, 3-month therapy with a GnRH agonist; if pain improves continue for 3 additional months, may consider hormonal add-back therapy

Surgery to evaluate for pathology if no improvement with GnRH agonist
    Excision/thermal ablation/laser of endometriotic lesions
    Excision of endometriomas
    ± Presacral neurectomy (for central pain)
    ± Hysterectomy and bilateral salpingo-oophorectomy

Endometriosis confirmed; hormonal management with one of following if pain persists/recurs following surgery:
    Continuous monophasic oral contraceptive pills to induce amenorrhea
    Progestins
        Medroxyprogesterone acetate (MPA) 30 mg p.o. q.d.
        Depot MPA 150 mg i.m. q.3mo.
        Megestrol 40 mg p.o. q.d.
        Norethindrone acetate 2–5 p.o. q.d.
    Danazol 400–800 mg p.o. q.d.
    GnRH agonist
        Nafarelin 200–400 µg intranasal b.i.d.
        Leuprolide 3.75 mg i.m. q.mo. or 11.25 mg i.m. q.3mo.
            ± add-back therapy with norethindrone 2–5 mg p.o. q.d. or conjugated/esterified estrogen 0.625 mg p.o. q.d. and MPA 2.5 mg p.o. q.d.

Multidisciplinary pain management – may be considered early in the management

Pelvic congestion

Pathophysiology The syndrome of pelvic congestion was first proposed in the 1950s by Taylor, who stated that autonomic nervous system dysfunction from emotional stress could cause smooth muscle spasm and congestion of the ovarian and uterine–pelvic venous plexes.[50] The pelvic venous system has a rich network of anastomoses in which most veins are without valves or may develop incompetent valves. Beard investigated the prevalence of pelvic venous congestion in a blinded study on patients with CPP with no obvious cause during laparoscopy. On transuterine pelvic venography, women with CPP had a larger (three times) mean ovarian vein diameter, delayed disappearance of contrast medium, and greater ovarian plexus congestion than in the control population.[51,52] In a small, single-blind, crossover study, the vasoconstrictor dihydroergotamine was found to decrease pelvic vein diameter by 35% and lead to significantly reduced pelvic pain.[53] Other substances may be important as well in controlling vascular tone and pain, including the local vasodilator peptide hormone substance P, which has been isolated to the endothelium of pelvic veins.[54]

Symptoms and signs Beard et al. reviewed the clinical presentation associated with pelvic congestion in 35 women documented to have pelvic congestion on venography compared with women with pelvic pain of classic pathology.[51] These women were more likely to present with:

- dull/aching lower pelvic pain (unilateral or bilateral) accentuated with postural changes and ambulation;
- pain exacerbated by menstruation and coitus;

- gastrointestinal symptoms not characteristic of irritable bowel syndrome;
- genitourinary symptoms without evidence of infection;
- significant emotional disturbance;
- vulvar varices;
- tenderness over the adnexa, uterus, parametria, and especially the uterosacral ligaments.[50,51]

Beard *et al.* found that the combination of abdominal tenderness over the ovarian point and history of postcoital ache was 94% sensitive and 77% specific for women with pelvic congestion.[51]

Diagnosis Prior to carrying out invasive measures, symptomatic treatment to differentiate gastrointestinal, genitourinary, or myofascial etiology of CPP should be performed. Different techniques are now available to diagnose pelvic congestion:

- Transuterine venogram: radio-opaque material is used to evaluate venous diameter, venous congestion, and time for contrast material to disappear.[52] Other techniques for venography include transfemoral ovarian vein catheterization and injection of vulvar varices.
- Transvaginal ultrasound: imaging associated with pelvic congestion includes uterine enlargement, thickened endometrium, cystic ovaries, and dilated pelvic veins. The response of pelvic vein diameter to vasoconstrictors can be monitored.[55,56]

- Magnetic resonance imaging (MRI).[57]
- Laparoscopy: pelvic pain patients with no evidence of pelvic pathology at laparoscopy may have pelvic congestion.[52] False negatives at the time of laparoscopy may occur secondary to elevated intra-abdominal pressure, Trendelenburg position associated with the procedure, and the retroperitoneal location of the vessels.

Treatment Hormonal suppression with medroxyprogesterone acetate (MPA) has been demonstrated to improve the symptoms of pelvic congestion.[58,59] One placebo-controlled study noted a 73% reduction in pain with MPA (30 mg daily for 4 months) compared with a 33% reduction with placebo.[58] Pain improvement was maintained at 1 year if cognitive–behavioral therapy was also utilized. Another study, although not controlled, demonstrated a 75% improvement in pain following treatment with MPA 30 mg daily for 6 months. The women noting improvement had a corresponding decrease in venous congestion documented by venography.[59] Oral contraceptive pills have not been proven to be effective in treatment of pelvic congestion.[60] Studies are needed to investigate the benefit of GnRH analogs.

Several small, noncontrolled studies have looked at transcatheter embolization of pelvic veins with good short-term success.[61–63] Further studies, however, are indicated to evaluate the risks and long-term benefits.

Surgical treatment often includes bilateral ovarian vein ligation and excision or ligation of collateral vessels, but long-term studies are not available. Hysterectomy with bilateral salpingo-oophorectomy may be considered in women who have failed medical management. In a prospective study, 12 of 36 women on hormone replacement therapy following a hysterectomy with bilateral salpingo-oophrectomy (for pelvic congestion) were noted to have residual pain at 1-year follow-up. One had continued pain severe enough to affect her daily activities.[64]

Ovarian remnant syndrome

Pathophysiology The ovarian remnant syndrome is a relatively rare complication resulting from ovarian cortical tissue being left *in situ* during a difficult hysterectomy and bilateral salpingo-oophorectomy, generally in the setting of extensive adhesions.[65,66] In this situation, the remnants of the ovarian tissue may become functional and cystic, producing symptoms of pelvic pain.[67]

Symptoms and signs Pelvic pain, usually arising 2–5 years after surgery, is often cyclic, accompanied by flank pain. The pain may be described as sharp and stabbing or as constant, dull, and nonradiating. Associated genitourinary and gastrointestinal symptoms may coexist.[68] Pelvic examination may reveal a tender mass in the lateral region of the pelvis.

Diagnosis The diagnosis is suspected on the basis of history, physical examination, and hormonal evalua-

tion.[65,69] Generally, these women have undergone multiple extensive pelvic–abdominal surgeries in the past for pelvic inflammatory disease, endometriosis, inflammatory bowel disease, and appendectomy.[69] In a patient who has had a bilateral salpingo-oophorectomy and is not on hormone replacement, premenopausal levels of estradiol and follicle-stimulating hormone (FSH) levels should be present, although on occasion the remaining ovarian tissue may not be active enough to suppress FSH levels. Clomiphene citrate may be used to stimulate ovarian tissue to enhance diagnosis by ultrasound. Computed tomography (CT) and MRI have not been extensively studied for their utility.

Treatment Hormonal therapy may be utilized to suppress the ovarian remnant. GnRH agonists have shown superior results over oral contraceptives, progestins, and danazol in providing relief. The patients who achieved relief with the GnRH agonist were also noted to have subsequent relief with surgery.[70]

Exploratory laparotomy is the method of choice for removal of residual ovarian tissue.[71] At the time of surgery, careful ureterolysis by retroperitoneal dissection should be performed to prevent ureteral damage during excision of the remnant tissue. Surgical management via laparoscopy is controversial given the presence of extensive adhesions and potential complications, including hemorrhage, ureteral, bladder, and bowel damage.[68] Recurrent remnants occur in 15% of cases.

Tumors and cysts of the reproductive organs/salpingo-oophoritis

Other gynecologic pathology that may present with symptoms of chronic discomfort include adnexal masses, uterine leiomyomata, or salpingo-oophoritis. Vague lower abdominal discomfort and fullness and bladder or gastrointestinal symptoms may be related to leiomyomata or an ovarian neoplasm. On examination, a pelvic mass is generally palpated, which is confirmed by ultrasound. A myomectomy or hysterectomy may be therapeutic for myomata, especially if associated with abnormal bleeding or if uterine size is greater than 14 cm.

Salpingo-oophoritis generally presents as an acute process. Chronic pelvic pain can develop secondary to past salpingo-oophoritis in the setting of adhesion formation, causing restriction of pelvic organs and stretching of the pelvic peritoneum.[72] Therefore, it is important to accurately diagnose and treat the acute process. Diagnosis is made by clinical criteria proposed by Sweet and Gibbs.[73] Two of the three must be present: lower abdominal pain as well as lower abdominal tenderness (with or without rebound), cervical motion tenderness, and adnexal tenderness. In addition, one of the following minor criteria must be present: (1) temperature greater than 38°C, leukocytosis (>10,500 white blood cells/mm^3); (2) culdocentesis fluid containing white cells and bacteria on Gram stain; (3) presence of an inflammatory mass; (4) elevated ESR; (5) a Gram stain from the endocervix revealing Gram-negative intracellular diplococci; or (6) a monoclonal smear from the endocervical secretions revealing *Chlamydia* or gonorrhea. However, clinical diagnosis leads to error in 50% of the cases,[73] and in repeated episodes of pain suggestive of salpingo-oophoritis laparoscopy may be performed to verify the diagnosis, cultures should be taken, and lysis of adhesions performed.

Gynecologic: cyclic pelvic pain

Cyclic pelvic pain is most commonly described as dysmenorrhea or painful menses. It is a common disorder of the female reproductive tract and affects approximately 50% of menstruating women.[74] Dysmenorrhea may be described as primary or secondary depending on its etiology. Primary dysmenorrhea refers to pain with menses in the absence of an underlying pathology; secondary dysmenorrhea refers to pain in the presence of an underlying disorder such as adenomyosis or endometriosis.

Pathophysiology
Several mechanisms likely exist to activate the thoracolumbar and pelvic afferents associated with dysmenorrhea. These include: (1) myometrial contractions leading to intense intrauterine pressure and uterine hypoxia; (2) hyperproduction of leukotrienes and other hormonal factors which increase afferent terminal excitability; (3) altered central nervous system (CNS) processing of the afferent barrage possibly mediated by opioid or γ-aminobutyric acid (GABA)-ergic mediations; and (4) environmental and behavioral factors.[75] In primary dysmenorrhea, an increase in endometrial prostaglandin production is also seen in the secretory phase of the cycle.[75]

Symptoms and signs
The diagnosis of cyclic pain often depends on the review of a daily pain and menstrual diary to confirm the cyclic nature of the pain. In primary dysmenorrhea, onset of pain generally occurs approximately 1 year following menarche when ovulatory cycles are established. The pain starts near or at the onset of menses, lasting for 48–72 h, is suprapubic and cramping, radiating to the lumbosacral region and anterior thighs. Associated gastrointestinal symptoms including nausea, vomiting, and diarrhea are common. In secondary dysmenorrhea, usually years after menarche, pain may occur up to 2 weeks prior to the onset of menses and last till the cessation of menses. Pain may further occur with anovulatory cycles after menarche. In primary dysmenorrhea, the physical examination is unremarkable, although at the time of dysmenorrhea some suprapubic and uterine tenderness is common. In secondary dysmenorrhea, careful pelvic examination may reveal abnormalities in adnexal structures, uterine size, contour, mobility and/or tenderness, and nodularity of the uterosacral ligaments and rectovaginal septum.

Diagnosis
Evaluation includes cervical cultures to rule out gonorrhea or *Chlamydia* infection, a complete blood count, and ESR. Transvaginal ultrasound may suggest a secondary disorder for the cyclic pain.

Treatment
The standard treatment for primary dysmenorrhea is prostaglandin synthetase inhibitors. Dosing requires around-the-clock administration every 6–8 h at the onset of menses or just prior to pain for the first few days of menses. Treatment is effective in up to 80% of the cases.[76] Further benefit may be obtained by adding an oral contraceptive pill with relief noted in more than 90%.[77] High-dose oral or depot progestins and GnRH agonists (with low-dose add-back therapy) are other forms of hormonal suppression.[78] If more aggressive medical therapy including narcotic analgesia is necessary, an operative procedure such as laparoscopy and, if indicated, hysteroscopy should be performed to evaluate for a possible secondary cause of pain. Other alternative forms of treatment include acupuncture or transcutaneous electrical nerve stimulation (TENS).[79–81] Kaplan and colleagues reported a 30% marked pain relief, 60% moderate pain relief, and 10% no relief in women with primary dysmenorrhea undergoing TENS.[81] Therefore, TENS may provide an adjuvant therapy to pharmacological intervention in treating primary dysmenorrhea. Again, if treatment fails, laparoscopy is warranted to rule out secondary dysmenorrhea, in particular endometriosis.

Surgical management should be implemented once conservative medical managements have failed or if an underlying disorder is anticipated. Surgical approaches to dysmenorrhea include laparoscopic uterosacral ligament ablation, presacral neurectomy, and, in selected cases of secondary dysmenorrhea, hysterectomy.[82,83] These interventions are further discussed later in this chapter.

Gastroenterologic causes of chronic pelvic pain

Gastrointestinal disease may mimic the features of chronic pelvic pain. Many of the patients referred to gynecologists with chronic pelvic pain actually have gastroenterologic pathology.[84,85] This stems from the common innervation tract (T10–L1) between the cervix, uterus, adnexa, and lower ileum, sigmoid colon, and rectum. It is therefore often difficult to determine whether lower abdominal pain is of gynecologic or of enterocolic origin.[86] In addition, as is true with other types of visceral pain, pain sensation from the gastrointestinal tract (GI) tract is often diffuse and poorly localized. The differential diagnosis and management of pain of enterocolic origin is presented in Chapter Ch42.[87–91]

Endometriosis affecting the bowel

Implantation of endometriotic lesions on the intestine can cause cyclic abdominal pain. In severe cases, partial or complete bowel obstruction may develop. Laparoscopy confirms the diagnosis. The incidence of a significant bowel involvement in women with endometriosis is approximately 5%.

Hernia

Although infrequent in the female population, the presence of an abdominal wall hernia in a patient with chronic pelvic pain should be included in the differential diagnosis.[92] These include inguinal (indirect or direct), femoral, spigelian, incisional, and umbilical. Symptoms and signs include history of a mass in the groin and pain or discomfort with an increase in intra-abdominal pressure. On examination, a mass may or may not be appreciated. If the history is suggestive, a diagnostic laparoscopy should be performed to evaluate for weakness in the peritoneum adjacent to the round ligament (indirect), at Hasselbach's triangle (direct), or just below the iliopubic tract above Cooper's ligament (femoral). Spigelian hernias result from a defect through the transversalis fascia, just lateral to rectus muscle at the level of the semicircular line of Douglas.[93] Incisional hernias occur generally at fascial defects with vertical incisions. Other types of hernias include sciatic hernias secondary to atrophy of the piriformis muscle, which may include the ipsilateral ovary in its hernia sac, and perineal hernias (cystocele, rectocele, and enterocele).[94] Treatment of abdominal hernias includes surgical repair through the laparoscope or through a skin incision. Perineal hernias are repaired surgically or a pessary may be used for more conservative management.

Urologic causes of chronic pelvic pain

Pathophysiology

Many chronic pelvic pain cases are primary urinary tract disorders.[84,95] Therefore, complete evaluation of chronic pelvic pain involves obtaining an in-depth history of urinary signs and symptoms. The overlap in clinical presentation in part relates to the close development and anatomic relationship of the urinary and genital tracts. The urethra bladder, vagina, and vestibule are all derived from the embryologic urogenital sinus and they have a similar neurologic innervation. In certain circumstances, one may see urologic symptoms stemming from a primary gynecologic cause, including bladder and ureteral involvement of endometriosis or external bladder compression with a uterine leiomyomata.

The differential diagnosis in urologic causes of chronic pelvic pain should include:

1 *Recurrent infectious cystitis* Complaints of suprapubic pain, dysuria, frequency, and urgency are the classic presentation of cystitis. Microscopic analysis with pyuria and a positive urine culture are diagnostic. In cases of recurrent infection, repeat culture will aid in diagnosis and management. Further history should be elicited to determine the etiology; if associated with intercourse, voiding following intercourse and prophylactic antibiotics may be used after coitus. Recurrent infections in peri- and postmenopausal women may benefit from vaginal estrogen cream by altering the vaginal pH and modifying the vaginal flora.[96] *Chlamydia* infection is responsible for about 25% of cases of pyuria and urethritis in women with a sterile urine culture.[95]

2 *Urethral syndrome*
   a *Etiology.* The diagnosis of urethral syndrome is one of exclusion. Its unknown etiology makes the diagnosis and treatment difficult. Subclinical infection, chronic inflammation of the periurethral glands, or urethral spasticity with periurethral muscle fatigue have been suggested as possible etiologies.
   b *Symptoms and signs.* Classically, urethral syndrome presents with irritative lower urinary tract symptoms – dysuria, suprapubic discomfort, urinary frequency, and dyspareunia.[95,97] Voiding dysfunction such as stranguria, the slow and painful discharge of urine, may occur. A careful physical examination should be performed to evaluate for possible structural causes of pain. The urethra should be evaluated for discharge, tenderness, or a mass suggestive or a urethral diverticulum or Skene's cyst.
   c *Diagnosis.* Diagnostic studies include urinalysis with urine culture and sensitivity urethral evaluation for *Chlamydia* or *Mycoplasma* infection and a wet mount for infectious or atrophic vaginitis.
   d *Treatment.* Treatment may consist of reeducation of voiding habits through pelvic floor muscle biofeedback,[95] antibiotic therapy with doxycycline or erythromycin for 10–14 days if *Chlamydia* is suspected, or chronic suppression with a 3- to 6-month low-dose course of broad-spectrum antibiotics. Urethral dilation has been performed in recalcitrant cases. In a prospective study, Bergman and colleagues assigned 60 women to serial urethral dilation, antibiotic treatment or placebo. Seventy-five percent of women in the urethral dilation group had absence of symptoms, which was significantly higher than in the placebo (20%) or tetracycline group (50%). Improvement in the uroflowmetry dynamics was also noted only in the dilation group.[97] Vaginal estrogen for peri- and postmenopausal women should also supplement treatment.[97] Other treatments have included muscle relaxants, α-antagonists (terazosin and doxazosin), and psychotherapy.

3 *Interstitial cystitis.* This is a symptom complex characterized by pelvic pain, urinary urgency, urinary frequency, and nocturia.[98]

a *Symptoms and signs.* Symptoms of dyspareunia and perimenstrual exacerbation with negative laboratory studies are consistent with both interstitial cystitis (IC) and urgency/frequency syndrome.[99] The NIH Consensus Criteria from 1988 for the diagnosis of IC includes at least two of the following: pain on bladder filling relieved by emptying; pain in the suprapubic, pelvic, urethral, vaginal, or perineal region; glomerulations on endoscopy or decreased compliance on cystometrogram.[100] Symptoms that do not meet IC criteria can be termed urgency/frequency syndrome.

b *Etiology.* The etiology of interstitial cystitis is unknown. However, it is likely multifactorial. Factors likely contributing to its pathogenesis include infections, autoimmune disorders, inflammatory conditions, alterations in the glycosaminoglycan layer of the bladder mucosa, and activated bladder sensory neuropeptides.[100]

c *Diagnosis.* Diagnostic evaluation involves cystoscopy with or without hydrodistension and biopsy under general or regional anesthesia. Petechial bladder mucosal hemorrhages (glomerulations) are characteristically seen. Hunner's ulcers and reduced bladder capacity (less than 850 cm³) are less common, but demonstrate more severe disease.

d *Treatment.* Treatment is empiric and for symptomatic improvement as most therapies are less than optimal. First-line therapy includes antihistamines, tricyclic antidepressants, or pentosan polysulfate sodium (PPS), which is Food and Drug Administration (FDA) approved for the treatment of IC.[101] Dimethyl sulfoxide (DMSO) is second-line therapy and is given intravesically, with or without hydrocortisone, heparin, bicarbonate, or lidocaine (lignocaine). Other intravesical therapies exist and include such agents as bacillus Calmette–Guerin (BCG), interferon, and hyaluronic acid (Systistat).[101] Other nonconventional therapies include a special bladder diet (Table 43.4), TENS, physical therapy, biofeedback to the pelvic floor muscles, sacral nerve stimulation, or repeated anesthetic blocks (hypogastric plexus).

4 *Carcinoma.* Infiltrating carcinomas of the bladder, cervix, uterus, or rectum may also present as severe suprapubic pain. These conditions should be apparent after performing the history, pelvic examination, urine analysis with cytology, and cystoscopy, although intravenous pyelogram (IVP) or CT urogram may be necessary.

Neurologic and musculoskeletal causes of chronic pelvic pain

Low back pain is a common complaint found in many different patient populations. In women with chronic pelvic pain, isolated back pain without pelvic pain is rarely

Table 43.4 *Diet for irritative voiding symptoms*

List A (foods to *avoid*)	List B (foods to substitute for list A foods)
All alcoholic beverages	Alcohol wines for flavoring
Apples	Almonds
Apple Juice	Apple, small
Avocados	Blueberries
Bananas	Carob
Beer	Coffee, no acid (Kava)
Brewer's yeast	Extracts, brandy, rum, etc.
Cantaloupe	French sauternes
Champagne	Imitation sour cream
Cheese	Onions, cooked
Chicken livers	Orange juice, reduced acid
Chillis/spicy foods	Peanuts
Chocolate	Pears
Citrus fruits	Pine nuts
Coffee	Processed cheeses, not aged
Corned beef	Spring water
Cranberries	Strawberries, ½ cup
Fava beans	Sun tea
Grapes	Tomatoes, low acid
Gauva	White chocolate
Lemon juice	Wines, late harvest
Lentils	Zest of orange or limes
Lima beans	Shallots, green onions
Mayonnaise	All other foods not on list A
NutraSweet	
Nuts	
Onions	
Peaches	
Pickled herring	
Pineapple	
Plums	
Prunes	
Raisins	
Rye bread	
Saccharine	
Sour cream	
Soy sauce	
Strawberries	
Tea	
Tomatoes	
Vinegar	
Vitamins buffered w/aspartate	
Yogurt	

a presentation of primary gynecologic pathology. Generally, the etiology of low back pain results from an imbalance of muscle groups related to repetitive movements, fatigue, or faulty posture (lordosis and kyphosis). Back pain may be caused by gynecologic, vascular, neurologic, psychogenic, or spondylogenic (related to the axial skeleton and its structures) pathology.[102,103]

Myofascial pain

Pathophysiology Reports of the prevalence of myofascial pain as a cause of pelvic pain vary from 15% to 89%.[13,84,104] This discrepancy in part reflects the overlap in innervation and referred pain sites in the musculoskeletal structures and the visceral pelvic structures. Whether pain is primarily myofascial or is a manifestation of referred pain is not known. Myofascial pain syndrome and fibromyalgia should be ruled out with history and physical examination.

Symptoms and signs Musculoskeletal pain typically presents as a dull aching pain that is difficult to localize. With respect to abdominopelvic pain, structures including the rectus muscle, iliopsoas, quadratus lambarum, piriformis, and obtutators, innervated via T12–L4, and levator ani, innervated via S2–4, can refer pain to the lower abdomen pelvis and vulva or vagina. This pain is further enhanced if there is a primary pelvic pathology or irritation, including bladder and colon activity, menses, and intercourse, as these organs also have a similar innervation of T10–S4.[13,103-105] Therefore, myofascial pain is often worse during menses. On digital examination of the abdominal, back, or vaginal dermatomes, pressure on a trigger point evokes local and referred pain. Performing a straight leg raising maneuver tensing the abdominal wall muscles exacerbates abdominal wall pain.

Treatment Physical therapy to evaluate posture, muscle length, strength, and flexibility as well as trigger point injections are critical in the treatment of myofascial pain. Psychological factors should also be assessed and treated. The comorbid factors of depression, anxiety, and maladaptive behavior may potentiate the pain.[13-105] Medications such as low-dose tricyclic antidepressants and anticonvulsants may also be useful.

Nerve entrapment or injury

Pathophysiology Injury to or cutaneous nerve entrapment of the ilioinguinal (T12, L1), iliohypogastric (T12, L1), and genitofemoral (L1, L2) nerves may result in chronic lower abdominal and perineal pain. Generally, this syndrome develops following a Pfannensteil skin incision or other lower abdominal skin incision which results in entrapment or damage to the abdominal cutaneous nerves.[106] This syndrome may also occur spontaneously by muscular impingement of the nerve between the transverse and internal oblique muscles from repetitive activity, physical trauma, or poor posture.

Symptoms and signs Stabbing, sharp pain, typically elicited by exercise and chronic dull aching pain that is relieved by bed-rest may reflect nerve entrapment.[106,107] In a series of 46 women with a clinical diagnosis of ilioinguinal nerve entrapment, 88% had hyperesthesiae and 53% dysesthesia.[108] The site of maximal pain with ilioinguinal or iliohypogastric nerve entrapment is along the lateral edge of the rectus margin and may radiate to the hip or sacroiliac region. Nerve entrapment is diagnosed by eliciting focal tenderness over the site of the nerve entrapment.[109] This is done by having the patient tense her abdominal muscles in the supine position by raising either her shoulders or legs while pressing with a single

finger medial and below the anteriosuperior iliac spine or along the course of the nerve. If the abdominal pain is secondary to nerve entrapment, the abdominal pain will worsen with this maneuver and is located in the characteristic dermatomal distribution for that nerve.[110]

Treatment Relief of pain with a peripheral nerve block is both diagnostic and therapeutic. Approximately 5 ml of bupivacaine 0.25% or other local anesthetic is injected into the tender point using a 22–26 gauge 1.5-inch-long needle. The needle is placed such that the fat pad is slowly penetrated until the needle tip reproduces the pain.[103-105,108] Initially, severe pain may occur; however, relief (5–10 min for onset of the local anesthetic) will follow and is continued by repeating biweekly injections, up to five, as needed. A depot corticosteroid may be included. Other forms of more long-standing treatment include cryoneurolysis and nerve transection. Hahn reported a 76% improvement in pain with surgical transection at 1 year of follow-up in 51 cases of treated trapped nerves.[108] As with all neurolytic techniques, however, there is a risk of painful neuroma formation and anesthesia dolorosa. Other therapeutic options include low-dose tricyclic antidepressants, anticonvulsants, physical therapy to strengthen muscles, and acupuncture. Narcotic mediations are usually ineffective.

Chronic pelvic pain without obvious pathology

The International Association for the Study of Pain (IASP) classification includes a category entitled chronic pelvic pain without obvious pathology. This category is useful because it allows the assignment of a diagnosis in situations where the etiology of the pain, even after an exhaustive evolution, remains elusive. This diagnosis should not imply, however, that the pain is psychogenic in nature. Yet unrecognized neurophysiologic or biochemical perturbations may in the future be identified in women with pelvic pain without obvious pathology. Dysmenorrhea, for example, was thought to be a neurotic affectation until the discovery of prostaglandins. The management of pelvic pain without obvious pathology is similar to that of any enigmatic pain process: multidisciplinary management including pharmacological and psychological interventions, although specific studies are lacking.

Central factors

Psychological factors in chronic pelvic pain

Psychological factors pay an important role in an individual's response to chronic pain (see Chapter Ch7). A pathophysiologic cause of CPP is often not identified while evaluating a complaint of CPP. Therefore, psycho-pathological causes are often considered to be the source of pain, i.e. personality and mood disturbances, childhood events such as sexual abuse, and sexual and relationship difficulties. The diathesis–stress model of pain integrates the neurobiological and psychological components of pain. In this model, a woman is more susceptible in certain social contexts to develop chronic pelvic pain based on her preexisting vulnerabilities (including cognitive, affective, biological, or behavioral).[111] A woman's response to an acute pain experience may therefore be more likely to progress to a chronic process based on a current or previous emotional experience, expectations, mechanism or thinking, and/or habits. This process likely involves alterations in central processing. The stimulus for these alterations and mechanisms underlying the maintenance of changes in central processing without an inflammatory stimulus or nerve damage are unknown. Other factors may include alterations in the hypothalamic–pituitary–adrenal axis and cortisol levels, as illustrated by Heim and colleagues.[112]

Personality profile

In chronic pelvic pain, studies using the Minnesota Multiphasic Personality Inventory (MMP) indicate that women with pelvic pain have a high prevalence of a convergence "V" profile (elevated scores on the hypochondriasis and hysteria scales and normal or lower scores on the depression scale).[113] This profile is independent of the presence or absence of a specific pathology such as endometriosis.[114] Furthermore, treatment resulting in a subjective improvement in pain severity and increased activity level produces a significant improvement in personality profile.[115]

Depression

Major depression and other dysthymic, panic, and somatization disorders have been associated with CPP of unknown etiology.[116,117] Higher depression scores and family histories of affective disorder were described in women with chronic pelvic pain without pathology than in women with chronic pelvic pain and pathology as established by laparoscopy.[116] Often, the depression preceded the onset of the pain; however, no prospective or outcome studies have been performed.[87,116,117]

Sexual and physical abuse

Women with chronic pelvic pain are generally thought to have a higher incidence of sexual and/or physical abuse in childhood and adulthood. Numerous studies have suggested an association with chronic pelvic pain and sexual or physical abuse with prevalence rates of approximately 50%.[117–121] Walling and colleagues compared women with CPP with women with nonpelvic chronic pain (headache) and pain-free women. A higher life time prevalence of major sexual abuse (56%), and physical abuse (50%) was found in the chronic pelvic pain group.[121] A history of sexual and physical abuse is generally considered an independent risk factor for chronic pelvic pain.[122] In addition to sexual or physical abuse, a higher incidence of substance abuse has been reported in the CPP population.[119] The prevalence and likely contributing factor of prior abuse to CPP makes eliciting this history important, in addition to evaluating for organic causes.[123]

CLINICAL PRESENTATION

History

Critical to the evaluation and management of CPP, one needs to elicit a detailed history of the onset, nature, and previous treatments. A pain questionnaire may assist in helping the patient express issues that she may otherwise be unable to verbally express.

The history should include:

- *The chronology of the pain.* In what context did the pain arise? Was there an eliciting event? Has the pain changed? What does the patient think is causing the pain?
- *The nature of the pain.* The character, intensity, location and radiation, aggravating and alleviating factors, and the effect of menses, exercise, work, stress, intercourse, and orgasm.
- *The severity of pain.* Zero to 10 on a visual analog-type reporting scale.
- *Associated somatic symptoms.* Specifically related to the:
  - Genital tract (abnormal vaginal bleeding, discharge, mittelschmerz, dysmenorrhea, dyspareunia, infertility).
  - Gastrointestinal tract (constipation, diarrhea, flatulence, tenesmus, alterations to pain before and after a bowel movement, blood, changes in color or caliber of stool).
  - Musculoskeletal system (pain distribution, radiation, association with injury, fatigue, postural changes, exercise, lifting).
  - Urologic tract (dysuria, urgency, frequency, suprapubic pain).
- *Prior evaluations for the pain, including treatment.* Operative and pathology reports should be obtained as well as side-effects/success or failure of prior treatments.
- *Impact on family, work, daily activities.* Is the degree of pain such that the pain prevents the patient from performing a family role or occupation? Is litigation or worker's compensation an issue? What is the attitude of the patient and family toward the pain and resultant behavior?
- *Past medical, surgical, gynecologic, obstetric history, and medication intake including pain medication.*
- *Current and past psychological history.* History of

past or current physical, sexual, and/or emotional abuse, history of hospitalization, suicide attempts, and chemical (drug or alcohol) dependence.

- *Patient's expectations.* What is the goal of treatment?

A detailed, prospective, daily pain diary to note the occurrence and intensity of pain, menstrual periods, and mood is important in the evaluation of CPP. Medication intake and aggravating and alleviating factors should be noted in the diary. A simple diary utilizes a visual analog scale from 0 (no pain) to 10 (most severe pain ever). The diary should be maintained for at least 2 months or two menstrual cycles.

CLINICAL FINDINGS

Examination

One should perform a complete physical examination, with particular attention to the abdomen, back, vagina, vulva, and pelvic floor muscles. Prior to the examination, the patient should point to the area(s) of pain, as this can help differentiate the source of pain. During the examination, the patient should be informed of what will take place and what to expect.

The examination should include evaluation of:

- *General.* The patient's general body habitus, posture while sitting, standing, and walking, and anxiety level.
- *Abdomen.* Evaluate for scars and sites of hypersensitivity at specific dermatome regions and for trigger points. A straight leg raising maneuver (active) should be performed to discern abdominal wall sources of pain, as abdominal wall pain is augmented and visceral pain is diminished with the above maneuver.[104,105,110] The quality of bowel sounds should be noted as well as distension, sites of tenderness to palpation, and guarding. While the patient is standing, evaluate visually and by palpation for hernias (inguinal, femoral, and Spigelian).
- *Musculoskeletal.* The patient should be evaluated for scoliosis, discrepancy in leg length, muscle strength, range of motion, and pelvic floor muscle tenderness. Trigger points should be elicited.
- *Gynecologic.* First assess the vulva for evidence of trauma and old scars (episiotomy). A cotton-tipped swab should then be used to evaluate for sites of hypersensitivity within the vulva and vestibule. A unidigital examination is then performed to palpate the urethra, bladder base, vaginal side-walls, levator ani, pubococcygeus, coccygeus, piriformis, abturator internus, cervix, and uterosacral ligament to elicit any tenderness. Evaluate for pelvic floor relaxation (cystocele, rectocele, enterocele) and vaginal atrophy. Bimanual examination may elicit uterine or adnexal tenderness, and/or abnormalities in size, shape, or

mobility. A rectal examination is then performed to further assess uterosacral tenderness, nodularity, and rectal disease/occult blood. Speculum examination should be performed to inspect visually for vaginal or cervical lesions, hypoestrogenization, and to rule out vaginitis. This examination may be difficult in the presence of levator ani spasm.

- *Neurologic.* Assessment of perineal and lower extremity strength, sensation, and reflexes.

DIAGNOSTIC CRITERIA

Diagnostic work-up includes a complete blood count (CBC), ESR, urinalysis and culture, cervical and urethral cultures (gonorrhea and *Chlamydia*), pregnancy test (if indicated), wet mount of vaginal secretions, Pap smear, stool guiacs, and, if diarrhea is present, stool culture. Ultrasound, CT, or MRI may be performed if pelvic examination is limited or if other pathology is suspected. Other studies (i.e. cystoscopy, colonoscopy) should be based on patient symptomatology or on consultation with other specialists (urologist, gastroenterologist, neurologist, orthopedist, and physical therapist). Surgical evaluation with diagnostic laparoscopy, hysteroscopy, or laparotomy may be considered if initial therapy fails or if pelvic examination is abnormal. Further evaluation is as outlined under the specific entities of pelvic pain.

EVIDENCE-BASED EVALUATION OF MANAGEMENT (WITH EVIDENCE SCORING)

Pharmacological**

Nonsteroidal anti-inflammatory drugs (NSAIDs), narcotics, antidepressants, and anticonvulsants have been utilized in the treatment of CPP as in other types of chronic pain. Only one randomized controlled trial has looked at the effect of a selective serotonin reuptake inhibitor on pelvic pain.[124] Engel and colleagues randomized 23 women in a double-blind crossover study to receive sertraline or placebo. Over a 14-week period (6 weeks placebo/sertraline, 2 weeks washout, 6 weeks sertraline/ placebo), no significant difference was appreciated in the measures of pain and functional disability studied.[124] Further investigation using larger numbers and duration of treatment is required to verify these results. No randomized controlled studies have evaluated the benefit of low-dose tricyclic antidepressants, anticonvulsants, NSAIDs, or narcotics, however all have been used successfully in pelvic pain patients. Treatment of CPP with narcotics should include a narcotic contract between provider and patient as well as regularly scheduled appointments for follow-up. Cyclic pelvic pain should respond to menstrual suppression with continuous oral contraceptive pills, high-dose progestins, or gonadotropin-releasing hormone agonists with hormone add-back therapy to minimize bone loss.

Physical*

No specific randomized studies have evaluated the benefits of physical therapy for the treatment of chronic pelvic pain. However, in the multidisciplinary approach of treatment for CPP, physical therapy is often incorporated in the management, especially in cases of myofascial syndrome. TENS and biofeedback are often used in conjunction by the physical therapist.[125] Transvaginal TENS provides electrical stimulation to the pelvic floor muscles and is also available.

Injection therapies*

Trigger point injections are felt to provide prolonged relief by interfering with transmission of the pain impulse and thus eliminating the positive feedback arc.[13] No randomized controlled studies have specifically looked at chronic pelvic pain and trigger point injections. One small, randomized, double-blind, crossover study compared trigger point injections in patients with myofascial syndrome with bupivacaine 0.5%, etidocaine 1%, or saline. Subjective improvement was noted with the local anesthetic treatment over saline.[126] Slocumb[13] studied the response of 122 women to trigger point injections, with abdominal pelvic pain characterized by dermatome hypersensitivity and trigger points: 89.3% reported relief or improvement in pain, such that no further therapy was required over the duration of the study (3–36 months). Of note, the response rate was related to the number of visits to the clinic for injections. A 94.8% response was noted with two visits or less, compared with a 66.7% response rate with six visits or more.[13] Trigger point injections can be repeated weekly or biweekly for up to five courses. Further management of myofascial pain is described in Chapter Ch44.

Anesthesia nerve blocks*

In some cases, a patient may have multiple trigger points at the vaginal wall, sacrum, and abdominal wall. In these cases, a caudal or epidural block may prove to be more fruitful in treating the pain than multiple trigger point injections.[13] Nerve blocks with local anesthetics may provide relief of neuralgia due to nerve injury. Arner *et al.* found prolonged pain relief in 25 of 38 patients following injection of 5–10 cm³ of 0.5% bupivacaine.[127] Prolonged partial pain relief may occur for weeks or months following one or more nerve blocks beyond the anticipated

duration of the local anesthetic. The initial pain relief is likely due to conduction block of nociceptive fibers in the nerve. The explanation for prolonged pain relief may be secondary to reduced capacity of the nerve to maintain repetitive impulses, the anti-inflammatory effects of the local anesthetic, decreased excitability of the nerve fiber, and systemic uptake of the anesthetic. Nerve blocks have also been used as a prerequisite for evaluating potential effectiveness prior to neurectomy.[128] Superior hypogastric plexus block by CT guidance and at the time of microlaparoscopy may provide further evaluation and management in chronic pelvic pain.[129,130] However, at this time, randomized controlled studies are lacking in the area of CPP.

Surgery

Very few randomized controlled trials exist which evaluate the surgical management of chronic pelvic pain.

Diagnostic laparoscopy**

Laparoscopy has an important role in the diagnosis and management of acute pelvic pain. Its exact role in the evaluation of patients with chronic pelvic pain is more controversial and limited. However, over 40% of laparoscopies are performed for evaluation of chronic pelvic pain.[3] Numerous epidemiological studies have investigated the presence of pathology at the time of diagnostic laparoscopy in CPP patients: 14–77% of patients have no obvious pathology and two-thirds of patients have findings of adhesions, which may or may not play a role in their pain.[34,131] In a review on the use of laparoscopy in chronic pelvic pain, Howard found that CPP patients had approximately twice the incidence of pelvic pathology compared with the 28% incidence of pathology in the non-CPP population.[3]

Indications

Prior to proceeding with laparoscopy, a thorough evaluation of the patient's pelvic pain should be carried out to exclude other nongynecologic etiologies of CPP, as outlined earlier in this chapter. An abnormal pelvic examination prior to laparoscopy is associated with pathology 70–90% of the time, and abnormal pathology is present in one-half of patients with normal preoperative pelvic examinations.[3] During the operative procedure, specific attention should be directed at sites of increased tenderness on physical examination. The exact time at which laparoscopy should be performed is controversial. CPP by classic definition is pain of 6 months' duration. However, waiting may lead to tissue damage and progression of the chronic pain process. Laparoscopy should be performed when one believes it will help in the management:

- Failure of medication (hormonal and analgesic) to relieve pain over a minimum of 2–3 months.

- Surgical management of adhesions, endometriosis, or hernias.[34,132]
- For pain mapping. Under conscious sedation and local anesthesia, direct visualization by minilaparoscopy can be performed to evaluate intra-abdominal sites associated with pelvic pain to help isolate sources of somatic and visceral pain. No outcome studies exist as to whether pain management guided by pain mapping is more efficacious. Performing a superior hypogastric block during this assessment may assess the potential effectiveness of a presacral neurectomy.[130]

At the time of laparoscopy, hysteroscopy may be performed to further evaluate for structural etiologies of dysmenorrhea such as cervical stenosis, endometrial polyps, and submucosal myomas.[133] However, further studies are needed to recommend routine hysteroscopy.

Contraindications
Known surgical risks that exceed the benefit of the procedure are contraindications. Laparoscopy may have a more limited role in posthysterectomy patients in whom dense adhesions or ovarian remnant syndrome are likely.[3]

Adverse effects
One may erroneously attribute the source of pain to "pathology" at the time of laparoscopy when a nongynecologic source such as irritable bowel syndrome, myofascial pain, or nerve entrapment may be the true etiology. The patient must also be clear that she may still have some degree of pain following the procedure. Surgical injury to bowel, bladder, ureter, vessels, and nerves are potential complications.

Evidence for efficacy**
The use of laparoscopy is controversial, as nonsurgical management of chronic pelvic pain is successful in 65–90% of patients regardless of the presence of "pathology."[13,43,134,135] The only randomized controlled evaluation of the use of laparoscopy is by Peters et al. in which 106 women with CPP were randomized to one of two treatment modalities.[135] The standard approach in 49 patients involved evaluation for a primary organic cause by routinely performing a laparoscopy. The other 57 patients underwent an integrated approach, including assessment of somatic, psychological, dietary, environmental, and physiotherapeutic factors. Laparoscopy was not routinely performed in this group.[135] Of the 49 patients in the standard group, 65% had no abnormality, 5% endometriosis, 18% had adhesions, and the remainder had myomata, ovarian cysts, or pelvic varices. The integrated approach was significantly more effective in the reduction of pelvic pain (75% vs. 41%, $P < 0.01$).[135] The authors concluded that laparoscopy provided too little a benefit to warrant its routine use in the management of CPP. Although there was a 35% incidence of pelvic pathology, these abnormalities overall were considered negligible and minimally additive to the preoperative diagnosis.[135] However, other

nonrandomized retrospective and prospective studies have suggested that diagnostic laparoscopy provides a positive psychological impact in the treatment of CPP.[136] At this time, the routine use of laparoscopy in the management of CPP remains controversial. Also, randomized studies are needed to determine whether laparoscopic conscious pain mapping is useful in the long-term alleviation of pain.

Hysterectomy*

Approximately 12% of hysterectomies are performed for the sole indication of CPP.[3] However, 30% of patients presenting to pelvic pain clinics have already undergone hysterectomy without experiencing relief of pain.[4] Reiter et al. noted a decline in the incidence of hysterectomy for the indication of CPP from 16.3% to 5.8% after the initiation of a multidisciplinary approach to the diagnosis and treatment of chronic pelvic pain.[134]

Indications
Patients with cyclic pain or dysfunctional uterine bleeding are excellent candidates for hysterectomy especially if they have relief of pain with hormonal suppression. The American College of Obstetricians and Gynecologists (ACOG) Criteria Set on hysterectomy for pelvic pain states the following as indications for hysterectomy:[137]

1 No remediable pathology found on laparoscopic examination.
2 Presence of pain for more than 6 months with negative effect on patient's quality of life.

In addition, prior to surgery, medical management should be tried, and other nongynecologic etiologies should be evaluated including the patient's psychological and psychosexual status.[137]

Contraindications
Desire for future fertility and known medical or psychological risks that exceed benefit.[137]

Adverse effects
Preoperatively, one needs to discuss with the patient the potential outcomes of the surgery – including the possibility of posthysterectomy pelvic pain – secondary to nerve entrapment, new trigger points, irritable bladder or bowel, postoperative adhesions, residual ovary, ovarian remnant, recurrent endometriosis, and vaginal cuff pain.[67]

Evidence of efficacy*
No randomized controlled trials have compared hysterectomy with no surgery in CPP patients. However, from the limited nonrandomized studies, one may estimate that one in four women will continue to have persistent pain following a hysterectomy for chronic pelvic pain.[137–140] The success rate of hysterectomy for the treatment of CPP is obviously better in women with cyclic pelvic pain. Stovall et al.,[139] in a retrospective study of

99 women, and Hillis *et al.*,[140] in a prospective cohort of 308 women, noted a 77% and 74% response rate, respectively, in woman who underwent hysterectomy for CPP felt to be of uterine origin. At 1-year follow-up, however, 25% of women in Stovall's group noted a persistence of worsening of pain. Hillis observed that persistent pain was associated with multiparity, prior history of pelvic inflammatory disease (PID), lack of pathology, and Medicare payer status.[140]

Presacral neurectomy/uterosacral transection**

Presacral neurectomy involves transection of the superior hypogastric plexus at the level of the sacrum. This differs from uterosacral transection (laparoscopic uterine nerve ablation; LUNA) in which the nerves are cut at the level of the uterus.

Indications

Cotte documented the use of presacral neurectomy or sympathectomy (PSN) as a treatment for intractable dysmenorrhea in 1937.[141] PSN has since been recommended as a surgical treatment for women with deep central pain secondary to primary dysmenorrhea or endometriosis. Afferent innervation from the cervix, uterus, and proximal fallopian tubes (T11–L12) travels through the superior hypogastric plexus as the presacral nerve. PSN interrupts the electrical transmission of pain from these organs by transection of these nerves.

In determining which patients with central pelvic pain may benefit from PSN or uterosacral transection, preoperative evaluation/requirements should include:

1 Failure in the past to respond to medical management.
2 Interference with daily activities secondary to the pain.
3 Assessment for structural abnormalities likely contributing to the pain.
4 Evaluation for somatic (nonvisceral) causes of pain.
5 Possible trial of paracervical or fluoroscopic guided hypogastric plexus blockade to assess whether surgery may benefit.
6 A discussion with the patient on the expectations/long-term relief of pain with the procedure.

Contraindications

Afferents from the adnexal structures travel with the sympathetic fibers along the infundibulopelvic ligament to enter the spinal cord at T9–T10. Therefore, lateralizing pain of visceral origin will not be relieved by PSN or LUNA.

Adverse effects

Discussion with the patient should also include risks of the procedure, including:

1 Vascular, bowel, bladder, and/or ureteral injury secondary to the close proximity of these structures necessitating laparotomy.[142]

2 Dysfunction of the bladder and rectum with PSN due to the common pathway of their sympathetic afferent nerves along the superior hypogastric plexus.[143] This is limited by normal micturition and defecation in part being dependent on an intact sacral autonomic nerve supply, which is unaffected by PSN.
3 With uterosacral nerve ablation, a theoretical risk of uterine prolapse exists.[144,145]

Evidence for efficacy**

Generally quoted statistics on the efficacy of PSN or LUNA report a 70–80% improvement in primary and less for secondary dysmenorrhea.[143,146–149] However, only three randomized controlled trials have looked at presacral neurectomy or uterosacral transection and relief of central pelvic pain:

1 Candiani and colleagues compared 71 patients with moderate or severe endometriosis with resection of endometriosis alone ($n=36$) or with PSN ($n=35$). Central pain was reduced, however there was no significant difference in pain at 6-month follow-up.[143]
2 Tjaden and colleagues performed a randomized controlled study with PSN and/or resection of moderate to severe endometriosis. In the group with PSN, 15/17 had no recurrence of pain with PSN versus no relief in the group without PSN. This study was prematurely terminated secondary to the significant benefits with PSN.[150]
3 Chen and colleagues compared laparoscopic PSN with LUNA for primary dysmenorrhea in 68 patients. Relief of pain at the 3-month follow-up was equal, however at the 12-month visit 82% in the PSN group compared with 51% in the LUNA group reported continued relief.[151]

In summary, one may consider the use of PSN in women who have failed conservative management; however, further controlled studies are required to truly determine its beneficial effect given the potential complications. PSN should be considered over uterosacral neurectomy (LUNA), however PSN is technically more difficult to perform and can require a laparotomy.

Psychological*

Emotional and psychological evaluation should be performed early in the evaluation of CPP. A psychologist familiar in the management of chronic pelvic pain can best serve the patient. Stress reduction, relaxation, and behavioral therapies should also be addressed. Issues often involve relationship dysfunction requiring family and marital therapy, presence of past or current physical or sexual abuse, and the negative effects on self-esteem and independence. Prolonged psychotherapy for these issues is generally not part of pain management but can be used in conjunction. No randomized controlled trials have assessed the effect of psychological approaches on chronic pelvic pain, however a randomized prospective trial of interdisciplinary management of CPP (which involves a component of psychological assessment and therapy) has been performed.[135] This studied demonstrated a significant improvement in pain in the multidisciplinary group over the standard gynecologic treatment group. Assessment should be designed to evaluate the pain complaint, its impact on life circumstances, controlling factors, and coping mechanisms. Standardized psychological testing is helpful to determine whether affective disturbance is present, as well as to establish a baseline against which to measure treatment response and guide treatment approaches.

Alternative medicine*

Nontraditional approaches to CPP include chiropractic treatment, hypnosis, and acupuncture.[79,152] In the medical literature, a single prospective study on chiropractic treatment in 18 CPP patients demonstrated significant improvement in pain and functioning over a 6-week treatment period of flexion/distraction and trigger point techniques.[152] Helms[153] in a randomized controlled study found a 90% (10 of 11 patients) improvement in dysmenorrhea with acupuncture compared with only 36% (4 of 11 patients) in the placebo acupuncture group. This improvement was associated with a 41% reduction in the use of analgesic medication. Further evaluation is needed to assess their utility, but nontraditional medicine may provide another option.

Multidisciplinary pain management***

Chronic pelvic pain therapy is often refractory to traditional medical and surgical approaches. However, numerous studies have demonstrated the utility of an interdisciplinary pain management program in treating chronic pelvic pain patients.[152,154,155] This approach involves simultaneous evaluation of somatic and psychological components of chronic pelvic pain by different health care specialists. Critical to this management is communication between the gynecologist, psychologist, and, if involved in the patient's care, the physical therapist, anesthesiologist, and dietitian. Therapeutic approaches include use of nonsteroidal anti-inflammatory medications, narcotics, tricyclic antidepressants, trigger point injections, and nerve blocks as indicated (i.e. pudendal, ilioinguinal, iliohypogastric, genitofemoral, and occasionally hypogastric are utilized). One program utilizing cognitive–behavioral therapy, acupuncture, and tricyclic antidepressants was successful in reducing pain by at least 50% in 85% of the subjects.[43,152] Other studies have suggested that similar results may be obtained with a multidisciplinary team.[134,135,154–156] In a prospective randomized, controlled study, the multidisciplinary approach combining the traditional gynecologic treatment with psychological, dietary, and physical therapy input was found to be more effective than traditional gynecologic (medical and surgical) management of cure.[135]

PROGNOSIS

Chronic pelvic pain is seldom cured but usually can be significantly ameliorated, with resultant improvement in mood, activity level, and overall quality of life. Traditional modes of therapy may result in multiple surgeries without significant improvement in pain. Successful management requires that the patient learns to live with a chronic process that may or may not have an obvious source. Pain reduction with an interdisciplinary approach may approach up to 85% and should be highly considered in the management of CPP.

VULVAR PAIN SYNDROME (VULVODYNIA)

Definition

Vulvodynia or vulvar pain is chronic vulvar discomfort characterized by burning, stinging, irritation, and/or rawness. Similar to chronic pelvic pain, it is a chronic medical problem that may have no apparent cause or may have multiple etiologies. Treatment is often long term and may require both medical and psychological components.

Within this syndrome, several clinical entities are classified – vulvar vestibulitis, vulvar dermatoses, cyclic vulvovaginitis, vestibular papillomatosis, and dysesthetic vulvodynia.[157] These conditions may coexist and are often difficult to distinguish completely from each other.

1 *Vulvar vestibulitis.* Entry dyspareunia with vestibule erythema and tenderness to light touch.
2 *Chronic vulvovaginitis.* Vulvar burning and itching. Vulvar erythema is diffuse and associated with vulvar swelling. The etiology is unclear, but candidiasis is often a contributing factor.
3 *Vulvar dermatoses.* The dermatoses includes lichen sclerosus, lichen planus, lichen simplex chronicus, and human papillomavirus (HPV) infection. Vulvar pain is noncyclic and associated with significant pruritus. On examination, hypopigmentation or hyperpigmentation is present with atrophic or hyperplastic tissue. A stenotic introitus, flattening of the labial folds, vulvar fissures, with white plaques and erythema may be present. Biopsy is required to make the diagnosis and eliminate a malignant process. The etiology for the vulvar dermatoses is unknown. Treatment depends on the specific dermatosis (high-potency topical corticosteroids, testosterone ointment).[158]
4 *Vestibular papillomatosis.* In vestibular papillomatosis, the mucosal surface at the medial labia minora is covered with multiple papillae, approximately 1 mm in diameter and 2–3 mm in length. Patients are generally asymptomatic, but may have pruritus or pain. On examination, vulvar papillae are present on the labia

minora. It is unclear whether the papillomatosis arises secondary to human papillomavirus (HPV) or an irritative agent.[158] Treatment options include trichloroacetic acid (TCA), topical 5-fluorouracil (5-FU), interferon, and laser therapy.

5 *Dysesthetic vulvodynia.* Generally considered a diagnosis of exclusion, it presents commonly in perimenopausal and postmenopausal women as non-specific superficial vulvar burning or perineal discomfort with intermittent, deep, aching pain. Patients deny entry dyspareunia. Physical examination is normal, with no tenderness on palpation. Pudendal neuralgia, hyperesthesiae, or hypoesthesiae in a saddle distribution extending from the mons pubis to the upper inner thighs and posteriorly across ischial tuberosities may be noted on examination.[159] The etiology may be secondary to an aberration in cutaneous nerve perception (pudendal nerve distribution S2–S4) at either the central or peripheral level. Amitriptyline or other tricyclic antidepressants starting at 10 mg q.d. to 40–60 mg q.d. may be of benefit in this condition.[157] Topical 5% lidocaine may provide additional benefit. Other reported treatments, although of unproven effectiveness, include acupuncture, pelvic floor muscle, physical therapy, TENS, regional nerve blocks, and capsaicin.[157]

Epidemiology

In the private gynecologic practice setting, the incidence of vulvodynia or vulvar vestibulitis may reach 15%.[160] These women are generally characterized as white, nulliparous, with a median age of 32,[161] although adolescents through postmenopausal women may be affected.

Etiology

Vulvar pain is multifactorial in many cases (Table 43.5) A detailed history and examination is therefore important to help direct diagnosis and treatment.[162]

Clinical presentation: history

Obtaining a thorough history is critical in the evaluation and management of vulvodynia. Pain symptoms must be well characterized to assess the onset, the type of pain (burning, stinging, irritation), timing (constant or cyclic), associated activities (i.e. intercourse), inciting agents (perfumes, lotions, detergents, clothing), and relieving factors (i.e. antifungal medications). A pain diary may better define these characteristics.

In addition, past or current infections (human papillomavirus, herpes, candida), medications, local and systemic dermatologic disorders, neurologic disorders (i.e.

Table 43.5 *Etiologies of vulvodynia*

Infections – Bartholin's gland abscess, vulvovaginal candidiasis, herpes, herpes zoster, human papillomavirus, molluscum contagiosum, *Trichomonas*

Trauma – sexual assault, prior vaginal deliveries, hymenectomy, vaginal surgery

Systemic illness – Bechet's disease, Crohn's disease, Sjögren syndrome, systemic lupus erythematosus

Neoplasia – vulvar intraepithelial neoplasia and invasive squamous cell carcinoma

Allergens/toxic medications – soaps, fabric softeners, bubble bath, sprays, douches, antiseptics, sanitary pads, suppositories, creams, laser treatment, podophyllin, trichloroacetic acid (TCA), 5-fluorouracil (5-FU)

Dermatological conditions – allergic and contact dermatitis, eczema, hidradenitis suppurativa, lichen planus, lichen sclerosus, pemphigoid, pemphigus, psoriasis, squamous cell hyperplasia

Urinary tract syndromes – interstitial cystitis and urethral syndrome

Neurological – referred pain from urethra, vagina, and bladder, dysesthesiae secondary to herpes zoster, spinal disk problems, specific neuralgias (pudendal, genitofemoral)

Psychological – sexual/physical abuse sexual history

herniated disks, herpes zoster, pudental or genitofemoral neuralgia), urologic disorders (interstitial cystitis, urethral syndrome), and physical trauma (vaginal deliveries, episiotomy, vaginal surgery) should be ascertained. Sexual history evaluating lubrication, ability to achieve orgasm, whether the pain is primary or secondary, and a history of sexual abuse should be assessed.

Clinical findings: examinations

In many cases, the vulva appears normal. However, careful inspection should be performed to evaluate for discoloration (erythema, hypopigmentation, or hyperpigmentation), lesions (ulcers and fissures) and atrophy (presence or absence of well-estrogenized tissue). On examination, tenderness (hyperesthesiae) at the periurethral or Bartholin's glands should be outlined using a cotton-tipped swab and scored (0, no pain, to 10, severe pain) and recorded. Tone and tenderness of the pelvic floor muscles (levator ani) should be assessed for vaginismus.

Vaginal pH, whiff test, and microscopic examination of vaginal secretions with potassium hydroxide (KOH) and normal saline can help evaluate for vaginitis. Vaginal fluid may be cultured for *Candida* (as microscopic evaluation may reveal candidiasis in only 50% of cases), bacterial culture, and immunoglobulin E (IgE) (to evaluate for local allergy).[161] All lesions or discolorations should be further evaluated by colposcopy. Acetowhite changes with application of 5% acetic acid should be biopsied as well as any distinct lesion to evaluate for an underlying dermatosis or infectious or neoplastic process.

Vulvar vestibulitis syndrome

Vulvar vestibulitis is a subset of vulvodynia. The vestibule is the nonpigmented, nonkeratinized, squamous epithelium of the vulva between the labia minora and the hymen. The ductal orifices from Bartholin's, Skene's, and the minor vestibular glands open onto the vestibule. Vulvar vestibulitis is characterized by three criteria:[160]

1 Introital pain on vestibular or vaginal entry (entry dyspareunia).
2 Vestibular erythema or inflammation of the vestibule, commonly involving the posterior fourchette.
3 Vestibular tenderness – pressure from a cotton-tipped applicator at the vestibule reproduces the pain.

This syndrome generally affects women in their twenties and thirties. It presents as persistent introital or contact-related burning. Urinary symptoms with a negative urine culture may be present in 11–44% of women.[161,163] The coexistence of interstitial cystitis and vestibulitis has been defined as the "urogenital sinus syndrome."[163] This may represent a disorder of the urogenital sinus-derived epithelium as the bladder, urethra, and vestibule arise from the urogenital sinus.

The etiology is often unknown. On biopsy, the subepithelial tissue often demonstrates a nonspecific, chronic inflammatory infiltrate, consisting predominately of lymphocytes without direct glandular inflammation.[164] In one study, 63% of women had a prior history of severe and repeated vulvovaginal candidiasis, 15% with pain onset within 6 weeks of vaginal surgery or delivery, and 12% with a history of sexual abuse.[160] However, the etiology may remain undetermined in up to one-third of cases.[161] It is controversial whether human papillomavirus (HPV) is an important factor in the etiology of vestibulitis. Older studies have often implicated HPV as an etiology; however, more current studies utilizing molecular techniques have not consistently demonstrated HPV infection and it is currently not considered a causative agent for vestibulitis.[165,166]

The underlying pathophysiologic disorder resulting in vulvar pain likely involves autonomic nerve dysfunction, resulting in altered immune function, increased tissue vascularity, vascular injury, and histamine release in the surrounding tissue (Fig. 43.1).[167,168] Treatment should therefore be based at all levels of the neuraxis.

EVIDENCE-BASED EVALUATION OF MANAGEMENT*

Few randomized controlled studies have evaluated the different treatment modalities for vulvodynia or vulvar vestibulitis. Most studies are retrospective, case-controlled studies with limited numbers.

The type of treatment ultimately depends on the etiology of the pain. Given the potential for multiple etiologies, successful treatment is often difficult. Success is usually defined by the patient's ability to have intercourse again or intercourse with decreased pain (Table 43.6).

Medical

Numerous medical options are available for treatment. Supportive measures, including sitz baths and topical 2% or 5% xylocaine gel or ointment should initially be utilized. Patients should be instructed on proper vulvar hygiene (cotton underwear, keeping area dry, avoidance of constrictive garments, prolonged sanitary pad usage, and irritating agents).

Antiviral agents, antifungal agents, antihistamines, topical steroids, or topical nonsteroidal anti-inflammatory agents or topical acetyl salicylic acid (5% aspirin cream) are frequently utilized but their efficacy in randomized controlled studies is lacking.

Pharmacological

Antivirals

Although it is not completely clear whether HPV is an inciting agent for vestibulitis, numerous antiviral agents (TCA, interferon, and 5-FU cream) have often been utilized to treat this disorder, especially when HPV has been identified on biopsy. Intralesional α-interferon, administered as 12, 1-million IU injections three times/week for 4 weeks in several small, case-controlled stud-

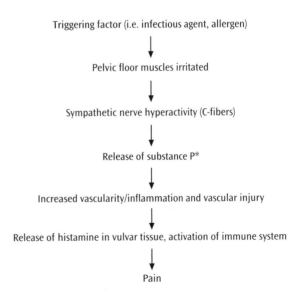

Triggering factor (i.e. infectious agent, allergen)
↓
Pelvic floor muscles irritated
↓
Sympathetic nerve hyperactivity (C-fibers)
↓
Release of substance P*
↓
Increased vascularity/inflammation and vascular injury
↓
Release of histamine in vulvar tissue, activation of immune system
↓
Pain

Figure 43.1 *Potential mechanisms of vulvodynia.*
*Important in the transmission and modulation of the pain response.

Table 43.6 *Treatment of vulvodynia*

Supportive measures – warm sitz baths, Burrow's solution, topical anesthetic agents (2% topical xylocaine gel or 5% ointment) and other lubricants with intercourse
Vulvar hygiene – cotton underwear, avoid constrictive garments
Treat underlying cause:
   Human papillomavirus (HPV)[a] – TCA 30%, topical 5-FU, interferon 1 million IU per injection to painful site with total of 12 injection sites over 4 weeks
   Candida – fluconazole 150 mg once a week for 6 weeks then once a month for 6 months
   Allergens – avoid agent (these patients should also avoid local creams and suppositories containing propylene glycol), hydroxyzine or other antihistamine, hydrocortisone 1% cream b.i.d., 5% aspirin cream q.i.d.
   Atrophy – topical estrogen vaginal cream, oral hormone replacement therapy
Diet modification – low-oxalate diet with calcium citrate 400 mg p.o. t.i.d.
Tricyclic antidepressants – amitriptyline, desipramine, nortriptyline, 10–50 mg h.s.
Psychological and behavioral pain management
Biofeedback
Surgery – vestibuloplasty, partial or total vestibuloectomy with vaginal advancement[a]

a. Current studies do not substantiate human papillomavirus as a causative factor in vulvodynia, however its treatment, in particular interferon, is still supported in the literature.
5-FU, 5-fluorouracil.

ies, report an 18–100% response rate.[161,162,169] One small, randomized controlled study observed a similar positive response using interferon when comparing total perineoplasty (six of nine patients) with subtotal perineoplasty plus interferon injections (seven of 10 patients).[170] In addition, fewer surgical complications were observed in the latter group. Further randomized trials are needed to evaluate the effectiveness of interferon. Application of topical 5-FU has not been consistently substantiated and may actually aggravate pain.

Antifungals

Vulvovaginal candidiasis has often been implicated in vulvodynia. Antifungals, including fluconazole 150 mg orally once a week for 6 weeks then once a month for 6 months, may provide relief in cases of cyclic monilial culture-positive vulvodynia. However, even in culture-positive cases of vulvar vestibulitis, improvement may not occur, as Ledger *et al*. reported only a 16% success.[161]

Antihistamines/corticosteroids

Allergens may also be an inciting agent for vulvodynia. In addition to avoiding the noxious substance, antihistamines (i.e. hydroxyzine) as well as topical corticosteroids (hydrocortisone 1% cream b.i.d.) may help alleviate the discomfort. Ledger *et al*. observed a 48% response to hydroxyzine, however no significant difference was noted between IgE-negative and -positive groups.[161] Although the histology revealing inflammatory changes suggests that an anti-inflammatory applied topically would be helpful, there are no data to support this approach. Steroid creams also thin tissue. However, we have anecdotally had positive treatment responses to 5% salicylic acid (aspirin) in a nonirritating base applied four times daily to the vestibule.

Estrogens

In cases of pain secondary to atrophied tissue which can occur postpartum, on low-dose oral contraceptives, or peri- or postmenopausally, estrogen vaginal cream or oral hormone replacement therapy as indicated should be utilized.

Tricyclic antidepressants

Tricyclic antidepressants in doses of 25–50 mg at night or at divided amounts throughout the day have been utilized in cases of vulvodynia. The lowest effective dose should be given to avoid the anticholinergic side-effects. McKay observed subjective improvement in patients with dysesthetic vulvodynia in a retrospective study, however no randomized trials have confirmed these findings.[157]

Capsaicin

Capsaicin is a cream used in the treatment of neuralgia, most commonly in herpes zoster and diabetic neuropathy. It functions as an analgesic agent, by initially stimulating and then depleting substance P release from pain-associated C-fibers. The net effect is desensitization. Few studies have examined the effect of capsaicin, especially on vulvar vestibulitis.[160,171,172] Further studies are indicated to evaluate its potential therapeutic role. The application of capsaicin is initially very painful as it is the active ingredient in hot chilli peppers.

Surgical

Perineoplasty

The Woodruff procedure, surgical excision of the vestibule or perineoplasty, is often performed in cases of severe vulvar vestibulitis recalcitrant to medical management.[173] The excision extends from the posterior fourchette to approximately 5 mm beneath and lateral to the urethra to a depth of approximately 2 mm. The adjacent vaginal tissue is then mobilized to cover the excised area. Woodruff noted major symptomatic relief in 14/14 patients treated surgically, of whom two noted intermittent discomfort and one noted recurrent urethral pain and urinary infection. In the literature, success rates based on nonrandomized, retrospective studies range from 47–100%. Success, however, diminishes as the length of follow-up increases.[161,162] To maximize the effect, surgery should include excision of the Bartholin's gland. Progressive introital dilation using vaginal dilators is also recommended by some and should be used for 6 weeks prior to intercourse.[161] As mentioned earlier, combining less aggressive surgery (subtotal perineoplasty) with interferon may be as effective as a total perineoplasty.[170] Subtotal or total perineoplasty is also recommended over vestibuloplasty (undercutting without excision of the vestibule to effect denervation) in one, small, randomized trial.[174]

CO$_2$ laser

Ablative techniques have shown less success in relieving pain secondary to scar formation from third-degree burns, however in one nonrandomized study 63% of patients experienced pain relief.[175] Laser treatment may also further aggravate pain, and has a prolonged healing time.[169]

Psychological and behavioral pain management

Although no longer felt to be primarily of psychological origin, these women may have confounding factors of depression and anxiety. Meana et al. observed that women with physical findings of vestibulitis did not have significant psychological findings. However, women with no apparent findings on examination were more likely to have psychological issues or relationship and sexual dysfunction.[176] One randomized trial observed a beneficial effect when behavioral treatment was incorporated either with or without surgical treatment.[177]

Diet modification

Hyperoxaluria has been implicated in aggravating vulvar pain through the formation of sharp oxalate crystals.[178] On contact with the skin, severe burning may occur. Baggish et al. in a prospective study noted a 10% objective (pain-free sexual intercourse) decrease in women following a low-oxalate diet (avoiding such foods as tea, coffee, cocoa, wine, chocolate, peanuts, peanut butter, all berries, prunes, all beans, eggplant, sweet potatoes, spinach, spicy food, vinegar, wheat germ, tofu) with calcium citrate (400 mg t.i.d.) to inhibit formation of calcium oxalate crystals.[179] Further investigation is needed as other studies report up to a 75% significant improvement on a low-oxalate diet and calcium citrate.[180] Long-term (6 months) compliance is required to optimize effect, and side-effects include abdominal bloating.

Biofeedback

Pelvic floor muscle irritability may aggravate the underlying cause of vulvar vestibulitis. Glazer et al. observed a decrease in subjective vulvar pain in 83% of women following 16 weeks of electromyographic biofeedback in a prospective, nonrandomized uncontrolled trial. A decrease in resting pelvic floor muscle tension and irritability was observed, with resumption of intercourse in 22 of 28 patients.[167] Pelvic floor muscle physical therapy may also be useful, although studies are lacking at this time.

Prognosis

Up to two-thirds of patients may be cured following a variety of treatments.[161] Recalcitrant cases even subsequent to surgery may occur resulting in continued dyspareunia. In these cases, further medical management should be pursued prior to intervening with additional surgical methods.[181]

Key points

- Chronic pelvic pain is pelvic pain that has persisted for 6 months or more. The amount of pain is greater than the degree of pathology.
- The prevalence of CPP is 12–15% in the general population and contributes greatly to the rising cost of health care.
- Knowledge of the innervation of the cutaneous, abdominal, and pelvic organs is critical in understanding the different etiologies of chronic pelvic pain.
- Gynecologic causes of CPP can be divided into noncyclic and cyclic in nature.
- Primary and secondary dysmenorrhea are cyclic in nature. Primary dysmenorrhea is best treated hormonally; treatment of secondary dysmenorrhea depends on the etiology.
- The most prevalent noncyclic gynecologic causes of CPP are adhesions and endometriosis.
- Adhesions are most common in women with previous surgery. Meticulous surgical technique is the only mechanism today to prevent formation of adhesions.
- The pain with endometriosis is most likely associated with deeply infiltrating lesions. Numerous medical and surgical techniques are available for treatment, however even following hysterectomy pain can still recur.

- In ovarian remnant syndrome, pain results from residual ovarian tissue being left *in situ*. Hormonal therapy may be used to suppress the remnant tissue, but surgical excision is the method of choice.
- Irritable bowel syndrome is the most prevalent gastroenterologic cause of CPP. It is characterized by alternating diarrhea and constipation, bloating, and pain relief with bowel movement.
- Pelvic pain, urinary urgency, urinary frequency, and frequent nocturia without evidence of urinary tract infection is suggestive of interstitial cystitis. Diagnosis is made with cystoscopy.
- Eliciting a trigger point is indicative of myofascial pain or nerve entrapment. Injection of local anesthetic can be therapeutic, as well as diagnostic.
- Psychological factors impact the perception of pelvic pain in CPP patients. Depression and a history of physical and/or sexual abuse are more common in this population and should be addressed by the appropriate professional.
- A detailed history of the pain characteristics as well as a pain diary using a visual analog scale should be utilized in the initial evaluation. Physical examination should encompass not only the gynecologic system, but also the musculoskeletal and neurologic systems. Diagnostic studies may be performed to further clarify the etiology.
- Management of CPP should involve a multidisciplinary approach for maximal benefit. Individual components of therapy may include:
  - NSAIDs, antidepressants, anticonvulsants and narcotics depending on the presumed etiology of the pain.
  - Physical therapy including TENS unit device in cases of suspected myofascial pain.
  - Trigger point injections and anesthetic nerve blocks may provide complete or prolonged relief of pain associated with a neurologic etiology such as nerve entrapment. Nerve transection surgery may be necessary, but may result in painful neuroma formation.
  - Surgery may include laparoscopy, presacral neurectomy, and/or hysterectomy with bilateral salpingo-oophorectomy.
  - Emotional and psychological evaluation (should be performed early in the management).
  - Alternative medicine such as chiropractic treatment, hypnosis, and acupuncture.
- Few randomized controlled studies exist to evaluate the effectiveness of the above treatment options. However, a multidisciplinary approach has been shown in a randomized controlled study to be effective in the management of CPP and should be considered in its treatment.
- Vulvodynia or vulvar pain is chronic vulvar discomfort characterized by burning, stinging, irritation, and/or rawness.
- Vulvar vestibulitis, vulvar dermatoses, cyclic vulvovaginitis, vestibular papillomatosis, and dysesthetic vulvodynia are subtypes of vulvodynia.
- The etiology of vulvodynia may be infectious, secondary to trauma, allergens, underlying dermatologic, neurologic, urologic, or systemic conditions.
- Physical examination should map areas of tenderness by using a cotton-tipped applicator.
- Vulvar vestibulitis is vulvar pain characterized by entry dyspareunia, vestibular erythema, and vestibular tenderness. The etiology is often unknown. Histopathology demonstrates a generalized subepithelial chronic inflammation without glandular involvement.
- Treatment for vulvodynia and vulvar vestibulitis is often empiric. Few randomized trials have evaluated the effectiveness of particular treatment modalities.
- Mainstay therapies include, depending on results of evaluation, antifungal agents, antivirals (interferon), antihistamines, topical corticosteroids, analgesics (lidocaine), and estrogen.
- Amitriptyline or other tricyclic antidepressants at low doses, biofeedback and physical therapy (of pelvic floor muscles), and behavioral therapy may enhance the above therapies.
- Surgical intervention (perineoplasty – total or subtotal) should be offered in cases of vulvar vestibulitis resistant to medical therapy.

REFERENCES

◆ 1. Mathias SD, Kuppermann M, Liberman RF, *et al*. Chronic pelvic pain: prevalence, health-related quality of life, and economic correlates. *Obstet Gynecol* 1996; **87**: 321–7.

2. Walker EA, Katon WJ, Katon WS, Alfrey H. The prevalence of chronic pain and irritable bowel syndrome in two university clinics. *J Psychosom Obstet Gynaecol* 1991; **12** (Suppl.): 66–9.

● 3. Howard FM. The role of laparoscopy in chronic pelvic pain: Promise and pitfalls. *Obstet Gynecol Surv* 1993; **48**: 357–87.

4. Reiter RC. A profile of women with chronic pelvic pain. *Clin Obstet Gynecol* 1990; **33**: 130–6.

5. Kumazawa T. Sensory innervation of reproductive organs. In: Cervero F, Morrison J eds. *Visceral Sensation*. New York, NY: Elsevier Science Publications, 1986: 115–31.

6. Cervero F, Tattersall JEH. Somatic and visceral sensory integration in the thoracic spinal cord. In: Cervero F, Morrison J eds. *Visceral Sensation*. New York, NY: Elsevier Science Publications, 1986: 189–205.

7. Procacci P, Zoppi M, Maresen M. Clinical Approach to Visceral Sensation. In: Cervero F, Morrison J, eds. *Visceral Sensation*. New York, NY: Elsevier Science Publications, 1986; 21–36.

8. Cervero F. Sensory innervation of the viscera: periph-

eral basis of visceral pain. *Physiol Rev* 1994; **74:** 95–138.

9. Berkley KJ. Communications from the uterus (and other tissues). In: Besson JM, ed. *Pharmacological Aspects of Peripheral Neurons Involved in Nociception, Pain Research and Clinical Management.* Amsterdam: Elsevier, 1994: 39–47.

10. Berkley KJ, Robbins A, Sato Y. Afferent fibres supplying the uterus in the rat. *J Neurophysiol* 1988; **59:** 142–63.

11. Wesselmann U, Lai J. Mechanisms of referred visceral pain: uterine inflammation in the adult virgin rat results in neurogenic plasma extravasation in the skin. *Pain* 1997; **73:** 209–317.

12. Giamberardina MA, Berkley KJ, Lezzi S, *et al.* Changes in skin and muscle sensitivity in dysmenorrheic vs normal women as a function of body site and monthly cycle. *Soc Neurosci* 1995; Abstract 1638.

◆ 13. Slocumb JC. Neurological factors in chronic pelvic pain: trigger points and the abdominal pelvic pain syndrome. *Am J Obstet Gynecol* 1984; **149:** 536–43.

14. Berkley KJ, Hubscher CH. Visceral and somatic sensory tracks through the neuroaxis and their relation to pain: Lessons from the rat female reproductive system. In: Beghart GF ed. *Visceral Pain, Progress in Pain Research and Management*, vol. 5. Seattle, WA: IASP Press, 1995: 195–216.

15. De Groat WC. Neurophysiology of the pelvic organs. In: Rushton DN ed. *Handbook of Neuro-Urology.* New York, NY: Marcel Dekker, 1994: 55–93.

16. Rogers Jr RM. Basic pelvic anatomy. In: Steege JF, Metzger DA, Levy BS eds. *Chronic Pelvic Pain: An Integrated Approach.* Philadelphia, PA: W. B. Saunders Company, 1998: 31–58.

17. Hughes JM. Psychological aspects of pelvic pain. In: Rocker I ed. *Pelvic Pain in Women. Diagnosis and Management.* London: Springer-Verlag, 1990: 13–20.

18. Rapkin AJ. Adhesions and pelvic pain: a retrospective study. *Obstet Gynecol* 1986; **68:** 13–15.

19. Kresch AJ, Seifer DB, Sachs LB, Barrese I. Laparoscopy in 100 women with chronic pelvic pain. *Obstet Gynecol* 1984; **64:** 672–4.

20. Lundberg WI, Wall JE, Mathers JE. Laparoscopy in the evaluation of pelvic pain. *Obstet Gynecol* 1973; **42:** 872–6.

21. Liston WA, Bradford WP, Downie J, Kerr MG. Laparoscopy in a general gynecologic unit. *Am J Obstet Gynecol* 1972; **113:** 672–7.

22. Keltz MD, Peck L, Liu S, *et al.* Large bowel-to-pelvic sidewall adhesions associated with chronic pelvic pain. *J Am Assoc Gynaecol Laparosc* 1995; **3:** 55–9.

23. Stovall TG, Elder RF, Ling FW. Predictors of pelvic adhesions. *J Reprod Med* 1989; **34:** 345–8.

24. Almeida OD, Val-Gallas JM. Conscious pain mapping. *J Am Assoc Gynecol Laparosc* 1997; **4:** 587–90.

25. Duffy DM, diZerega GS. Adhesion controversies; pelvic pain as a cause of adhesions, crystalloids on preventing them. *J Reprod Med* 1996; **41:** 19–26.

26. Saravelos HG, Li T-C, Cooke ID. An analysis of the outcome of microsurgical and laparoscopic adhesiolysis for chronic pelvic pain. *Hum Reprod* 1995; **10:** 2895–901.

27. Chan CLK, Wood C. Pelvic adhesiolysis: the assessment of symptom relief by 100 patients. *Aust NZ J Obstet Gynaecol* 1985; **25:** 295–8.

28. Fayez JA, Clark RR. Operative laparoscopy for the treatment of localized chronic pelvic-abdominal pain caused by postoperative adhesions. *J Gynecol Surg* 1994; **10:** 79–83.

29. Daniell JP. Laparoscopic enterolysis for chronic abdominal pain. *J Gynecol Surg* 1989; **5:** 61–6.

◆ 30. Peters AAW, Trimbos-Kemper GCM, Admiral C, Trimbos JB. A randomized clinical trial on the benefit of adhesiolysis in patients with intraperitoneal adhesions and chronic pelvic pain. *Br J Obstet Gynaecol* 1992; **99:** 59–62.

31. Steege JF, Scott AL. Resolution of chronic pelvic pain after laparoscopic lysis of adhesions. *Am J Obstet Gynecol* 1991; **165:** 278–83.

32. Monk BJ, Berman ML, Montz FJ. Adhesions after extensive gynecologic surgery: clinical significance, etiology, and prevention. *Am J Obstet Gynecol* 1994; **170:** 1396–403.

● 33. Steege JF. Adhesions and pelvic pain. In: Steege JF, Metzger DA, Levy BS eds. *Chronic Pelvic Pain – an Integrated Approach.* Philadelphia, PA: W. B. Saunders Company, 1998: 115–25.

34. Reese KA, Reddy S, Rock JA. Endometriosis in an adolescent population: the Emory experience. *J Pediatr Adolesc Gynecol* 1996; **9:** 125–8.

35. Martin DC, Hubert GD, VanderZwaag R. Laparoscopic appearances of peritoneal endometriosis. *Fertil Steril* 1989; **51:** 63.

36. Chatman DL, Ward AB. Endometriosis in adolescents. *Obstet Gynecol* 1982; **27:** 186–90.

37. Eskenazi B, Warner ML. Epidemiology of endometriosis. *Obstet Gynecol Clin North Am* 1997; **24:** 235–58.

● 38. D'Hooghe TM, Hill JA. Endometriosis. In: Berek JS, Adashi EY, Hillard PA eds. *Novak's Gynecology,* 12th edn. Baltimore, MD: Williams & Wilkins, 1996: 887–914.

● 39. Hurd, WJ. Criteria that indicate endometriosis in the cause of chronic pelvic pain. *Obstet Gynecol* 1998; **92:** 1029–32.

40. Redwine DB. Age-related evolution on colour appearance of endometriosis. *Fertil Steril* 1987; **48:** 1062–3.

41. Cornillie FJ, Oosterlynck D, Lauweryns JM, *et al.* Deeply infiltrating pelvic endometriosis: histology and clinical significance. *Fertil Steril* 1990; **53:** 978–83.

42. Sutton CJ, Pooley AS, Ewen SP, Haines P. Follow-up report on a randomized controlled trial of laser laparoscopy in the treatment of pelvic pain associated with minimal to moderate endometriosis. *Fertil Steril* 1997; **68:** 1070–4.

43. Bergqvist A, Bergh T, Hogstrom L, *et al.* Effects of trip-

torelin versus placebo on the symptoms of endometriosis. *Fertil Steril* 1998; **69:** 702–8.

◆ 44. Hornstein MD, Surrey ES, Weisberg GW, Casino LA. Leuprolide acetate depot and hormonal add-back in endometriosis: a 12-month study. *Obstet Gynecol* 1998; **91:** 16–24.

45. Waller KG, Shaw RW. Gonadotropin-releasing hormone analogues for the treatment of endometriosis: long-term follow-up. *Fertil Steril* 1993; **59:** 511–15.

◆ 46. Rapkin AJ, Kames LD. The pain management approach to chronic pelvic pain. *J Reprod Med* 1987; **32:** 323–7.

47. Fukaya T, Hoshiai H, Yajima A. Is pelvic endometriosis always associated with chronic pain? A retrospective study of 618 cases diagnosed by laparoscopy. *Am J Obstet Gynecol* 1993; **169:** 719–22.

48. Vercellini P, Trespidi L, De Giorgi O, *et al*. Endometriosis and pelvic pain: relation to disease stage and localization. *Fertil Steril* 1996; **65:** 299–304.

49. Stovall DW, Bowser LM, Archer DF, Guzick DS. Endometriosis-associated pelvic pain: evidence for an association between the stage of the disease and a history of chronic pelvic pain. *Fertil Steril* 1997; **68:** 13–18.

50. Taylor Jr JC. Pelvic pain based on a vascular and autonomic nervous system disorder. *Am J Obstet Gynecol* 1954; **67:** 1177–96.

51. Beard RW, Reginald PW, Wadworth J. Clinical features of women with chronic lower abdominal pain and pelvic congestion. *Br J Obstet Gynaecol* 1988; **95:** 153–61.

◆ 52. Beard RW, Highman JH, Pearce S, Reginald PW. Diagnosis of pelvic varicosities in women with chronic pelvic pain. *Lancet* 1984; **2:** 946–9.

53. Reginald PW, Beard RW, Kooner JS, *et al*. Intravenous dihydroergotamine to relieve pelvic congestion with pain in young women. *Lancet* 1987; **2:** 351–3.

54. Stones RW, Loesch A, Beard RW, Burnstock G. Substance P: endothelial localization and pharmacology in the human ovarian vein. *Obstet Gynecol* 1995; **85:** 273–8.

55. Stones RW, Rae T, Rogers V, *et al*. Pelvic congestion in women: evaluation with transvaginal ultrasound and observation of venous pharmacology. *Br J Radiol* 1990; **63:** 710–11.

56. Adams J, Reginald PW, Franks S, *et al*. Uterine size and endometrial thickness and the significance of cystic ovaries in women with pelvic pain due to congestion. *Br J Obstet Gynaecol* 1990; **97:** 583–7.

57. Gupta A, McCarthy S. Pelvic varices as a cause for pelvic pain: MRI appearance. *Magn Reson Imaging* 1994; **12:** 679–81.

58. Farquhar CM, Rogers V, Frank S, *et al*. A randomized controlled trial of medroxyprogesterone acetate and psychotherapy for the treatment of pelvic congestion. *Br J Obstet Gynaecol* 1989; **96:** 1153–62.

59. Regional PW, Adams J, Franks S, *et al*. Medroxyprogesterone acetate in the treatment of pelvic pain due to venous congestion. *Br J Obstet Gynaecol* 1989; **96:** 1148–52.

60. Allen WM. Chronic pelvic congestion and pelvic pain. *Am J Obstet Gynecol* 1971; **109:** 198–202.

61. Sichlau MJ, Yao JST, Vogelzang RL. Transcatheter embolotherapy for the treatment of pelvic congestion syndrome. *Obstet Gynecol* 1994; **83:** 892–6.

62. Capasso P, Simons C, Trotteur G, *et al*. Treatment of symptomatic pelvic varices by ovarian vein embolization. *Cardiovasc Intervent Radiol* 1997; **20:** 107–11.

63. Tarazov PG, Prozorovskij KV, Ryzhkov VK. Pelvic pain syndrome caused by ovarian varices. Treatment by transcatheter embolization. *Acta Radiol* 1997; **38:** 1023–5.

64. Beard RW, Kennedy RG, Gangar KF, *et al*. Bilateral oophorectomy and hysterectomy in the treatment of intractable pelvic pain associated with pelvic congestion. *Br J Obstet Gynaecol* 1991; **98:** 988–92.

● 65. Steege JF. Ovarian remnant syndrome. *Obstet Gynecol* 1987; **70:** 64–7.

66. Siddall-Allum J, Rae T, Rogers V, *et al*. Chronic pain caused by residual ovaries and ovarian remnants. *Br J Obstet Gynaecol* 1994; **101:** 979–85.

● 67. Steege JF. Pain after hysterectomy. In: Steege JF, Metzger DA, Levy BS eds. *Chronic Pelvic Pain – an Integrated Approach*. Philadelphia, PA: W. B. Saunders Company, 1998: 135–44.

68. Lafferty HW, Angioli R, Rudolph J, Penalver MA. Ovarian remnant syndrome: experience at Jackson Memorial Hospital, University of Miami, 1985 through 1993. *Am J Obstet Gynecol* 1996; **174:** 641–5.

● 69. Price FV, Edwards R, Buchsbaum HJ. Ovarian remnant syndrome: difficulties in diagnosis and management. *Obstet Gynecol Surv* 1990; **45:** 151–6.

70. Carey MP, Slack MC. GnRH analogue in assessing chronic pelvic pain in women with residual ovaries. *Br J Obstet Gynaecol* 1996; **103:** 150–3.

71. Pettit PD, Lee RA. Ovarian remnant syndrome. Diagnostic dilemma and surgical challenge. *Obstet Gynecol* 1988; **71:** 580–3.

72. Lipscomb GH, Ling FW. Relationship of infection and chronic pelvic pain. *Obstet Gynecol Clin North Am* 1993; **20:** 699–708.

73. Sweet RL, Gibbs RS. Pelvic inflammatory disease. In: Sweet RL, Gibbs RS eds. *Infectious Diseases of the Female Genital Tract*. Baltimore, MD: Williams & Wilkins, 1990; 241–66.

● 74. The American College of Obstetricians and Gynecologists. Dysmenorrhea. *ACOG Technical Bulletin* 1983; 68.

75. Rapkin AJ, Rasgon NL, Berkley KJ. Dysmenorrhea. In: Yaksh TL, Lynch C, Zapol WM *et al*. eds. *Anesthesia: Biologic Foundations*. Philadelphia, PA: Lippincott-Raven, 1997: 785–93.

76. The Medical Letter: drugs for dysmenorrhea. *Med Lett Drugs Ther* 1979; **21:** 81–4.

77. Chan WY, Dawood MY. Prostaglandin levels in menstrual fluid of non-dysmenorrheic and of dysmenorrheic subjects with and without oral contraceptive

or ibuprofen therapy. *Adv Prostaglandin Thromb Res* 1980: **8:** 1443–7.

● 78. Smith RP. Cyclic pelvic pain and dysmenorrhea. In: Ling FW ed. *Obstetrics and Gynecology Clinics of North America*, vol. 4. Philadelphia, PA: W. B. Saunders Company, 1993: 753–64.

79. Helms JM. Acupuncture for the management of primary dysmenorrhea. *Obstet Gynecol* 1987; **69:** 51–6.

80. Mannheimer JS, Whaler EC. The efficacy of transcutaneous electrical nerve stimulation in dysmenorrhea. *Clin J Pain* 1985; **1:** 75–83.

81. Kaplan B, Peled Y, Pardo J, *et al*. Transcutaneous electrical nerve stimulation (TENS) as a relief for dysmenorrhea. *Clin Exp Obstet Gynecol* 1994; **21:** 87–90.

82. Malinak, LR. Operative management of pelvic pain. *Clin Obstet Gynecol* 1980; **23:** 191–9.

83. Doyle IB. Paracervical uterine denervation by transection of the cervical plexus for the relief of dysmenorrhea. *Am J Obstet Gynecol* 1955; **70:** 1–16.

◆ 84. Reiter RC. Occult somatic pathology in women with chronic pelvic pain. *Clin Obstet Gynecol* 1990; **33:** 154–60.

85. Walker EA, Gelfand AN, Gelfand MD, *et al*. Chronic pelvic pain and gynecological symptoms in women with irritable bowel syndrome. *J Psychosomat Obstet Gynecol* 1996; **17:** 39–46.

● 86. Rapkin AJ, Mayer EA. Gastroenterologic causes of chronic pelvic pain. In: Ling FW ed. *Obstetrics and Gynecology Clinics of North America: Contemporary Management of Chronic Pain*. Philadelphia, PA: W. B. Saunders Company, 1993: 663–84.

◆ 87. Thompson WG. Irritable bowel syndrome: pathogenesis and management. *Lancet* 1993; **341:** 1569–72.

88. Whitehead WE, Cheskin LJ, Heller BR, *et al*. Evidence for exacerbation of irritable bowel syndrome during menses. *Gastroenterology* 1990; **98:** 1485–9.

◆ 89. Longstreth GF, Preskill DB, Youkeles L. Irritable bowel syndrome in women having diagnostic laparoscopy or hysterectomy. Relation to gynecologic features and outcome. *Dig Dis Sci* 1990; **35:** 1285–90.

● 90. Drossman DA, Thompson WG. The irritable bowel syndrome. Review and a graduated multicomponent treatment approach. *Ann Intern Med* 1992; **116:** 1009–16.

91. Lee AW, Bell RM, Griffen Jr WO, Hagihara P. Recurrent appendiceal colic. *Surg Gynecol Obstet* 1985; **161:** 21–4.

92. Hightower NC, Roberts JW. Acute and chronic lower abdominal pain of enterologic origin in chronic pelvic pain. In: Renaer MR ed. *Chronic Pelvic Pain in Women*. New York, NY: Springer-Verlag, 1981: 110–37.

93. Spangen L. Spigelian hernia. *Surg Clin North Am* 1984; **64:** 351–66.

94. Miklos JR, O'Reilly MJ, Saye WB. Sciatic hernia as a cause of chronic pelvic pain in women. *Obstet Gynecol* 1998; **91:** 998–1001.

● 95. Summit RL. Urogynecologic causes of chronic pelvic pain. In: Ling FW ed. *Obstetrics and Gynecology Clinics of North America: Contemporary Management of Chronic Pain*. Philadelphia, PA: W. B. Saunders Company, 1993; 685–98.

◆ 96. Raz R, Stamm WE. A controlled trial on intravaginal estriol in postmenopausal women with recurrent urinary tract infections. *N Engl J Med* 1993; **329:** 753–6.

97. Bergman A, Karram M, Bhatia NN. Urethral syndrome: a comparison of different treatment modalities. *J Reprod Med* 1989; **34:** 157–60.

◆ 98. Nigro DA, Wein AJ, Foy M, *et al*. Associations among cystoscopic and urodynamic findings in women enrolled in the Interstitial Cystitis Data Base (ICDB) Study. *Urology* 1997; **49** (Suppl. 5AS): 86–92.

99. Karram MM. Frequency, urgency, and painful bladder syndrome. In: Walters MD, Karram MM eds. *Clinical Urogynecology*. St Louis, MO: Mosby, 1993: 285–98.

◆100. Gillenwater JY, Wein AJ. Summary of the National Institute of Arthritis, Diabetes, Digestive and Kidney Diseases Workshop on Interstitial Cystitis. National Institutes of Health, Bethesda, MD, August 28–29. *J Urol* 1988; **140:** 203–6.

●101. Sant GR. Interstitial cystitis – a urogynecologic perspective. *Contemp OB/GYN* 1998; **June:** 119–30.

102. Morscher E. Low back pain in women. In: Renaer MR ed. *Chronic Pelvic Pain in Women*. New York, NY: Springer-Verlag, 1981: 137–54.

●103. Baker PK. Musculoskeletal origins of chronic pelvic pain. In: Ling FW ed. *Obstetrics and Gynecology Clinics of North America: Contemporary Management of Chronic Pain*. Philadelphia, PA: W. B. Saunders Company, 1993: 719–42.

●104. Slocomb JC. Chronic somatic myofascial and neurogenic abdominal pelvic pain. In: Porreco RP, Reiter RC eds. *Clinical Obstetrics and Gynecology*. Philadelphia, PA: J. B. Lippincott & Co, 1990: 145–53.

105. Travell J. Myofascial trigger points. Clinical view. *Adv Pain Res Ther* 1976; **1:** 919–26.

106. Sippo WC, Burghardt A, Gomez AC. Nerve entrapment after pfannensteil incision. *Am J Obstet Gynecol* 1987; **157:** 420–1.

◆107. Hammeroff SR, Carlson GL, Brown BR. Ilioinguinal pain syndrome. *Pain* 1981; **10:** 253–7.

108. Hahn L. Clinical findings and results of operative treatment in ilioninguinal nerve entrapment syndrome. *Br J Obstet Gynaecol* 1989; **96:** 1080–3.

●109. MacDonald JS. Management of chronic pain. In: Ling FW ed. *Obstetrics and Gynecology Clinics of North America: Contemporary Management of Chronic Pain*. Philadelphia, PA: W. B. Saunders Company, 1993: 817–39.

110. Thomson H, Francis DMA. Abdominal-wall tenderness: a useful sign in the acute abdomen. *Lancet* 1977; **1:** 1053.

111. Jacobs MC. Psychological issues. In: *An Integrated Approach to the Management of Chronic Pelvic Pain*. Killingworth: Pharmedica Press, 1997: 8–14.

112. Heim C, Ehlert U, Hanker JP, Hellhammer DH. Abuse-related posttraumatic stress disorder and alterations of the hypothalamic–pituitary–adrenal axis in women with chronic pelvic pain. *Psychosom Med* 1998; **60:** 309–18.

113. Castelnuova-Tedesco P, Krout BM. Psychosomatic aspects of chronic pelvic pain. *Psychiatr Med* 1970; **1:** 109–26.

●114. Renaer M, Vertommen H, Nijs P, *et al*. Psychosocial aspects of chronic pelvic pain in women. *Am J Obstet Gynecol* 1979; **134:** 75–80.

115. Duleba AJ, Jubanyik KJ, Greenfeld DA, Olive DL. Changes in personality profile associated with laparoscopic surgery for chronic pelvic pain. *J Am Assoc Gynecol Laparosc* 1998; **5:** 389–95.

◆116. Magni G, Salmi A, deLeo D, Ceola A. Chronic pelvic pain and depression. *Psychopath* 1984; **17:** 132–6.

117. Walker E, Katon W, Harrop-Griffiths J. Relationship of chronic pelvic pain of psychiatric diagnoses and childhood sexual abuse. *Am J Psych* 1988; **145:** 75–80.

118. Gross RJ, Doerr H, Caldirola D, *et al*. Borderline syndrome and incest in chronic pelvic pain patients. *Intern J Psychiatr Med* 1980; **10:** 79–96.

119. Harrop-Griffiths J, Katon W, Walker E, *et al*. The association between chronic pelvic pain, psychiatric diagnoses and childhood sexual abuse. *Obstet Gynecol* 1988; **71:** 589–94.

120. Rapkin AJ, Kames LD, Darke LL. History of physical and sexual abuse in women with chronic pelvic pain. *Obstet Gynecol* 1990; **76:** 90–6.

121. Walling MK, Reiter RC, O'Hara MW, *et al*. Abuse history and chronic pain in women. 1. Prevalence of sexual abuse and physical abuse. *Obstet Gynecol* 1994; **84:** 193–9.

122. Abramson LY, Seligman MEP, Teasdale JD. Learned helplessness in human: critique and reformation. *Abnorm Psychol* 1978; **87:** 49–74.

123. Toomey TC, Hernandez JT, Gittelman DF, Hulka JF. Relationship of sexual and physical abuse to pain and psychological assessment variables in chronic pelvic pain patients. *Pain* 1993; **53:** 105–9.

◆124. Engel Jr CC, Walker EA, Engel AL, *et al*. A randomized, double-blind crossover trial of sertraline in women with chronic pelvic pain. *J Psychosom Res* 1998; **44:** 203–7.

125. Morris L, Newton RA. Use of high voltage pulsed galvanic stimulation for patients with levator ani syndrome. *Phys Ther* 1987; **67:** 265.

126. Hammeroff SR, Crago BR, Blitt CD, *et al*. Comparison of bupivacaine, etidocaine, and saline for trigger point therapy. *Anesth Analg* 1981; **60:** 752–5.

127. Arner S, Lindblom U, Meyerson BA, Molander C. Prolonged relief of neuralgia after regional anaesthetic blocks. A call for further experimental and systemic clinical studies. *Pain* 1990; **43:** 287–97.

128. Starling JR, Harms BA. Diagnosis and treatment of genitofemoral and ilioinguinal neuralgia. *World J Surg* 1989; **13:** 586–91.

129. Wechsler RJ, Maurer PM, Halpern EJ, Frank ED. Superior hypogastric plexus block for chronic pelvic pain in the presence of endometriosis: CT techniques and results. *Radiology* 1995; **196:** 103–6.

130. Steege JF. Superior hypogastric block during microlaparoscopic pain mapping. *J Am Assoc Gynecol Laparosc* 1998; **5:** 265–7.

131. Stout AL, Steege JF, Dodson WC, Hughes CL. Relationship of laparoscopic findings to self-report of pelvic pain. *Am J Obstet Gynecol* 1991; **164:** 73–9.

132. Baker PN, Symonds MD: The resolution of chronic pelvic pain after normal laparoscopy findings. *Am J Obstet Gynecol* 1992; **166:** 835–6.

133. Nezhat F, Nezhat C, Nezhat CH, *et al*. Use of hysteroscopy in addition to laparoscopy for evaluating chronic pelvic pain. *J Reprod Med* 1995; **40:** 431–4.

◆134. Reiter RC, Gambone JC, Johnson SR. Availability of a multidisciplinary pelvic pain clinic and frequency of hysterectomy for pelvic pain. *J Psychosomat Obstet Gynaecol* 1991; **12** (Suppl.): 109.

◆135. Peters AA, Van Dorst E, Jellis B, *et al*. A randomized clinical trial to compare two different approaches in women with chronic pelvic pain. *Obstet Gynecol* 1991; **77:** 740–4.

136. Elcombe S, Gath D, Day A. The psychological effects of laparoscopy on women with chronic pelvic pain. *Psychol Med* 1997; **27:** 1041–50.

137. ACOG criteria set. Hysterectomy, abdominal or vaginal for chronic pelvic pain. Number 29, November 1997. Committee on Quality Assessment. American College of Obstetricians and Gynecologists. *Int J Gynaecol Obstet* 1998; **60:** 316–17.

138. Carlston KJ, Miller BA, Fowler Jr FJ. The Main women's health study. II. Outcomes of nonsurgical management of leiomyomas, abnormal bleeding, and chronic pelvic pain. *Obstet Gynecol* 1994; **83:** 566–72.

139. Stovall TG, Ling FW, Crawford DA. Hysterectomy for chronic pelvic pain of presumed uterine etiology. *Obstet Gynecol* 1990; **75:** 676–9.

140. Hillis SD, Marchbanks PA, Peterson HB. The effectiveness of hysterectomy for chronic pelvic pain. *Obstet Gynecol* 1995; **86:** 941–5.

141. Cotte G. Resection of the presacral nerves in the treatment of obstinate dysmenorrhea. *Am J Obstet Gynecol* 1937; **33:** 1034–40.

142. Chen F-P, Soong Y-K. The efficacy and complications of laparoscopic presacral neurectomy in pelvic pain. *Obstet Gynecol* 1997; **90:** 974–7.

143. Candiani GB, Fedele L, Vercellini P, *et al*. Presacral neurectomy for the treatment of pelvic pain associated with endometriosis: a controlled study. *Am J Obstet Gynecol* 1992; **167:** 100–3.

144. Davis GD. Uterine prolapse after laparoscopic uterosacral transection in nulliparous airborne trainees. A report of three cases. *J Reprod Med;* 1996; **41:** 279–80.

145. Good MC, Copas Jr PR, Doody MC. Uterine prolapse after laparoscopic uterosacral transection. A case report. *J Reprod Med* 1992; **37:** 995–6.

146. Ingersoll FM, Meigs JV. Presacral neurectomy for dysmenorrhea. *N Engl J Med* 1948; **238:** 357–60.

147. Polan ML, DeCherney A. Presacral neurectomy for pelvic pain in infertility. *Fertil Steril* 1980; **34:** 557–60.

148. Vercellini P, Fedele L, Bianchi S, Candiani GB. Pelvic denervation for chronic pain associated with endometriosis. Fact or fancy? *Am J Obstet Gynecol* 1991; **165:** 745–9.

149. Nezhat CH, Seidman DS, Nezhat FR, Nezhat CR. Long-term outcome of laparoscopic presacral neurectomy for the treatment of central pelvic pain attributed to endometriosis. *Obstet Gynecol* 1998; **91:** 701–4.

150. Tjaden B, Schlaff WD, Kimball A, Rock JA. The efficacy of presacral neurectomy for the relief of midline dysmenorrhea. *Obstet Gynecol* 1992; **167:** 100–3.

151. Chen FP, Chang SD, Chu KK, Soong YK. Comparison of laparoscopic presacral neurectomy and laparoscopic uterine nerve ablation for primary dysmenorrhea. *J Reprod Med* 1996; **41:** 463–6.

◆152. Kames LD, Rapkin AJ, Naliboff BD, *et al.* Effectiveness of an interdisciplinary pain management program for the treatment of chronic pelvic pain. *Pain* 1990; **41:** 41–6.

153. Helms JM. Acupuncture for the management of primary dysmenorrhea. *Obstet Gynecol* 1987; **69:** 51–6.

154. Hawk C, Long C, Azad A. Chiropractic care for women with chronic pelvic pain: a prospective single-group intervention study. *J Man Physiol Ther* 1997; **20:** 73–9.

◆155. Milburn A, Reiter RC, Rhomberg AT. Multidisciplinary approach to chronic pelvic pain. In: Ling FW ed. *Obstetrics and Gynecology Clinics of North America: Contemporary Management of Chronic Pelvic Pain*. Philadelphia, PA: W. B. Saunders Company, 1993: 643–61.

◆156. Gambone JC, Reiter RC. Nonsurgical management of chronic pelvic pain: a multidisciplinary approach. *Clin Obstet Gynecol* 1990; **33:** 205–11.

157. McKay M. Dysesthetic ("essential") vulvodynia – treatment with emitriptyline. *J Reprod Med* 1993; **38:** 9–13.

●158. Wilkinson EJ. Vulvar nonneoplastic epithelial disorders. *ACOG Educ Bull* 1997; **241:** 1–7.

●159. Turner MLC, Marinoff SC. Pudental neuralgia. *Am J Obstet Gynecol* 1991; **165:** 1233–6.

◆160. Friedrich EG. Vulvar vestibulitis syndrome. *J Reprod Med* 1987; **32:** 110–15.

◆161. Ledger WJ, Kessler A, Leonard GH, Witkin SS. Vulvar vestibulitis – a complex clinical entity. *Infect Dis Obstet Gynecol* 1996; **4:** 269–75.

●162. Baggish MS, Miklos JR. Vulvar pain syndrome: a review. *Obstet Gynecol Surv* 1995; **50:** 618–27.

163. McCormack WM. Two urogenital sinus syndromes. Interstitial cystitis and focal vulvitis. *J Reprod Med* 1990; **35:** 873–6.

◆164. Pyka RE, Wilkinson EJ, Friedrich Jr EG, *et al.* The histopathology of vulvar vestibulitis syndrome. *Int J Gynecol Pathol* 1998; **7:** 249–57.

165. Bergeron C, Moyal-Barracco M, Pelisse M, *et al.* Vulvar vestibulitis: lack of evidence for human papillomavirus etiology. *J Reprod Med* 1994; **39:** 936–8.

166. Bornstein J, Shapiro S, Goldshmid N, *et al.* Polymerase chain reaction search for vital etiology of vulvar vestibulitis syndrome. *Am J Obstet Gynecol* 1996; **175:** 139–44.

167. Glazer HI, Rodke G, Swencionis C, *et al.* Treatment of vulvar vestibulitis syndrome with electromyographic biofeedback of pelvic floor musculature. *J Reprod Med* 1995; **40:** 283–90.

168. Stewart EG, Berger BM. Parallel pathologies? Vulvar vestibulitis and interstitial cystitis. *J Reprod Med* 1997; **42:** 131–4.

169. Mann MS, Kaufman RH, Brown D, Adam E. Vulvar vestibulitis: significant clinical variables and treatment options. *Obstet Gynecol* 1992; **79:** 122–5.

170. Bornstein J, Abramovici H. Combination of subtotal perineoplasty and interferon for the treatment of vulvar vestibulitis. *Gynecol Obstet Invest* 1997; **44:** 53–6.

171. Rumsfield JA, West DP. Topical capsaicin in dermatologic and peripheral pain disorders. *DICP Ann Pharmacother* 1991; **25:** 381–7.

172. Sonni L, Cattaneo A, De Marco A, *et al.* Idiopathic vulvodynia – clinical evaluation of the pain threshold with acetic acid solutions. *J Reprod Med* 1995; **40:** 337–41.

◆173. Woodruff JD, Parmley TH. The infection of the minor vestibular glands. *Obstet Gynecol* 1983; **62:** 609–12.

174. Bornstein J, Zarfati D, Goldik Z, Abramovici H. Perineoplasty compared with vestibuloplasty for severe vestibulitis. *Br J Obstet Gynaecol* 1995; **102:** 652–5.

175. Davis GD. The management of vulvar vestibulitis syndrome with the carbon dioxide laser. *J Gynecol Surg* 1989; **5:** 87–91.

176. Meana M, Yitzchak MB, Samir K, Cohen D. Biopsychosocial profile of women with dyspareunia. *Obstet Gynecol* 1997; **90:** 583–9.

177. Schultz WC, Gianotten WL, van der Meijden WI, *et al.* Behaviour approach with or without surgical intervention to the vulvar vestibulitis syndrome: a prospective randomized and intervention to the vulvar vestibulitis syndrome: a prospective randomized and non-randomized study. *J Psychosom Obstet Gynaecol* 1996; **17:** 143–8.

178. Solomon CC, Melmed MH, Heitler SM. Calcium citrate for vulvar vestibulitis. *J Reprod Med* 1991; **36:** 879–82.

179. Baggish MS, Sze EHM, Johnson R. Urinary oxalate excretion and its role in vulvar pain syndrome. *Am J Obstet Gynecol* 1997; **177:** 507–11.

180. Melmed HM. A low calcium oxalate diet and calcium citrate administration are effective treatments for vulvar pain syndrome. *J Gynecol Surg* 1996; **12:** 217–18.

181. Bornstein J, Goldik Z, Alter Z, *et al.* Persistent vulvar vestibulitis: the continuing challenge. *Obstet Gynecol Surv* 1998; **53:** 39–44.

44

Myofascial pain and fibromyalgia: mechanisms to management

JAMES R FRICTON

Myofascial pain (MFP) and fibromyalgia (FM) are pain disorders characterized by localized soft tissue tenderness and pain. MFP is the most common cause of persistent regional pain such as back pain, shoulder pain, tension-type headaches, and facial pain, whereas FM is one of the most common causes of widespread pain in the body.

Two studies of pain clinic populations have revealed that MFP was cited as the most common cause of pain, being responsible for 54.6% of a chronic head and neck pain population[1] and 85% of a back pain population.[2] In addition, Skootsky et al.[3] studied MFP in a general internal medicine practice and found that among those patients who presented with pain 29.6% were found to have MFP as the cause of the pain. Symptoms of FM also appear to be prevalent in the general population, with up to 5% of the population exhibiting them, and are more prevalent in patients with chronic fatigue, estimated to be at least 20%.[4] Because of a lack of objective findings and diagnostic criteria for these disorders, they are often overlooked as common causes of persistent pain.[1,2,5*,6*,7–9] The purpose of this chapter is to discuss the most recent information on diagnostic criteria, clinical characteristics, proposed pathophysiology, and treatment strategies for MFP and FM.

CLINICAL PRESENTATION

Diagnostic criteria for myofascial pain

The clinical characteristics of MFP include trigger points (TrP) in muscle bands, pain in a zone of reference, occa-

sional associated symptoms, and the presence of contributing factors (Table 44.1). A TrP is defined as localized deep tenderness in a taut band of skeletal muscle that is responsible for the pain in the zone of reference; if treated, it will resolve the resultant pain.[10–15] The zone of reference is defined as the area of perceived pain referred by the irritable TrP. The pain is usually located over the TrP or spreads out from the TrP to a distant site (Fig. 44.1). There are generally no neurologic deficits associated with the disorder unless a nerve entrapment syndrome with weakness and diminished sensation coincides with the muscle TrPs.[14] Blood and urine studies are generally normal unless a concomitant medical disorder is present. Imaging studies, including radiographs and magnetic resonance imaging, do not reveal any pathologic changes in the muscle or connective tissue.

The affected muscles may also display an increased fatigability, stiffness, subjective weakness, pain on movement, and slightly restricted range of motion.[11–15] The muscles are painful when stretched, causing the patient to protect the muscle through poor posture and sustained contraction.[16] For example, a study of jaw range of motion in patients with MFP and no joint abnormalities demonstrated a slightly diminished range of motion (approximately 10%) compared with normal subjects and pain in full range of motion.[17] This is considerably less limitation than was found with joint locking due to a temporomandibular joint (TMJ) internal derangement.[17] This restriction may perpetuate the TrP and develop other TrPs in the same muscle and agonist muscles. As mentioned earlier, this can cause multiple TrPs with overlapping areas of pain referral and changes in pain patterns as TrPs are inactivated.

Trigger points in taut band of muscle	Pain in zone of reference
Tenderness on palpation	Constant dull ache
Consistent points of tenderness	Fluctuates in intensity
Palpation alters pain locally or distally	Consistent patterns of referral
	Alleviation with extinction of trigger point
Associated symptoms	*Contributing factors*
Otologic	Traumatic and whiplash injuries
Paresthesiae	Occupational and repetitive strain injuries
Gastrointestinal distress	Physical disorders
Visual disturbances	Parafunctional muscle tension-producing
Dermatographia	habits
	Postural and repetitive strains
	Disuse
	Metabolic/nutritional
	Sleep disturbance
	Psychosocial and emotional stressors
	direct

Table 44.1 *Clinical characteristics of myofascial pain*

Although routine clinical electromyographic (EMG) studies show no significant abnormalities associated with TrPs, some specialized EMG studies reveal differences.[5,18–20] Needle insertion into the TrP can produce a burst of electrical activity that is not produced in adjacent muscle fibers.[21] In two experimental EMG studies of TrPs, Simons[20] and Fricton *et al.*[18] found abnormal electrical activity associated with the local muscle twitch response when specifically snapping the tense muscle band containing a myofascial TrP. The consistency of soft tissues over the TrPs has been found to be higher than adjacent muscles.[22,23] Skin overlying the TrPs in the masseter muscle appears to be warmer when measured by infrared emission.[24,25] Although each of these findings is, by and large, the result of a solitary study, together they provide preliminary evidence of a broad range of objective characteristics that may prove important in the future diagnosis of MFP.

MFP, particularly in the head and neck, is frequently overlooked as a diagnosis because it is often accompanied by signs and symptoms other than pain, such as coincidental pathology conditions and behavioral and psychosocial problems.[11] The signs and symptoms of MFP may appear to mimic many other conditions, such as joint disorders, including arthritis, fibromyalgia, migraine headaches, neuralgias, temporal arteritis, causalgia, TMJ disorders, spinal disk disease, sinusitis, and other pathologies causing confusion in diagnosis.

On the other hand, the characteristics of MFP also appear to accompany many other pain disorders. For example, TrPs often develop in association with joint pathology, such as disk derangements, osteoarthritis, and subluxation.[11,26] MFP has also been reported to be found with systemic or local infections of viral or bacterial origin; with lupus erythematosis, scleroderma, and rheumatoid arthritis; and along segmental distribution of nerve

injury, nerve root compression, or neuralgias. Pathology of specific viscera has been observed with the development of specific TrPs and patterns of pain referral, such as TrPs in the pectoralis major found with acute myocardial infarction.[19]

Diagnostic criteria for fibromyalgia

Fibromyalgia (FM) is a common rheumatic pain syndrome that resembles MFP and is characterized by widespread pain and tenderness on palpation at definable classic locations on the neck, trunk, and extremities (Table 44.2). The prevalence of fibromyalgia in the general population ranges from 3.7% to 20%.[27,28] Other characteristics of FM are divided into the frequency at which they occur. The characteristics that occur in more than 75% of FM patients include chronic fatigue, stiffness, and sleep disturbance, whereas a variety of associated symptoms that occur in less that 25% of FM patients include irritable bowel, headaches, psychologic distress, Raynaud's phenomena, swelling, paresthesiae, and functional disabilities.[29,30] It has been shown that central nervous system-modulating factors such as stress, sleep disorders, and depression play some role in FM.[31–34] Sleep abnormalities have been well documented, but it is unproven whether these are the primary abnormality or whether they are an associated or secondary abnormality. Over 75% of fibromyalgia patients are women aged 30–60 years.[35] Because FM commonly occurs with other medical conditions, it is possible that the reported age of onset is artificially high. Therefore, FM should be suspected in any person presenting with widespread pain since the consequences of prolonged, undiagnosed pain can be considerable.

Figure 44.1 *Examples of Trigger points with associated patterns of referral in the head and neck.*

 Trigger point

Referral pattern

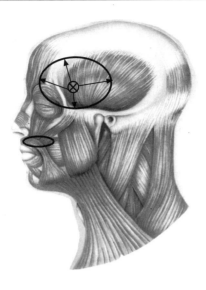

Pain source: Temporalis muscle

Pain site: Temple
                  Frontal
                  Retro-orbital
                  Maxillary anterior teeth

Associated
symptoms: Dental hypersensitivity

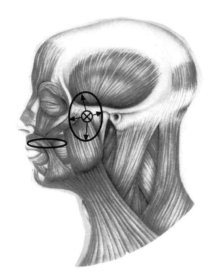

Pain source: Deep masseter

Pain site: Preauricular
                  Earache
                  Maxillary posterior teeth

Associated
symptoms: Dental hypersensitivity

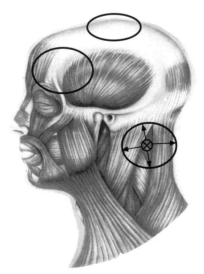

Pain source: Splenius capitus

Pain site: Frontal
                  Occipital
                  Posterior neck
                  Vertex

Associated: Migraine trigger

Table 44.2 *Clinical characteristics of fibromyalgia as defined by the American College of Rheumatology 1990 criteria*

1 *History of widespread pain*
   Definition
   Pain is considered widespread when all of the following are present: pain in the left side of the body, pain in the right side of the body, pain above the waist, pain below the waist. In addition, axial skeletal pain (cervical spine or anterior chest or thoracic spine or low back) must be present. In this definition, shoulder and buttock pain is considered as pain for each involved side. Low back pain is considered lower segment pain

2 *Pain in 11 of 18 tender point sites on digital palpation*
   Definition
   Pain on digital palpation must be present in at least 11 of the following 18 tender point sites:

Occiput	Bilateral, at the suboccipital muscle insertion
Low cervical	Bilateral, at the anterior aspect of the intertransverse spaces at C5–C7
Trapezius	Bilateral, at the midpoint of the upper border
Supraspinatus	Bilateral, at origins above the medial border of the scapular spine
Second rib	Bilateral, upper surfaces just lateral to the costochondral junctions
Lateral epicondyle	Bilateral, 2 cm distal to the epicondyles
Gluteal	Bilateral, in upper outer quadrants of buttocks in anterior fold of muscle
Greater trochanter	Bilateral, posterior to the trochanteric prominence
Knee	Bilateral, at the medial fat pad proximal to the joint line

Digital palpation should be performed with a force of 4 kg. For a tender point to be considered "positive," the subject must state that the palpation was painful. "Tender" is not to be considered "painful"

Note that for classification purposes patients will be said to have fibromyalgia if both criteria are satisfied. Widespread pain must have been present for at least 3 months. The presence of a second clinical disorder does not exclude the diagnosis of fibromyalgia.

Clinical findings: examination for tenderness

Tenderness in the soft tissues is the primary clinical and diagnostic characteristic in both MFP and FM. Tenderness in FM is termed a tender point (TeP) whereas in MFP it is termed a trigger point (TrP).

TrPs in MFP consist of 2- to 5-mm-diameter points of increased hypersensitivity in palpable bands of skeletal muscle, tendons, and ligaments with decreasing hypersensitivity as one palpates the band further away from the TrP. The points may be active or latent.[15] Active TrPs are hypersensitive and display continuous pain in the zone of reference that can be altered with specific palpation. Latent TrPs display only hypersensitivity with no continuous pain. This localized tenderness, elicited with both manual palpation and pressure algometers, has been found to be a reliable indicator of the presence and severity of MFP.[26] However, the presence of taut bands appears to be a characteristic of skeletal muscles in all subjects regardless of the presence of MFP.[36]

Palpating the active TrP with sustained deep, single-finger pressure on the taut band will elicit an alteration of the pain (intensification or reduction) in the zone of reference (area of pain complaint) or cause radiation of the pain toward the zone of reference. This can occur immediately or be delayed a few seconds. The pattern of referral is both reproducible and consistent with patterns seen in other patients with similar TrPs (Fig. 44.1). This enables a clinician to use the zone of reference as a guide to locate the TrP for the purposes of treatment. TePs, on the other

hand, require a standardized palpation at 18 predefined sites, as noted in Fig. 44.2 and Table 44.2.

Many of the TePs seen in the diagnosis of FM are in similar locations to the TrPs in MFP. For example, Simons[37] points out that 16 of the 18 TeP sites in FM lie at well-known TrP sites. Many of the clinical characteristics of FM such as fatigue, morning stiffness, and sleep disorders can also accompany MFP. Bennett[38] has compared these two disorders and concludes that they are two distinct disorders but that they may have the same underlying pathophysiology. Fibromyalgia is characterized by more common central nervous system-generated contributing factors such as sleep disorders, depression, and stress. Myofascial pain, on the other hand, is distinguished by more common regional contributing factors such as localized trauma, posture, and muscle tension habits. Generally, MFP has a better prognosis for treatment than FM.

The patient's behavioral reaction to this firm palpation is a distinguishing characteristic of MFP and FM and is termed a "jump sign." This reaction may include withdrawal of their head, wrinkling of their face or forehead, or a verbal response such as "that's it" or "Oh, yes." The "jump sign" should be distinguished from the "local twitch response" in MFP that can also occur with palpation. This latter response can be elicited by placing the muscle in moderate passive tension and snapping the band containing the TrP briskly with firm pressure from a palpating finger moving perpendicularly across the muscle band at its most tender point. This pressure can produce a reproducible shortening of the muscle band

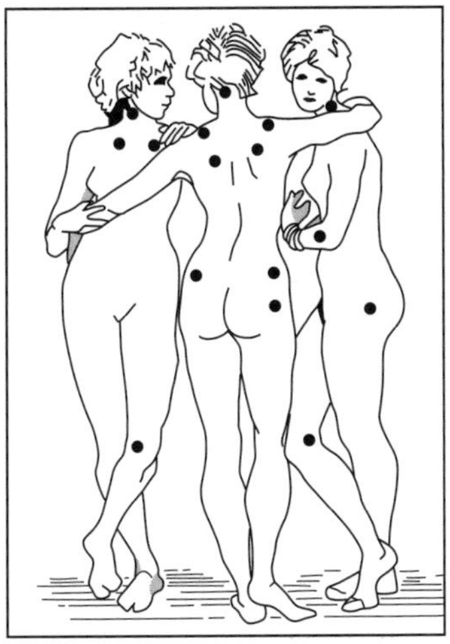

Figure 44.2 *Fibromyalgia tender points.*

1 Widespread aching and pain (pain in all four quadrants: right, left, above and below waist)

2 Eleven or more tender points out of a total of 18 (pressure of about 4 kg with thumb over nine paired locations)

(visible in larger muscles) and associated electromyographic changes that are characteristic of the "local twitch response" described later.[5,18–20] In locating an active TrP, the "jump sign" should be elicited and, if possible, alteration of the patient's complaint by the palpation.

TePs require direct pressure of about 4 kg/cm^2 over the site instead of the snapping palpation with TrPs. Begin by palpating the TeP by pressure over neutral areas such as the middle of the forehead. This gives the examiner an appreciation of the individual's pain threshold and provides a standard pressure to be placed directly over the TeP sites. The TeP will then elicit a pain directly over the site of the tenderness without the radiation of pain that often characterizes MFP TrPs.

Clinical findings: pain

The regional pain found with MFP needs to be distinguished from the widespread muscular pain associated with fibromyalgia (FM) (Table 44.3). In both cases, the pain is often described as a "chronic, dull, aching pain" and is central to the diagnosis of both disorders. These two disorders have many similar characteristics and may represent two ends of a continuous spectrum.

There is evidence that the pain of MFP is related to and/or generated by the TrP, particularly if it is distant from the TrP. For example, clinical examination of TrPs demonstrates that in accessible muscles palpation of the active TrPs will alter, usually by intensifying, the referred pain. In addition, injections of local anesthetic into the active TrP will reduce or eliminate the referred pain and the tenderness.[39–41] Treatments such as spray and stretch, exercise, or massage directed at the muscle with the TrP will also predictably reduce the referred pain.[42] Other evidence to confirm the relationship includes the use of pressure algometry to show a positive correlation between the scope of tenderness and the severity of pain.[43] In addition, the change in scope of tenderness in response to treatment positively correlates with the change in symptom severity ($r = 0.54$).[43]

The pain in FM is relatively stable and consistent; this is in contrast to pain in MFP, which can vary in intensity and location depending on which muscles are involved. Patients with FM most often have pain in the low back, neck, shoulders, and hips.[29,44,45] These are areas that are also frequently affected in MFP, reflecting the overlap between the two disorders. These studies have also shown that the pain in FM is considerably more severe over a larger body area than that seen in patients with other nonlocalized rheumatic disease syndromes.

Relationship to other muscle pain disorders

Many of the characteristics of MFP and FM are also found in other muscle pain disorders such as tension-type headaches, myositis, muscle spasm, and chronic fatigue syndrome, as described in the literature. Perhaps the most pragmatic taxonomy related to differentiating muscle pain disorders is in the Academy of Orofacial Pain's guidelines for diagnosis and management of orofacial pain.[46] In this classification, different muscle disorders are descriptively defined by their characteristics and classified as MFP (regional pain and localized TrP tenderness), fibromyalgia (widespread pain with TePs), myositis (regional pain and diffuse tenderness), muscle spasm (brief painful contraction with limited range of motion), contracture (longstanding limited range of motion from muscle fibrosis), and muscle splinting (regional pain and localized tenderness accompanying a joint problem). Other terms used in the past for the broad category of muscle pain syndromes, such as fibrositis, myofascial pain dysfunction (MPD), myelogelosen, interstitial myofibrositis, musculofascial pain dysfunction, TMJ dysfunction, nonarticular rheumatism, and myalgia, are poorly defined and confusing and should be avoided.

	Fibromyalgia	Myofascial pain
Sex (male–female ratio)	1:10	1:7
Pain	3/4 quadrants	Regional, related to muscle involved
Tender point pain	Local	Referred
Tender point distribution	Widespread	Regional in muscle involved
Tender point	Muscle/tendon	Muscle belly
Stiffness	Widespread	Regional
General fatigue	Debilitating	Usually absent
Prognosis	Seldom cured	Usually good

Table 44.3 *Some differences between fibromyalgia and myofascial pain*

Contributing factors

As with all chronic pain conditions, concomitant social, behavioral, and psychologic disturbances often precede or follow the development of MFP and FM.[43] Patients report psychologic symptoms such as frustration, anxiety, depression, and anger if acute cases become chronic. Maladaptive behaviors such as pain verbalization, poor sleep and dietary habits, lack of exercise, poor posture, bruxism, other tension-producing habits, and medication dependencies can also be seen when pain becomes prolonged. Each of these may complicate the clinical picture by perpetuating the pain, preventing compliance with the treatment program, and causing self-perpetuating chronic pain cycles to develop.

Parafunctional muscle tension-producing habits such as back bracing, neck tensing, and teeth clenching can be generated as a form of tension release as well as a learned behavioral response. The relationships between stress and MFP and between stress and FM are difficult to assess because stress is difficult to define and major methodologic problems exist in studying stress. Although no evidence suggests a direct causal relationship between stress and FM or MFP, some studies suggest that a correlation does exist between them. There is a higher than normal incidence of psychophysiologic disorders such as migraine headaches, backache, neck pain, nervous asthma, and ulcers in patients with MFP and FM, which suggests similar etiologic factors.[47,48] Also, higher than normal levels of urinary concentrations of catecholamines and 17-hydroxysteriods, which are commonly associated with a high number of stressful events, have been found in a group of myofascial pain dysfunction syndrome patients.[49] In addition, stress management interventions frequently provide significant benefit for patients with MFP and FM.

Poor muscle health caused by repetetive strain, lack of exercise, muscle disuse, or poor posture has also been suggested to predispose the muscle to the development of TrPs and TePs.[50,51] These points often arise after muscles have been weakened through immobilization caused by, for example, the prolonged use of cervical collars or extended bedrest. Postural discrepancies may also contribute to joint displacement and abnormal functional patterns, which can contribute to abnormal proprioceptive input and sustained muscle contraction in an attempt to correct the poor postural relationships and allow better neuromuscular function. Poor posture caused by a unilateral short leg, small hemipelvis, increased cervical or lumbar lordosis, noncompensated scoliosis, occlusal abnormalities, and poor positioning of the head or tongue have also been implicated.[52]

ETIOLOGY AND PATHOPHYSIOLOGY

Research suggests that an explanatory model can account for the mechanisms of the development of myalgia, from its onset to increasing severity, that are found in clinical and chronic cases. It is apparent that both central and peripheral mechanisms are associated with this process, but peripheral factors may play a more prominent role in MFP whereas central factors may occur more in FM.

The nature of the peripheral neuropathologic and/or dysfunctional processes of MFP TrPs or FM TePs and the peripheral changes associated with the pain are still not fully understood. A number of histologic and biochemical studies have been carried out on biopsies of tender muscle sites in patients with both generalized and regional muscle complaints. These studies suggest that there are localized progressive increases in oxidative metabolism, particularly in muscle fiber type I, with depleted energy supply, increased metabolic byproducts, and resultant muscle nociception at the periphery. This results in local and referred pain in the central nervous system (CNS) that can be altered by a central biasing mechanism which either amplifies or suppresses the pain.

Injury to muscle fiber type I

Each skeletal muscle has different proportions of muscle fiber types that are grouped into three broad categories: type I, type IIA, and type IIB (Table 44.4).[53] (Types IIC and IIM are involved in development and are not frequently seen in the adult skeletal muscles.) Type I muscle fibers are functionally associated with static muscle tone and posture. They are slow twitch, fatigue-resis-

Table 44.4 *Characteristics of muscle fiber types I, IIA, and IIB in skeletal muscles*

	Major fiber types		
	Type I (red)	Type IIA (pink)	Type IIB (white)
Staining	Weak: ATPase (light pink)	Strong: ATPase (light pink)	Strong: ATPase (light pink)
	Strong NADH-TR (dark pink)	Strong NADH-TR (dark pink)	Weak NADH-TR (dark pink)
Contraction speed and fatigue	Slow twitch; without fatigue; gradual recruitment to maximal force	Fast twitch; fatigue resistant; higher threshold to recruitment	Slow twitch; fatigue resistant; develops highest muscle tension
Cellular characteristics	Low glycogen; high number of mitochondria; high oxidative enzymes; slow myosin	Low glycogen; low number of mitochondria; low oxidative enzymes; fast myosin	Rich in glycogen; low number of mitochondria; low oxidative enzymes; fast myosin
Morphology	1 Less in deep masseter with short face	1 More in deep masseter with short face	1 Hypertrophy with long face
	2 More with loss of teeth	2 Less with loss of teeth	2 Less with loss of teeth
Function	Posture; sustained low force contraction; increase muscle length does not alter function or morphology	Long-term use; sustained high force contraction; increased muscle length does not alter function or morphology	Strength; brief high force contraction; increased muscle length does not alter function or morphology
Response to electrical stimulation	At 50 Hz: type I to II; increased glycogen; decreased mitochondria	At 10 Hz: type II to I; decreased glycogen; increased mitochondria	At 10 Hz: type II to I; decreased glycogen; increased mitochondria
Metabolism	Oxidative phosphorylation	Glycolytic	Glycolytic

Types IIC and IIM are primarily involved in growth and development and are not often seen in skeletal muscles.[100]

tant fibers with a high number of mitochondria, which are needed for oxidative phosphorylation used in energy metabolism. Type II fibers are functionally associated with increased velocity and force of contraction over brief periods. They are fast twitch fibers that fatigue easily, are rich in glycogen, and use anaerobic glycolysis for energy metabolism. These fiber types can transform from one type to another depending on the demands placed on a muscle. For example, Uhlig and colleagues found signs of fiber transformation from type I to type IIC fibers in cervical muscles associated with pain and dysfunction after spondylodesis.[54] This is consistent with the transformation associated with prolonged inactivity due to the injury. Furthermore, Mayo and colleagues found decreases in the cross-sectional diameter of muscle fiber types I and II in the masticatory system in rhesus monkeys undergoing maxillomandibular fixation.[55]

Thus, transformation owing to inactivity and pain can decrease both the percentage and size of type I fibers available to maintain normal postural and resting muscle activity. On the other hand, an increase in the demands of postural muscle activity may result in an increase in type I fibers and a decrease in type II fibers, as found by Bengsston and colleagues in muscle pain patients.[7,8] If the increased demand placed on the type I fibers by repetitive strain from activities such as clenching or shoulder tensing is beyond normal physiologic parameters, the intra-

cellular components of these fibers will be damaged. This will result in hyperpolarization outside the muscle due to high levels of K^+ from sustained motor unit activity and K^+ pump damage, damage to the actin and myosin myofilaments, disruption of the sarcoplasmic reticulum and the calcium pump, and a decrease in local blood flow. Specific factors that are important in initiating this process include both direct macrotrauma and indirect microtrauma from repetitive muscle strain factors.[56]

Metabolic distress at the motor endplates

In explaining the local nature of myofascial pain TrPs, Simons[57] suggests that the damage to the muscle occurs primarily at the motor endplates, creating an energy crisis at the TrP.[57] He also suggests that this crisis occurs from a grossly abnormal increase in acetylcholine release at the endplate and generation of numerous miniature endplate potentials. This results in an increase in energy demand, sustained depolarization of the postjunction membrane, and mitochondrial changes. Other studies support this mechanism.[58-61] For example, Hubbard and Berkoff found spontaneous EMG activity at the TrP,[61] Hong found that the EMG characteristics of the local twitch response are generated locally without input from the CNS,[59] and Hong and Torigoe found that botulism A toxin injections that act on the neuromuscular junction are also effective in MFP TrPs.[58]

Histologic studies also provide some support for this mechanism. They have demonstrated myofibrillar lysis, moth-eaten fibers, and ragged red type I fibers with deposition of glycogen and abnormal mitochondria, but there is little evidence to support the cellular inflammation hypothesis.[7,62] Studies of muscle energy metabolism found a decrease in the levels of adenosine triphosphate (ATP), adenosine diphosphate (ADP), and phosphoryl creatine, and abnormal tissue oxygenation in muscles with TrPs.[63] El-Labban and colleagues demonstrated histologically that TMJ ankylosis will result in degenerative changes in the masseter and temporalis muscles.[64] It has been hypothesized that these changes represent localized progressive increases in oxidative metabolism and depleted energy supply in type I fibers. This may result in progressive abnormal muscle changes that initially include reactive dysfunctional changes occurring within the muscle, particularly in muscle fiber type I and surrounding connective tissue.[62]

Activation of muscle nociceptors

Whether they are caused by a high potassium concentration and hyperpolarization outside the muscle as a result of K^+ pump damage, by a high calcium concentration owing to damage to the sarcoplasmic reticulum, or by inflammatory mediators from tissue damage, the metabolic byproducts resulting from damage can result in peripheral sensitization of nociceptors and muscle fatigue and disuse.[65] Localized tenderness and pain in the muscle involve type III and IV muscle nociceptors and have been shown to be activated by noxious substances, including K^+, bradykinin, histamine, and prostaglandins that can be released locally from the damage and trigger tenderness.[66–71] It is important to note that K^+ activates more type IV muscle nociceptors than other agents, providing support that localized increases in K^+ at the neuromuscular junction may be responsible for some sensitization of nociceptors. This peripheral sensitization is thought to play a major role in local tenderness and pain that, together with central sensitization, produces hyperalgesia in patients with persistent muscle pain.

Transmission of pain to the central nervous system

The afferent inputs from type III and IV muscle nociceptors in the body are transmitted to the CNS through cells such as those of the laminae I, V, and possibly IV of the dorsal horn on the way to the cortex, resulting in perception of local pain.[72,73] In the trigeminal system, these afferent inputs project to the second-order neurons in the brain stem regions, including the superficial laminae of the trigeminal subnucleus caudalis as well as its more rostral laminae such as interpolaris and oralis.[74,75] These neurons can then project to neurons in higher levels of the CNS, such as the thalamus, cranial motor nuclei, or the reticular formation.[76] In the thalamus, the ventrobasal complex (VB), the posterior group of nuclei (PO), and parts of the medial thalamus are involved in receiving and relaying somatosensory information.[77] These inputs can also converge with other visceral and somatic inputs from tissues such as the joint or skin and be responsible for referred pain perception.[76]

Modification of central nociceptive input

Both FM and MFP need to be considered as primary disorders of central pain perception. Although nociceptive inputs from the periphery do occur, they have been shown to be modified by multiple factors in their transmission to the CNS. For example, low- and high-intensity electrical stimulation of sensory nerves or noxious stimulation of sites remote from the site of pain will suppress nociceptive responses of the trigeminal brain stem neurons and related reflexes.[75] This provides support for the theory that afferent inputs can be *inhibited* by multiple peripherally or centrally initiated alterations in neural input to the brain stem through various treatment modalities such as cold, heat, analgesic medications, massage, muscular injections, and transcutaneous electrical stimulation.[68]

Likewise, persistent peripheral or central nociceptive activity can result in an increase in abnormal neuroplastic changes in cutaneous and deep neurons. These neuroplastic changes may include prolonged responsiveness to afferent inputs, increased receptive field size, and spontaneous bursts of activity.[78–80] Thus, peripheral inputs from muscles may also be *facilitated or accentuated* by multiple peripherally or centrally initiated alterations in neural input with further sustained neural activity such as persistent joint pain, sustained muscle activity habits or postural tension, or CNS alterations such as depression and anxiety that can support the central sensitization, further perpetuating the problem. This sensitization may be subserved by a number of neuropeptides including, for example, substance P, serotonin, acetylcholine, and endorphins. Serotonin (5-hydroxytryptamine) is a CNS neurotransmitter that has been shown to have an inverse relationship to fibromyalgic pain and has also been shown, with substance P, to be elevated in the cerebral spinal fluid in FM patients.[81,82]

These biochemical changes underlie an integrated "central biasing mechanism" in the CNS that will dampen or accentuate peripheral input.[68] This mechanism may explain many of the characteristics of MFP and FM, including the broad regions of pain referral, the recruitment of additional muscles in chronic cases, the interrelationship between muscle and joint pain, and the ability of many treatments, including medication, spray and stretch, massage, and TrP injections, to reduce the pain for longer than the duration of action.

There is also evidence that patients with FM may have an abnormality associated with their immune system that may distinguish them from MFP patients and that may support the more systemic nature of FM. Several studies have found that most patients with chronic fatigue and immune dysfunction syndrome (CFIDS) fulfill the criteria for FM and that they may have several serum abnormalities of the immune function.[83-85] It is suggested that, in some FM patients, an infectious process led to chronic disturbances in both the immune system functioning and the mechanisms of sleep and pain regulation.

EVIDENCED-BASED MANAGEMENT

Treatment of MFP can range from simple cases with transient single-muscle syndromes to complex cases involving multiple muscles and many interrelating contributing factors, including the presence of FM. Many authors have found success in the treatment of MFP and FM using a wide variety of techniques such as exercise, trigger point injections, vapocoolant spray and stretch, transcutaneous electrical nerve stimulation (TENS), biofeedback, posture correction, tricyclic antidepressants, muscle relaxant and other medications, and addressing perpetuating factors.[10*,12***,14***,15***,43*,86*,87*,88***] However, the difficulty in management lies in the critical need to match the level of complexity of the management program with the complexity of the patient. Failure to address the entire problem, including all involved muscles, concomitant diagnoses, and contributing factors, may lead to failure to resolve the pain and perpetuation of the pain. The worse prognosis for outcome in patients with FM (only 5% of patients have sustained remission after treatment) is another factor that distinguishes MFP and FM.

Although there are no controlled studies examining progression of chronic pain syndromes, results from clinical studies reveal that patients with MFP and/or FM have seen many clinicians and have received numerous medications and multiple other singular treatments for years without receiving more than temporary improvement. In one study of 164 MFP patients, the mean duration of pain was 5.8 years for males and 6.9 years for females, with a mean of 4.5 past clinicians seen for the study.[11*] In another study of 102 consecutive TMJ and craniofacial pain patients that included 59.8% MFP patients, the mean duration of pain was 6.0 years, with 28.8 previous treatment sessions, 5.1 previous doctors, and 6.4 previous medications.[43*]

These and other studies of chronic pain suggest that, regardless of the pathogenesis of muscular pain, a major characteristic of some of these patients is the failure of traditional approaches to resolve the problem. Each clinician confronted with a patient with MFP or FM needs to recognize and address the whole problem to maximize the potential for a successful outcome. Treating only those patients whose complexity matches the treatment strategy available to the clinician can improve success. Simple cases with minimal behavioral and psychosocial involvement can typically be managed by a single clinician. Complex patients should be managed within an interdisciplinary pain clinic setting that uses a team of clinicians to address different aspects of the problem in a concerted fashion.

Management includes muscle exercises, therapy to TrPs, and reducing all contributing factors. The short-term goal is to restore the muscle to normal length, posture, and full joint range of motion with exercises and trigger point therapy. This is followed long term with a regular muscle stretching, postural, and strengthening exercise program as well as control of contributing factors.

Long-term control of pain depends on patient education, self-responsibility, and development of long-term doctor–patient relationships. This often requires shifting the paradigms implicit in patient care and listed in Table 44.5. The difficulty in long-term management often lies not in treating the TrPs but rather in the complex task of changing the identified contributing factors since they can be integrally related to the patient's attitudes, lifestyle, and social and physical environment. Interdisciplinary teams integrate various health professionals in a supportive environment to accomplish both long-term treatment of illness and modification of these contributing factors. Many approaches, such as habit-reversal techniques, biofeedback, and stress management have been used to achieve this result within a team approach.

Muscle exercises

The most useful exercise techniques for muscle rehabilitation include muscle stretching, posture, strengthening

Table 44.5 *Shifting the doctor–patient paradigms involves each member of the team following the same concepts by conveying the same messages implicit in their dialogue with the patient*

Concept	Statement
Self-responsibility	You have more influence on your problem than we do
Self-care	You will need to make daily changes in order to improve your condition
Education	We can teach you how to make the changes
Long-term change	It will take at least 6 months for the changes to have an effect
Strong doctor–patient relationship	We will support you as you make the changes
Patient motivation	Do you want to make the changes?

exercises, and, particularly for FM, cardiovascular fitness. In patients with both MFP and FM, a home program of active and passive muscle-stretching exercises will reduce the activity of TrPs while postural exercises will reduce the likelihood of TrPs being reactivated by physical strain. Strengthening and cardiovascular fitness exercises will improve circulation, strength, and durability of the muscles.[89]**

Evaluating the present range of motion of muscles is the first step in prescribing a set of exercises to follow. For example, in the head and neck, a range of motion should be determined for the jaw and neck at the initial evaluation. A limited mandibular opening in the jaw will indicate whether there are any TrPs within the elevator muscles: temporalis, masseter, and medial pterygoid. If mandibular opening is measured as the interincisal distance, the maximum range of opening is generally between 42 and 60 mm or approximately the width of three knuckles (nondominant hand). A mandibular opening with TrPs in the masseter will be approximately 30–40 mm or the width of two knuckles.[90] If contracture of masticatory muscles is present, the mandibular opening can be limited to 10–20 mm. Other causes of diminished mandibular opening include structural disorders of the temporomandibular joint, such as ankylosis, internal derangements, and gross osteoarthritis.

Passive and active stretching of the muscles will increase the opening to the normal range as well as decrease the pain. Passive stretching of the masticatory muscles during counterstimulation of the TrP can be accomplished through placing a properly trimmed and sterile cork, tongue blades, or other object between the incisors while the spray and stretch technique is accomplished. It must be emphasized that rapid jerky stretching or overstretching of the muscle must be avoided in order to reduce potential injury to the muscle.

Postural exercises are designed to teach the patient mental reminders to hold the body in a balanced relaxed position and to use the body in positions that afford the best mechanical advantage. This includes static postural problems such as unilateral short leg, small hemipelvis, occlusal discrepancies, and scoliosis or functional postural habits such as forward head, jaw thrust, shoulder phone bracing, and lumbar lifting. In a study of postural problems in 164 head and neck MFP patients, Fricton and Kroening[11] found poor sitting/standing posture in 96%, forward head in 84.7%, rounded shoulders in 82.3%, lower tongue position in 67.7%, abnormal lordosis in 46.3%, scoliosis in 15.9%, and leg length discrepancy in 14.0%. In improving posture, specific skeletal conditions such as structural asymmetry or weakness of certain muscles need to be considered. In the masticatory system, the patient should be instructed to place the tongue gently on the roof of the mouth and keep the teeth slightly apart. In the cervical spine, a forward or lateral head posture must be corrected by guiding the chin in and the head vertex up. The shoulders will naturally fall back if

the thorax is positioned up and back with proper lumbar support. Patients need to be instructed in the proper posture for each position – sitting, standing, and lying down – as well as in movements that are carried out repetitively throughout the day such as lifting or turning the head to the side. Sleeping posture on the side or back is particularly important for patients who wake up with soreness.

Improved posture is also facilitated by regular physical conditioning. Patients need to be placed on a conditioning program to facilitate increased aerobic capacity and strength. Aerobic programs such as becoming involved in an exercise class, regular running, walking, cycling, or swimming will improve comfort, endurance, and functional status of patients with MFP.[15]*

Muscle therapy

There are many methods suggested for providing repetitive stimulation to tender muscles. Massage, acupressure, and ultrasound provide noninvasive mechanical disruption to inactivate the TrPs. Moist heat applications, ice packs, fluorimethane, and diathermy provide skin and muscle temperature change as a form of counterstimulation. Transcutaneous electrical nerve stimulation, electroacupuncture, and direct current stimulation provide electric currents to stimulate the muscles and TrPs. Acupuncture and TrP injections of local anesthetic, corticosteroids, or saline cause direct mechanical or chemical alteration of TrPs. The two most common techniques for treating a TrP – spray and stretch technique and injections – will be discussed here.

With the spray and stretch technique, an application of a vapocoolant spray such as fluorimethane over the muscle with simultaneous passive stretching can provide immediate reduction of pain, although lasting relief requires a full management program.[14]* The technique involves directing a thin stream of fluorimethane spray from the finely calibrated nozzle toward the skin directly overlying the muscle with the TrP. A few sweeps of the spray are first passed over the TrP and zone of reference before adding sufficient manual stretch to the muscle to elicit pain and discomfort. The muscle is put on a progressively increasing passive stretch while the jet stream of spray is directed at an acute angle from 30–50 cm (1–1.5 feet) away. It is applied in one direction – from the TrP toward its reference zone – in slow, even sweeps over adjacent parallel areas at a rate of about 10 cm/s. This sequence can be repeated up to four times if the clinician warms the muscle with his or her hand or warm moist packs are used to prevent overcooling after each sequence. Frosting the skin and excessive sweeps should be avoided because it may lower the underlying skeletal muscle temperature, which tends to aggravate TrPs. The range of passive and active motion can be tested before and after spraying as an indication of the responsiveness to therapy. Failure to reduce TrPs with spray and stretch may be due to: (1) inability to secure full muscle length because of bone or joint abnormalities, muscle contracture, or the patient avoiding voluntary relaxation; (2) incorrect spray technique; or (3) failure to reduce perpetuating factors. If spray and stretch fails with repeated trials, direct needling with TrP injections may be effective.

TrP injections have also been shown to reduce pain, increase the range of motion, increase exercise tolerance, and increase the circulation in muscles.[39*,40*,41**] The pain relief may last from the duration of the anesthetic to many months, depending on the chronicity and severity of the TrPs and the degree of reducing perpetuating factors. As the critical factor in relief appears to be the mechanical disruption of the TrP by the needle, precision in needling of the exact TrP and the intensity of pain during needling appear to be the major factors in TrP inactivation.[19*] TrP injections with local anesthetic are generally more effective and comfortable than dry needling or injecting other substances such as saline, although acupuncture may be helpful for patients with chronic TrPs in multiple muscles. The effect of needling can be complemented with the use of local anesthetics in concentrations less than those required for a nerve conduction block. This can markedly lengthen the relative refractory period of peripheral nerves and limit the maximum frequency of impulse conduction. Local anesthetics can be chosen for their duration, safety, and versatility. Three percent chlorprocaine (short acting) and 5% procaine (medium acting) without vasoconstrictors are suggested.

Pharmacotherapy

Pharmacotherapy is a useful adjunct to the initial treatment of MFP and FM. The most commonly used medications for pain are classified as non-narcotic analgesics (nonsteroidal anti-inflammatories), narcotic analgesics, muscle relaxants, tranquilizers (ataractics), sedatives, and antidepressants. Analgesics are used to allay pain, as muscle relaxants, and as tranquilizers for anxiety, fear, and muscle tension; sedatives are used to enhance sleep; and antidepressants are used for pain, depression, and enhancing sleep.[91***]

Randomized clinical trials on nonsteroidal anti-inflammatory drugs (NSAIDs) such as ibuprofen or piroxicam suggest that, for myalgia, short-term use of these medications for analgesic and/or anti-inflammatory effects certainly can be considered as a supplement to overall management.[92**] Chronic long-term use should be viewed with caution because of the long-term systemic and gastrointestinal effects. However, the recently available cyclo-oxygenase 2 (COX-2) inhibitors (e.g. rofecoxib, Vioxx) may prove to be safer than NSAIDs for long-term use and may have fewer gastrointestinal toxic effects. If some therapeutic result is not apparent after 7–10 days, or if the patient develops any side-effects,

especially gastrointestinal symptoms, the medication should be discontinued.

For MFP, especially with a limited range of motion, benzodiazepines, including diazepam and clonazepam, have been shown to be effective.[92**] Experience suggests that these are best used before bedtime to minimize sedation while awake. In clinical trials of myalgia, cyclobenzaprine has been shown to be efficacious in reducing pain and improving sleep[92**] and can be considered when a benzodiazepine is too sedating. These medications, with or without NSAIDs, can also be considered for a 2- to 4-week trial with minimal habituation potential. However, long-term use has not been adequately tested.

Research on medications for FM, especially with sleep disturbances, indicates that tricyclic antidepressants, such as amitriptyline, have a significant impact on sleep disturbances, anxiety, and pain in FM. As such, these medications can be used in appropriate cases in the long term.[93*] However, the side-effects with amitriptyline can be significant; nortriptyline is an analogous medication with fewer side-effects. Typically, the dosage for either of these medications for patients with FM but without depression is in the 25- to 75-mg range at bedtime. The use of selective serotonin reuptake inhibitors (SSRIs) has been suggested for depression and pain but these may also have the common side-effect of increasing muscle tension and aggravating pain.

For chronic pain conditions that are resistant to interventions, use of opioids can be considered. Tramadol has been shown to be effective in FM.[94] However, there are no randomized, controlled trials (RCTs) evaluating the appropriateness of opioids in the long-term treatment of chronic pain. At this time, chronic opioid use is mainly indicated for patients with chronic intractable severe pain conditions that are refractory to all other reasonable treatments because of their side-effects, including constipation, sedation, potential for dose escalation, and the unknown effects with long-term use.

Despite the advantages of medications for pain disorders, there exists an opportunity for problems to occur as a result of their misuse. The problems that can occur from the use of medications include chemical dependency, behavioral reinforcement of continuing pain, inhibition of endogenous pain relief mechanisms, side-effects, and adverse effects from the use of polypharmaceuticals. For this reason, use of medication should proceed with caution.

Control of contributing factors

One of the common causes of failure in managing MFP and FM is the failure to recognize and subsequently control contributing factors that may perpetuate muscle restriction and tension. As noted earlier, postural contributing factors, whether behavioral or biologic, perpetuate muscle pain if not corrected. In general, a muscle is more predisposed to developing problems if it is held in a sustained contraction in the normal position, especially if it is in an abnormally shortened position. Such a situation exists with structural problems such as loss of posterior teeth, an excessive lordosis of the cervical spine, a unilateral short leg, or a small hemipelvis. An occlusal imbalance can be corrected with an occlusal stabilization splint, also termed a flat plane or full coverage splint. Other postural factors that can be corrected include a foot lift for a unilateral leg-length discrepancy, a pelvic lift for a small hemipelvis, and proper height of arm rests in chairs for short upper arms.

Behavioral factors causing sustained muscle tension can also occur with habits such as a receptionist cradling a phone between the head and shoulder for hours each day, a laborer lifting with lumbar strain, a student studying with the head forward for hours at a time, or bruxism, clenching, gum-chewing, or other oral parafunctional habits. Correcting poor habits through education and long-term reinforcement is essential to preventing a reduced TrP from returning. Biofeedback, meditation, hypnosis, stress-management counseling, psychotherapy, anti-anxiety medications, antidepressants, and even placebos have been reported to be effective in treating MFP and FM.[43***,86*,87*] Many of these treatments are directed toward reducing muscle tension-producing habits such as bruxism or bracing of muscles. Teaching control of habits is a difficult process because of the relationship that muscle tension may have to psychosocial factors. Simply telling a patient to stop the habits may be helpful with some, but with others it may result in noncompliance, failure, and frustration. An integrated approach involving education, increased awareness, and other treatments such as behavior modification, biofeedback, hypnosis, or drug therapy may prove to be more successful.

Pain clinic team management

Although each clinician may have limited success in managing the "whole" patient alone, the assumption behind a team approach is that it is vital to address different aspects of the problem with different specialists in order to enhance the overall potential for success.[2***,43***,95,96*] Although these programs provide a broader framework for treating the complex patient, they have added another dimension to the skills needed by the clinician: working as part of a coordinated team. Failure to adequately integrate care may result in poor communication, fragmented care, distrustful relationships, and eventually confusion and failure in management. However, team coordination can be facilitated by a well-defined evaluation and management system that clearly integrates team members.

A prerequisite to a team approach is an inclusive medical model and conceptual framework that places the physical, behavioral, and psychosocial aspects of illness on an equal and integrated basis.[97,98] With an inclusive theory of human systems and their relationship to illness, a patient can be assessed as a whole person by different clinicians from diverse backgrounds. Although each clinician understands a different part of the patient's problem, they can integrate them with other clinicians' perspectives and see how each part is interrelated in the whole patient. For example, a physician or dentist will evaluate the physical diagnosis, a physical therapist will evaluate poor postural habits, and a psychologist will evaluate behavioral problems or social stressors. Each factor will become part of the problem list to be addressed in the treatment plan. In the process, the synergism of each factor in the etiology of the disorder can become apparent to clinicians. For example, social stressors can lead to anxiety; anxiety can lead to poor posture and muscle tension; and the poor posture and muscle tension can lead to myofascial pain syndrome; the pain contributes to more anxiety and a cycle continues. Likewise, a reduction of each factor will work synergistically to improve the whole problem. Treatment of only one factor may improve the problem, but relief may be partial or temporary. Treatment of all factors simultaneously can have a cumulative effect that is greater than the effects of treating each factor individually.

The problem list for a patient with a specific chronic illness includes both a physical diagnosis and a list of contributing factors. In establishing the problem list, the clinician needs to determine whether the patient is complex and requires a team approach. Recommended criteria for determining complexity include any one of the following: multiple diagnoses, persistent pain for longer than 6 months, significant emotional problems (depression, anxiety), frequent use of health care services or medication, daily oral parafunctional habits, and significant lifestyle disturbances. The use of a screening instrument questionnaires can readily elicit the degree of complexity of a case at initial evaluation.[43,99] The more complex the case is, the greater the need for a team approach. The decision to use a team must be made at the time of evaluation and not part way through a failing singular treatment plan. If a team approach is needed, the broad understanding of the patient is then used to design a long-term management program that both treats the physical diagnosis and helps reduce the contributing factors.

The primary goals of the program include reducing the symptoms and their negative effects while helping the patient to return to normal function without the need for future health care. The patient first participates in an educational session with each clinician to learn about the diagnoses and contributing factors, why it is necessary to change these factors, and how to do it. The dentist or physician is responsible for establishing the physical diagnosis, providing short-term medical or dental care, and monitoring medication and patient progress. The health psychologist is responsible for providing instruction about contributing factors; diagnosing, managing, or referring for primary psychologic disturbances; and establishing a program to support the patient and family in making changes. The physical therapist is responsible for providing support, instruction, and a management program, such as an exercise and posture program, that is based on specifically assigned and common contributing factors. Depending on the therapist's background and the patient's needs, this person may also provide special care such as physical therapy modalities or occupational therapy. Each clinician is also responsible for establishing a trusting, supportive relationship with the patient while reaffirming the self-care philosophy of the program, reinforcing change, and assuring compliance. The patient is viewed as responsible for making the changes (Table 44.4). The team meets weekly to review current patient progress and discuss new patients.

SUMMARY

Myofascial pain (MFP) is a regional muscle pain disorder that is characterized by localized muscle tenderness and pain and is one of the most common causes of persistent regional pain. Fibromyalgia (FM) is a widespread pain disorder characterized by widespread tenderness at specific TePs, decreased pain threshold, sleep disturbance, fatigue, and often psychologic distress. The affected muscles in both disorders may also display an increased fatigability, stiffness, subjective weakness, pain in movement, and slightly restricted range of motion that is unrelated to joint restriction. They are frequently overlooked as a diagnosis because they are often accompanied by other signs and symptoms in addition to pain, such as coincidental pathology conditions and behavioral and psychosocial problems. As these disorders persist, chronic pain characteristics often precede or follow their development.

Management of both disorders includes exercise, therapy to the TrPs, and reducing all contributing factors. The difficulty in managing both MFP and FM lies in the critical need to match the level of complexity of the management program to the complexity of the patient. Failure to address the entire problem through a team approach, if needed, may lead to failure to resolve the pain and perpetuation of a chronic pain syndrome.

REFERENCES

1. Arlen H. The otomandibular syndrome: a new concept. *Ear Nose Throat J* 1977; **56** (2): 60–2.
2. Aronoff GM, Evans WO, Enders PL. A review of follow-up studies of multidisciplinary pain units. *Pain* 1983; **16:** 1–11.
3. Skootsky S, Jaeger B, Oye RK. Prevalence of myofascial pain in general internal medicine practice. *West J Med* 1989; **151:** 157–60.
4. Wolfe F. Fibromyalgia. In: Sessle BJ, Bryant PS, Dionne RA eds. *Temporomandibular Disorders and Related Pain Conditions. Progress in Pain Research and Management,* vol. 4. Seattle, WA: IASP Press, 1995: 31–46.
5. Arroyo Jr P. Electromyography in the evaluation of reflex muscle spasm: simplified method for direct evaluation of muscle-relaxant drugs. *J Fla Med Assoc* 1966; **53:** 29–31.
6. Awad EA. Interstitial myofibrositis: hypothesis of the mechanism. *Arch Phys Med Rehabil* 1973; **54:** 449–53.
7. Bengtsson A, Henriksson KG, Jorfeldt L, *et al*. Primary fibromyalgia: a clinical and laboratory study of 55 patients. *Scand J Rheumatol* 1986; **15:** 340–7.
8. Bengtsson A, Henriksson KG, Larsson J. Reduced high-energy phosphate levels in the painful muscles of patients with primary fibromyalgia. *Arthritis Rheum* 1986; **29:** 817–21.
9. Braun B, DiGiovann A, Schiffman E, *et al*. A cross-sectional study of temporomandibular joint dysfunction in post-cervical trauma patients. *J Craniomandibular Disord Oral Facial Pain* 1992; **6:** 24–31.
10. Bonica JJ. Management of myofascial pain syndrome in general practice. *JAMA* 1957; **164:** 732–8.
11. Fricton JR, Kroening R. Practical differential diagnosis of chronic craniofacial pain. *Oral Surg Oral Med Oral Pathol* 1982; **54:** 628–34.
◆ 12. Simons DG. Muscle pain syndromes. Part I. *Am J Phys Med* 1975; **54:** 289–311.
13. Simons DG. Traumatic fibromyositis or myofascial trigger points. *West J Med* 1978; **128:** 69–71.
14. Travell J. Myofascial trigger points: clinical view. In: Bonica JJ, Albe-Fessard DD eds. *Advances in Pain Research and Therapy.* New York, NY: Raven Press, 1976: 919–26.
15. Travell J, Simons DG. *Myofascial Pain and Dysfunction: The Trigger Point Manual.* Baltimore, MD: Williams & Wilkins, 1983: 63–158.
16. Travell J. Identification of myofascial trigger point syndromes: a case of atypical facial neuralgia. *Arch Phys Med Rehabil* 1981; **62:** 100–6.
17. Fricton JR, Kroening R, Haley D, Siegert R, Myofascial pain and dysfunction: a review of clinical characteristics of 164 patients. *Oral Surg* **57:** 615–27.
18. Fricton J, Auvinen MD, Dykstra D, Schiffman E. Myofascial pain syndrome: electromyographic changes associated with local twitch response. *Arch Phys Med Rehabil* 1985; **66:** 314–17.
19. Lewit K. The needle effect in the relief of myofascial pain. *Pain* 1979; **6:** 83–90.
20. Simons DG. Electrogenic nature of palpable bands and "jump sign" associated with myofascial trigger points. In: Bonica JJ, *et al*. eds. *Advances in Pain Research and Therapy.* New York, NY: Raven Press, 1976: 913–18.
21. Dexter JR, Simons DS. Local twitch response in human muscle evoked by palpation and needle penetration of trigger point. *Arch Phys Med Rehabil* 1981; **62:** 521–2.
22. Fischer AA. Tissue compliance meter for objective,

quantitative documentation of soft tissue consistency and pathology. *Arch Phys Med Rehabil* 1987; **68:** 122–5.

23. Fischer A. Documentation of myofascial trigger points. *Arch Phys Med Rehabil* 1988; **69:** 286–91.

24. Berry DC, Yemm R. A further study of facial skin temperature in patients with mandibular dysfunction. *J Oral Rehabil* 1974; **1:** 255–64.

25. Berry DC, Yemm R. Variations in skin temperature of the face in normal subjects and in patients with mandibular dysfunction. *Br J Oral Surg* 1971; **8:** 242–7.

26. Schiffman EL, Fricton JR. Epidemiology of TMJ and craniofacial pain: an unrecognized societal problem. In: Fricton JR, Kroening RJ, Hathaway KM eds. *TMJ and Craniofacial Pain: Diagnosis and Management*, 1st edn. St Louis, MO: Ishiyaku EuroAmerica, 1988: 1–10.

27. Wolfe F, Cathey MA. Prevalence of primary and secondary fibrositis. *J Rheumatol* 1983; **10:** 965–8.

28. Yunus MB, Masi AT, Calabro JJ, *et al.* Primary fibromyalgia (fibrositis): clinical study of 50 patients with matched normal controls. *Semin Arthritis Rheum* 1981; **11:** 151–71.

29. McCain GA, Scudds RA. The concept of primary fibromyalgia (fibrositis): clinical value, relation and significance to other chronic musculoskeletal pain syndromes. *Pain* 1988; **33:** 273–87.

30. Eriksson PO, Lindman R, Stal P, Bengtsson A. Symptoms and signs of mandibular dysfunction in primary fibromyalgia syndrome (PSF) patients. *Swed Dent J* 1988; **12** (4): 141–9.

31. Kudrow L, Sutkus BJ. MMPI pattern specificity in primary headache disorders. *Headache* 1979; **19:** 18–24.

32. Rugh JD, Solberg WK. Psychological implications in temporomandibular pain and dysfunction. *Oral Sci Rev* 1976; **7:** 3–30.

33. Greene CS, Olson RE, Laskin DM. Psychological factors in the etiology, progression, and treatment of MPD syndrome. *J Am Dent Assoc* 1982; **105:** 443–8.

● 34. Roberts AH, Reinhardt L. The behavioral management of chronic pain: long-term follow-up with comparison groups. *Pain* 1980; **8:** 151–62.

35. Wolfe F. Fibromyalgia: the clinical syndrome. *Rheum Dis Clin North Am* 1989; **15:** 1–18.

36. Fricton J, Dall'Arancio, D. Myofascial pain of the head and neck: controlled outcome study of an interdisciplinary pain program. *J Musculoskeletal Pain* 1994; **2:** 81–99.

37. Simons DG. Myofascial trigger points and the whiplash syndrome. *Clin J Pain* 1989; **5:** 279.

38. Bennett R. Myofascial pain syndromes and the fibromyalgia syndrome: a comparative analysis. In: Fricton J, Awad EA eds. *Myofascial Pain and Fibromyalgia*. New York, NY: Raven Press, 1990: 43–66.

39. Cifala J. Myofascial (trigger point pain) injection: theory and treatment. *Osteopath Med* 1979; **April:** 31–6.

40. Cooper AL. Trigger point injection: its place in physical. *Arch Phys Med* 1961; **42:** 704–9.

41. Jaeger B, Skootsky, SA. Double blind, controlled study of different myofascial trigger point injection techniques. *Pain* 1987; **4** (Suppl.): S292.

◆ 42. Jaeger B, Reeves JL. Quantification of changes in myofascial trigger point sensitivity with the pressure algometer following passive stretch. *Pain* 1986; **27:** 203–10.

43. Fricton JR, Hathaway KM, Bromaghim C. Interdisciplinary management of patients with TMJ and craniofacial pain: characteristics and outcome. *J Craniomandibular Disord* 1987; **1:** 115–22.

44. Leavitt F, Katz RS, Golden HE, *et al.* Comparison of pain properties in fibromyalgia patients and rheumatoid arthritis patients. *Arthritis Rheum* 1986; **29:** 775–81.

45. Wolfe F, Cathey MA, Kleinheksel SM. Fibrositis (fibromyalgia) in rheumatoid arthritis. *J Rheumatol* 1984; **11:** 814–18.

46. Okeson JP. *Orofacial Pains*. Chicago, IL: Quintessence, 1995.

47. Berry DC. Facial pain related to muscle dysfunction. *Br J Oral Surg* 1967; **4:** 222–6.

48. Gold S, Lipton J, Marbach J, Gurion B. Sites of psychophysiological complaints in MPD patients. II. Areas remote from orofacial region. *J Dent Res* 1975; abstract 480: 165.

49. Evaskus DS, Laskin DM. A biochemical measure of stress in patients with myofascial pain-dysfunction syndrome. *J Dent Res* 1972; **51:** 1464–6.

50. Glyn JH. Rheumatic pains: some concepts and hypotheses. *Proc R Soc Med* 1971; **64:** 354–60.

51. Kendall HO, Kendall F, Boynton D. *Posture and Pain*. Huntington, NY: R.E. Krieger, 1970: 15–45.

52. Simons D. Muscular pain syndromes. In: Fricton J, Awad EA eds. *Myofascial Pain and Fibromyalgia*. New York, NY: Raven Press, 1990: 1–43.

53. Eriksson PO, Thornell LE. Histochemical and morphological muscle-fibre characteristics of the human masseter, the medial pterygoid, and the temporal muscles. *Arch Oral Biol* 1983; **28:** 781–90.

54. Uhlig Y, Weber BR, Grob D, Muntener M. Fiber composition and fiber transformation in neck muscles of patients with dysfunction of the cervical spine. *J Orthop Res* 1995; **13:** 240–9.

55. Mayo KH, Ellis III E, Carlson DS. Histochemical characteristics of masseter and temporalis muscles after 5 weeks of maxillomandibular fixation: an investigation in Macaca mulatta. *Oral Surg Oral Med Oral Pathol* 1988; **66:** 421–6.

56. Schiffman E, Fricton JR, Haley D. The relationship of occlusion, parafunctional habits and recent life events to mandibular dysfunction in a non-patient population. *J Oral Rehabil* 1992; **19:** 201–23.

57. Simons DG. Myofascial trigger points: the critical experiment. *J Musculoskeletal Pain* 1997; **5:** 113–18.

58. Cheshire WP, Abashian SW, Mann JD. Botulinum toxin in the treatment of myofascial pain syndrome. *Pain* 1994; **59:** 65–9.

59. Hong C-Z. Persistence of local twitch response with loss

of conduction to and from the spinal cord. *Arch Phys Med Rehabil* 1994; **75:** 12–16.

60. Hong C-Z, Torigoe Y. Electrophysiological characteristics of localized twitch responses in responsive taut bands of rabbit skeletal muscle. *J Musculoskeletal Pain* 1994; **2** (2): 17–43.

61. Hubbard DR, Berkoff GM. Myofascial trigger points show spontaneous needle EMG activity. *Spine* 1993; **18:** 1803–7.

62. Yunus M, Kalyan-Raman UP, Kalyan-Raman K, Masi AT. Pathologic changes in muscle in primary fibromyalgia syndrome. *Am J Med* 1986; **81** (3A): 38–42.

63. Larsson H, Lindberg U. The effect of divalent cations on the interaction between calf spleen profilin and different actins. *Biochim Biophys Acta* 1988; **953:** 95–105.

64. El-Labban NG, Harris M, Hopper C, Barber P. Degenerative changes in masseter and temporalis muscles in limited mouth opening and TMJ ankylosis. *Oral Pathol Med* 1990; **19:** 423–5.

65. Mao J, Stein RB, Osborn JW. Fatigue in human jaw muscles: a review. *J Orofacial Pain* 1993; **7:** 135–42.

66. Kniffki K, Mense, S, Schmidt, RF. Responses of group IV afferent units from skeletal muscle to stretch, contraction and chemical stimulation. *Exp Brain Res* 1978; **31:** 511–22.

67. Lim R, Guzman F, Rodgers DW. Note on the muscle receptors concerned with pain. In: Barker D ed. *Symposium on Muscle Receptors*. Hong Kong: Hong Kong University Press, 1962: 215–19.

68. Melzack R. Myofascial trigger points: relation to acupuncture and mechanisms of pain. *Arch Phys Med Rehabil* 1981; **62:** 114–17.

69. Mense S. Nervous outflow from skeletal muscle following chemical noxious stimulation. *J Physiol* 1977; **267:** 75–88.

70. Pomeranz B, Wall PD, Weber WV. Cord cells responding to fine myelinated afferents from viscera, muscle and skin. *J Physiol* 1968; **199:** 511–32.

71. Selzer M, Spencer WA. Convergence of visceral and cutaneous afferent pathways in the lumbar spinal cord. *Brain Res* 1969; **14:** 331–48.

72. Dubner R. Hyperalgesia in response to injury to cutaneous and deep tissues. In: Fricton J, Dubner R eds. *Orofacial Pain and Temporomandibular Disorders*. New York, NY: Raven Press, 1995: 61–71.

73. Dubner R, Bennett GJ. Spinal and trigeminal mechanisms of nociception. *Annu Rev Neurosci* 1983; **6:** 381–418.

74. Sessle BJ, Dubner R. Presynaptic hyperpolarization of fibers projecting to trigeminal brain stem and thalamic nuclei. *Brain Res* 1970; **22:** 121–5.

75. Sessle B. Brainstem mechanisms of orofacial pain. In: Fricton J, Dubner R eds. *Orofacial Pain and Temporomandibular Disorders*. New York, NY: Raven Press, 1995: 43–60.

76. Sessle BJ. Masticatory muscle disorders: basic science perspectives. In: Sessle BJ, Bryant PS, Dionne RA eds.

Temporomandibular Disorders and Related Pain Conditions. Progress in Pain Research and Therapy, vol. 4 Seattle, WA: IASP Press, 1995: 47–61.

77. Willis WD. *The Pain System*. Basel: Karger, 1985.

78. Mense S. Nociception from skeletal muscle in relation to clinical muscle pain. *Pain* 1993; **54:** 241–89.

79. Guilbaud G. Central neurophysiological processing of joint pain on the basis of studies performed in normal animals and in models of experimental arthritis. *Can J Physiol Pharmacol* 1991; **69:** 637–46.

80. Dubner R. Neuronal plasticity in the spinal dorsal horn following tissue inflammation. In: Inoki R, Shigenaga Y, Tohyama M eds. *Processing and Inhibition of Nociceptive Information*. Tokyo: Excerpta Medica, 1992: 35–41.

81. Russell IJ, Michalek JE, Vipraio GA, Fletcher EM. Serum amino acids in fibrositis/fibromyalgia syndrome. *Arthritis Rheum* 1989; **32** (S47): abstract.

82. Vaerøy H, Helle R, Førre O, *et al*. Elevated CSF levels of substance P and high incidence of Raynaud's phenomenon in patients with fibromyalgia: new features for diagnosis. *Pain* 1988; **32:** 21–6.

◆ 83. Goldenberg DL, Simms RW, Gieger AG, Komaroff AL. Most patients with chronic fatigue syndrome have fibromyalgia. *Arthritis Rheum* 1989; **32** (S47): abstract.

84. Komaroff AL, Goldenberg D. The chronic fatigue syndrome: definition, current studies and lessons for fibromyalgia research. *J Rheumatol* 1989; **19** (Suppl.): 23–7.

85. Moldofsky H. Non-restorative sleep and symptoms after a febrile illness in patients with fibrositis and chronic fatigue syndrome. *J Rheumatol* 1989; **16** (Suppl. 19): 150–3.

86. Clarke NG, Kardachi BJ. The treatment of myofascial pain–dysfunction syndrome using the biofeedback principle. *J Periodontol* 1977; **48:** 643–5.

87. Graff-Radford SB, Reeves JL, Jaeger B. Management of chronic head and neck pain: effectiveness of altering factors perpetuating myofascial pain. *Headache* 1987; **27** (4): 186–90.

● 88. Felson DT, Goldenberg DL. The natural history of fibromyalgia. *Arthritis Rheum* 1986; **29:** 1522–6.

89. McCain GA, Bell DA, Mai F, Halliday PD. A controlled study of the effects of a supervised cardiovascular fitness training program on the manifestations of the primary fibromyalgia syndrome. *Arthritis Rheum* 1988; **31:** 1135–41.

90. Miehlke K, Schulz G. So called muscular rheumatism. *Internist* 1961; **2:** 447–53.

91. Fields HL, Liebeskind JC eds. *Pharmacological Approaches to the Treatment of Chronic Pain: New Concepts and Critical Issues*. Seattle, WA: IASP Press, 1994.

92. Singer E, Dionne R. A controlled evaluation of ibuprofen and diazepam for chronic orofacial muscle pain. *J Orofacial Pain* 1997; **11:** 139–46.

93. Wedel A, Carlsson GE. Sick-leave in patients with functional disturbances of the masticatory system. *Swed Dent J* 1987; **11:** 53–9.

94. Bennett R. Fibromyalgia, chronic fatigue syndrome, and myofascial pain. *Curr Opin Rheumatol* 1998; **10:** 95–108.

95. Ng LKY ed. *New Approaches to Treatment of Chronic Pain: a Review of Multidisciplinary Pain Clinics and Pain Centers*. NIDA Research 36 Monograph Series. Washington, DC: US Government Printing Office, 1981.

96. Nielson WR, Walker C, McCain GA. Cognitive behavioral treatment of fibromyalgia syndrome: preliminary findings. *J Rheumatol* 1992; **19:** 98–103.

97. Rodin J. Biopsychosocial aspects of self management. In: Karoly P, Kanfer FH eds. *Self Management and Behavioral Change: from Theory to Practice*. New York, NY: Pergamon Press, 1974.

98. Schneider F, Kraly P. Conceptions of pain experience: the emergence of multidimensional models and their implications for contemporary clinical practice. *Clin Psychol Rev* 1983; **3:** 61–86.

99. Turk DC, Rudy TE, Salovey P. The McGill Pain Questionnaire reconsidered: confirming the factor structure and examining appropriate uses. *Pain* 1985; **21:** 385–97.

100. Miller A. *Craniomandibular Muscles: Their Role in Function and Form*. Boca Raton, FL: CRC Press, 1991.

45

Psychiatric diagnosis and chronic pain

STEVEN A KING

Many mental disorders, in addition to the depressive and the somatoform disorders, are associated with chronic pain.[1] This chapter will review these other disorders and other psychiatric problems commonly encountered among patients with chronic pain.

MEDICAL CONDITIONS, MENTAL DISORDERS, AND PAIN

Trying to elucidate the degree to which physical and psychological factors are involved in pain can be difficult:

- Many studies have shown that the presence of identifiable physical changes often do not correlate with the presence or severity of pain.
- Gore et al.[2] reported that there was no relationship between radiological findings and the severity of neck pain experienced.
- In a study in which magnetic resonance imaging of the lumbar spine was performed on asymptomatic subjects, Jensen et al.[3] found that 64% had at least one abnormal lumbar disk and 38% had two or more.

One of the major revisions of how pain is dealt with appears in The Diagnostic and Statistical Manual of Mental Disorders, 4th edn (DSM-IV), but not in the previous editions of the DSM. This revision was the creation of the diagnosis of "pain disorder associated with both psychological factors and a general medical condition."[4] This was the first DSM diagnosis to recognize that, in many cases of pain, both physical and psychological issues are of importance and need to be addressed.[5]

For many years, researchers and clinicians have sought to develop methods for determining whether the etiology of a patient's pain is physical or psychological. Much of the focus has been on various instruments of psychological testing that will be discussed elsewhere in this volume.

The most well known of the other efforts to assist health care professionals in clarifying the etiology of pain are the five signs described by Waddell et al.,[6] which they believed indicated that low back pain was of nonorganic origin:

1. tenderness that is superficial or nonanatomic in distribution;
2. pain brought on by movements that should not cause pain but are simulations of those that will;
3. the disappearance of positive physical signs when the patient is distracted;
4. regional disturbances involving weakness or sensory deficits that are nonanatomic in origin;
5. overreaction by the patient during the examination.

Although the presence of one or more of these signs has often been considered to indicate that psychological factors are predominant, the authors noted that they are subject to a range of interpretations on the part of clinicians and may be invalid for certain connective tissue disorders.

Main and Waddell[7] have since highlighted that these signs should be employed with a high degree of caution and that they should be considered to be a psychological "yellow flag" to indicate that a comprehensive assessment of the role that psychosocial factors may be playing in the pain should be undertaken.

ANXIETY DISORDERS

Anxiety disorders occur frequently in patients with both chronic and acute pain.[8] Of the anxiety disorders, panic disorder and its association with chest pain has been the most studied:

- In the DSM-IV, panic disorder is defined as the presence of recurrent, unexpected panic attacks followed by at least 1 month of persistent concern about having another attack, worry about the possible implications or consequences of the attack, or a significant behavioral change related to the attacks.
- Panic attacks involve a discrete period of intense fear or discomfort accompanied by at least 4 of 13 symptoms, including chest pain, palpitations, sweating, shortness of breath, nausea or abdominal distress, dizziness, and paresthesiae.

The literature indicates that approximately 30% of patients with chest pain and normal angiograms fit the criteria for panic disorder.[9] Unfortunately, it appears that most of these cases go undiagnosed and untreated. Fleet et al.[10] found that 98% of patients with panic disorder presenting to an emergency department for chest pain were not so diagnosed by treating physicians:

- These patients often receive multiple evaluations of their physical status with no improvement in symptoms because the true etiology is not addressed.
- Panic disorder has also been reported to be associated with other pain syndromes, including:
  - fibromyalgia; Epstein et al.[11] reported that functional impairment in patients with fibromyalgia appeared to be correlated with their level of anxiety;
  - irritable bowel syndrome.[12]

Post-traumatic stress disorder (PTSD) appears to be another anxiety disorder in which pain may be a common complaint. Beckham et al.[13] found that 80% of patients with combat-related PTSD suffered chronic pain.

FACTITIOUS DISORDER, MALINGERING, AND SOMATIZATION DISORDER

Three disorders that are sometimes confused are factitious disorder, malingering, and somatization disorder. In all three, there is no physical condition present to explain the patient's symptoms:

- In factitious disorder and malingering, patients consciously fabricate symptoms and may even physically injure themselves in order to produce observable changes denoting an illness.
- The major difference between these two is the patient's motivation:

  - In malingering, the object is to obtain some concrete goal such as financial gain or avoiding undesired duties.
  - In factitious disorder, the most severe form of which has also been called Münchhausen syndrome, the only apparent reason for the patient's dishonesty is to obtain medical care. Vomiting, diarrhea, and abdominal pain are among the most common presenting symptoms of factitious disorder.

Etiology of malingering and factitious disorder

Although the reasons for malingering are usually clear and obvious, the etiology of factitious disorder remains mysterious. It is among the most difficult mental disorders to study because once patients with it are confronted with evidence of their dishonesty they often discharge themselves and seek medical help elsewhere.

Patients with factitious disorder often have worked in the medical field or have a close relative or acquaintance who has done so. However, it is unclear whether this medical background is involved in the etiology of the disorder or whether the association reflects the fact that patients who are knowledgeable about medicine are able to provide more believable stories regarding illnesses and are therefore more likely to receive the treatment they seek.

Health care professionals who care for children should also be aware of factitious disorder by proxy. In this disorder, a person, usually a parent, reports that another person, usually a child, is suffering physical complaints and may actually cause physical changes in order to mimic the presentation of an illness. Again, the only apparent motivation is to obtain involvement in the health care system.

Etiology of somatization disorder

In contrast to malingerers and those with factitious disorder, patients with somatization disorder present a true picture of their symptoms.

Diagnostic criteria for somatization disorder include:

- pain in at least four different body parts or organ systems;
- two gastrointestinal and one genitourinary symptom other than pain;
- a pseudoneurological condition such as vision changes, paralysis, or weakness.

The symptoms suffered by these patients are as real to them as those associated with any physical condition.

Unfortunately, by the time patients with somatization disorder come to the attention of a mental health professional, they may have real physical problems secondary to the many treatments they have received.

Obviously, it is of paramount importance to carefully evaluate patients for the presence of a physical disorder and for other mental disorders before diagnosing malingering or factitious disorders.

In countries such as the USA, where patients who develop pain as the result of an injury may receive some financial compensation if the problem is severe enough to impair work-related activities, concerns about malingering are often paramount. Unfortunately, these concerns have reached such a degree that it is not uncommon for patients involved in workers' compensation and disability systems or in some form of litigation surrounding their pain to, at some point, be suspected of malingering.

Although patients may exaggerate symptoms and the extent of disability in order to obtain financial gains, such exaggerations usually occur after the presence of the injury or illness that initiated the pain is established.

There are many anecdotal reports of malingering, but the few studies that have been performed on this problem indicate that it is a relatively infrequent problem.

The US Social Security Administration's Commission on the Evaluation of Pain explored the issue of malingering in great depth and reported that:

1 There did not appear to be many malingerers among social security disability applicants.
2 Honest, legitimate, health care professionals are able to detect most cases of malingering.[14]

Leavitt and Sweet[15] similarly found malingering to be rare in individuals complaining of low back pain.

SEXUAL PAIN DISORDERS

The sexual pain disorders identified in the DSM-IV include:

- Dyspareunia: recurrent or persistent genital pain associated with sexual intercourse in males and females.
- Vaginismus: recurrent or persistent involuntary spasm of the musculature of the outer third of the vagina that interferes with sexual intercourse.

As with other DSM-IV disorders, the symptoms must cause marked distress or interpersonal difficulty and are not better accounted for by a general medical condition or substance use.

SUBSTANCE ABUSE AND DEPENDENCE

The extent of the problems of substance abuse and dependence among patients with pain, especially those with chronic pain, remains controversial.

Some confusion appears to exist because of the DSM-IV terminology. In DSM-IV, substance dependence is defined as a maladaptive pattern of substance use and is essentially considered to be synonymous with addiction. This is in contrast to physiological dependence. However, signs of physiological dependence, including tolerance and withdrawal, are also considered by the DSM-IV to be criteria for dependence. But, in order for this diagnosis to be made, the patient must also demonstrate at least one sign or symptom indicative of psychological problems, including interference with social, occupational, or recreational activities; a persistent desire or unsuccessful efforts to reduce substance use; or use of the substance for a longer period or in larger amounts than was intended.

There are limited studies on the problem of substance use among pain patients. One of the most controversial areas is the problem of iatrogenic substance abuse, i.e. patients abusing medications prescribed by physicians to manage their pain, especially opioids, or for other comorbid problems such as sleep difficulties, for which benzodiazepines are often prescribed.

Generally, it appears that patients with acute pain or those who are terminally ill are at very low risk for abusing or developing a psychological dependence on opioid analgesics.

There is less clarity of this issue with regard to chronic pain. Some of the studies most widely cited to demonstrate that opioid abuse and dependence is an infrequent problem among chronic pain patients without a history of substance use problems have marked methodological flaws. For example, an often cited letter from Porter and Jick reported that only four out of 11,882 patients without a history of addiction who received at least one narcotic during hospitalization developed addiction and appears to have also included many patients who had acute pain or who were terminally ill.[16]

Other studies have failed to account for the fact that patients may obtain medications from multiple sources and not inform each source of the presence of the others.[17]

In one of the most comprehensive studies on the problems of iatrogenic opioid abuse and dependence, Bouckams et al. reported that, of 59 patients with chronic nonmalignant pain and without a history of substance abuse problems who were treated with narcotics and followed for an average of 36 months, 24% developed narcotic addiction.[18] Hoffmann et al. found that 12.6% of 414 chronic pain patients developed psychological dependency on analgesics, and an additional 2.9% were in remission for this problem.[19]

Although abuse of opioids is often considered to be the major substance use problem among patients with pain, other commonly prescribed medications also appear to be misused.

King and Strain reported that 38% of patients with chronic pain presenting to a pain management service were chronic users of benzodiazepines despite literature indicating that these drugs are generally contraindicated for this patient cohort.[20] Because benzodiazepine withdrawal, in contrast to opioid withdrawal, can be a life-threatening problem, it is especially important to recognize misuse of this class of medications and to formulate appropriate detoxification schedules.

PERSONALITY DISORDERS

Although studies have examined personality traits among chronic pain patients, the prevalence of personality disorders remain unclear.

In their review of 27 studies applying DSM criteria to patients with pain, King and Strain found that only five patients were diagnosed with a personality disorder.[21] Of these five studies, three reported that more than 40% of patients suffered a personality disorder. The frequency of the various personality disorders differed among these studies.

Russ *et al.*[22] studied the pain experiences of patients with borderline personality disorder – a mental disorder often associated with self-injury including multiple suicide attempts. They reported that patients with borderline personality disorder who did not experience pain during self-injury may actually not experience pain in the same way as other people and that this may be due to a combination of a possible cognitive impairment that makes it difficult to distinguish between situations associated with various levels of pain and dissociative mechanisms.

SLEEP DISORDERS

One of the most common comorbid complaints of patients with chronic pain is difficulty sleeping. Delayed sleep onset, frequent awakenings, nonrestorative sleep, and decreased sleep time are often reported by these patients.[23]

Because of literature indicating that problems with sleep can exacerbate and perhaps even precipitate pain, it is important to address sleep problems rather than simply discounting them as an expected part of the pain experience.[24]

SUICIDE AND CHRONIC PAIN

Although there are limited studies on suicide among patients with chronic pain, those that have been performed indicate that these patients are at increased risk for taking their own lives. Increases in suicide attempts and ideation have been reported among migraine headache and chronic abdominal and back pain sufferers.[25–27]

How much these increased rates are the result of the depression suffered by many chronic pain patients and how much is the result of the pain itself remains unclear.

Although both pain and depression probably play significant roles, it is interesting to note that Magni *et al.*[26] found that patients with chronic abdominal pain who were not depressed had elevated levels of suicidal ideation and attempts.

This indicates that it is of vital importance for physicians and other health care professionals who evaluate and treat these chronic pain patients to assess them for suicide potential. Certainly, all patients should be asked whether they have had any thoughts of killing themselves or whether they wish their lives would end. Patients who have had such thoughts require a more extensive evaluation, including:[28]

1 Patients should be asked if they have thought of any specific ways to end their life. The presence of such thoughts increases the likelihood of suicide.
2 The potential lethality of the method should be assessed. Although all methods may be lethal, those from which the patient has less of a chance of being rescued, such as shooting, hanging, or jumping off a building or bridge, are considered to be of heightened concern in contrast to an overdose of drugs or cutting oneself.
3 Substance abuse or dependence: the use of central nervous system (CNS)-active substances can impair judgment and substance abusers are often impulsive.
4 Past history of suicide attempts: previously attempting suicide markedly increases the risk for future attempts.

CHRONIC PAIN SYNDROME

A diagnosis that is commonly applied to patients with chronic pain for which no physical cause can be identified is chronic pain syndrome.

Because it is not contained in the formal diagnostic classification systems for pain, the criteria for this diagnosis are variable depending on the user. Most clinicians appear to employ Black's criteria:[29]

> Intractable, often multiple pain complaints, which are usually inappropriate to existing somatogenic problems; multiple physician contacts and many nonproductive diagnostic procedures; excessive preoccupation with the pain problem; [and] an altered behavior pattern with some of the features of depression, anxiety, and neuroticism.

Owing to the subjective nature of many of the criteria, the validity of this diagnosis is questionable. Furthermore, some of the factors, such as the overuse of diagnostic procedures, may be related as much to limitations in health care professionals' knowledge about pain as to patient behavior.

Because of these limitations, the perjorative connotations that have surrounded its use, and because its use may lead health care professionals to ignore the physical and mental disorders involved in the pain that they should be addressing, the diagnosis of chronic pain syndrome is best avoided.

CONCLUSION

It is clear that chronic pain is frequently associated with mental disorders and psychological problems. The presence of these in no way invalidates patients' complaints of pain nor do they eliminate the possibility that a general medical condition may also be playing a role in the pain. All patients with chronic pain deserve a careful psychological evaluation to determine whether a mental disorder is present and, if so, to have a treatment plan initiated that addresses it.

REFERENCES

● 1. King SA. Pain disorders. In: Hales RE, Yudofsky SC, Talbott eds. *American Psychiatric Press Textbook of Psychiatry*, 3rd edn. Washington, DC: American Psychiatric Press, 1999: 1003–21.

2. Gore DR, Septic SB, Garner GM, Murray MP. Neck pain: a long-term follow-up of 205 patients. *Spine* 1987; **12:** 1–5.

3. Jensen MC, Brant-Zawadzki, Obuchowki N, *et al*. Magnetic resonance imaging of the lumbar spine in people without back pain. *N Engl J Med* 1994: **331:** 69–73.

4. American Psychiatric Association. *Diagnostic and Statistical Manual of Mental disorders*, 4th edn. Washington, DC: American Psychiatric Association, 1994.

● 5. King SA. DSM-IV and pain. *Clin J Pain* 1995; **11:** 171–6

6. Waddell G, McCulloch JA, Kummel E, Venner RM. Nonorganic physical signs in low back pain. *Spine* 1980; **5:** 117–25.

7. Main CJ, Waddell G. Spine update: behavioral responses to examination: a reappraisal of the interpretation of "nonorganic signs." *Spine* 1998; **23:** 2367–71.

8. Gureje O, Von Korff M, Simon GE, Gater R. Persistent pain and well-being. *JAMA* 1998; **280:** 147–51.

9. Fleet RP, Dupuis G, Marchand A, *et al*. Panic disorder in coronary artery disease patients with noncardiac chest pain. *J Psychosm Res* 1998; **44:** 81–90.

10. Fleet RP, Dupuis G, Marchand A, *et al*. Panic disorder in emergency department chest pain patients: prevalence, comorbidity, suicidal ideation, and physician recognition. *Am J Med* 1996; **101:** 371–80.

11. Epstein SA, Kay G, Clauw D, *et al*. Psychiatric disorders in patients with fibromyalgia. *Psychosomatics* 1999; **40:** 57–63.

12. Maunder RG. Panic disorder associated with gastrointestinal disease: a review and hypotheses. *J Psychosom Res* 1998; **44:** 91–105.

13. Beckham JC, Crawford AL, Feldman ME, *et al*. Chronic posttraumatic stress disorder and chronic pain Vietnam combat veterans. *J Psychosom Res* 1997; **43:** 379–89.

14. US Department of Health and Human Services. *Report of the Commission on the Evaluation of Pain*. U.S. Department of Health and Human Services, Social Security Administration, Office of Disability. Publication no. 64-031, 1987.

15. Leavitt F, Sweet JJ. Characteristics and frequency of malingering among patients with low back pain. *Pain* 1986; **25:** 357–74.

16. Porter J, Jick H. Addiction rare in patients treated with narcotics. *N Engl J Med* 1980; **302:** 123.

17. King SA. Formal treatment agreements and opioids in nonmalignant pain. *J Pain Symptom Manage* 1996; **12:** 206–7.

18. Bouckoms AJ, Masand P, Murray GB, *et al*. Chronic nonmalignant pain treated with long-term oral narcotic analgesics. *Ann Clin Psychiatry* 1992; **4:** 185–92.

19. Hoffmann NG, Olofsson O, Salen B, Wickstrom L. Prevalence of abuse and dependency in chronic pain patients. *Int J Addict* 1995; **30:** 919–27.

20. King SA, Strain JJ. Benzodiazepine use by chronic pain patients. *Clin J Pain* 1990; **6:** 143–7.

● 21. King SA, Strain JJ. Somatoform pain disorder. In: Widiger TA, Francis AJ, Pincus HA *et al*. eds. *DSM-IV Source Book*, vol. 2. Washington, DC: American Psychiatric Press, 1996: 915–31.

22. Russ MJ, Clark WCC, Cross LW, *et al*. Pain and self-injury in borderline patients: sensory decision theory, coping strategies, and locus of control. *Psychiatry Res* 1996; **63:** 57–65.

23. Moffitt PF, Kalucy EC, Baum FE, Cooke RD. Sleep difficulties, pain, and other correlates. *J Intern Med* 1991; **230:** 245–9.

24. Moldofsky H, Scarisbrick P. Induction of neurasthenic musculoskeletal pain syndrome by selective sleep stage deprivation. *Psychosom Med* 1976; **38:** 35–44.

25. Breslau N, Davis GC, Andreski P. Migraine, psychiatric disorders, and suicide attempts; an epidemiologic study of young adults. *Psychiatr Res* 1991; **37:** 11–23.

26. Magni G, Rigatti-Luchini S, Fracca F, Merskey H. Suicidality in chronic abdominal pain: an analysis of the Hispanic health and nutrition examination survey (HHANES). *Pain* 1998; **76:** 137–44.

27. Pentitten J. Back pain and risk of suicide among Finnish farmers. *Am J Public Health* 1995; **85:** 1452–3.

28. Ghosh TB, Victor BS. Suicide. In: Hales RE, Yudofsky SC, Talbott JA eds. *American Psychiatric Press Textbook of Psychiatry*, 3rd edn. Washington, DC: American Psychiatric Press, 1999.

29. Black RG. The chronic pain syndrome. *Surg Clin North Am* 1975; **55:** 999–1011.

46

Chronic pain in children

PATRICK McGRATH, ROSS HETHERINGTON, AND G ALLEN FINLEY

Chronic and recurrent pain occurs in about 15–20% of children and adolescents.[1] However, most of these individuals do not seek care, and only a small group has significant disability from pain.[2] Children and adolescents frequently continue to attend school and function in their daily lives, but there is often a significant decline in their functioning.[3] Pediatric chronic and recurrent pains are important because of the burden of suffering and because lifelong patterns in the way individuals manage their pain may be established during this period.

The last 15 years have seen a dramatic increase in research and clinical experience in pediatric chronic pain. Pediatric pain is now covered quite well in pediatric and pain journals and in pain and anesthesia texts. Chronic pain clinics or services have been initiated in many specialized children's facilities, and clinical knowledge and experience has increased. Although much more remains to be learned, we now have a good corpus of scientific and clinical knowledge to guide treatment.

Chronic and recurrent pain that is due to a well-characterized disease such as arthritis, inflammatory bowel disease, or cancer will not be discussed because these problems are usually treated by management of the underlying disease. In contrast, because the major treatments for sickle cell pain are symptomatic, it will be included here.

This chapter will review the most common chronic and recurrent pediatric pain problems. For each problem, we will examine the diagnostic criteria, the prevalence, and the treatment. We will evaluate the scientific evidence for each treatment that we discuss. Although pediatric pain research has grown rapidly in the past few years, it

still remains an area that is primarily guided by clinical judgment or less than ideal research.

HEADACHES

Headaches are very common and can have a wide variety of causes. Fortunately, most headaches are not from serious pathology but are from transient causes such as a cold. The most common recurrent headaches are migraine and tension headaches. There is evidence that these headaches are increasing in prevalence.[4] The literature on pediatric headache is much less extensive than that on adult headache. However, compared with most pediatric pains, headaches are well researched. The psychosocial but not the physiological aspects of pediatric migraine and tension headaches have been quite extensively investigated[5] and many treatments have been evaluated.[6]

Headache prevalence begins at a low rate and gradually increases during childhood. At puberty, the rate of headache increases sharply[7] and girls tend to have both a higher rate of headache and more severe pain.[8]

Diagnostic criteria for headache have been developed by the International Headache Society (IHS).[9] The classification works well for communication with other scientists and for conveying research results. However, headaches that do not fit the classification system are just as important. The care that a child deserves and the anguish that he or she suffers are similar whether they have classifiable headaches or not.

Migraine

The most common migraines are migraine with aura and migraine without aura. Migraines with aura used to be called classic migraine and migraines without aura were known as common migraine. Auras are usually visual and often consist of holes in the vision (scotoma) or bright lines that look like a many-sided star or an eighteenth-century fort (fortification spectra). Auras develop gradually over a few minutes. However, they can consist of any other focal hemispheric or brainstem dysfunction that precedes the headache. They may consist of more than one symptom, but are always fully reversible within an hour.

Migraines are often unilateral, often have pulsating pain, and are usually made worse by physical activity. They are typically of moderate or severe intensity. Common symptoms during the headache include nausea, vomiting, and sensitivity to light or sound. In children and adolescents, migraines are often shorter in duration (i.e. less than 2 h) than is typical in adults.[10,11]

The prevalence of migraine headaches in children and adolescents is between 2.5% and 10%.[12] As in headaches in general, the occurrence of migraine is low in younger school-age children and increases sharply at puberty.[7] Before puberty, boys are slightly more affected, but, after puberty, girls are much more likely to have migraine.[8]

Bille[13] carried out a long-term follow-up of a sample of children with "pronounced migraine," i.e. fairly severe migraine more often than once a month. He found that about one-third were migraine free as adults. One-third lost their migraine for some time but later regained it, and about one-third had migraine throughout the 40-year follow-up period. He found that males were more likely to lose their migraine than females.

Metshonkala[14] found that prepubertal children with migraine (aged 8–9 years) had a poor 2- to 3-year prognosis, with boys worse off than girls. Overall, about 80% of children still had migraine, 10% did not have migraine but had tension headaches, and only 10% were headache free.

There is no doubt that migraine is a genetically transmitted disorder. Twin studies suggest that early onset migraine may have a higher genetic loading than later onset migraine.[15,16] About 40–60% of the likelihood of developing migraine has been estimated to be genetic.[12] There are no good estimates for relationships between frequency and severity of attacks and genetic inheritance. Advances in brain imaging and the development of drugs with specific antimigraine effects have improved our understanding of the pathophysiology of migraine as a complex neurogenic and vascular disorder. These studies have been conducted on adults and, although there are clear developmental differences in the expression of migraine, it appears that the basic pathophysiology of migraine is similar in children, adolescents, and adults. Recent summaries of this rapidly changing literature are provided in *The Headaches*.[17]

Although claims of a specific migraine personality have not been borne out,[18] it is clear that there is a higher rate of depressive feelings in young people with migraine[19] and that stress is a frequent precipitant of individual attacks. Migraine is best viewed as a biopsychosocial disorder rather than only as a biological disorder.

The first line of treatment of migraine consists of the avoidance of known triggers, the most common being missing meals. However, no trials have been performed to evaluate avoidance of triggers. The second strategy is the use of over-the-counter (OTC) analgesics. In many countries, aspirin is not used because of the concern with Reye syndrome.[20] Surprisingly few studies have been carried out evaluating analgesic approaches. In one of the few studies, ibuprofen was shown in a well-designed randomized trial to be more effective than acetaminophen (paracetamol).[21]**

Most adolescents,[22] like most adults,[22] delay taking analgesics for about 1 h after a headache begins.

Sumatriptan and the other triptans are widely used and have been evaluated in adults, but have had mixed results in children and adolescents. Some well-designed studies have not shown an effect,[23] but a recent trial[24] has shown excellent results with intranasal sumatriptan in a randomized, double-blind crossover trial with 14 children with migraine. Similarly, Winner and colleagues[25] in a randomized, double-blind, single attack trial of 653 adolescents with migraine found that nasal sumatriptan was superior to placebo. However, the difference between placebo and sumatriptan was modest: significant pain relief at 2 h was 63% versus 53% for placebo (significant) and complete relief at 2 h was 36% for the 20-mg dose of sumatriptan versus 25% for the placebo (not significant).[25]**

The best-validated treatments for migraine in adolescents are behavioral treatments, including relaxation training and finger temperature biofeedback. Holden and colleagues[6] recently reviewed the evidence and concluded that, according to the criteria developed by the American Psychological Association, relaxation was "effective" for headaches and that temperature biofeedback and cognitive therapy "showed promise." They did not differentiate between migraine and tension headache in their review.[6]***

The typical treatment program consists of 8–10 sessions during which a psychologist teaches the child or adolescent self-management skills in order to change his or her responses to stress. A typical program is outlined in Table 46.1. The same treatment – delivered mostly by manuals, audiotapes, and a telephone therapist with only minimal direct therapist contact – has been shown to be as effective as treatment delivered face to face by a therapist.[26]

In spite of the evidence for the effectiveness of behavioral treatments, most migraine sufferers do not have access to these treatments. Most children and adolescents

Table 46.1 *Typical 10-session migraine treatment program*

1	Rationale for treatment, review of baseline diaries, and explanation of program
2	Relaxation with tension
3	Introduction to cognitive therapy
4	Distraction strategies, relaxation without tension
5	Imagery, behavioral rehearsal, relaxation with imagery
6	Assertion training
7	Differential relaxation, minirelaxation
8	Problem solving
9	Combining relaxation strategies
10	Summary and review

with migraine manage their headaches without missing much school and without the benefit of any professional assistance. They do, however, suffer from a significant reduction in their quality of life[27] because of their headaches.

Tension headaches

Tension headaches, although more frequent than migraine, have been much less extensively investigated. The criteria for tension-type headaches have only recently begun to be applied to studies. However, the headaches studied in many of the earlier studies of nonmigraine headache are likely to have been tension-type headache.

To meet IHS criteria for tension headaches,[9] the headaches must last from 10 min to 7 days, must not be accompanied by vomiting or moderate or severe nausea, and must have two of the following pain characteristics: pressing or tightening quality; mild or moderate intensity; bilateral or variable location; not aggravated by physical activity. Sensitivity to light or sound can occur but not both.

Most children and adolescents with tension headache have the episodic variety. Chronic tension headache, in which pain occurs more than 50% of the time, is the least-studied variant, but may be more resistant to treatment and may have more impact on the patient's quality of life.[27]

The prevalence of tension headaches, as defined by the IHS criteria, has not been well studied. Pothman and colleagues[28] found that about 50% of children had tension headache and that the rate increased in adolescence. Chronic tension headache in which pain occurs on more than 180 days a year was found in one study to occur in 1% of school-age children.[29]

The persistence of tension headache has been investigated in a few studies. A Swedish study found that about half of the children who suffered from unspecified weekly recurrent headaches that were probably tension-type headaches improved within 1 year.[30] In a study from Finland, more than 50% of 8- to 9-year-old children continued to experience nonmigrainous headache when

they were 11–13 years old. About one-third developed migraine, and only 1 in 10 were headache free.[31] With the limited evidence that we have, it appears that the prognosis for untreated tension-type headaches is poor.

There has been very limited work on the etiology of tension-type headaches in children and adolescents. The genetic contribution is not clear. Research studies have found that children and adolescents with tension headaches have more stress, fear of failure, and problems with others,[32] are more likely to have been bullied by others,[31] have more stress symptoms and feelings of being pressured and frustrated,[33] and are more likely to be in a larger class at school.[34]

Analgesics, especially over-the-counter (OTC) analgesics (acetaminophen and ibuprofen), are the most common treatment, but no trials have been carried out with children or adolescents with tension headache. Most adolescents do not take medication until headaches are well established, and some do not take a full dose of medication.[35] Children and adolescents who have chronic tension headache may be at risk of overuse of analgesics and subsequent analgesic rebound headaches. Opioids are seldom recommended.

Larsson and colleagues have conducted a series of well-designed trials[36-41] showing that treatment with relaxation training delivered in a group at school or by a telephone therapist is effective. The studies by Larsson et al.[36-41] in the school setting using nonpsychologists as therapists have provided a model of cost-effective treatment. The previously mentioned review of treatments on pediatric headache covered tension headache as well as migraine.[6]***

Tension headaches are prevalent, and if they are not well managed by OTC medication there are often few options. Much work needs to be done to improve this situation, and what is known needs to be available to the children who need help. In particular, the effective behavioral treatments should be made more available.

Chronic tension headache is a significant problem for a small but important number of children and adolescents.[42] Some of these problems may be from overuse of medication, but there is virtually no research on pediatric chronic tension headaches.

RECURRENT ABDOMINAL PAIN

It has long been recognized that many children have recurrent abdominal pain that has no known organic cause. Although infrequent or mild abdominal pain may not interfere with normal activities, for some children pain significantly interferes with normal activities. Apley and Naish's criteria,[43] which are widely used, require at least three episodes of pain that are severe enough to interfere with activities and that occur over a period of not less than 3 months. Recently, these criteria have been challenged as lacking specificity.[44] Children with abdominal pain vary in their symptoms, but little research has been carried out to determine whether different symptoms require different treatments.

Apley and Naish's early epidemiological study of 1,000 children in the UK[43] found that the prevalence of recurrent abdominal pain was about 10% and that it was most common in girls in middle childhood. Data from a national survey on the health and development of a population-based cohort born in 1946 carried out by the UK's Medical Research Council have been examined to determine the correlates of recurrent abdominal pain.[45] Because a preexisting cohort was used, the data could not exactly follow the Apley and Naish criteria. It was found that about 20% of children had abdominal pain at 7 years, 19% at 11 years and 17% at 15 years. Two-fifths of the children had abdominal pain during at least one of the three time periods, 10% during at least two, and 2.1% during all three.[45]

The long-term follow-up studies of children with recurrent abdominal pain have found mixed results. Some follow-up studies found an increased rate of somatic symptoms in adulthood.[46–49] This increase was usually in vague somatic symptoms and was sometimes interpreted as somatization or irritable bowel syndrome. However, a population-based cohort study[51] found that children with recurrent abdominal pain had more psychiatric disorders but did not have increased risk for physical symptoms[45] in adulthood.

Pain from a known disease or disorder is usually not included in this classification, and few children who have significant pathologies are misdiagnosed. Biological and psychological etiologies have been identified in recurrent abdominal pain. Increased visceral sensitivity and slowed bowel motility have been identified as the most common biological factors.[50,51] Subtypes of recurrent abdominal pain with possible differences in biological factors have been suggested. Walker,[44] for example, has suggested grouping recurrent abdominal pain as: (1) functional dyspepsia, with pain in the upper abdomen; (2) irritable bowel syndrome, characterized by pain that is relieved by defecation and associated with changes in stool frequency or consistency; (3) functional constipation, characterized by fecal retention; and (4) functional abdominal pain characterized by peri-umbilical abdominal pain unrelated to food intake or bowel habits. There has been insufficient experience with subgroupings to know whether they are useful in predicting the course of the problem or the response to treatment.

Psychological issues that have been linked to recurrent abdominal pain include a high level of negative life events in the family and low social competence,[52] and a passive style of coping[53] has been linked to continuation of pain. Most commonly, increased levels of child and parent depression,[54] anxiety, and other psychological problems[45] as well as family stress have been suggested as important.

Two treatment strategies have been shown to be effective in randomized trials with recurrent abdominal pain.

First, supplementary dietary corn fiber[55] was demonstrated to reduce abdominal pain in a sample of children with recurrent abdominal pain who were recruited from primary care physicians. About 50% of the children obtained more than a 50% reduction in pain from the fiber treatment. Placebo response was half as effective.[55]**

Second, studies from Australia[56–58] demonstrated that cognitive behavior therapy is effective in reducing pain. For example, in one study, 44 children aged 7–14 years were randomly assigned to receive standard care or family cognitive behavior therapy.[58] The therapy consisted of a six-session package of education about recurrent abdominal pain, contingency management for parents, and self-management for children.[58]**

In the clinic, treatment is matched to the assessment of the individual patient. So, a child with recurrent abdominal pain and separation anxiety is likely to be treated differently from a child with recurrent abdominal pain who appears to be constipated. As research accumulates, it is likely that clearly defined subgroups of patients with recurrent abdominal pain that have adequate diagnostic criteria and evidence of different treatment effectiveness will emerge. Unfortunately, there have been few well-designed treatment trials on recurrent abdominal pain and, as a result, most treatment decisions are not evidence based.

MUSCULOSKELETAL PAIN

Musculoskeletal pains are common and include pains in the limbs, back, and neck as well as diffuse pains. In a survey of musculoskeletal pain in 1,756 third- and fifth-grade children,[59] 564 or 32% reported weekly musculoskeletal pain in at least one area. One year later, 50% of those reporting pain in the original survey were still suffering pain.[60] Girls had more persistent pain than boys, and persistent pain increased with age. Neck pain was the most persistent pain. Daytime tiredness and the belief that one was disabled also predicted persistence of pain.

Widespread pain or fibromyalgia and back pain have received the most attention and will be reviewed now.

Fibromyalgia

The diagnosis of fibromyalgia has often been one that is given little credibility. The American College of Rheumatology (ACR) has adopted diagnostic criteria for fibromyalgia.[61] Fibromyalgia is characterized by widespread pain accompanied by fatigue, poor sleep, and other nonmusculoskeletal symptoms.

Two diagnostic systems have been used for fibromyalgia in children and adolescents. The ACR criteria were developed for adults but have been applied to children and adolescents.[61] A second set of criteria were developed by Yunus and Masi[62] specifically for children.

The prevalence of fibromyalgia has been examined in few studies. An Israeli study[63,64] used ACR criteria and found that 6% of 338 students aged 9–15 years had fibromyalgia. A Scandinavian study[59] found that 22 of 1,756 (1.25%) children in third and fifth grade with an average age of 10 years met ACR criteria for fibromyalgia. The age of onset has been suggested to be as low as 5 years, but there may be an increase in prevalence with age. Females predominate in the clinical setting in children and adults.

The prognosis of fibromyalgia is unclear in children. Buskila in his Israeli school study[64] found that most children had spontaneously remitted by the 30-month follow-up. On the other hand, in a tertiary care, clinical, follow-up study of children who were primarily fibromyalgia sufferers, 61% had not improved on follow-up an average of 27 months later.[65]

The etiology of fibromyalgia is unknown. There are many etiological theories, including psychological theories, none of which have strong research support. At this point in time, it is best to consider fibromyalgia as a disorder or disorders of unknown etiology.

Only a few treatment studies have been performed with children and adolescents with fibromyalgia. Two uncontrolled studies[66*,67*] found that many patients showed improvement with cyclobenzaprine. Cognitive behavioral treatment was examined in a clinical series of five girls aged 8–17 years.[68] In this study, four out of five were completely well and one was much improved after cognitive behavioral treatment.[68*] There is no good evidence for effective treatments in this disorder. Unfortunately, the adult literature is not much help as there are no clearly effective treatments for fibromyalgia in adults.

Back pain

Previously, it was thought that most children and adolescents with back pain were likely to have serious disorders.[69] This was an error that was probably based on referral bias. Children with "normal" back pain did not make it to the specialist clinics. It is now evident that most back pain in the pediatric age group does not signify serious pathology.

No standard diagnostic criteria have been developed for back pain in young people. Pain is usually described by location and by the presence or absence of any neurological signs such as radiation of pain that may indicate nerve involvement. Standard criteria could be of help in research communication about back pain in children and adolescents.

Back pain is common and increases with age. For example, Taimela et al.[70] examined 1,171 children aged 7–16 years and found an overall prevalence of low back pain in the previous month of 10.1% in boys and 9.4% in girls. An Icelandic study[71] found that 11% of 11- to 12-year-olds were reported to have back pain once a month and 7.6% once a week. Older children, aged 15–16 years, had more back pain (once a month 29.5%; once a week 11.9%). Girls may have more back pain than boys.[8] It is unknown how much disability there is from pediatric back pain.

Back pain in children and adolescents often recurs. For example, Taimela et al.[70] found that 26% of boys and 30% of girls had recurrent pain, and 3% of girls had continual back pain. In general, other studies from several different countries have found a small number of adolescents reporting constant pain, but about half report recurrent pain lasting a few years.[72]

Several studies have investigated correlates of back pain. Anthropometric dimensions, spinal mobility, trunk muscle strength, and sociodemographic, familial, psychological, and lifestyle factors have been implicated in back pain. Unfortunately, most studies are retrospective or cross-sectional and the direction of causality cannot be ascertained. For example, although some studies have found that watching television for more than 2 h a day is related to having back pain,[73] it may be that some children watch more television because of back pain as well as television watching contributing to back pain. Prospective and experimental studies are needed to begin to disentangle causal factors from results and simply associated factors in adolescent back pain.

Most children with back pain do not seek medical advice.[74] Even in children with frequent and severe back pain, most do not go to the doctor.[73] Children, as do adults, treat their pain with analgesics obtained over the counter and with reduction or change of activity.[73*] No reasonably well-designed treatment trials of back pain in children or adolescents could be found.

Although the epidemiology of back pain has been well studied, other studies, especially treatment studies, are lacking. These studies are important both because of the suffering of children and because treating back pain in children and adolescents may help to prevent adult back pain.

NEUROPATHIC PAIN

Neuropathic pain includes pain due to damage to nerves, which includes central pain from stroke or spinal cord injury, polyneuropathies from metabolic or other causes, mononeuropathies from entrapment or trauma, neuralgias, phantom limb pain, and sympathetic pain of both the reflex sympathetic dystrophy type (complex regional pain syndrome type I; CRPS-I) and the causalgia type (complex regional pain syndrome type II; CRPS-II). There are very few studies on neuropathic pain in children and adolescents compared with the data available on adults. Fortunately, neuropathic pain may be less frequent in children than in adults.

Phantom limb pain and CRPS-I have been best researched and will be the focus of this section. CRPS-I has previously been most commonly known as reflex sympathetic dystrophy or Sudeck's dystrophy.

Phantom limb pain

Phantom limb pain occurs in a limb absent because of traumatic or surgical removal or because of congenital abnormality. Pain is often described as tingling, pins and needles, burning, cramping, or shooting. Pain may begin within days of the amputation. Pain usually reduces over time. Not all phantom sensation is painful, and phantom sensation is more common than pain.[75] Residual limb pain is not considered to be phantom pain.

Most studies of phantom limb pain in children and adolescents have very small sample sizes and almost all have recruited from hospital clinics. Wilkins and colleagues[75] surveyed 60 child and adolescent amputees, aged 8–18 years, recruited from all children in seven provinces in Canada who were in community-based programs for child amputees. They found that 29% reported phantom pain. Less than 4% of the congenital amputees reported phantom pain whereas 49% of the surgically amputated children had phantom pain. Phantom pain was associated with residual limb pain and was triggered by a variety of physical and psychological triggers. None of the children reported phantom pain that significantly interfered with their lives.

Cross-sectional studies have shown that phantom limb pain tends to decline with time after amputation.[75] The etiology of phantom limb pain is unknown. Melzack[76,77] has proposed that the neuromatrix in the brain provides a map of sensations that persists despite congenital lack of a limb or amputation. Katz[78] has argued that a sympathetic component may also be important.

Because of the lack of trials, treatment of phantom pain in children and adolescents has been based on theory and clinical experience. Aggressive preemptive pain management prior to amputation is often recommended.* Phantom limb pains, like other neuropathic pains, are typically treated with low-dose antidepressants, for example amitriptyline, nortriptyline, or desipramine, that are titrated up.* Treatment is switched to another antidepressant if significant side-effects occur before pain relief. Because of concern with cardiac antidepressant effects, especially prolonged QT syndrome, baseline electrocardiograms (ECGs), monitoring of vital signs, and serial ECGs as the dose escalates are mandatory. The selective serotonin reuptake inhibitors (SSRIs) appear to be less effective. When tricyclic antidepressants are withdrawn, it should be done gradually.

Anticonvulsants have been shown to be effective in adult studies of neuropathic pain. The major anticonvulsants used with children are gabapentin and carbazepine, but no trials have been published.* Numerous other approaches including transcutaneous electrical nerve stimulation (TENS) and massage are useful in individual cases.*

In summary, although there are some possible treatments of phantom pain in children, no treatments have been demonstrated to be effective.

Complex regional pain syndrome type I

Complex regional pain syndrome type I (CRPS-I) often occurs following a minor injury in a limb, but sometimes no injury is noted. The pain is often burning, there is allodynia and hyperpathia, and the limb shows signs of sympathetic involvement, especially temperature changes.

The prevalence of CRPS-I in the pediatric age range has not been well researched. Clinics usually report that the disorder is most common in the lower limbs of girls and onset is often in the early teenage years. There are very few data on the prognosis of CRPS-I in adolescents, but the prognosis for children and adolescents may be better than that for adults.

The cause of CRPS-I is not understood, but it is thought to be related to endogenous localized triggering of pain and the sympathetic nervous system. The common belief that CRPS-I is caused by psychological factors has not been supported.[79]

There are no controlled trials of CRPS-I treatment in children and adolescents.

The best evidence (which is weak), at this time, is obtained from clinical series in children[80,81] and suggests that conservative treatment by means of education, physiotherapy, and systemic pharmacotherapy (most commonly amitryptyline and gabapentin) with behavioral psychotherapy is often effective.* If these are not effective, epidural sympathetic neural blockade has been reported to have been used.[82]*

SICKLE CELL PAIN

Sickle cell disease (SCD) is often accompanied by pain. The frequency and severity of recurrent pain varies from absent or very mild to frequent and severe, requiring hospitalization with narcotic analgesia.[83] Thus, the lives of many children and adolescents with sickle cell disease are punctuated by episodes of excruciating musculoskeletal pain that can result in frequent school absences, require medical intervention, promote depression or anxiety, limit participation in leisure activities, impair peer relations, and increase family stress.[84,85]

SCD is a recessively transmitted group of disorders involving a single-base mutation in the β-gene on chromosome 11. The disorder directly affects hemoglobin, which periodically changes from the typical plate-like shape to a crescent or sickle shape. Diagnosis is made on the basis of hematological laboratory analysis. SCD has

in school children: a study of sociodemographic differences. *Eur J Pediatr* 1996; **155:** 984–6.

◆ 72. McGrath PJ, Breau L. Musculoskeletal pain. In: Finley GA, McGrath PJ eds. *Chronic and Recurrent Pain in Children and Adolescents*. Seattle, WA: IASP Press, 1999: 173–97.

73. Balague F, Dutoit G, Waldburger M. Low back pain in schoolchildren: an epidemiological study. *Scand J Rehabil Med* 1988; **20:** 175–9.

74. Newcomer K, Sinaki M. Low back pain and its relationship to back strength and physical activity in children. *Acta Paediatr* 1996; **85:** 1433–9.

75. Wilkins KL, McGrath PJ, Finley GA, Katz J. Phantom limb sensations and phantom limb pain in child and adolescent amputees. *Pain* 1998; **78:** 7–12.

76. Melzack R. Phantom limbs, the self and the brain (the D. O. Hebb memorial lecture). *Can Psychol* 1989; **30:** 1–16.

◆ 77. Melzack R. Phantom-limb pain and the brain. In: Bromm B, Desmedt JE eds. *Pain and the Brain: From Nociception to Cognition*. New York, NY: Raven Press, 1995: 73–82.

78. Katz J. Psychophysiological contributions to phantom limbs. *Can J Psychiatry* 1992; **37:** 282–98.

◆ 79. Lynch ME. Psychological aspects of reflex sympathetic dystrophy: a review of the adult and paediatric literature. *Pain* 1992; **49:** 337–47.

80. Sherry DD, Wallace CA, Kelley C, *et al.* Short and long term outcomes of children with complex regional pain syndrome type I treated with exercise therapy. *Clin J Pain* 1999; 15 (3): 218–23.

◆ 81. Wilder RT, Berde CB, Wolohan M, *et al.* Reflex sympathetic dystrophy and follow-up of seventy patients. *J Bone Joint Surg* 1992; **74:** 910–19.

82. Olsson GL. Neuropathic pain in children. In: Finley GA, McGrath PJ eds. *Chronic and Recurrent Pain in Children and Adolescents*. Seattle, WA: IASP Press, 1999: 75–98.

83. Walco GA, Dampier CD. Pain in children and adolescents with sickle cell disease: a descriptive study. *J Pediatr Psychol* 1990; **15:** 643–58.

84. Hurtig AL, Koepke D, Park KB. Relation between severity of chronic illness and adjustment in children and adolescents with sickle cell disease. *J Pediatr Psychol* 1989; **14:** 117–32.

85. Beyer JE, Simmons LE, Woods GM, Woods PM. A chronology of pain/comfort in children with sickle cell disease. *Arch Pediatr Adolesc Med* 1999; **153:** 913–20.

86. Platt OS, Thorington BD, Brambilla DJ, *et al.* Pain in sickle cell disease: rates and risk factors . *N Engl J Med* 1991; **325:** 11–16.

◆ 87. The Genetic Resource. *Proceedings of the Conference on Sickle Cell Disease Related Pain: Assessment and Management*, special issue. New England Regional Genetics Group (NERGG), 1994.

88. American Pain Society. Guidelines for the management of acute and chronic pain in sickle cell disease. Glenview, IL: American Pain Society, 1999 (electronic copies are not available, but ordering information is on the American Pain Society website: www.ampainsoc.org).

◆ 89. Allen KD, Shriver MD. Role of parent-mediated pain behavior management strategies in biofeedback treatment of childhood migraines. *Behav Ther* 1998; **29:** 477–90.

90. Ramsden R, Friedman B, Williamson DA. Treatment of childhood headache reports with contingency management procedures. *J Clin Child Psychol* 1983; **12:** 202–6.

91. Osborne RB, Hatcher JW, Richtsmeier AJ. The role of social modeling in unexplained pediatric pain. *J Pediatr Psychol* 1989; **14:** 43–61.

92. Goodman JE, McGrath PJ. Modelling of pain behavior by mothers in an experimental pain paradigm. Manuscript submitted.

93. Mathews JR, McGrath PJ, Pigeon H. Assessment and measurement of pain in children. In: Schechter NL, Berde CB, Yaster M eds. *Pain in Infants, Children, and Adolescents*. Baltimore, MD: Williams & Wilkins, 1993: 97–112.

94. McGrath PJ, Mathews JR, Pigeon H. Assessment of pain in children: a systematic psychosocial model. In: Bond MR, Charlton JE, Woolf CJ eds. *Proceedings of the Vth World Congress on Pain*. Elsevier, 1991: 509–26.

95. Dunn-Geier BJ, McGrath PJ, Rourke BP, *et al.* Adolescent chronic pain: the ability to cope. *Pain* 1986; **26:** 23–32.

96. Jensen TS, Turner JA, Wiesenfeld-Hallin Z eds. *Aggregation of Pain Complaints and Pain-related Disability and Handicap in a Community Sample of Families*. Seattle, WA: IASP Press, 1997.

97. Schanberg LE, Keefe FJ, Lefebvre JC, *et al.* Social context of pain in children with juvenile primary fibromyalgia syndrome: parental pain history and family environment. *Clin J Pain* 1998; **14:** 107–15.

98. Aasland A, Flato B, Vandvik IH. Psychosocial factors in children with idiopathic musculoskeletal pain: a prospective, longitudinal study. *Acta Paediatr* 1997; **86:** 740–6.

● 99. Coderre TJ, Katz J. Peripheral and central hyperexcitability: differential signs and symptoms in persistent pain. *Behav Brain Sci* 1997; **20:** 404–19.

47

Chronic pain in the elderly

ROBERT D HELME AND BENNY KATZ

All societies are aging.[1] The population of the world will age much faster in the next half century than in the past. In this time, the proportion of people over 60 years of age is projected to more than double to 22% of the world's population, and those over 80 years of age will increase by about sixfold. Although occurring later, developing countries are aging at a more rapid rate than developed countries. The reduction in mortality in old age has been achieved through postponement of the lethal consequences of chronic diseases associated with middle age, rather than by a reduction in the incidence of degenerative conditions found in old age. Pain is one of the most common symptoms associated with the increased burden of pathology observed with the aging process.

Aging of the population has created a demand to attend to a wide range of issues of concern to older people, such as accommodation, retirement age, income support, environmental conditions and hazards, use of discretionary time, spirituality, and health. Within the health domain, there is increasing interest in cost-effective health systems, management of age-associated diseases, and health maintenance. Research into the biology of aging is providing a means to understand both why and how we age.

Pain as it affects older people is no exception to this general interest in aging. Recent summary publications on this topic include the volume *Pain in the Elderly* by the International Association for the Study of Pain,[2] clinical practice guidelines on the management of chronic pain in older persons under the auspices of the American Geriatrics Society,[3] and chapters in recent texts on geriatric medicine[4,5] which contain many pertinent references.

Many clinicians are now familiar with the general principles of management of pain and other health problems in older individuals. Despite this increased awareness of the problem of chronic pain, too often we find this problem is ignored or managed in a suboptimal manner. Particular issues covered in this chapter include the principles of aged care medicine as a framework in which to consider optimal pain management for older people, the reasons underlying the discrepancy between an increase in pain-associated pathology with no increase in pain complaint over age 65, variations to pain assessment and management dictated by comorbidities, including their effects on physical and psychosocial function, and a brief discussion on the problem of pain management in the patient with dementia.

PRINCIPLES OF AGED CARE MEDICINE

There has been considerable debate as to whether geriatric medicine is a discrete medical specialty. The increased demand for health services as individuals age results in most clinicians dealing with a large number of older persons. Aged care medicine is characterized by the prominence of recurrent or persistent clinical syndromes such as cognitive impairment, impairment of mobility, falls and fractures, and incontinence. These syndromes may be aggravated by association with visual impairment and hearing loss. Reduced physiological reserve results in previously well older individuals decompensating following a relatively trivial stressor, which in itself may go unrecognized. Iatrogenic factors, such as adverse drug reactions, frequently contribute to these presentations. Unlike other branches of medicine, the common presenting symptoms in the older individual are not organ specific, and usually do not help to identify the underlying disease. Comprehensive evaluation identifies multiple factors contributing to the presenting syndrome. The degree of diagnostic certainty following any step in the evaluation process tends to be less, because of the frequency of abnormal findings in asymptomatic older persons. For example, computed tomographic and magnetic resonance imaging studies of the lumbar spine in asymptomatic individuals over 60 years of age reveal more than 80% with abnormal findings, and 21% with spinal canal stenosis.[6]

Age is best considered as a surrogate which is highly correlated with functional impairment, and this becomes more obvious in people over 75 as physiologic reserves decline. As a group, however, when any single parameter is being considered, the range of normality of older individuals is more diverse than in any other age group. Aged care medicine requires the assessment and management of impairment, disability, and handicap in a heterogeneous population. The therapeutic approach is often aimed at stabilization of treatable processes, rehabilitation of residual disability, and facilitation of support services to minimize handicap. Cure is a less frequent outcome. A multidisciplinary approach to assessment and management is a common characteristic of aged care medicine and pain management.

Regardless of age, the optimal approach to the management of pain or any other problem is to treat the underlying cause. However, many of the problems diagnosed in older people are irreversible and demand a symptomatic rather than a curative approach. Older people often prefer maintenance of functional capacity to prolongation of the course of an incurable disease, or may decline definitive intervention such as surgery because they fear further disability from associated complications. There is also a paucity of evidence of the efficacy for many treatments we employ with older people, as they have generally only been studied in younger cohorts. For example, Rochon et al.[7]*** reviewed randomized studies of non-steroidal anti-inflammatory drugs, and found that only 207 patients aged over 65 years had been included among almost 10,000 patients in 83 trials, and no one 85 years or older was studied.

In summary, aged care medicine requires knowledge and skills in the management of age-associated syndromes, including disease processes and their interactions, impairment, disability, and handicap. It places more emphasis on optimizing quality of life than maximizing duration of life. It has a commitment to improving the health status of older people by addressing the broader issues of disease prevention, health promotion, disease screening, eradicating obstacles within the health service system, leadership, advocacy, education, and research.

There is an obvious overlap of these issues with those of pain medicine.

EPIDEMIOLOGY OF PAIN IN OLDER PEOPLE

One of the most quoted prevalence studies of pain in which the effect of age was examined is that by Crook et al.[8] This was a telephone survey of a random sample obtained from a group general practitioner list and had a gratifying 95% response rate. It was one of the first studies to clearly demonstrate increased pain complaint with increasing age and highlighted the importance of pain as a frequent problem for a large number of older people. There were very few participants over the age of 80, a problem common to most community-based studies that seek to explore issues relevant to older people. The questions asked in this study regarding the temporal nature of pain did not follow the usual pattern of description for acute and chronic pain, which means their classification of pain as temporary or persistent is not easily compared with other studies. It was intriguing that temporary pain had the same prevalence at all ages, and this remains the only study in the literature that has reported age-related prevalence figures for acute pain of any type.

However, other studies have not necessarily replicated these results.[9,10] Collectively, the studies suggest a peak or plateau in the prevalence of pain by age 65, and a decline in reported pain in those over 80 years of age. This is surprising given an age-related increase in disease prevalence, which continues into the seventh, eighth, and ninth decades of life. When severity of disease is taken into account, it appears that the very old report lower levels of pain.[11-13] One notable exception is a report by Donahue et al.[14] addressing the incidence of postherpetic neuralgia in patients enrolled in a health maintenance organization. They reported a sharp increase with age in the incidence of postherpetic neuralgia, continuing to rise in those over 75 years of age. Any generalized interpretation of the data must be somewhat guarded, however, as each study has its limitations.

Many reasons can be put forward why reported prevalence figures for pain in older people vary so widely.[15] They include methodological variations such as the source of data acquisition, whether it be by personal or proxy interview, telephone interview, or postal survey (age effects of postal surveys have, for example, been shown to have a selection bias toward the more healthy older person); the number of subjects in each age group; response rates, especially for the oldest old; and the unreliability of memory for pain, especially in older people for whom the effects of age-associated memory impairment and incipient dementia become frequent enough to seriously affect the data acquired in a large-scale prevalence survey. Perhaps the most likely reason for the variation in absolute prevalence figures, however, is the nature of the questions asked: the pain time interval, the time in pain within this interval, the severity or interference of the pain in daily life, often recorded as whether the pain is "troubling" or "bothersome," and the effect of cueing (e.g. specifically asking about back pain, neck pain, headache, etc.).

A number of studies have examined pain at particular body sites, and some consistent trends have emerged. The prevalence of articular joint pain more than doubles in adults over 65 years compared with young adult samples.[16–19] Conversely, the prevalence of headache shows a progressive decrease with increasing age after a peak prevalence at 45–50 years of age.[16,18] The frequency of facial/dental pain and abdominal/stomach pain also appears to diminish during old age.[20] Chest pain probably peaks during late middle age at the time of the peak of ischemic heart disease presentation, but declines thereafter despite the continuing high mortality from this disease.[16] The findings are more equivocal with respect to back pain with reports of both an increase[16,17] and decrease in back pain with advancing age.[18] A summary view is that age is associated with an increase in the prevalence of chronic pain up to age 65, but not acute pain. Pain in the head, abdomen, and chest is reduced among older people, and joint pain is increased.

REASONS FOR AGE-RELATED CHANGES IN PAIN PREVALENCE

The overriding factor contributing to increased pain complaint with age is pathological load. Many illnesses increase in prevalence with advancing age, and the interplay of multiple diseases in an individual case is the hallmark of aged care medicine. Older patients with occasional or regular pain are more likely to suffer from a circumscribed list of diseases, including cancer, osteoarthritis, osteoporosis, fractures of the spine or limbs, peripheral vascular disease, peripheral neuropathy, stroke, polymyalgia rheumatica, temporal arteritis, gout, and postherpetic neuralgia.

Reasons for the relative decline in pain report among older people are more numerous, but also more speculative.[15] First, there are issues related to sample bias. For instance, those older persons with painful disease may be sequestered into institutional care where pain rates up to 80% have been reported, thereby reducing pain prevalence estimates in community-dwelling older persons. Furthermore, the response rates among the very old remaining in the community may be poor, especially for those who are disabled by disease and hence more likely to suffer from pain. The very old, those over 85 years, also represent a select sample of survivors, and these individuals may experience less pain-causing disease. The report of pain by an older individual may also be suppressed by more significant life events such as the death of a spouse,

concern regarding loss of independence, fear that pain report will lead to unwanted investigations, treatments, or the finding of serious pathology. There is a general perception that older persons are more stoic, cautious in attribution, and more likely to misattribute pain symptoms to the aging process itself. They may not even use the term pain, preferring discomfort, hurting, or aching. Furthermore, pain may not be present at the time of questioning, for instance patients are usually questioned while seated – a position likely to ease arthritic pains. Last, there remains the possibility of age-related changes in the function of nociceptive pathways, thereby leading to reduced pain sensitivity during senescence.

PAIN PHYSIOLOGY AND AGE

Most psychophysical studies have shown a progressive decrease in pain sensitivity with advancing age. An exception is when the stimulus is electrical in nature.[9,21] A recent study using differential nerve fiber blockade has shown that older persons rely on less well-localized C-fiber activation before reporting the presence of pain, whereas younger adults utilize the additional information from Aδ nociceptive fibers.[22] Moreover, when Aδ-fiber input was blocked in young adults, the observed age-associated differences in pain threshold and subjective ratings of pain quality essentially disappeared. Age differences in the temporal summation of nociceptive input also varies as a function of nociceptive fiber type,[21] and such differential age effects on Aδ- and C-fiber function may help to explain some of the disparity in psychophysical findings. On the other hand, diminished physiologic reserve in descending inhibitory pathways[23] may also lead to reduced pain tolerance in older people.

Studies of clinical pain states have also indicated that older persons may exhibit a relative absence of pain in the presentation of certain visceral disease states such as ischemic heart pain and abdominal pain associated with acute infection.[24–29] Unfortunately, most of the clinical studies are difficult to interpret because the severity of pathology is seldom known, although controlled investigations of myocardial pain during exercise-induced ischemia generally support the view of a clinically significant decrease in ischemic pain perception with advancing age.[26,30,31]

In summary, limited evidence from physiological studies, psychophysical investigations, and age variations in disease presentation all suggest age-related alterations in the function of peripheral and central nervous system (CNS) nociceptive pathways. These changes are likely to influence the sensitivity to painful sensation and would be expected to contribute to a decline in pain report in persons of advanced age. However, most of the evidence of age differences in nociceptive function is indirect and the clinical relevance of reduced pain sensitivity to experimental pain stimuli is still the subject of considerable debate. It seems likely that pain report does decline as a consequence of age-related changes in nociceptive function, but more definitive studies on physiological changes in nociceptive pathways are needed in order to fully resolve this issue.

PAIN ASSESSMENT IN OLDER PEOPLE

Despite an age-related increase in prevalence up to the age of 65, pain should not be regarded as a normal consequence of the aging process. Pain is always due to pathology, either physical or psychologic. Acute pain usually settles spontaneously, with or without symptomatic approaches, or requires specific therapy targeted at the cause of the pain. Chronic pain, on the other hand, persists for longer than the expected time-frame for normal healing, or is related to progressive pathology. In some individuals, chronic pain is not associated with any obvious tissue damage or antecedent injury. The successful management of chronic pain in an older person relies on a comprehensive assessment of all factors that contribute to pain, suffering, and disability. Adequate time needs to be given to take a history of symptoms often extending over decades and to review previous assessments, investigations, procedures, and the response to current and past interventions. The reliability of the history may be affected by the chronicity of the pain, side-effects of interventions, and any coexisting cognitive impairment. A collaborative history may need to be obtained. Physical examination is often slow and laborious, but the individual should not be hurried. The assessment may need to take place over several consultations and should ideally include a functional assessment in the individual's normal environment. One must be vigilant for the effects that coexisting diseases will have on the therapeutic options, and the impact these diseases have on pain report and disability. Care is required so as not to falsely attribute drug side-effects to underlying pathology.

Treatment must be tailored to meet the needs of the individual. Whenever possible, it should be directed at the cause of pain, taking into consideration comorbidities and the preference of the patient. Treatment of specific conditions is discussed in detail in other chapters. Although eradication of chronic nonmalignant pain is possible, it is also infrequent. When remedial therapy is not possible, the primary focus should then be directed at symptom management. In most patients, the combination of oral analgesia together with simple physical therapies is sufficient. However, in cases where initial treatment efforts fail, there is no justification for allowing pain and suffering to continue. Multidisciplinary pain-management clinics have been shown to be effective for older individuals and should be utilized.

MEASUREMENT OF PAIN, SUFFERING, AND DISABILITY

Older people can successfully complete validated self-report measures of pain, mood, activity, and disease impact as long as adequate time is allowed to complete the task and other factors such as visual impairment, hearing loss, and physical disability of the hands are taken into account.[32] Older persons are more likely to spend time deliberating over a question, rather than responding in an impulsive manner as is often observed in younger individuals.

Behavioral indicators of pain include measures of medication use, number of different treatments, and visits to physicians and other health care providers. Another category of behavioral measures includes motor activities that indicate pain complaint, such as moaning, limping, rubbing, and facial expressions. Other measures include the use of walking aids, collars, and cushions. Functional measures such as sleep duration, up-time,[33] mobility, self-care, and recreational activity are also relevant and can be reliably assessed in older people. The influence of comorbidities on these measures is obvious. There is a preference for behavioral indicators to be performance measures undertaken during direct observation rather than self-report. Behavioral measures have been shown to be objective, sensitive to treatment effects, and clinically relevant. However, such measures are often time-consuming and are strongly influenced by social context. Inter- and intraobserver reliability for these measures is strong if observer training has been undertaken. Behavioral methods may be especially useful for pain evaluation in adults with cognitive impairment or communication problems.[34] Psychologic assessment should seek to identify the extent to which symptoms of depression and anxiety are present.[35] When selecting questionnaire measures of psychopathology for older patients, it is worth remembering that some measures include common somatic items, such as insomnia and fatigue in order to index feelings of depression or anxiety. Owing to the high incidence of physical disease in older persons, such measures may be less appropriate. There is also some evidence to suggest that older adults may under-report negative mood states, thereby emphasizing the need for age-appropriate norms.[36] A more comprehensive psychologic assessment should include attention to the cognitive coping style of the older person as well as assessment of pain beliefs and degree of somatic preoccupation. Unfortunately, standardized age-specific instruments for monitoring these domains have yet to be developed.

Several options exist for the measurement of activity levels and disability, including performance measures of timed "up and go,"[37] and direct observation of activity performance through to self-report measures, such as activity diaries and standardized questionnaires. Traditional scales used with geriatric populations to measure self-care independence, such as the Barthel or Katz Activities of Daily Living (ADL) indices and instrumental ADL measures [e.g. Lawton and Brody, Clifton Assessment Procedures for the Eldery (CAPE)], may be useful,[38] although they fail to monitor higher function discretionary activities which are more likely to be affected in community-dwelling older persons with chronic pain. These may then be replaced by measures such as the human activity profile and quality-of-life measures. Again, one must be careful with the interpretation of activity measures, whether they be self-report or observational, as activity restriction may occur because of comorbid medical problems rather than as a consequence of pain. In this regard, it may be better to use a measure which evaluates the self-perceived impact of pain on functional abilities. The Sickness Impact Profile (SIP) has been shown to be useful in patients with chronic pain, has been validated for elderly populations,[39] and can demonstrate distinct pain clinic cohorts with high pain impact.[18] A simple question asking what the patient would do if they had no pain can often help to determine goals of therapy as well as identify misattributions of pain-associated pathology. Common concomitants of pain in older people are depression, decreased socialization, sleep disturbance, and impaired ambulation. The SIP monitors fundamental physical functions (e.g. ambulation, sleep and rest, mobility, and self care), discretionary activities such as home maintenance, recreation, and pastimes, as well as activities which occur in a social context (social interaction and communication).

MANAGEMENT

A careful evaluation of the individual is likely to identify the likely pathophysiological basis of chronic pain in the older person, whether nociceptive, neuropathic, or psychogenic. This in turn leads to the selection of an appropriate management regimen and is helpful in determining prognosis. In clinical practice, most chronic pain in the elderly is related to nociceptive factors, in particular degenerative musculoskeletal disease.

The reader is referred to other chapters for details of management of specific conditions which occur with higher frequency in older people.

MEDICATIONS

Simple analgesics

Simple analgesics are the mainstay of most interventions for pain, whether self-initiated or prescribed. Most patients will have self-medicated with simple analgesics prior to seeking attention for ongoing pain. This is often the most convenient and cost-effective approach, but has led to an overemphasis on pharmacologic approaches.

Pharmacologic therapy is most effective when combined with nonpharmacologic strategies. All pharmacologic therapies carry a balance of benefits and burdens. Although older people are more likely to experience adverse reactions to medications, analgesic drugs can be used safely and effectively. The clinician should be aware, however, that patients may use multiple proprietary preparations that contain the same generic analgesic, particularly acetaminophen (paracetamol), which may result in inadvertent toxicity. Selection of appropriate drug therapy for the older patient needs to take into consideration age-related pharmacokinetic and pharmacodynamic changes, and coexisting diseases which may be adversely affected by the new treatment. Many medications, such as simple analgesics, can be prescribed without dose adjustment. Many of the medications used for pain management do, however, have neuropsychiatric or anticholinergic side-effects and hence should be used with caution in older individuals. In general, it is best to commence at a lower than normal therapeutic dose, commonly half the adult dose, and titrate upwards as tolerated. Fear of adverse side-effects should induce caution when prescribing, but should not leave the individual suffering unnecessarily. The timing of medication is as important as the choice of medication. Pain which is persistent is better managed with regular dosing of medication. For intermittent pain which can be predicted, such as pain induced by activity, analgesics should be taken prior to the precipitating activity.

Acetaminophen is the preferred analgesic for older people for many indications, particularly in noninflammatory musculoskeletal conditions, as it is effective, has relatively few side-effects in standard doses, and dose adjustment is seldom required. However, despite its widespread use, and relative safety compared with other analgesics, acetaminophen should not be assumed to be completely safe for older individuals. Hepatotoxicity may occur with massive overdose, or with therapeutic doses in susceptible individuals such as chronic alcohol users, those with poor nutritional status, and concomitant use of medications associated with hepatic microsomal induction such as anticonvulsants. Despite these cautions, it must be emphasized that hepatotoxicity with therapeutic doses of acetaminophen is rare.

When pain relief is insufficient with acetaminophen alone, codeine may be added in combination. Combining two different analgesics avoids increasing the dose of either drug, and reduces the likelihood of side-effects from either medication. The analgesic effect of codeine is believed to be mediated through hepatic O-methylation to morphine. Therapeutic doses of either medication do not influence the pharmacokinetics of the other component. The combination of codeine with acetaminophen confers greater analgesia, but is associated with more side-effects with sustained usage. Common side-effects in older people include nausea, constipation, drowsiness, and dizziness. No controlled trials of the most common dose combination used in the UK and Australasia [8 mg codeine with acetaminophen 500 mg (Panadeine)] have been reported. This combination is likely to be less efficacious but to have fewer side-effects than the 30- to 60-mg codeine doses that have been used to good effect in most studies.[40,41]

Nonsteroidal anti-inflammatory drugs

The majority of individuals prescribed nonsteroidal anti-inflammatory drugs (NSAIDs) are over 65 years old. The major life-threatening complications of NSAIDs are gastrointestinal bleeding and perforation. At least 10–20% of patients will have dyspepsia while taking a NSAID.[42] The occurrence of warning symptoms is not predictive, and as many as 80% of NSAID users have no symptoms before bleeding or perforation. The risk of NSAIDs increases linearly with age. In individuals over 60 years of age, the risk of serious gastrointestinal events while taking NSAIDs is more than five times that of controls, whereas the risk for younger patients is slightly more than 1.5-fold.[43] The use of enteric-coated preparations and rectal suppositories of NSAIDs has failed to prevent the development of ulcers. Coadministration of misoprostol with the NSAID has been demonstrated to reduce the upper gastrointestinal complication rate of nonselective NSAIDs, but it is not always well tolerated.[44**] Omeprazole and high-dose famotidine have also been shown to confer protection and may be better tolerated; H_2 blockers in standard doses are less effective.

The options for management of patients with NSAIDs who are at high risk of serious upper gastrointestinal events are to use either a nonselective NSAID with gastroprotective therapy or a cyclo-oxygenase 2-specific inhibitor (COX-2-specific inhibitor).

The two currently available COX-2 inhibitors, celecoxib and rofecoxib, have been shown to have significantly lower incidence of gastrointestinal toxicity than nonselective NSAIDs.[45***] This benefit is attenuated by the coadministration of low-dose aspirin.[45] COX-2 inhibitors appear to affect renal function in a similar fashion to nonselective NSAIDs, and particular care is required in patients with renal impairment or in those taking diuretics and angiotensin converting enzyme (ACE) inhibitors. COX-2 inhibitors may diminish the antihypertensive effects of ACE inhibitors and diuretic effects of frusemide and thiazides. Celecoxib inhibits cytochrome P_{450} (CYP2C9) enzyme and thus may cause elevation of plasma concentrations of drugs metabolized by this enzyme, such as some β-blockers, antidepressants, and antipsychotics.

Opioids

An expert panel of the American Geriatrics Society acknowledged that the use of opioid analgesia for the management of chronic nonmalignant pain remains controversial, but suggested that it is probably underutilized in older people.[3] Opioid dependency and illicit drug use in the older population is uncommon. Fear of drug dependency and addictive behaviors does not justify failure to relieve pain. Opioids should not be used, however, as an alternative to a comprehensive care program. Doses of opioids needed for nonmalignant pain in the elderly are often quite small. The elderly are thought to be more sensitive to equivalent doses and blood levels of opioids,[46***] and often receive greater and more prolonged pain relief. In the low doses of opioids used for nonmalignant pain management in the elderly, neurologic and psychologic side-effects such as sedation, loss of concentration, and ability to drive are probably more important than hypoxia, myoclonus, and pruritus observed when higher doses are used for other indications.

Adjuvant analgesics

Medications not formally classified as analgesics, but those that are effective in certain painful conditions are known as adjuvant analgesics. In some situations, these medications enhance the effectiveness of conventional analgesics, but in others they are used as the principal analgesic agent. The largest body of literature concerns the use of tricyclic antidepressants. Newer antidepressant classes such as the selective serotonergic reuptake inhibitors (SSRIs) have proven to be better tolerated for older, depressed patients as they have few serious side-effects.[47***] However, SSRIs have not been proven to be as effective as the tricyclic antidepressants for analgesia, and mianserin is no more effective than placebo.[48**] Controlled trials have demonstrated an analgesic response to tricyclics in a variety of painful disorders, including postherpetic neuralgia, diabetic neuropathy, tension and migraine headache, atypical facial pain, rheumatoid arthritis, chronic low back pain, and cancer. Approximately one-third of patients with diabetic neuropathy and postherpetic neuralgia can expect to achieve 50% pain relief with tricyclic antidepressants. The analgesic effects of tricyclic antidepressants are independent of the antidepressant effects and occur more rapidly and at a lower dose than used in depression, with a median dose in the 50–75 mg range. The sedating side-effects may be used to advantage for individuals with pain-related insomnia. Older patients are prone to sedation, constipation, postural hypotension, falls, and urinary retention induced by these agents. A low starting dose is recommended, for instance amitriptyline or nortriptyline 10 mg at night, increasing every 3 or 4 days as tolerated to 75 mg.[47***,49***]

Anticonvulsants are widely used in neuropathic pain states despite limited evidence for their efficacy in controlled studies. The best evidence supports the use of carbamazepine in trigeminal neuralgia, gabapentin in postherpetic neuralgia, and gabapentin, carbamazepine and phenytoin in painful diabetic neuropathy.[47,49] They may be used alone or combined with antidepressants, however the combination increases the potential for adverse effects. A troublesome side-effect of carbamazepine in older people, even in small doses, is ataxia and dizziness, leading to falls. The recommended starting dose in the elderly is carbamazepine 50–100 mg daily. This may be increased after 3 or 4 days as tolerated. Gabapentin has a superior side-effect profile, although its efficacy appears to be similar to other anticonvulsants. As gabapentin is excreted unchanged by the kidneys, the dose needs to be modified according to age-related changes in renal function. Other anticonvulsants may be selected according to side-effect profile. The elderly are particularly susceptible to the sedating effects of clonazepam, which is rarely indicated. The response to one adjuvant analgesic agent within a class is not predictive of the analgesic effect of other agents within the same class. If one adjuvant analgesic does not prove effective, it is not unreasonable to consider a second or even third agent or a combination of agents.

Topical preparations

Topical preparations have rarely been subject to controlled trials. Based on their widespread use, liniments and topical NSAIDs are probably effective and do not appear to have any serious adverse effects in older people. Topical capsaicin is of proven benefit for painful diabetic neuropathy, but its use in other situations has generally been disappointing.

Compliance

Problems with medication compliance are not unique to the older population, but, given their higher medication usage, compliance is an important issue. It has repeatedly been shown to be a problem when more than four medications are prescribed for older individuals. Poor compliance may be deliberate or nondeliberate. An example of deliberate noncompliance is when an individual elects not to take a medication because of side-effects. Nondeliberate poor compliance is more likely to occur when a drug regimen is too complex for the individual to follow, for instance because of confusion with multiple medications or unclear instructions. Strategies shown to be of benefit include counseling, written instructions, supervision, and diary packaging. The problems associated with polypharmacy and compliance must be balanced against the likelihood that a combination of analgesics in low dose is more likely to have fewer side-effects than high doses of single agents. Care should be taken when prescribing combination analgesics to individuals whose pain is not well controlled.

NONPHARMACOLOGIC APPROACHES

Nonpharmacologic approaches encompass a broad range of physical and other treatment modalities. They tend to be underutilized in the elderly. Nonpharmacologic approaches, either alone or used in combination with medications, should be an integral part of the care plan for older patients with chronic pain. They often have the advantage of being relatively inexpensive and free of serious side-effects, even if proof of efficacy may be absent for some.

Physical therapies

Physical therapies may be aimed at improving general fitness and feelings of well-being, or focused upon the pain or the cause of pain. Older people with chronic pain are often physically deconditioned. Regular physical activity increases fitness, enhances a feeling of well-being and confidence, and may have a beneficial effect on reducing the impact of pain. Simple adjustments in posture and daily routines, such as preparing meals in a seated position, breaking up the housework, or the provision of a walking aid can reduce the impact of pain on daily life. The use of a walking frame that causes a mild degree of lumbar flexion will ease the pain of vertebral canal stenosis, or ease the weight load through an arthritic joint. Attention to posture may also improve back and neck pain. Hot water bottles and heat packs warmed in the microwave oven are simple measures which are often very helpful. Hydrotherapy should be considered when weight-bearing exercises aggravate pain. The buoyancy of water reduces effective weight, thus allowing joints to be moved with minimal effort through a full range, and warm water decreases pain and muscle spasm. Hydrotherapy programs also have a beneficial socializing aspect. Specific exercises targeted at muscles around weight-bearing joints have also been used in older people.

Transcutaneous electric nerve stimulation (TENS) is a popular method of symptom relief for a wide range of painful nociceptor and neuropathic pain conditions, yet the response is unpredictable. In a randomized trial of patients over 60 years of age with chronic back pain, both TENS and acupuncture improved pain scores and was associated with a reduction in analgesic consumption for up to 3 months.[50]** Previous nonresponders to TENS can sometimes obtain benefit with prolonged use or altered stimulus parameters on a subsequent trial. Response to TENS is more likely to be achieved if supervised by an experienced health care professional. TENS has the benefit of being portable, safe, and inexpensive. Most older individuals adapt well to TENS, although some find electronic devices daunting. They should be encouraged to experiment with electrode placement and settings over a period of time, before declaring it an ineffective therapy. Other physical therapies include massage and cold. The mechanisms by which benefits accrue remain largely obscure. The available evidence would suggest that older people respond as well to these therapies as do younger cohorts. In light of the safety of these techniques, and their low cost, individuals should be encouraged to use them alone or in conjunction with pharmacologic therapies. There is no evidence that spinal manipulative therapy or chiropractic is better than placebo for the management of chronic pain in older people.

Psychologic approaches

Psychologic factors may contribute to the cause and maintenance of pain. Regardless of the pathophysiological basis of chronic pain, psychologic strategies have a role in management.

The most fundamental psychologic approach is that of patient education. It should form part of each consultation, and may be enhanced with written information. Education of patients and carers concerning the causes of pain, realistic expectations of treatment, and prognosis of pain are all important. Self-management programs have been shown to be cost-effective in reducing pain severity and number of medical visits for patients with chronic rheumatologic conditions, including older patients. The effective size of these interventions is modest, and in the order of that bestowed by NSAIDs.

The clinician needs to ensure that the patient is accepting a pain-management approach, rather than seeking disease cure or total eradication of pain. In the absence of a consensus approach, satisfaction with outcome is likely to be suboptimal. The essence of pain management is to establish appropriate pain coping strategies and discourage behaviors which may perpetuate the pain syndrome. Cognitive strategies are aimed at attenuating pain and suffering by modifying belief structures, attitudes, and thoughts. Although it may not be expressed, older individuals often fear that persistent pain is indicative of serious organic pathology, such as cancer. An awareness of this concern and a careful explanation as to the cause of the pain, and of what is not causing the pain, often reassure the patient.

Other treatment strategies include distraction therapy, relaxation, biofeedback, and hypnosis. The patient is encouraged to take an active role and accept some responsibility for the way they feel, rather than being a passive victim of pain. Cognitive strategies have been used to good effect in older people.

Poor sleep patterns may be the result of unrelieved pain or psychologic factors. Whatever the cause, improved sleep often helps patients to cope with pain. Sleep hygiene includes reduction of stimulants such as caffeinated beverages, relaxation used at bedtime, a bedroom which is quiet and comfortable, and discouragement from activities such as watching television while in bed. Reliance on hypnosedatives for anything but short-term use should be discouraged, as they are associated with adverse effects on daytime alertness and cognition and increase the risk of falls in the elderly. In situations where insomnia coexists with a painful condition for which an adjuvant analgesic is indicated, one may consider sedating agents such as amitriptyline or clonazepam, but they should not be prescribed primarily for this indication. Nonpharmacologic approaches are preferred to pharmacologic approaches for insomnia.

Cognitive strategies are usually combined with a behavioral approach. Respondent behavior refers to the responses elicited by a noxious stimulus, whereas operant behavior is that which becomes reinforced by subsequent environmental, social, and interpersonal influences. These behaviors may become reinforced through gaining attention, concern, and social contact that may not otherwise have been available.[51]*** Invalidism and abnormal pain behavior may persist even in the absence of continuing noxious stimulation. Behavioral operant conditioning discourages inappropriate pain behaviors. Usually, in conjunction with the patient's relatives, positive reinforcement is provided for behavior unrelated to pain and for successfully achieving preset goals. Family members, health professionals, and others are encouraged to ignore abnormal pain behaviors. A number of studies have demonstrated increased activity, reduced analgesic consumption, and improved mood in middle-aged adults, with some reporting benefit for older patients with chronic pain.[51,52]***

MULTIDISCIPLINARY MANAGEMENT

There has been a steady proliferation of multidisciplinary–interdisciplinary treatment facilities for the management of complex chronic pain problems over the past 25 years. This trend reflects the increasing recognition that single-modality treatment approaches are inadequate in addressing the multidimensional impact of chronic pain for many patients. Recent evidence supports this approach, and it has rapidly become the treatment of choice for the management of more complex chronic pain problems, particularly when conventional strategies have failed.[53]*** This approach sits well with the principles of aged care medicine.

One might reasonably expect that older patients would constitute a sizable proportion of the client population at multidisciplinary clinics, yet this does not appear to be the case. Exclusion may result from the specification of age-related entry requirements, such as vocational restoration as a treatment goal, the need for third-party payment (e.g. workers' compensation), or the presence of comorbid medical conditions which would interfere with standard treatment protocols. Some clinics enforce upper age limits because of the belief that older patients will impact negatively on program success rates and ageist community attitudes may contribute to a negative referral bias. It is possible, of course, that the elderly complain less of pain and avoid activities which aggravate pain. Regardless of the exact reasons, it is evident that a large segment of the older population is currently not receiving the benefits of multidisciplinary treatment approaches to pain management.

Special considerations in the multidisciplinary treatment of older adults

At present, there are very few multidisciplinary pain clinics specifically for older persons, and several authors have noted the importance of modifying standard multidisciplinary treatment protocols in order to accommodate their needs.[32★★★,54★★★] Perhaps the most fundamental consideration relates to the specific objectives of the multidisciplinary treatment plan. The more generic treatment goals such as rationalization of medication use, targets for physical activity, and decreased pain are likely to be similar, but specific objectives will vary as a function of age. For instance, occupational rehabilitation and restoration of full physical function are likely to be important for young adults, whereas a resumption of recreational, spiritual, and social interaction as well as maintenance of functional independence within a community setting are likely to be of greater priority for older people.

It is always important to solicit the patients' beliefs about their ability to successfully complete assigned tasks. This is particularly true when dealing with older people. Targets for a reduction in medication or increased activity may appear simple from the perspective of the therapist, yet totally unrealistic from the patient's point of view. Some older people have poor self-efficacy, and cohort differences in the doctor–patient relationship may contribute to a greater reticence on their part to discuss instructions or to consider challenging the doctor's authority. The goal is active participation and empowerment.

Clinics with significant numbers of older patients should have clinicians who have specific expertise in the management of the elderly. There are a number of specific medical issues which may affect successful multidisciplinary pain management in older persons that require the expertise of an experienced physician. First and foremost is the effect of comorbidity on the diagnosis and treatment of pain and the patient. Complications may result from a failure to take into consideration conditions which may be asymptomatic until a new medication is introduced. Second, there are specific pain-causing pathologies which are more common in older people. The team also needs to involve the carer in all aspects of the management program. The role of family members and other concerned individuals needs to be considered in undertaking the assessment, counseling, and delivering therapies. Perhaps more than any other age group, there is a need to assess the whole patient, including their social and physical environment, and not just the pain condition. It is likely that group therapy programs will be more effective if members share similar life experiences, have similar objectives and aspirations, and face similar problems.

Some comment should be made on any unintentional endorsement of negative stereotypes of the aged as being frail, incompetent, and suffering from multiple physical impairments. It is worth remembering that a large majority of older people within the community are able to manage pain by themselves or with minimal assistance from their general practitioner. Patients who attend pain clinics represent a select group, and in some cases the older patient who attends will be frail and suffering from multiple comorbid medical conditions.[39] The intention is not to endorse negative stereotypes but rather to emphasize the diverse range of treatment options required to deal with older individuals, who tend to be the most heterogeneous cohort within the population. This will require the clinic to cater for the individuals who require a considerable increase in the time for assessment, repetition of instructions, and more simple and structured explanations of treatment approaches. However, most will be able to manage without the need for these modifications.

Outcome studies of multidisciplinary pain treatment for older people

The literature on treatment outcome reveals overwhelming support for multidisciplinary treatment of older chronic pain patients.[9★★★,53★★★,54★★★] However, no study has used appropriate control groups or randomization procedures in the evaluation of treatment efficacy. There is a lack of standardized measurement tools for documenting disease and disability. It is not always clear whether the outcome measures have been validated for use with older people, and the sample size in evaluation studies is often small. Despite these limitations, there are more than 10 independent studies which show clear benefits for many older chronic pain patients, and on the basis of this evidence it would appear that age should not be a barrier to the introduction of multidisciplinary pain management. The goals for success, however, may not necessarily include reduced pain. Older people will often prefer to increase ambulation and socialization rather than rest to decrease pain. Others will accept pain if it allows independence in their own home, rather than opting for less pain in the sedentary environment of an old age home.

PAIN IN PATIENTS WITH DEMENTIA

The prevalence rate of dementia doubles every 5 years from age 60 to 2% at 65, 4% at age 70, and to 30% and higher after the age of 85 years; Alzheimer's disease accounts for 65–75% of cases.[55] It is therefore likely that pain and dementia will coexist in many older individuals. The extent of this problem will increase with the aging of the population. The range of cognitive and behavioral impairments in patients with dementing illnesses is extremely wide, extending from the imperceptibly subtle to profound impairment requiring institutional care. It is quite possible that an older individual presenting for pain management may have a degree of cognitive impairment, or even dementia not previously recognized. Early diagnosis of dementia is important as patients may present with nonspecific physical complaints that prompt costly work-ups and unnecessary treatments. If uncertain about a patient's cognitive status, a screening instrument such as the minimental status examination should be employed, or the individual referred for further evaluation.[56] A brief cognitive screen can be completed in 5 min.

When a patient appears to have a dementia, the two most important entities to exclude are depression and delirium. The association of chronic pain and depression is well recognized by clinicians experienced in pain management; however, in the elderly depression may be much harder to diagnose. The complexity may be further compounded by the presence of a degree of cognitive impairment. Depressive symptoms are present in up to 86% of patients with Alzheimer's disease, and about 10–20% have a diagnosable depressive disorder. One clue to the presence of depression may be that the subjective complaints of cognitive impairment exceed neuropsychologic deficits. Delirium may be equally difficult for the inexperienced clinician to differentiate from dementia. Unlike the acute delirium seen in childhood, delirium in the elderly can be subacute, stretching over weeks or months, and may coexist with a dementia. Medications are among the most common causes of delirium, including those frequently used in pain management such as narcotics, benzodiazepines, and those with anticholinergic effects, e.g. tricyclic antidepressants. Individuals with cognitive impairment tend to be more sensitive to the neuropsychiatric side-effects of medications.

In most cases, the neuropathological changes of dementia progress over the course of the illness, requiring frequent monitoring and reevaluation of the appropriateness of therapy. Nonpharmacologic treatment approaches should not be ignored, as many medications have adverse effects on cognitive function. Patients should be encouraged to be active participants in their care and decision-making for as long as possible. Emotion-orientated psychotherapy, reminiscence therapy, and stimulation-orientated therapy such as music, art, and pet therapy and exercise may be helpful in individual cases.

Dementia is one of the major factors leading to residential care admission, particularly in the advanced stages of the disease. Surveys in residential care settings have frequently demonstrated that patients with dementia are more likely to have a painful condition that is unrecognized or undertreated.[57] The interaction between the pathology causing dementia and the perception of pain in these individuals has been reviewed.[58] A major clinical distinction is between individuals who maintain communicative skills and those who have lost them, particularly in the advanced stages of Alzheimer's disease. Verbal patients with even severe dementia can report pain consistently using a variety of psychometric instruments, although simple word descriptors such as the present pain intensity of the McGill Pain Questionnaire appear to have greater clinical utility. Nonverbal patients may come to attention because of changes in behavior, such as agitation, diminished physical activity, or the appearance of distress. Apart from pain, altered behavior may be due to related factors, including urinary infection, constipation, decubitus ulcers, depression, and reactions to medications. Careful evaluation is required, followed by one or multiple therapeutic trials, perhaps commencing with a safe analgesic such as acetaminophen. This may lead to the conclusion that the altered behavior was likely due to pain.

Individuals with dementia appear to report less pain than cognitively intact individuals. There are some case reports, however, where increased pain report was considered to be an early manifestation of the onset of dementia. Experimental evidence shows that pain threshold is unaltered in dementia.[59] However, the definitions of pain and dementia both contain references to cognition and affect. When these entities coexist, it is changes in the cognitive and affective domains that are observed. This has been illustrated experimentally by showing a blunted heart rate response preceding venipuncture in demented patients compared with those who are cognitively intact.[60] The specificity of behavioral observation is, however, poor as other nonpainful conditions may present with the same symptoms.

Pain management in patients with dementia is a complex matter often requiring specific training and expertise. There is an enhanced duty of care for the clinician dealing with a patient who is no longer competent, ensuring that basic human rights such as relief of pain and suffering are adequately addressed. Selection of investigations and treatments must take into consideration the way the individual will tolerate these interventions, together with an understanding of the attitudes or beliefs of the individual prior to the onset of dementia, and those of the person responsible for implementing management decisions. A great deal more research is required in the assessment and management of pain in the setting of dementia, which will assume increasing clinical importance as the population ages.

CONCLUSIONS

Pain is a common complaint of older people. It should be assessed and managed in the same way as for younger people, but with close attention to the impact of underlying diseases on the pain experience before and after treatment. There is evidence that the pain experience of older people is different, but this pertains more to the experimental laboratory than to the clinic. Most older individuals are well managed in normal services. Selection of therapy needs special consideration in the elderly. Acetaminophen is an appropriate starting point for most musculoskeletal pain. The elderly are at increased risk of side-effects from NSAIDs, especially in relation to the gastrointestinal tract. Opioids and adjuvant analgesics are more likely to cause side-effects than in the young. If used, they should be started in small doses and increased slowly. Nonpharmacologic approaches, such as psychologic and physical therapies, are probably underemployed in the elderly, and may be used separately or in combination with pharmacologic therapy.

There is a subset of older individuals, often with multiple medical and functional problems including dementia, who are perhaps best managed by specialists in aged care. Advanced age poses special challenges in pain management, but age *per se* should not be a barrier to good pain management. If pain persists, and continues to affect the enjoyment of life, then consideration should be given to referral to a multidisciplinary pain-management clinic. It has been observed that the older segments of the population are currently underrepresented in state-of-the-art pain treatment facilities. Services offered by multidisciplinary pain clinics must, however, be relevant to the needs of the individuals who are being treated. Age differences exist in relation to specific treatment goals, the pace of assessment and treatment protocols, and self-efficacy. The general social milieu of the pain-management service needs to be sensitive to these issues. The available literature on treatment outcome would suggest that older people can show considerable benefit from multidisciplinary pain management and exhibit a similar magnitude of improvement to younger patients.

REFERENCES

1. United Nations. http://www.popin.org/pop1998/8.htm
◆ 2. Ferrell BR, Ferrell BA eds. *Pain in the Elderly: Task Force on Pain in the Elderly*. Seattle, WA: IASP Press, 1996.
3. American Geriatrics Society. Clinical practice guidelines: the management of chronic pain in older persons. *J Am Geriatr Soc* 1998; **46**: 635–51.
4. Helme RD, Katz B. Control of pain. In: Pathy MSJ ed. *Principles and Practice of Geriatric Medicine*, 3rd edn. Chichester: John Wiley and Sons,1998: 954–61.
● 5. Katz B, Helme RD. Pain problems in old age. In: Brocklehurst J, Tallis R, Fillit H eds. *Textbook of Geriatric Medicine and Gerontology*, 6th edn. London: Churchill Livingstone, 2001.
6. Wiesel SW, Tsourmas N, Feffer HL. The incidence of pos-itive CAT scans in an asymptomatic group of patients. *Spine* 1984; **9**: 549–51.
7. Rochon PA, Fortin PR, Dear KBG, *et al*. Reporting of age data in clinical trials of arthritis. *Arch Intern Med* 1993; **153**: 243–8.
8. Crook J, Rideout E, Browne G. The prevalence of pain complaints in a general population. *Pain* 1984; **18**: 299–314.
9. Gibson SJ, Helme RD. Age differences in pain perception and report: a review of physiological, psychological, laboratory and clinical studies. *Pain Rev* 1995; **2**: 111–37.
10. Helme RD, Gibson SJ. Pain in older people. In: Crombie IK, Croft PR, Linton SJ, *et al*. eds. *Epidemiology of Pain*. Seattle, WA: IASP Press, 1999: 103–11.
11. Miller PF, Sheps DS, Bragdon EE, *et al*. Aging and pain perception in ischemic heart disease. *Am Heart J* 1990; **120**: 22–31.
12. Moss MS, Lawton MP, Glicksman A. The role of pain in the last year of life of older persons. *J Gerontol* 1991; **46**: 51–7.
13. Lasch H, Castell DO, Castell JA. Evidence for diminished visceral pain with ageing: studies using graded intra-esophageal balloon distension. *Am J Physiol* 1997; **272**: G1–G3.
14. Donahue JG, Choo PW, Manson JAE, Platt R. The incidence of herpes zoster. *Arch Intern Med* 1995; **155**: 1605–9.
15. Helme RD, Gibson SJ. Pain in the elderly. In: Jensen TS, Turner JA, Wiesenfeld-Hallin Z eds. *Proceedings of the 8th World Congress on Pain, Progress in Pain Research and Management*. Seattle, WA: IASP Press, 1997: 919–44.
16. Harkins SW, Price DD, Bush FM, Small RE. Geriatric pain. In: Wall PD, Melzack R eds. *Textbook of Pain*. New York, NY: Churchill Livingstone, 1994: 769–84.
17. Von Korff Dworkin SF, LeResche L Graded chronic pain status: an epidemiologic study. *Pain* 1990; **40**: 279–91.
18. Sternbach RA. Survey of pain in the United States: the Nuprin Pain Report. *Clin J Pain* 1986; **2**: 49–53.
19. Barberger-Gateau P, Chaslerie A, Dartigues J, *et al*. Health measure correlates in a French elderly community population: the PAQUID study. *J Gerontol* 1992; **472**: S88–S95.
20. Kay L, Jorgensen T, Schultz-Larsen K. Abdominal pain in a 70-year old Danish population. *J Clin Epidemiol* 1992; **45**: 1377–82.
21. Harkins SW, Davis MD, Bush FM, Kasberger J. Suppression of first pain and slow temporal summation of second pain in relation to age. *J Gerontol* 1996; **51**: M260–5.
22. Chakour MC, Gibson SJ, Bradbeer M, Helme RD. Effect of age on A-delta fibre modulation of thermal pain perception. *Pain* 1996; **64**: 143–52.
23. Washington LJ, Gibson SJ, Helme RD. Age related differences in endogenous analgesia to repeated cold water immersion in human volunteers. *Pain* 2000; **89**: 89–96.

24. MacDonald JB, Ballie J, Williams BO, Ballantyne D. Coronary care in the elderly. *Age Ageing* 1983; **12:** 17–20.

25. Solomon CG, Lee TH, Cook EF, *et al.* Comparison of clinical presentation of acute myocardial infarction in patients older than 65 years of age to younger patients: the multicenter chest pain study experience. *Am J Cardiol* 1989; **63:** 772–6.

26. Miller PF, Sheps DS, Bragdon EE, *et al.* Age and pain perception in ischemic heart disease. *Am Heart J* 1990; **120:** 22–30.

27. Norman DC, Yoshikawa TT. Intra-abdominal infections in the elderly. *J Am Geriatr Soc* 1983; **31:** 677–84.

28. Albano W, Zielinski CM, Organ CH. Is appendicitis in the aged really different? *Geriatrics* 1975; **30:** 81–8.

29. Clinch D, Banjeree AK, Ostick G. Absence of abdominal pain in elderly patients with peptic ulcer. *Age Ageing* 1984; **13:** 120–3.

30. Ambepitiya GB, Iyengar EN, Roberts ME. Silent exertional myocardial ischaemia and perception of angina in elderly people. *Age Ageing* 1993; **22:** 302–7.

31. Ambepitiya GB, Roberts M, Ranjadayalan K, Tallis R. Silent exertional myocardial ischemia in the elderly: a quantitative analysis of anginal perceptual threshold and the influence of autonomic function. *J Am Geriatr Soc* 1994; **42:** 732–7.

● 32. Helme RD, Katz B, Gibson SJ, *et al.* Multidisciplinary pain clinics for older people: do they have a role? *Clin Geriatr Med* 1996; **12:** 563–82.

33. Tran P-V, Schwarz J, Gorman M, Helme RD. Validation of an automated up-timer for measurement of mobility in older adults. *Med J Aust* 1997; **167:** 434–6.

34. Farrell MJ, Katz B, Helme RD. The impact of dementia on the pain experience. *Pain* 1996; **67:** 7–15.

35. Gibson SJ, Katz B, Corran TC, *et al.* Pain in older persons. *Disabil Rehabil* 1994; **16:** 127–39.

36. Gibson SJ. The measurement of mood states in older adults. *J Gerontol* 1997; **52:** P167–74.

37. Podsiadlo D, Richardson S. The timed "up and go": a test of basic functional mobility for frail elderly persons. *JAGS* 1991; **39:** 142–8

38. Kane RA, Kane RL. *Assessing the Elderly: a Practical Guide to Measurement.* Lexington, MA: Lexington Books, 1981.

39. Farrell MJ, Gibson SJ, Helme RD. The effect of medical status on the activity of elderly pain clinic patients. *J Am Geriatr Soc* 1995; **43:** 102–7.

40. de Craen AJM, Di Giulio G, Lampe-Schoenmaeckers AJEM, *et al.* Analgesic efficacy and safety of paracetamol–codeine combinations versus paracetamol alone: a systematic review. *Br Med J* 1996; **313:** 321–5.

41. Moore A, Collins S, Carroll D, McQuay H. Paracetamol with and without codeine in acute pain: a quantitative systematic review. *Pain* 1997; **70:** 193–201.

42. Wolfe MM, Lichtenstein DR, Singh G. Gastrointestinal toxicity of nonsteroidal antiinflammatory drugs. *N Engl J Med* 1999; **340:** 1888–99.

43. Lanza FL. A guideline for the treatment and prevention of NSAID-Induced ulcers. *Am J Gastroenterol* 1998; **93:** 2037–46.

44. Silverstein FE, Graham DY, Senior JR, *et al.* Misoprostol reduces serious gastrointestinal complications in patients with rheumatoid arthritis receiving nonsteroidal anti-inflammatory drugs. *Ann Intern Med* 1995; **123:** 241–9.

45. Silverstein FE, Faich G, Goldstein JL, *et al.* Gastrointestinal toxicity with celecoxib vs nonsteroidal anti-inflammatory drugs for osteoarthritis and rheumatoid arthritis. The CLASS study: a randomized controlled trial. *JAMA* 2000; **284:** 1247–55.

◆ 46. Forman WB. Opioid analgesic drugs in the elderly. *Clin Geriatr Med* 1996; **12:** 489–500.

47. Collins SL, Moore A, McQuay HJ, Wiffen P. Antidepressants and anticonvulsants for diabetic neuropathy and postherpetic neuralgia: a quantitative systematic review. *J Pain Symptom Manage* 2000; **20:** 449–58.

48. McQuay HJ, Moore RA. Antidepressants and chronic pain. *Br Med J* 1997; **314:** 763–4.

49. Sindrup SH, Jensen TS. Efficacy of pharmacological treatments of neuropathic pain: an update and effect related to mechanisms of drug action. *Pain* 1999; **83:** 389–400.

50. Grant DJ, Bishop-Miller J, Winchester DM, *et al.* A randomised comparative trial of acupuncture versus transcutaneous electrical nerve stimulation for chronic back pain in the elderly. *Pain* 1999; **82:** 9–13.

51. Fordyce WE. Evaluating and managing chronic pain. *Geriatrics* 1978; **33:** 59–62.

52. Puder RS. Age analysis of cognitive–behavioral group therapy for chronic pain outpatients. *Psychol Aging* 1988; **3:** 3204–7.

◆ 53. Gibson SJ, Farrell MJ, Katz B, Helme RD. Multidisciplinary management of chronic non-malignant pain in older adults. In: Ferrell BR, Ferrell BA eds. *Pain in the Elderly.* Seattle, WA: IASP Press, 1996, 81–9.

54. Ferrell BA, Ferrell BR. Pain in the nursing home. *J Am Geriatr Soc* 1990; **38:** 409–14.

55. Richards SS, Hendrie HC. Diagnosis, management, and treatment of Alzheimer's disease. *Arch Intern Med* 1999; **159:** 789–98.

56. Folstein MF, Folstein SE, McHugh PR. Mini mental state: a practical method for grading the cognitive state of patients for the clinician. *J Psychiatr Res* 1975; **12:** 189–98.

57. Ferrell BA, Ferrell BR. Pain in cognitively impaired nursing home patients. *J Pain Symptom Manage* 1995; **10:** 591–8.

◆ 58. Farrell MJ, Katz B, Helme RD. The impact of dementia on the pain experience. *Pain* 1996; **67:** 7–15.

59. Bendetti F, Vighetti S, Ricco C, *et al.* Pain threshold and tolerance in Alzheimer's disease. *Pain* 1999; **80:** 377–82.

60. Porter FL, Malhtra KM, Wolf CM, *et al.* Dementia and response to pain in the elderly. *Pain* 1996; **68:** 413–21.

Index

Page numbers in **bold** refer to tables or boxes; page numbers in *italic* refer to figures. Abbreviations: CBT, cognitive–behavioral therapy; CPRP, comprehensive pain rehabilitation program; CRPS, complex regional pain syndrome; CT, computed tomography; MRI, magnetic resonance imaging; NSAIDs, nonsteroidal anti-inflammatory drugs; PHN, postherpetic neuralgia; TENS, transcutaneous electrical nerve stimulation; TMJ, temporomandibular joint.